Department of International Economic and Social Affairs

Population Studies   No.100

Fertility Behaviour in the Context of Development

Evidence from the World Fertility Survey

United Nations   New York, 1987

NOTE

The designations employed and the presentation of the material in this document do not imply the expression of any opinion whatsoever on the part of the Secretariat of the United Nations concerning the legal status of any country, territory, city or area or of its authorities, or concerning the delimitation of its frontiers or boundaries.

Where the designation "country or area" is used in the text, it covers, as appropriate, countries, territories, cities or areas.

The designations "developed" and "developing" economies are intended for statistical convenience and do not, necessarily, express a judgement about the stage reached by a particular country or area in the development process.

The views expressed in signed papers do not imply the expression of any opinion on the part of the United Nations Secretariat. Papers have been edited and consolidated in accordance with United Nations practice and requirements.

ST/ESA/SER.A/100

UNITED NATIONS PUBLICATION

Sales No. E.86.XIII.5

04750

ISBN 92-1-151161-5

PREFACE

The World Fertility Survey (WFS) programme had as one of its objectives the collection of internationally comparable data. The Population Division of the Department of International Economic and Social Affairs of the United Nations Secretariat has had a 40-year tradition of undertaking global comparative studies of demographic phenomena. Thus, it was natural and appropriate that the data arising from this international survey programme should form the basis of a major research programme in the Population Division.

The United Nations Working Group on Comparative Analysis of World Fertility Survey Data was set up in mid-1977 by the Population Division with financial support from the United Nations Fund for Population Activities (UNFPA) in order to establish guidelines for and maintain close co-ordination with the United Nations Programme of Comparative Analysis of World Fertility Survey Data.[1] The members of the Group represented all the regional commissions, as well as the International Labour Organisation (ILO), the United Nations Educational, Scientific and Cultural Organization (UNESCO) and the World Health Organization (WHO). The Population Division took the lead in designing comparative analyses of the data from the developing countries to be undertaken in parallel at the global and regional levels. For analysis of the data from the developed countries, the Economic Commission for Europe (ECE) took the lead with the assistance of the United Nations Working Group on Social Demography, which included experts involved in the national surveys.

At the first meeting of that Working Group in 1977, a two-phased plan of research was adopted. The first phase, to include data from 20 developing countries, was to be experimental in nature. For this phase, the Minimum Research Programme included a range of topics on fertility and its determinants which were of common interest to the Group. The Group met subsequently (1978, 1979, 1980, 1982) to review and discuss work in progress with respect to the Minimum Research Programme. Most members of the Working Group submitted background papers based on this analysis to the Expert Group Meeting on Fertility and the Family, held at New Delhi in January 1983 in preparation for the International Conference on Population, 1984 (see references, section B). A series of publications deriving from the Minimum Research Programme appeared during these years (see references, section C). During the same period, a series of short summary papers based on the findings from the developed countries and prepared by ECE were published in the WFS Comparative Studies series (see references, section D).

The sixth and last meeting of the United Nations Working Group was held in October 1984 to finalize plans for the second stage of the work. For the Population Division at United Nations Headquarters, this stage included publication of the present study on the WFS findings, as well as publications concerning policy implications related to WFS, women's employment and fertility and data quality in the surveys (see references, section E).

The present report is the culmination of the United Nations comparative analysis of the WFS data, including both regional and global perspectives. The chapters in parts one and two were prepared by the Population Division with the aid of two consultants, Susheela Singh for chapters III and VI, and Ann Blanc for chapter IX. These chapters present analyses of levels and differentials in fertility and its major components based on data from surveys in 38 developing countries roughly evenly divided between the three major regions (12 from Africa, 13 from Latin America and the Caribbean, and 13 from Asia and Oceania).[2] Part three presents regional perspectives, three of which were prepared by the population divisions of the Economic and Social Commission for Asia and the Pacific, the Economic Commission for Latin America and the Caribbean, and the Economic Commission for Africa, using data from countries within their regional mandates. The fourth was prepared by a consultant, Samir Farid; it covers the countries of Western Asia and Northern Africa not included in the preceding chapters. Part four provides an overview of fertility and family planning in the developed countries, prepared by the Population Division of ECE. The concluding chapter, prepared in collaboration with a consultant, Elise Jones, brings the findings from the developed and developing countries together in order to draw some conclusions about the state of knowledge of fertility at the conclusion of the WFS programme.

The research undertaken for this report was partially supported by UNFPA through project support to the Population Division and to the regional commissions. The publication of the report was financed by UNFPA. The support of all countries whose WFS data were analysed in this report is gratefully acknowledged. Through their goodwill, the data tapes from these surveys were made available to the Population Division for this comparative analysis project.

NOTES

[1] Described in detail in Acsádi, 1980.
[2] The countries covered are:
Africa: Benin, Cameroon, Côte d'Ivoire, Egypt, Ghana, Kenya, Lesotho, Mauritania, Morocco, Senegal, Sudan, Tunisia;
Latin America and the Caribbean: Colombia, Costa Rica, Dominican Republic, Ecuador, Guyana, Haiti, Jamaica, Mexico, Panama, Paraguay, Peru, Trinidad and Tobago, Venezuela;
Asia and Oceania: Bangladesh, Fiji, Indonesia, Jordan, Malaysia, Nepal, Pakistan, Philippines, Republic of Korea, Sri Lanka, Syrian Arab Republic, Thailand, Yemen.

REFERENCES

A. *Background of research programme*

Acsádi, George T. (1980). Research plan for comparative analysis of WFS data of the Population Division of the United Nations; Review of characteristics, measures and other indicators (variables considered for use in Comparative Analysis of World Fertility Survey Data in the Frame of the United Nations Minimum Research Programme); and Research objectives, hypotheses and minimum tabulation plan (relevant to the United Nations Minimum Research Programme for Comparative Analysis of World Fertility Survey Data). In *The United Nations Programme for Comparative Analysis of World Fertility Survey Data*, a project of the United Nations carried out in collaboration with the United Nations Fund for Population Activities. New York: United Nations Fund for Population Activities, 3-26, 27-62, 63-89.

B. *Background papers for Expert Group Meeting on Family and Fertility, New Delhi, 5-11 January 1983*

United Nations Headquarters

United Nations Secretariat. Department of International Economic and Social Affairs. Population Division. Comparative analysis of fertility levels and trends as assessed from twenty world fertility surveys. IESA/P/ICP.1984/EG.I/11.

_____. Relationships between fertility and education: a comparative analysis of WFS data for 22 developing countries. IESA/P/ICP.1984/EG.I/18.

_____. The impact of population structure on crude fertility measures. IESA/P/ICP.1984/EG.I/22.

_____. Marital status and fertility: summary report of an analysis of WFS data. IESA/P/ICP.1984/EG.I/25.

_____. Some relationships between marital unions and fertility in six countries of the West Indies. IESA/P/ICP.1984/EG.I/27.

Regional commissions

Economic Commission for Europe. Socio-economic determinants of achieved fertility in some developed countries; a multivariate analysis based on World Fertility Survey data. IESA/P/ICP.1984/EG.I/6.

Economic and Social Commission for Asia and the Pacific. A report on levels and trends of fertility in the ESCAP region; comparative analysis of WFS data. IESA/P/ICP.1984/EG.I/9.

_____. Differentials in urban-rural fertility in the countries of the ESCAP region. IESA/P/ICP.1984/EG.I/10.

_____. Marital status composition and fertility; a comparative analysis of WFS data. IESA/P/ICP.1984/EG.I/23.

Economic Commission for Latin America and the Caribbean. Latin American Demographic Centre (Centro Latinoamericano de Demografía). Family planning and fertility. IESA/P/ICP.1984/EG.I/4.

_____. Marital status composition and fertility; a methodological approach applicable to a comparative analysis of fertility surveys data. IESA/P/ICP.1984/EG.I/14.

Economic Commission for Africa. Marriage and fertility in Africa. IESA/P/ICP.1984/EG.I/17.

Specialized agencies

United Nations Educational, Scientific and Cultural Organization. Women's education and fertility relationships in 14 World Fertility Survey countries. IESA/P/ICP.1984/EG.I/20.

World Health Organization. Some health-related aspects of fertility. IESA/P/ICP.1984/EG.I/8.

C. *Publications and documents deriving from the Minimum Research Programme*

United Nations Headquarters

United Nations Secretariat (1981). Department of International Economic and Social Affairs. Population Division. *Some Factors Affecting Fertility and Fertility Preferences in Developing Countries*. Non-sales publication ST/ESA/SER.R/37.

_____ (1981). *Variations in the Incidence of Knowledge and Use of Contraception: A Comparative Analysis of World Fertility Survey Results for Twenty Developing Countries*. Non-sales publication ST/ESA/SER.R/40.

_____ (1981). A proposed occupational classification system for women to be used in the International Comparative Analysis of World Fertility Survey data. Working paper ESA/P/WP/70.

_____ (1981). An educational coding system construction for application in the United Nations Programme of Comparative Analysis of World Fertility Survey data. Working paper ESA/P/WP/71.

_____ (1982). *The Impact of Population Structure on Crude Fertility Measures: A Comparative Analysis of World Fertility Survey Results for Twenty-one Developing Countries*. Non-sales publication ST/ESA/SER.R/49.

_____ (1983). *Marital Status and Fertility: A Comparative Analysis of World Fertility Survey Data for Twenty-one Countries*. Non-sales publication ST/ESA/SER.R/52.

_____ (1983). *Relationships Between Fertility and Education: A Comparative Analysis of World Fertility Survey Data for Twenty-two Developing Countries*. Non-sales publication ST/ESA/SER.R/48.

_____ (1983). *Fertility Levels and Trends as Assessed from Twenty World Fertility Surveys*. Non-sales publication ST/ESA/SER.R/50.

_____ (1984). *Some Relationships Between Nuptiality and Fertility in Countries of the West Indies*. Non-sales publication ST/ESA/SER.R/46.

United Nations Fund for Population Activities (1980). *The United Nations Programme for Comparative Analysis of World Fertility Survey Data*, a project of the United Nations carried out in collaboration with UNFPA. New York.

_____ (1980). *Some Factors Affecting Fertility in Eight Developing Countries: An Analysis of WFS Survey Data*. New York.

Economic and Social Commission for Asia and the Pacific

Economic and Social Commission for Asia and the Pacific (1984). Population Division. The influence of infant and child mortality on fertility in the countries of the ESCAP region: an analysis of data from the World Fertility Survey. Paper submitted to the Sixth Meeting of the United Nations Working Group on Comparative Analysis of World Fertility Survey Data, New York, 22-25 October 1984. UN/UNFPA/WFS.VI/5.

Economic Commission for Latin America and the Caribbean/Latin American Demographic Centre

Arguëllo, Omar (1980). Variables socio-económicas y fecundidad. *Notas de Población* 8(23):123-148.

Baldión W., Edgar (1981). Mortalidad infantil en relación al nivel de fecundidad. Santiago, Chile; Centro Latinoamericano de Demografía (mimeographed).

Bartlema, Jan (1978). *La fecundidad en la República Dominicana, 1960-1975: calculada a partir de los datos de la Encuesta Nacional de Fecundidad*. CELADE Series A, No. 157. Santiago, Chile: Centro Latinoamericano de Demografía.

Bocaz, Albino (1975). Confiabilidad de las muestras: análisis comparativo de fecundidad (mimeographed).

Conning, Arthur M., and Albert A. Marckwardt (1982). *Analysis of WFS Data in Colombia, Panama, Paraguay and Peru: Highlights from the CELADE Research and Training Seminar*. World Fertility Survey Occasional Papers, No. 25. Voorburg, The Netherlands: International Statistical Institute.

Economic Commission for Latin America and the Caribbean (1982). Estructura matrimonial y fecundidad. Paper prepared for the Fifth Meeting of the United Nations Working Group on Comparative Analysis of World Fertility Survey Data, Geneva, 26-29 January 1982.

González, G. and V. Ramírez (1980). Differenciales socioeconómicas de la fecundidad en América Latina. Santiago, Chile: Centro Latinoamericano de Demografía.

Gougain, Laura (1983). *Fecundidad y participación laboral femenina en Panamá*. CELADE series D, No. 105. Santiago, Chile: Centro Latinoamericano de Demografía.

Guerra G., Federico. Relación entre mortalidad infantil y fecundidad en Panamá. Santiago, Chile: Centro Latinoamericano de Demografía (mimeographed).

Mostajo, Nelly (1981). *Actitudes de la mujer frente a la fecundidad y uso de métodos anticonceptivos*. CELADE Series D, No. 107. Santiago, Chile: Centro Latinoamericano de Demografía.

Ramírez, Nelson, and others (1977). La Encuesta Nacional de Fecundidad: procedimientos empleados y problema principales encontrados. Paper prepared for the Reunión General de la Encuesta Mundial de Fecundidad para Latinoamérica, México (mimeographed).

Rodríguez V., Virginia (1978). La fecundidad en Costa Rica según la Encuesta Nacional de Fecundidad. San José, Costa Rica: Centro Latinoamericano de Demografía.

Rosero Bixby, Luis (1978). Nupcialidad y exposición al riesgo de embarazo en Costa Rica. *Notas de Población* 6(17):33-62.

Schoemaker, Juan Francisco (1981). *Participación laboral femenina y fecundidad en Paraguay*. CELADE Series D, No. 99. Santiago, Chile: Centro Latinoamericano de Demografía.

Taucher, Erica (1982). Efectos del descenso de la fecundidad sobre los niveles de mortalidad infantil: un estudio basado en datos de cinco países latinoamericanos. Santiago, Chile: Centro Latinoamericano de Demografía.

Vlassoff, Michael (1986). Tendencias y diferenciales de la fecundidad en América Latina: un análisis con los datos de la Encuesta Mundial de Fecundidad. *Notas de Población* 14(41).

Westoff, Charles F. (1981). Fecundidad no deseada en seis países en vías de desarrollo: perspectivas internacionales en planificación familiar. Santiago, Chile: Centro Latinoamericano de Demografía.

Economic Commission for Africa

Economic Commission for Africa (1983). Population Division. *Nuptiality and Fertility: A Comparative Analysis of WFS Data*. African Population Studies Series, No. 5. E/ECA/SER.A/3. Addis Ababa.

_____(1985). Regional Review Seminar on Analysis of Infant and Child Mortality.

_____(1985). Niveaux, tendances et déterminants de la fécondité au Cameroun, au Kenya et au Sénégal. ECA/PD/WP/1985/4.

_____(1985). Croissance démographique et évaluation des programmes de planification familiale en Afrique: Egypte, Ghana, Kenya, Maroc, Tunisie. ECA/PD/WP/1985/14.

_____(1985). Interrelationship between infant and child mortality, socio-economic factors and fertility in Africa. ECA/PD/WP/1985/16.

_____(1985). Estimation de niveaux actuels de la fécondité dans quelques pays africains: analyse comparative des données de l'EMF. In *Dynamique de la population afrique*. Addis Ababa. E/ECA/PSD.4/29.

_____(1986). Structure des ménages et fécondité en Afrique sub-Saharienne: Cameroun, Côte d'Ivoire, Ghana, Kenya, Lesotho, Nigeria. ECA/POP/85/2.3.

_____(forthcoming). Impact démographique de l'évolution du rôle de la femme. Analyse du rapport entre le statut de la femme et les niveaux de fécondité dans cinq pays de l'Afrique de l'Ouest: Benin, Côte d'Ivoire, Ghana, Nigeria, Sénégal. ECA/TP/POP/86/2.3(a).

_____(forthcoming). Socio-economic determinants of infant and childhood mortality in Africa based on WFS data. ECA/WFS/POP/87/2.2.

_____(forthcoming). Trends in infant and childhood mortality and their implications for population growth in African countries. ECA/TP/POP/87/2.5.

_____(forthcoming). Structure des ménages et fécondité dans les pays arabes: Egypte, Maroc, Mauritanie, Tunisie, Soudan. ECA/TP/POP/87/2.2.

D. Economic Commission for Europe: reports on developed countries

Berent, Jerzy (1982). *Family Planning in Europe and USA in the 1970s*. World Fertility Survey Comparative Studies, No. 20; ECE Analyses of WFS Surveys in Europe and USA. Voorburg, The Netherlands: International Statistical Institute.

_____. *Family Size Preferences in Europe and USA: Ultimate Expected Number of Children*. World Fertility Survey Comparative Studies, No. 26; ECE Analyses. Voorburg, The Netherlands: International Statistical Institute.

_____. Elise F. Jones and M. Khalid Siddiqui (1982). *Basic Characteristics. Sample Designs and Questionnaires*. World Fertility Survey Comparative Studies, No. 18; ECE Analyses. Voorburg, The Netherlands: International Statistical Institute.

Ford, Kathleen (1984). *Timing and Spacing of Births*. World Fertility Survey Comparative Studies, No. 38; ECE Analyses. Voorburg, The Netherlands: International Statistical Institute.

Jones, Elise F. (1982). *Socio-economic Differentials in Achieved Fertility*. World Fertility Survey Comparative Studies, No. 21; ECE Analyses. Voorburg, The Netherlands: International Statistical Institute.

E. Recent United Nations reports concerning the World Fertility Survey

United Nations (1985). Department of International Economic and Social Affairs. Population Division. *Women's Employment and Fertility: A Comparative Analysis of World Fertility Results for 38 Developing Countries*. Population Studies, No. 96.
Sales No. E.85.XIII.5.

_____(1986). *Policy Relevance of Findings of the World Fertility Survey for Developing Countries*. Non-sales publication ST/ESA/SER.R/59.

_____(forthcoming). *A Comparative Evaluation of Data Quality in 38 World Fertility Surveys*. Non-sales publication ST/ESA/SER.R/50/Rev.1.

CONTENTS

	Page
PREFACE	iii
EXPLANATORY NOTES	xix
INTRODUCTION	1
Background	1
Conceptual framework	2
Characteristics of study countries	4
Characteristics of the data	9
Plan of analysis	13

PART ONE. FERTILITY AND ITS PROXIMATE DETERMINANTS IN THE DEVELOPING COUNTRIES

Chapter

I. LEVELS AND TRENDS IN FERTILITY ... 19
    A. The data ... 20
    B. Recent fertility ... 22
    C. Cumulative fertility ... 27
    D. Fertility trends ... 28
    E. Adolescent fertility ... 34
    F. Childlessness ... 34
    G. Conclusion ... 35
    Annex. Comparative assessment of data quality ... 38

II. FERTILITY PREFERENCES ... 48
    A. The data ... 50
    B. Size preferences ... 51
    C. Sex preferences ... 61
    D. Unwanted fertility ... 68
    E. Conclusion ... 72

III. NUPTIALITY ... 76
    A. Marital status of women ... 77
    B. Fertility according to time spent married ... 85
    C. Age at marriage and fertility ... 90
    D. Marriage and childbearing among adolescents ... 98
    E. Summary and conclusions ... 100

IV. BREAST-FEEDING AND RELATED ASPECTS OF POST-PARTUM REPRODUCTIVE BEHAVIOUR ... 104
    A. Data and methodology ... 106
    B. General characteristics ... 108
    C. Breast-feeding and family limitation ... 116
    D. Other aspects of reproductive behaviour associated with the breast-feeding period ... 119
    E. Conclusion ... 126

V. CONTRACEPTIVE PRACTICE ... 129
    A. The data ... 130
    B. An overview of levels of contraceptive knowledge and use ... 132
    C. Differentials in use of any method ... 137
    D. Knowledge and use of specific contraceptive methods ... 147
    E. Contraceptive discontinuation and method-switching ... 155
    F. Summary and conclusions ... 160

VI. THE MAJOR PROXIMATE DETERMINANTS AND THEIR CONTRIBUTION TO FERTILITY ... 165
    A. The Bongaarts model of proximate determinants ... 166
    B. Aggregate indices and their components ... 167
    C. Relationships for age groups ... 175

Chapter		Page
D.	Conclusion	180
	Annex. Measurement of components of the model	183

PART TWO. SOCIO-ECONOMIC FACTORS AFFECTING FERTILITY IN THE DEVELOPING COUNTRIES

VII.	RURAL OR URBAN RESIDENCE AND FERTILITY		187
	A.	Measures of residence	190
	B.	Preliminary analysis	192
	C.	Multivariate analysis	204
	D.	Summary and conclusions	208
VIII.	EDUCATION AND FERTILITY		214
	A.	Measures of education	217
	B.	Preliminary analysis	221
	C.	Multivariate analysis	238
	D.	Summary and conclusions	247
IX.	WOMEN'S EMPLOYMENT AND FERTILITY		255
	A.	Data and measurement	257
	B.	Level and pattern of women's work	259
	C.	Women's work and fertility	265
	D.	Women's work and intermediate variables	272
	E.	Conclusion	277
Annex to Part Two.	The multivariate marital fertility model		280

PART THREE. REGIONAL PERSPECTIVES FROM THE DEVELOPING COUNTRIES

X.	A REVIEW OF THE FERTILITY SITUATION IN COUNTRIES IN THE REGION OF THE ECONOMIC AND SOCIAL COMMISSION FOR ASIA AND THE PACIFIC		
	Economic and Social Commission for Asia and the Pacific		283
	A.	The data	284
	B.	Levels and patterns of fertility	284
	C.	Analysis of fertility change	287
	D.	Determinants of fertility	289
	E.	Summary and discussion	296
	F.	Policy implications	297
XI.	A REVIEW OF THE FERTILITY SITUATION IN COUNTRIES IN THE REGION OF THE ECONOMIC COMMISSION FOR LATIN AMERICA AND THE CARIBBEAN		
	Economic Commission for Latin America and the Caribbean		299
	A.	Levels and trends in fertility	300
	B.	Levels and trends in some variables related to fertility	302
	C.	Some socio-economic determinants of fertility	305
	D.	Differentials in proximate determinants of fertility	313
	E.	Contributions of proximate determinants to fertility reduction	317
	F.	Conclusion	319
XII.	COMPARATIVE ANALYSIS OF WORLD FERTILITY SURVEY DATA: AFRICA, SOUTH OF THE SAHARA		
	Economic Commission for Africa		324
	A.	Background	325
	B.	Marriage and types of marital unions	326
	C.	Fertility	330
	D.	Post-partum non-susceptible period	334
	E.	Desired family size and knowledge and use of contraception	336
	F.	Summary and policy implications	336
XIII.	A REVIEW OF THE FERTILITY SITUATION IN THE ARAB COUNTRIES OF WESTERN ASIA AND NORTHERN AFRICA		
	Samir Farid		340
	A.	Fertility	341
	B.	Nuptiality	346
	C.	Breast-feeding	348
	D.	Fertility preferences	349
	E.	Family planning	350
	F.	Conclusion	352

Chapter		Page

PART FOUR. COMPARISONS WITH DEVELOPED COUNTRIES

XIV. FERTILITY AND FAMILY PLANNING IN THE DEVELOPED COUNTRIES
    Economic Commission for Europe 357
    A. Basic characteristics of the surveys 358
    B. Data and methodology of the comparative analysis 360
    C. Summary of findings 360
    D. Concluding remarks 369
    Annex. Variables selected for the Economic Commission for Europe comparative analysis 370

XV. A GLOBAL PERSPECTIVE 371
    A. Fertility 373
    B. Proximate determinants 375
    C. Socio-economic differentials 378
    D. Conclusion 381

LIST OF TABLES

No.
1. World Fertility Survey countries by major region and subregion, and percentage of regional/subregional developing-country population represented 5
2. Indicators of development and their index values for 38 World Fertility Survey countries, around 1975 6
3. Index of development and rank values for 38 World Fertility Survey countries, around 1975 7
4. Four development indices and rank values for 38 World Fertility Survey countries, around 1975 8
5. Family planning programme effort scores and grouping of World Fertility Survey countries according to interpolated scores 9
6. Cross-classification of countries participating in the World Fertility Survey, by strength of family planning programme effort, level of development and region 10
7. Timing of the World Fertility Survey in countries selected for study 11
8. Characteristics of population and sample covered by the World Fertility Survey, by region and country 12
9. Number of countries classified by assessment of quality of recent fertility estimates and fertility trends, by region and level of development 22
10. Population estimates, crude birth rates and total fertility rates for the five years preceding the survey date, by region and country 23
11. Crude birth rates and total fertility rates, by level of development and strength of family planning programme effort 24
12. Age-specific fertility rates and total fertility rates for the five years preceding the survey date, by region and country 24
13. Age-specific marital fertility rates for the five years preceding the survey date, by region and country 26
14. Mean numbers of children ever born, by age of woman and by region and country 28
15. Mean numbers of living children, by age of woman and by region and country   29
16. Total fertility rates for women aged 15-44 and percentage change in total fertility rates for the periods from 10-14 to 0-4 years prior to the survey date, by region, 19 countries 30
17. Trends in total fertility rates for women aged 15-44 and percentage change in total fertility rates for the periods from 10-14 to 0-4 years prior to the survey date, by level of development and strength of family planning programme effort, 19 countries 31
18. Percentage change in age-specific fertility rates for women aged 15-39 from 10-14 to 0-4 years prior to the survey date, by region, 19 countries 31
19. Percentage change in marital age-specific fertility rates for women aged 15-39 from 10-14 to 0-4 years prior to the survey date, by region, 16 countries . 32
20. Percentage change in marital age-specific fertility rates for women aged 15-39 from 10-14 to 0-4 years prior to the survey date, by level of development and strength of family planning programme effort, 16 countries 33
21. Age-specific fertility rates for women aged 15-19 for the period 0-4 years prior to the survey date, by region and country 33

No.		Page
22.	Percentage of women with no living children and percentage with no fertile pregnancies among currently married women aged 30-44 and married for at least a total of five years, by region and country	35
23.	Indicators of the quality of World Fertility Survey age data	38
24.	Indicators of the quality of World Fertility Survey marital history data	39
25.	Overall quality of enumeration of recent births from the World Fertility Survey	41
26.	Overall quality of recent age-specific fertility rates and recent marital age-specific fertility rates	43
27.	Overall quality of trends in birth from the World Fertility Survey	44
28.	Overall quality of 15-year trends in age-specific fertility rates and marital age-specific fertility rates	46
29.	Percentage of non-numerical responses, mean desired family size and proportions who desired exactly i children among ever-married women aged 15-49	52
30.	Mean percentage of non-numerical responses, by level of development and strength of family planning programme effort	53
31.	Mean desired family size, by level of development and strength of family planning programme effort	55
32.	Mean desired family size, by number of living children, including current pregnancy, among ever-married women aged 15-49	56
33.	Percentage of currently married, fecund women who wanted no more children, by number of living children, including current pregnancy	59
34.	Observed and standardized percentages of currently married, fecund women who wanted no more children: averages by level of development and strength of family planning programme effort	61
35.	Percentage who wanted no more children at parities 2, 4 and 6 for age groups 15-24, 25-34 and 35-39	62
36.	Preferences for sex of next child and preference ratio among currently married, fecund women who wanted another child	63
37.	Preferences for sex of next child and preference ratio among currently married, fecund women who wanted another child, by level of development	64
38.	Preferences for sex of next child, by family composition among currently married, fecund women who wanted another child	65
39.	Preferences for sex of next child, by level of development and family composition	66
40.	Percentage who wanted no more children, by family composition among currently married, fecund and non-pregnant women with from two to four living children	67
41.	Measures of unwanted and wanted fertility	69
42.	Total fertility rate, wanted and unwanted total fertility rate and proportion of unwanted fertility, by level of development and strength of family planning programme effort	71
43.	Percentage of women never married in five-year current age groups and singulate mean age at marriage, by region, country and level of development	78
44.	Percentage married by exact age 20, according to five-year current age group, by region, country and level of development	80
45.	Estimates of mean age at marriage, based on the Coale-McNeil model, for five-year age groups, by region and level of development	82
46.	Percentage of women's reproductive years expected to be spent in various marital states, by region, country and level of development	83
47.	Percentage distribution of ever-married women by status of first marriage, based on women aged 40-49, by region, country and level of development	84
48.	Percentage distribution of births in the five years preceding the survey, according to marital status of the mother at the time of birth, by region, level of development and strength of family planning programme effort	87
49.	Total fertility rates for the five years preceding the survey and total fertility rates standardized for proportion currently married in each age group, by country, region and level of development	88
50.	Mean number of children ever born to ever-married women aged 40-49, according to status of first marriage, by region, level of development and strength of family planning programme effort	90
51.	Cumulative percentage of women having a first birth within specific periods since first marriage, according to age at first marriage, by region and level of development	91
52.	Age-specific marital fertility rates, according to age at first marriage, by region, level of development and strength of family planning programme effort	93

No.		Page
53.	Mean number of children ever born to ever-married women aged 40-49, according to age at first marriage, by region, country and level of development	96
54.	Percentage of ever-married women aged 40-49 who were childless, according to age at first marriage, by region and level of development	97
55.	Percentage who had married or had given birth by specific ages, based on women aged 20-24, by country, region, level of development and strength of family planning programme effort	99
56.	Summary measures of marriage patterns and fertility, by region and level of development	100
57.	Mean, median, first and third quartiles of breast-feeding duration for all births and mean breast-feeding duration only for births that were breast-fed	108
58.	Incidence of breast-feeding, by level of development and strength of family planning programme effort	110
59.	Percentage of women who were still breast-feeding at various durations from birth	111
60.	Mean duration of breast-feeding, by level of development and strength of family planning programme effort	111
61.	Prevalence and average duration of breast-feeding by sex of children, using current status data	113
62.	Incidence and mean duration of breast-feeding by age of mother, using current status data	114
63.	Mean duration of breast-feeding of children by age of mother: averages by level of development and strength of family planning programme effort	115
64.	Incidence and average duration of breast-feeding by birth order, using current status data	115
65.	Average difference in mean duration of breast-feeding by birth order	116
66.	Mean duration of breast-feeding of children by birth order of child: averages by level of development and strength of family planning programme effort	116
67.	Incidence and mean duration of breast-feeding among women who had used or had not used contraception during last closed birth interval	117
68.	Percentage of women currently using contraception among those still breast-feeding at the time of the survey	119
69.	Percentage of women using contraception among those still breast-feeding at the time of the survey: averages by level of development and strength of family planning programme effort	120
70.	Duration of full breast-feeding, post-partum amenorrhoea and post-partum sexual abstinence, using current status data	121
71.	Difference in durations of general and full breast-feeding and mean duration of full breast-feeding, by age of mother and use of contraception: data for last closed birth interval	125
72.	Difference in durations of general breast-feeding and post-partum amenorrhoea: data for last closed birth interval	125
73.	Difference in durations of general breast-feeding, post-partum amenorrhoea and post-partum abstinence: data for last closed birth interval	126
74.	Percentages of currently married women aged 15-49 who knew any contraceptive method, knew a family planning outlet, had ever used a method and were currently using modern and traditional methods, by country	131
75.	Average percentages of women who knew any contraceptive method, had ever used a method and were currently using modern and traditional methods, by region, level of development and strength of family planning programme effort	133
76.	Percentage who knew of contraception and percentage who had ever used a method, single and currently married women	134
77.	Percentage of currently married women who were currently using contraception, by age group	135
78.	Percentage of currently married women who were currently using contraception, by number of living children	138
79.	Ever-use and current use of contraception by exposed women, by desire for more children	141
80.	Percentage of currently married women aged 15-49 who knew specific contraceptive methods	144
81.	Percentage of currently married women and current contraceptive users aged 15-49 who were currently using each method	145
82.	Average demographic characteristics of women at first use of contraception and at interview, for women who had ever used contraception, nine countries	156

No.		Page
83.	Selected indicators of first use and current use of specific contraceptive methods, nine countries	157
84.	Percentage who were currently using the first method and percentage using any method, by time since first use, nine countries	157
85.	Selected indicators of contraceptive continuation and use of multiple methods	159
86.	The three indices and the total fertility rate, by region and country, level of development and strength of family planning programme effort	168
87.	Proportion of variance explained, direction of relationship and orthogonal regression coefficients for pairs of indices, for all countries, by region, level of development and strength of family planning programme effort	172
88.	Relative percentage contribution of each of the proximate determinants to the difference between the total fecundity rate and the total fertility rate, by region, level of development and strength of family planning programme effort	173
89.	Components of the indices of marriage and contraception, by region and country, level of development and strength of family planning programme effort	174
90.	Total fertility rate, total marital fertility rate, total natural marital fertility rate and total fecundity rate, by region and country, level of development and strength of family planning programme effort	174
91.	Means and standard deviations of the indices, by age group	175
92.	Average fertility rates by age group and percentage of difference between actual and potential fertility rates explained by three proximate determinants	176
93.	Age patterns of observed and standard fecundity rates: ages 25-44 expressed as a proportion of rate for ages 20-24, by groups of countries	180
94.	Percentage distribution of ever-married women aged 15-49, according to current type of place of residence, by country, region and level of development	191
95.	Percentage distribution of ever-married women aged 15-49, according to category of constructed residence variable, by country, region and level of development	192
96.	Total fertility rate and mean number of children born to all women aged 40-49, by current type of place of residence, for countries and groups	193
97.	Percentage of children ever born who were still alive at interview and mean number of living children, for ever-married women aged 40-49, according to type of place of residence: averages by region and level of development	194
98.	Percentage of ever-married women aged 15-49 who gave a non-numerical response to the question on desired family size, by type of place of current residence, selected countries	196
99.	Mean desired family size, ever-married women aged 15-49, according to current residence, by country, region and level of development	197
100.	Percentage of ever-married women aged 40-49 with more living children than the number desired, according to type of place of residence: averages by region and level of development	198
101.	Singulate mean age at marriage, by current residence	199
102.	Singulate mean age at marriage and reported mean age at marriage among women aged 40-49, according to current residence: averages by region and level of development	199
103.	Mean duration of breast-feeding, by residence	200
104.	Percentage of currently married women aged 15-49 who were currently using contraception, by current residence	202
105.	Description of regression models	204
106.	Summary of partial regression coefficients according to residence group, by region, level of development and strength of family planning programme effort: dependent variable = children ever born/duration of marriage	205
107.	Summary of partial regression coefficients according to residence group, by region and level of development: dependent variable = desired family size	207
108.	Summary of partial regression coefficients according to residence group, by region, level of development and strength of family planning programme effort: dependent variable = percentage who were currently using contraception	209
109.	Percentage distribution of ever-married women and their husbands according to number of years of education completed, mean number of years for ever-married women, all women and husbands; and correlation between husband's and wife's education	218
110.	Mean number of years of education for all women interviewed, by current age group, and difference in mean educational attainment between husbands of women aged 25-29 years and 45-49 years	220

No.		Page
111.	Percentage of women literate, according to number of years of education, by country, region and level of development	222
112.	Measures of current and cumulative fertility according to respondent's education: total fertility rate for ages 15-49; total marital fertility rate for durations 0-24; and mean number of children ever born to women aged 40-49	224
113.	Percentage of children ever born who were still alive at interview and mean number of living children, by respondent's education, for ever-married women aged 40-49: averages by region and level of development	227
114.	Mean number of children ever born to ever-married women aged 40-49, according to husband's education, by country and region	228
115.	Mean desired family size for ever-married women aged 15-49, according to respondent's education, by country and averages by region and level of development	229
116.	Percentage of ever-married women aged 15-49 who gave a non-numerical response to question on desired family size, by respondent's education, selected countries	230
117.	Percentage of ever-married women aged 40-49 with more living children than the number desired, by respondent's education: averages by region and level of development	231
118.	Percentage of women aged 40-49 never married, according to respondent's education, by regions and for selected countries	232
119.	Singulate mean age at marriage, according to respondent's education, by country, region and level of development	233
120.	Selected indicators of trend in average age at marriage, by respondent's education: mean values for 23 countries	234
121.	Mean duration of breast-feeding, according to respondent's education, by country, region and level of development	235
122.	Percentage of currently married women aged 15-49 currently using contraception, according to respondent's education, by country, region, level of development and strength of family planning programme effort	237
123.	Description of regression models	239
124.	Summary of partial regression coefficients for categories of respondent's education, models 1-4; and for categories of husband's education, model 3, by region and level of development: dependent variable = children ever born/ duration of marriage	240
125.	Summary of partial regression coefficients for categories of respondent's education, models 5-8: by region and level of development: dependent variable = desired family size	246
126.	Summary of partial regression coefficients for categories of respondent's education, models 9-11, by region and level of development: dependent variable = current use of contraception	248
127.	Percentage of women aged 25-49 who were currently working: estimates of the World Fertility Survey and the International Labour Organisation	259
128.	Percentage distribution according to current or most recent occupation since marriage, ever-married women aged 15-49 and women who had worked since marriage, by country, region and level of development	264
129.	Mean age at marriage, according to occupation before marriage, adjusted for education, by country, region and level of development	265
130.	Mean number of children ever born to ever-married women aged 40-49, according to respondent's occupation since marriage, by region and level of development	266
131.	Partial regression coefficients for occupation variables, women married three or more years: dependent variable = children ever born/duration of marriage	268
132.	Partial regression coefficients for occupation variables, women married three or more years, by region and level of development: dependent variable = children ever born/duration of marriage	269
133.	Summary of partial regression coefficients according to respondent's occupational group, by region and level of development: dependent variable = desired family size	273
134.	Percentage of currently married women who were currently using any contraceptive method, according to current occupation, by country, region and level of development	275
135.	Percentage who reported themselves infecund, by type of occupation since marriage and by region	277
136.	Percentage distribution of ever-married women aged 30-49, by number of children ever born, for five-year age groups, countries in the ESCAP region	285

No.		Page
137.	Mean number of children ever born to ever-married women, by current age group, countries in the ESCAP region	286
138.	Mean number of children ever born to all ever-married women, by number of years since first marriage, countries in the ESCAP region	286
139.	Total fertility rate and total marital fertility rate for the five years preceding the survey, countries in the ESCAP region	287
140.	Live birth rates by age group and total fertility rates for the five years preceding the survey, selected countries in the ESCAP region	288
141.	Marital fertility rates by age group and total marital fertility rates for the five years preceding the survey, selected countries in the ESCAP region	288
142.	Trends in live birth rates by age group and in total fertility rates in selected countries in the ESCAP region, periods 0-4, 5-9 and 10-14 years prior to the survey	288
143.	Trends in marital fertility rates by age group and in total marital fertility rates in selected countries in the ESCAP region, periods 0-4, 5-9 and 10-14 years prior to the survey	290
144.	Mean number of children ever born to ever-married women, by age at first union, countries in the ESCAP region	292
145.	Mean number of children ever born to ever-married women aged 45-49, by age at first marriage, countries in the ESCAP region	292
146.	Mean number of children ever born to ever-married women aged 40-49, by continuity of first marriage and whether remarried, countries in the ESCAP region	292
147.	Duration of breast-feeding and percentage of children ever breast-fed, countries in the ESCAP region	293
148.	Contraception index and its components, countries in the ESCAP region	293
149.	Age-specific marital fertility rates, by current residence, 1975-1980, countries in the ESCAP region	294
150.	Age-specific marital fertility rates, by respondent's education, 1975-1980, countries in the ESCAP region	295
151.	Age-specific marital fertility rates, by respondent's work status, 1975-1980, countries in the ESCAP region	296
152.	Measures of childlessness and behavioural infecundity for various age groups, countries in the ECLAC region	303
153.	Levels and trends of infant and child mortality, countries in the ECLAC region	305
154.	Percentage who were currently using contraception among women with two living children, by sex composition of living children, countries in the ECLAC region	305
155.	Recent fertility, by current residence and respondent's education, countries in the ECLAC region	306
156.	Recent marital fertility, by husband's occupation and respondent's work status, countries in the ECLAC region	309
157.	Regression coefficients for log-linear model with children ever born as dependent variable and union duration, age at first union and child-death experience as independent variables, countries in the ECLAC region	310
158.	Predicted cumulative fertility at 8 and 25 years of marital duration, by residential status of respondents, countries in the ECLAC region	312
159.	Predicted cumulative fertility at 8 and 25 years of marital duration, by years of education, countries in the ECLAC region	314
160.	Median age at first union and differentials in singulate mean age at marriage, by residence and years of education, countries in the ECLAC region	316
161.	Percentage of ever-users of contraception among currently married women and percentage using modern methods, by current residence, countries in the ECLAC region	316
162.	Percentage of ever-users of contraception among currently married women and percentage using modern methods, by years of education, countries in the ECLAC region	317
163.	Mean duration of breast-feeding for surviving children, by current residence and years of education, countries in the ECLAC region	318
164.	Relative contributions of three proximate determinants to differentials in recent fertility between residence and educational groups, countries in the ECLAC region	319
165.	Percentage distribution of ever-married women aged 15 or over, by level of education, countries in sub-Saharan Africa	325

No.		Page
166.	Percentage distribution of ever-married women aged 20-29 and 30-39, by level of education, countries in sub-Saharan Africa	326
167.	Proportion of women ever married, by age group, and singulate mean age at marriage, countries in sub-Saharan Africa	327
168.	Proportion of women married by specified ages for selected cohorts, countries in sub-Saharan Africa	328
169.	Age-specific proportions of women ever married and singulate mean age at marriage, by place of residence, eight countries in sub-Saharan Africa	329
170.	Proportion of women ever married in selected age groups and singulate mean age at marriage, by level of education, seven countries in sub-Saharan Africa	330
171.	Distribution of ever-married women by current marital status, selected age groups, countries in sub-Saharan Africa	331
172.	Proportion of ever-married women in polygamous unions, by level of education, countries in sub-Saharan Africa	331
173.	Proportion of women's reproductive years expected to be spent in various marital states, countries in sub-Saharan Africa	332
174.	Crude birth rates and total fertility rates for the five years preceding the survey date, countries in sub-Saharan Africa, and averages compared with other regions	332
175.	Average age-specific fertility rates for ever-married women during the five years preceding the survey, sub-Saharan Africa, Latin America and the Caribbean, and Asia and Oceania	333
176.	Percentage contribution to total fertility rates of all women aged under 20, 20-29 and 30-49 years, countries in sub-Saharan Africa	333
177.	Trends in fertility levels in the recent past, countries in sub-Saharan Africa	333
178.	Mean number of children ever born to women aged 40 or over, by current marital status, countries in sub-Saharan Africa	334
179.	Mean number of live births to ever-married women as a proportion of mean number of live births to women married and with no co-wives, women aged 40 or over, countries in sub-Saharan Africa	334
180.	Proportion of all ever-married women aged 40 or over who were childless, by type of marital union, countries in sub-Saharan Africa	335
181.	Total fertility rate, by type of place of current residence, countries in sub-Saharan Africa	335
182.	Total fertility rate for ages 15-49, by respondent's education, eight countries in sub-Saharan Africa	335
183.	Mean duration of breast-feeding, post-partum amenorrhoea, abstinence and non-susceptibility, selected age groups and all ages, eight countries in sub-Saharan Africa	336
184.	Desired family size, countries in sub-Saharan Africa	337
185.	Selected demographic indicators for six Arab countries in Western Asia and Northern Africa	341
186.	Mean number of children ever born to ever-married women, by current age, six Arab countries in Western Asia and Northern Africa	342
187.	Age-specific fertility rates and total fertility rates for the period 0-4 years prior to the survey, six Arab countries in Western Asia and Northern Africa	342
188.	Estimated total fertility rates for five-year periods prior to the survey, calculated from birth history data, six Arab countries in Western Asia and Northern Africa	343
189.	Cumulative fertility to marital duration 15-19 years, by age at marriage, six Arab countries in Western Asia and Northern Africa	344
190.	Age-specific fertility rates and total fertility rates, by current residence, six Arab countries in Western Asia and Northern Africa	345
191.	Current levels of fertility according to current residence, six Arab countries in Western Asia and Northern Africa	345
192.	Current levels of fertility, by wife's level of education, six Arab countries in Western Asia and Northern Africa	346
193.	Proportions ever married, by age group and sex, and singulate mean age at marriage, six Arab countries in Western Asia and Northern Africa	347
194.	Median age at first marriage for cohorts of women aged 15-49, six Arab countries in Western Asia and Northern Africa	348
195.	Age-specific percentages of ever-married women and singulate mean age at marriage, by type of residence, six Arab countries in Western Asia and Northern Africa	348
196.	Age-specific percentages of ever-married women and singulate mean age at marriage, by level of education, Jordan, Morocco and Syrian Arab Republic	349

No.		Page
197.	Levels of ever-use and current use of contraception among currently married women, six Arab countries in Western Asia and Northern Africa	351
198.	Levels of ever-use and current use of contraception among currently married women, by type of place of residence, six Arab countries in Western Asia and Northern Africa	351
199.	Levels of ever-use and current use of contraception among currently married women, by educational level, six Arab countries in Western Asia and Northern Africa	352
200.	Percentage distribution of currently married fecund women according to intentions concerning fertility and contraceptive use, six Arab countries in Western Asia and Northern Africa	352
201.	Some characteristics of surveys of 16 developed countries	359
202.	Levels of fertility and family planning, 16 developed countries: selected indicators	362
203.	Selected indicators of fertility and family planning for 11 developed countries, around 1970 and around 1975	363
204.	Average ultimate expected fertility and median number of months between marriage and first birth, by marriage cohort, selected developed countries	364
205.	Current use of modern and traditional methods, by marriage cohort, selected developed countries	364
206.	Average number of live births standardized by marriage duration, by wife's education, residence and work history, selected developed countries	366
207.	Average ultimate expected number of children standardized by marriage duration, by wife's education, residence and work history, selected developed countries	366
208.	Median number of months between marriage and first birth, by wife's education, residence and work history, selected developed countries	367
209.	Cumulative probability of a first birth seven months after first marriage, by wife's education and work history, selected developed countries	367
210.	Current use of modern methods of contraception, by wife's education, residence and work history, selected developed countries	368
211.	Current use of traditional methods of contraception, by wife's education, residence and work history, selected developed countries	368
212.	Selected marriage indicators for Europe: subregional averages	376

LIST OF FIGURES

1.	Relationship between survey design, country setting and data comparability	11
2.	Age-specific fertility rates, by region	25
3.	Age-specific fertility rates, by level of development and strength of family planning programme effort	25
4.	Marital age-specific fertility rates, by region, level of development and strength of family planning programme effort	27
5.	Age-specific fertility rates for the periods 10-14 and 0-4 years prior to the survey date, by level of development and strength of family planning programme effort, 19 countries	30
6.	Mean number of children ever born and living, by age group of woman and level of development	32
7.	Adolescent fertility rates, by age of woman and by region, level of development and strength of family planning programme effort	34
8.	Mean desired family size, by region, level of development and strength of family planning programme effort	54
9.	Percentage of ever-married women, by number of children desired, regional groups	56
10.	Mean number of children desired, by number of living children, for regions	58
11.	Percentage who wanted no more children, by number of living children, for regions	60
12.	Percentage who wanted no more children, by number of living children, various levels of development	60
13.	Percentage who wanted no more children, by number of living children, for strength of family planning programme effort	60
14.	Singulate mean age at marriage, by region and level of development	79
15.	Percentage married by exact age 20, five-year current age groups, by region and level of development	81

No.		Page
16.	Percentage of women currently married, by age group, for regions and selected countries	82
17.	Percentage ever remarried among women aged 40-49 whose first marriage had been dissolved, by percentage of all first marriages ever dissolved, selected countries	85
18.	Age-specific fertility rates for all women and marital age-specific fertility rates, averaged for all countries and for regions	86
19.	Average age-specific fertility rates and average rates within and outside marriage, by region	87
20.	Total fertility rates, by percentage of reproductive years married	88
21.	Age at marriage and family size	89
22.	Age-specific marital fertility rates, by age at marriage and by region, level of development and strength of family planning programme effort	94
23.	Percentage of women who had never breast-fed, by country	109
24.	Proportion of women who were still breast-feeding after specified intervals from birth, by region	112
25.	Proportions who were breast-feeding, full breast-feeding, amenorrhoeic and abstaining, using current status data	122
26.	Percentage of currently married women currently using contraception and percentage who had ever used, by age: averages by region	136
27.	Percentage who wanted no more children and percentage who were using contraception, according to current family size, selected countries	139
28.	Percentage of currently married women currently using contraception and percentage who had ever used, by number of living children: averages by region	140
29.	Index of contraceptive use for birth-spacing, by percentage of women who had breast-fed for at least six months	143
30.	Average pattern of current contraceptive use, by age and family size, adjusted for other variables	143
31.	Percentage of currently married women aged 15-49 currently using specific contraceptive methods: extreme values for 38 countries and 25th, 50th and 75th percentiles	148
32.	Current use of specific contraceptive methods, by age group and number of living children: average distributions for 38 countries	150
33.	Age differences in percentage of current contraceptive users employing specific methods, individual countries	151
34.	Percentage of currently married women using sterilization, the pill and other methods, by age: Egypt and Panama	152
35.	Average percentage of current contraceptive users employing the pill, sterilization and other methods, by age and family size, adjusted for other variables	153
36.	Average percentage of exposed women and current contraceptive users employing specific methods, by desire for more children	154
37.	Percentage currently using the first method and percentage using any method, by years since first use of contraception	158
38.	Contraceptive continuation ratio, by percentage of women who had ever used contraception, for exposed women who wanted no more children	159
39.	Summary distribution of values of the three C indices	169
40.	Distribution of the three C indices within regional and development groups	170
41.	Scatter-plot of indices for marriage, C_m, and contraception, C_c, for 38 World Fertility Survey countries	171
42.	Scatter-plot of indices for contraception, C_c, and post-partum infecundability, C_i, for 38 World Fertility Survey countries	171
43.	Scatter-plot of indices for marriage, C_m, and post-partum infecundability, C_i, for 38 World Fertility Survey countries	171
44.	Age-specific fertility rates, by region, level of development and strength of family planning programme effort	177
45.	Percentage of difference between actual and potential fertility rates explained by three proximate determinants, by age group, according to region, level of development and strength of family planning programme effort	178
46.	Total fertility rate and mean number of children ever born to ever-married women aged 40-49, according to current residence, by region and level of development	195
47.	Singulate mean age at marriage by residence, all countries	198
48.	Mean duration of breast-feeding, according to residence, by region and level of development	201

No.		Page
49.	Percentage of currently married women aged 15-49 currently using contraception, by residence, all countries	203
50.	Percentage currently using contraception, by residence: averages by strength of family planning programme effort within development groups	203
51.	Adjusted difference in marital fertility, *CEB/D*, between long-term rural and long-term urban residents, by level of development	206
52.	Adjusted difference in desired family size between long-term rural and long-term urban residents, by level of development	208
53.	Adjusted difference between percentage currently using contraception among long-term rural and long-term urban residents, by level of development	210
54.	Hypothesized relationship between fertility and education at different levels of development	216
55.	Mean number of children ever born to women aged 40-49 and total fertility rate: extreme values and quartiles for all countries with data available, by respondent's education	223
56.	Average values of total fertility rate and children ever born, according to education, by region, level of development and strength of family planning programme effort	226
57.	Mean number of children ever born to ever-married women aged 40-49 years, by husband's and respondent's education: averages by region	229
58.	Mean desired family size, by respondent's education, for sub-Saharan Africa and for other regions combined	230
59.	Singulate mean age at marriage, by respondent's education	233
60.	Mean duration of breast-feeding, according to respondent's education, by region and level of development	236
61.	Percentage currently using contraception, by respondent's education	237
62.	Percentage using contraception, by respondent's education: averages by strength of family planning programme effort within development groups	238
63.	Partial regression coefficients for categories of respondent's education, model 2: dependent variable = *CEB/D*	241
64.	Partial regression coefficients for categories of respondent's education, rural and urban areas of selected countries: dependent variable = *CEB/D*	243
65.	Adjusted difference in marital fertility, *CEB/D*, at zero and at 10 or more years of respondent's and husband's education, model 3, by level of development	245
66.	Adjusted difference in number of children desired at zero and at 10 or more years of education, model 7, by region and level of development	247
67.	Adjusted difference in percentage of currently married women currently using contraception at zero and at 10 or more years of respondent's education, model 10, by region and level of development	249
68.	Age patterns of current work, selected countries	260
69.	Percentage of ever-married women currently working, by region and type of place of residence	261
70.	Current work, by years of education, selected countries	262
71.	Ratio of proportion of women formerly married and currently working to proportion currently married and currently working, by overall level of female labour force participation	263
72.	Partial regression coefficients of occupation variables, by level of socio-economic development	270
73.	Partial regression coefficients of variable indicating work in a modern occupation, by gross enrolment ratio for females, 1975	271
74.	Partial regression coefficients of variable indicating work in a modern occupation, by family planning programme effort	272
75.	Differential in contraceptive use between designated occupational group and "no work" category, by level of development	274
76.	Age-specific and duration-specific fertility rates, by educational category, selected countries in the ECLAC region	308
77.	Children ever born to ever-married women, by current age and educational level, Guyana and Mexico	310
78.	Number of children ever born according to union duration, by child-death experience and age at first union, countries in the ECLAC region: predicted values from regression models	311
79.	Predicted number of children ever born, by duration of union for residential-educational groups, Mexico and Paraguay	313
80.	Predicted number of children ever born according to duration of union, by years of education: Jamaica and Peru	315

No.		Page
81.	Percentage of currently married women currently using contraception, by number of living children: selected developing and developed countries	378

Explanatory Notes

Symbols of United Nations documents are composed of capital letters combined with figures. Mention of such a symbol indicates a reference to a United Nations document.

Reference to "dollars" ($) indicates United States dollars, unless otherwise stated.

Reference to "tons" indicates metric tons, unless otherwise stated.

The term "billion" signifies a thousand million.

Annual rates of growth or change refer to annual compound rates, unless otherwise stated.

A hyphen (-) between years, e.g., 1984-1985, indicates the full period involved, including the beginning and end years; a slash (/) indicates a financial year, school year or crop year, e.g., 1984/85.

A point (.) is used to indicate decimals.

The following symbols have been used in the tables:

Two dots (. .) indicate that data are not available or are not separately reported.

A dash (—) indicates that the amount is nil or negligible.

A hyphen (-) indicates that the item is not applicable.

A minus sign (−) before a number indicates a deficit or decrease, except as indicated.

Details and percentages in tables do not necessarily add to totals because of rounding.

The following abbreviations have been used:

ASFECR	age-specific fecundity rate
ASFR	age-specific fertility rate
ASMFR	age-specific marital fertility rate
ASNFR	age-specific natural fertility rate
CBR	crude birth rate
CEB	children ever born
CEB/D	children ever born/duration of marriage
ECA	Economic Commission for Africa
ECE	Economic Commission for Europe
ECLAC	Economic Commission for Latin America and the Caribbean
ESCAP	Economic Commission for Asia and the Pacific
FOTCAF	factors other than contraception affecting fertility
GDP	gross domestic product
GNP	gross national product
ILO	International Labour Organisation
IMR	infant mortality rate
IUD	intra-uterine device
SMAM	singulate mean age at marriage
TF	total fecundity rate
TFR	total fertility rate
TMFR	total marital fertility
TN	total natural marital fertility rate
UNESCO	United Nations Educational, Scientific and Cultural Organization
UNFPA	United Nations Fund for Population Activities
WFS	World Fertility Survey
WHO	World Health Organization

INTRODUCTION

ABSTRACT

The purpose of this publication, which represents the final output of a long project, is to further the understanding of fertility behaviour through a systematic analysis of its determinants, using the roughly comparable data available from the World Fertility Survey (WFS) programme. Most of the study focuses on 38 developing countries (fairly evenly divided between Africa, Latin America and the Caribbean, and Asia and Oceania), but many of the participating developed countries also are included in one part of the book.

The conceptual framework described in this introduction is designed to elucidate the relative importance of three societal-level variables in determining the course of the demographic transition in different countries: (*a*) level of socio-economic development; (*b*) regional or geographical setting; and (*c*) government population policy. Thus, in this report, data on various aspects of reproductive behaviour—not only fertility but fertility preferences, nuptiality, breast-feeding and contraceptive practice—are grouped into broad categories with respect to these three variables; and observed patterns are described and analysed with respect to both demographic and socio-economic differentials. Trends for certain variables also are assessed and compared between groups of countries.

This introduction explains the measurement of these societal characteristics and examines their distribution according to the countries studied. The index of socio-economic development adopted was constructed from measures of its four broadly accepted components: (*a*) economic product; (*b*) current educational enrolment; (*c*) health; and (*d*) extent of communications. Government population policy is measured as a composite index of strength of family planning programme effort adjusted to correspond roughly to the survey date in each country. While the WFS data for the developing countries were found to be broadly comparable, certain incomparabilities arose due not just to differences in questionnaire design but to certain conditions within the countries which influenced the way in which questions were presented by the interviewers and perceived by the respondents. These differences are highlighted in this introduction because they affect the cross-country comparability of nuptiality measures and socio-economic characteristics.

The organization of the book reflects not only the topics covered by the World Fertility Survey questionnaire but the organization of work on the comparative analysis of the WFS data within the United Nations system. The first two parts, prepared at United Nations Headquarters, provide a broad perspective on patterns within the developing countries and their differences. Part three provides regional perspectives on related topics prepared by the regional commissions or regional experts, and part four presents comparisons with the developed countries and a global perspective.

BACKGROUND

In the decade between the two major population conferences, held at Bucharest in 1974 and at Mexico City in 1984, there was an explosion of information on fertility from every region of the world, largely generated through the special surveys conducted under the auspices of the World Fertility Survey (WFS) programme. This international survey programme was developed in collaboration with the United Nations and in co-operation with the International Union for the Scientific Study of Population and was run under the aegis of the International Statistical Institute. The programme was funded by a number of national and international agencies, including the United Nations Fund for Population Activities, the United Kingdom Office of Development Assistance and the United States Agency for International Development. Its objective was defined as being "to assist a large number of interested countries, particularly the developing countries, in carrying out nationally representative, internationally comparable, and scientifically designed and conducted surveys of human fertility behaviour" (Grebenik, 1981, p. 11).

Beginning in 1972, the work of the programme was given a strong impetus by the recommendations of the World Population Plan of Action, which include broad support for data collection and analysis as well as a specific invitation to all countries to co-operate with the World Fertility Survey (United Nations, 1975).

The timing of the WFS programme was closely linked with a growing global awareness of population problems. The countries in Latin America and the Caribbean and in Asia and Oceania that joined the programme in the first few years included those such as Jamaica, Panama, Malaysia, the Republic of Korea, Sri Lanka and Thailand, where fertility change was already well under way; and others, such as Bangladesh and Pakistan, where fertility decline was not apparent but was urgently sought. These first countries had an established tradition of data collection and previous experience with demographic surveys. In later years, the countries that joined the programme were more often those with less of a tradition of data collection, without firmly articulated population goals and at an earlier stage in their economic development and demographic transition. Thus, the final set of surveys provides an extremely heterogeneous selection of countries with respect to many of the key factors differentiating countries according to phases of the demographic transition. Under the WFS programme in the years between the conferences at Bucharest and Mexico City, surveys were completed and reports published in 40 developing countries[1] and 21 developed countries.

Prior to this programme, comparative demographic analysis had to rely upon data drawn from different sources which, although based on similar methods of data collection (i.e., census, survey and vital registration) and certain international guidelines (United Nations, 1969), were collected independently and often for different purposes. Thus, comparative demographic analysis was restricted to comparisons of broad national characteristics and trends and to descriptive discussions of variations in national experiences. With the WFS programme, in contrast, national surveys were undertaken with guidance from a single organization which had data comparability as one of its principal goals.[2] The resulting data sets available to the international community for analysis provide the opportunity to study and to compare in depth the multiple dimensions of demographic relationships in a way not previously possible.[3] The availability of these data proved to be invaluable in undertaking the review and appraisal of the World Population Plan of Action 10 years after the Conference at Bucharest (United Nations, 1986), and the findings of the WFS data were referred to repeatedly in the subsequent international debate at Mexico City.

The International Conference on Population was held at Mexico City in August 1984—the same month in which the World Fertility Survey was formally terminated. At that time, full comparative analysis of the WFS data, including all major regions, was just beginning because many of the data tapes for Africa had just recently become available. While much comparative data had been published for Latin America and the Caribbean and for Asia—in the WFS Cross-National Summaries series, in the Minimum Research Programme of the United Nations described in the preface and in selected comparative analyses—a global perspective was not yet possible.

The objective of this study is the further understanding of fertility behaviour through a systematic analysis of its determinants using roughly comparable data from a diverse range of countries. As many participating countries as possible were included in the analysis. However, certain organizational constraints as well as timing considerations prevented the inclusion of data from all countries. In the African region, data from Nigeria had to be excluded because they were not available in time to complete necessary data tabulations. Although data from the Turkish survey were published in its *First Country Report*, the tabulations for this study required the standard recode tape, which was not yet available for comparative analysis. The Economic Commission for Europe (ECE) took responsibility for analysis of the data for developed countries. However, the data from the fertility surveys in Israel and Japan were excluded because, among other things, the available material was limited in scope and because as non-European countries they were at the periphery of the geographical focus of the comparative study. In addition, data from Portugal, Sweden and Switzerland were excluded because they were not available in sufficient time. Therefore, the analyses included in this report are based on 38 data sets from developing countries (parts one, two and three) and 16 data sets from developed countries (part four).

This study emphasizes primarily the findings from developing countries because a separate report on the findings from developed countries is being published (Economic Commission for Europe, forthcoming). It was, however, considered useful to include here a summary of the developed-country findings (chapter XIV) so that comparisons could be made and conclusions drawn with respect to the new knowledge of fertility behaviour (chapter XV). In the introductory material that follows, the conceptual framework for this study is discussed. Then an overview of certain characteristics of the participating countries, as well as certain features of the data, is presented to provide some background for the subsequent study. Lastly, the plan of analysis and the organization of the study are explained.

CONCEPTUAL FRAMEWORK

The conceptual framework adopted for this study was designed to elucidate certain broad issues of global policy significance. The international debate on population issues and, in particular, on the determinants of fertility decline centres on the relative importance of level of socio-economic development, regional or geographical setting and government population policy in determining the course of the demographic transition for a particular country. Although the debate may be partially ideological, it is not entirely so. To an important extent, it derives from a lack of knowledge which can only be overcome through a systematic study of a broad range of national experiences. Within this debate, several key questions can be identified, the first two relating to the existence and universality of a development-fertility relationship and the third relating to the feasibility and efficacy of government intervention. For example, current discussions of the appropriate design of population policy in Africa centre on the question whether Africa rests on one end of a development-fertility continuum or whether its situation is unique when viewed in either a historical context or a contemporary comparative context. If the former view is largely correct, policy designed for the African context can draw largely on experience in Latin America and the Caribbean and in Asia and Oceania, while if the latter view is closer to reality, new and imaginative approaches must be designed after careful study of the African context.

Such questions are not new to demographic research. Cross-national studies have had a long tradition. Simple and parsimonious multivariate relationships have been estimated between various aggregate measures of economic development (as well as other relevant variables) and crude measures of fertility with each country representing one observation (Adelman, 1963; Russett and others, 1964; Friedlander and Silver, 1967). More recently, the increasing availability of data on fertility trends as well as on various economic and social statistics at a national level has permitted cross-national studies to measure the relationship between economic trends and birth-rate trends in different policy settings (Mauldin and Berelson, 1978; Cutright, 1983; Lapham and Mauldin, 1984; Boulier, 1985). Not only do such studies show a strong relationship between economic development (however measured) and fertility but recent studies incorporating measures of policy intervention almost universally show that within groups of countries at similar levels of development, fertility decline is greatest in those countries which are thought to have the most aggressive family planning programmes. It is always difficult to be certain that non-programme influences on fertility have been adequately controlled in analyses of this type (Demeny, 1979; Hernandez, 1981). However, controlled experiments and studies focusing on differential access to contraception within countries, as well as a variety of analytical specifications applied to cross-national data, suggest that family planning programmes have accelerated the fertility decline in developing countries to an important degree (Boulier, 1985). Building on past research, the present study examines fertility in the context of socio-economic development and directs attention also to relationships between fertility and family planning programme effort.

While the WFS data provide many new opportunities for analysis because of their comparability and scope, their modest inventory of social and economic information, as contrasted with a heavy emphasis on demographic measurement, presents certain limitations on the range of policy questions that can be addressed. The WFS core questionnaire was not based on any one explicit theory of fertility determinants. Instead, its goal was to serve as an instrument for the accurate and thorough description of fertility and its primary components. The vast array of WFS publications (in particular, the individual First Country Reports and the Comparative Studies and Scientific Reports series) attest to the success of the programme in achieving its main objective. The participating countries represent a range of points on the development spectrum and a diversity of cultural settings, and the many WFS publications document a high degree of variability between countries in all aspects of fertility.

Basically, these data can address three broad sets of questions in a comparative framework: (*a*) the extent and range of inter-country differences in demographic variables and their differentials according to several social characteristics; (*b*) the general applicability of certain reproductive models at the individual level through the comparison of country-level findings; and (*c*) the relationship between macro-level differences between countries in culture, economic development and population policy and micro-level reproductive processes, sometimes called the "multi-level approach". Behavioural models of fertility cannot be properly tested with WFS data because information is lacking on variables required by their predictive theoretical frameworks. In the case of economic models, these variables would include most importantly individual earnings and household income.[4] The testing of sociological theories, such as Caldwell's (1982) theory of intergenerational wealth flows, would require not only more economic data than WFS has to offer but information on intra-familial relations of power and deference and on household structure. Although information about household structure is available in some WFS household surveys, such data have not been systematically linked to the individual data and cannot be used for comparative analysis. Structural theories of fertility (such as McNicoll, 1980) emphasize the importance of social and administrative organizations as intermediary factors which shape the course of the demographic transition in different settings. Again, although community data on the presence of certain local institutions were collected in a few settings by WFS, the results have been less revealing than originally hoped (Casterline, 1985); and, in any case, the restricted availability and non-standard content of the community surveys preclude their use for comparative analysis.

Because the WFS questionnaire was atheoretical in its design, the vast majority of comparative research findings fall into the first category of questions mentioned in the preceding paragraph. These include the descriptive findings published by WFS in the Cross-National Summaries series, the World Fertility Survey Reports published by the Population Reference Bureau and the Minimum Research Programme of the United Nations Working Group on Comparative Analysis (United Nations, 1981, 1981a, 1982, 1983, 1983a, 1983b, 1984). The distinction between "theoretical" and "descriptive" aims is not, however, a clear-cut one. Although WFS was not specifically designed to test any particular theoretical view, the social and economic factors measured—primarily type of place of residence, education, type of work and, in some countries, religion and ethnicity—were chosen with the expectation that they would divide the population in ways related to fertility and the other demographic factors that were the primary focus of the surveys. Such descriptive results provide abundant material from which existing theories can be reassessed and new hypotheses developed. Despite the lack of economic information and the cross-sectional design of the survey, the WFS results can be used to re-examine traditional thinking about the demographic transition (Cleland, 1985).

The comparative analysis of WFS data has also contributed to advancing the modelling of reproductive processes. Widespread application of the Bongaarts (1978) proximate determinants model has proved it to be a useful way of relating the major intermediate variables to fertility (Casterline and others, 1984). The findings emerging from these applications have the potential for laying the base for further theoretical development with respect to not only the reproduction process itself but the channels through which psychological, social and economic factors may operate on fertility. They are also likely to lead to further empirical probing in order to identify more precisely some of the major sources of unexplained variation. Other models of the reproductive process have been tested using WFS data, in particular some focusing on the determinants of birth-interval length and the pace of reproduction (see Hobcraft and Casterline, 1983; and Rodríguez and others, 1984). Some of the provocative and surprising findings that have emerged from these analyses will force demographers to re-examine former assumptions about the effect of achieved parity on subsequent reproductive behaviour.

The other major area where comparative analysis of the WFS data has the potential to contribute to the understanding of country differences is multi-level analysis—an approach in which individual variations in fertility are seen to depend not only upon individual characteristics but upon key features of the environment in which these women are living. This approach was chosen for this study. While the approach is not new, the availability of WFS data makes it possible to apply it systematically.

Several scholars at the University of Michigan have pioneered in the statistical application of this approach (Hermalin and Mason, 1980; Hermalin, 1986; Mason, 1986) and have used WFS data to illustrate its applicability to a model of family-building at different phases of a woman's life cycle (Entwisle and Mason, 1985). Using sophisticated multivariate estimating procedures and specially designed computer programs, Entwisle and Mason (1985) quantified the relationship between gross national product, family planning programme effort and children ever born, controlling for respondent's education and residence based on data from 15 WFS countries (primarily drawn from Asia and Oceania and Latin America and the Caribbean). Their approach is based on several assumptions. The first is that the relationship between macro-level country characteristics and individual-level reproductive behaviour has a stable underlying structure which is quantifiable. The second is that the sampling error with which that relationship is estimated can be contained within reasonable bounds. The distinct advantage of this approach is that it allows an estimate of the interaction between gross national product (GNP) and family planning effort in its effect on micro-socio-economic fertility differentials. However, it would be difficult in this approach to test for a non-monotonic relationship between the level of development and fertility differentials—a relationship that might be expected based on transition theories. In addition, it would be difficult to achieve a sufficient sample of countries to test the stability of the estimated relationships across culturally distinct regions.

In this study, the multi-level approach has been applied in a simpler and more descriptive form in order to avoid some of the problems inherent in the more statistically rigorous application described above. The framework is used to explore various aspects of reproductive behaviour —not only fertility but fertility preferences, nuptiality, breast-feeding and contraceptive practice. This approach is, none the less, systematic. The strategy adopted here is to group country findings in broad categories according to region, socio-economic development and strength of family planning programme effort and to use the simple descriptive device of comparing unweighted group averages to denote patterns and relationships between country characteristics and various aspects of individual reproductive behaviour. An unweighted average allows each country to have an equal weight in the analysis (regardless of population size or sample size). Attention is centred on the broad differences between groups of countries and on the degree of heterogeneity or homogeneity among countries within these groups, rather than on the specific patterns observed for individual countries.

The patterns to be examined include not only descriptive measures of various aspects of overall national reproductive behaviour according to developmental setting (for example) but socio-economic differentials in fertility and related behaviour. Although cross-sectional findings can only be suggestive with respect to the process of demographic transition, trends for certain variables can also be assessed and compared between groups of countries. Thus, the detailed information available for individual women in each country is utilized while at the same time the large number of individual country findings are made more digestible.

This approach can shed light on the development-fertility relationship as it is observed in different cultural and policy settings. However, findings emerging from this study cannot be used to predict future trends in reproductive behaviour in any individual country in the course of development or as a consequence of family planning programme initiatives. Indeed, the finding of a negative relationship between family planning programme effort and fertility across countries could reflect not only the effect of development on fertility but the effect of fertility levels on policy implementation, with countries with lower fertility having a greater demand for services (Lloyd, 1974; Demeny, 1979). In the same vein, a negative relationship between development levels and fertility could partially reflect the positive effect of lower fertility on economic growth per capita.

It should also be stressed that although many aspects of reproduction are examined here, this report by no means represents an exhaustive analysis of WFS data. It is complementary to, and is not a substitute for, country-specific studies. First, a comparative approach by its very nature stresses aspects of the data that have been measured in a reasonably standard way for all or most countries. Secondly, given the enormous volume of information gathered in WFS, it has been necessary to select among topics and to limit the amount of detail that can be considered for any one country. Thirdly, the comparative approach directs attention to the identification of patterns that are typical of countries with certain socio-economic or cultural characteristics. Further analyses, beyond the scope of the present volume, are required to understand the reasons that certain countries diverge from the usual patterns. Comparative studies set the stage for such work by helping to establish which patterns are usual and therefore likely to have similar causes in a variety of settings, and which patterns may need to be explained by involving historical or cultural features unique to a particular society.

CHARACTERISTICS OF STUDY COUNTRIES

As mentioned above, the three country characteristics chosen as macro variables are region, level of socio-economic development and strength of family planning programme effort. The developed countries were analysed separately but since they form a very distinct group with respect to all three characteristics, these countries are considered one group whose experience is contrasted with the developing countries. For each of the three characteristics chosen, countries are grouped in broad categories. In the case of region, the groups are based on a country's location within one of three major regions and wherever appropriate (when there is substantial within-region variability) subregional groups are also presented. As concerns family planning programme effort and socio-economic development, the determination of groups was more complex, and it required the weighting of multiple factors and the ranking of countries to form broad and reasonably distinct groups. In the discussion here, the groups and the factors considered in their construction are discussed for each characteristic.

Region

The distribution of the developing countries participating in the WFS programme, according to United Nations regional groups, is shown in table 1. The 38 countries for which data have been included in this study are evenly distributed among the regions: 12 in Africa; 13 in Latin America and the Caribbean; and 13 in Asia and Oceania. While the surveys in Africa and in Latin America and the Caribbean covered roughly 30 and 44 per cent of the resident populations, respectively, only 22 per cent of the population of Asia and Oceania was covered, largely because several very populous countries in Asia, notably China and India, did not participate.

TABLE 1. WORLD FERTILITY SURVEY COUNTRIES BY MAJOR REGION AND SUBREGION, AND PERCENTAGE OF REGIONAL/SUBREGIONAL DEVELOPING-COUNTRY POPULATION REPRESENTED

Region and subregion	Countries in subregion	Percentage of developing-country population included[a]
Africa		
Eastern Africa	Kenya	12
Middle Africa	Cameroon	17
Northern Africa	Egypt, Morocco, Sudan, Tunisia	79
Southern Africa	Lesotho	4
Western Africa	Benin, Côte d'Ivoire,[b] Ghana, Mauritania, Senegal	21
	ALL AFRICA	30
Latin America and the Caribbean		
Caribbean	Dominican Republic, Haiti, Jamaica, Trinidad and Tobago	51
Central America	Costa Rica, Mexico, Panama	80
Temperate South America	—	0
Tropical America	Colombia, Ecuador, Guyana, Paraguay, Peru, Venezuela	34
	ALL LATIN AMERICA AND THE CARIBBEAN	44
Asia and Oceania[c]		
Asia[c]		
East Asia[c]	Republic of Korea	22
South Asia		
South-eastern Asia	Indonesia, Malaysia, Philippines, Thailand	72
Southern Asia	Bangladesh, Nepal, Pakistan, Sri Lanka	22
Western Asia	Jordan, Syrian Arab Republic, Yemen	19
Oceania[c]	Fiji	12
	ALL ASIA AND OCEANIA	22

Source: Based on United Nations (1985).
[a] Population estimates for 1985.
[b] Formerly called the Ivory Coast.
[c] Percentages based on regional population excluding developing countries: Japan; Australia; New Zealand.

Within each regional group, the countries are very unevenly distributed, as can be seen in table 1. Thus, the broad regional groups disguise the heavy weight given to certain subregions (e.g., Northern Africa, the Caribbean, Central America and South-eastern Asia). None the less, the broad regional groups were chosen as a useful way to categorize countries because of their convenience and because of some of the geographical, cultural and historical characteristics that they share. It should be kept in mind, however, that certain subregions, such as sub-Saharan Africa and the Arab countries of Northern Africa and Western Asia, do form distinct groups from the perspective of culture, religion and history; and it is useful to look at them separately in certain circumstances. In fact, as mentioned in the last section of this introduction, the Arab countries of Northern Africa and Western Asia are discussed separately in part three of this study.

Socio-economic development

The 38 developing countries included in the analysis were grouped into four broad development groups using macro-data for each country, drawing on sources independent of the WFS data. It was found that alternative composite indices of socio-economic development (Mauldin and Berelson, 1978; Fabri, 1977; Morris, 1979), which had been previously developed using a variety of indicators and weighting schemes, produced roughly similar groups of the countries included in this report. No one of these indices, however, has received the general endorsement of the international community and none of those which included a range of modernization measures was available for the mid-1970s or for all 38 countries of concern here (i.e., the indices developed by Mauldin and Berelson and by Fabri). Thus, for the purposes of this report, a simple index was constructed for 1975 using four broadly accepted components: (*a*) economic production based on gross domestic product (GDP) per capita; (*b*) education based on the gross enrolment ratio for males and females for the primary and secondary levels of schooling combined; (*c*) health based on the infant mortality rate; and (*d*) communication based on ownership ratios of passenger motor cars, television sets and radios.

Broadly speaking, development can be viewed as a multi-dimensional phenomenon; some of its major dimensions include level of economic production, level of education, level of health services, degree of urbanization, status of women, level of nutrition, quality of housing, distribution of goods and services, and access to communication. However, many of the categories listed above are problematical. For example, no suitable measure of housing quality is available for the 38 countries under study. Nutrition, on the other hand, is too complex a concept to yield one single measure. There is no general agreement about a "normal" daily calorie intake, given cross-country differences in average body weight. Furthermore, the issue of protein requirement is much more complex. Because of these problems, it was decided to focus on only four components in constructing a development index: economic production; education; health; and communications.

Of the many choices available for measuring economic production, GDP per capita is the most widely accepted and universally available indicator. The problem of the international comparability of GDP, however, is generally acknowledged; and a joint World Bank/United Nations project is undertaking the task of measuring GDP in terms of equivalent purchasing power (Kravis and others, 1975). The work is so arduous, unfortunately, that data for selected countries only have been incorporated into the project to date and results are not available for many of the WFS countries. None the less, a measure has been devised which makes use of the results currently available from the World Bank/United Nations project and avoids the use of nominal GDP per capita, evaluated at artificial rates of exchange (Kravis and others, 1978). The method estimates real GDP per capita by regression techniques using nominal GDP and measures of the importance of international trade in the national product based on the degree of price isolation and openness of the national economy. Although this measure of GDP is an estimate based on regression parameters derived from the comparability project mentioned above, it is expected that a much more realistic idea of GDP, in comparative terms, is achieved in this way than by using nominal GDP per capita in dollars as derived from the actual exchange rate. Economic production for the present purposes, therefore, is taken as real GDP per capita from the study by Kravis and others (1978).[5] Estimates for 1974 are used.[6] Real GDP per capita, shown in table 2, column (1), is transformed into an index with values from 0 to 100 (see column (7)). The lowest observed GDP per capita, $212 per annum in Bangladesh, was chosen as the lower limit of the index (= 0) and $3,356 (the highest, Venezuela) as the upper limit (= 100). The index numbers of GDP per capita are given in table 2, column (7).

TABLE 2. INDICATORS OF DEVELOPMENT AND THEIR INDEX VALUES FOR 38 WORLD FERTILITY SURVEY COUNTRIES, AROUND 1975

Country	GDP (1)	ENROL (2)	IMR (3)	TVS (4)	CARS (5)	RADIOS (6)	IGDP (7)	IENROL (8)	IIMR (9)	ICOM (10)	IDEV (11)	RANK (12)
Bangladesh	212	50	150	(0.5)	0.4	6	0	47	15	1	63	32
Benin	265	32	166	0.1	4.0	53	2	25	3	8	38	35
Cameroon	584	57	137	..	6.0	62	12	56	25	17	110	28
Colombia	1 274	74	67	(70)	11.0	117	34	77	79	50	240	11
Costa Rica	1 585	79	51	76	23.0	76	44	83	92	57	276	8
Côte d'Ivoire[a]	922	40	143	(3)	10.0	118	23	35	21	23	102	29
Dominican Republic	1 446	65	84	49	10.0	41	39	65	66	32	202	17
Ecuador	1 035	75	100	46	5.0	325	26	78	54	55	213	14
Egypt	670	59	130	28	4.0	133	15	58	31	29	133	22
Fiji	1 499	91	47	..	22.3	494	41	98	95	88	322	4
Ghana	842	54	117	3.7	5.0	100	20	52	41	15	128	23
Guyana	962	75	58	..	25.0	367	24	78	86	81	269	10
Haiti	429	35	135	2.9	3.0	21	7	28	27	5	67	31
Indonesia	425	53	112	8	2.0	36	7	51	45	8	111	27
Jamaica	1 871	77	42	56	39.0	337	53	80	98	86	317	5
Jordan	710	85	87	55	7.0	179	16	90	64	48	218	13
Kenya	450	65	117	4.0	9.0	36	8	65	41	12	126	24
Lesotho	304	72	130	..	2.0	23	3	74	31	5	113	26
Malaysia	1 406	69	40	60	25.0	154	38	70	100	62	270	9
Mexico	1 758	77	55	84	24.0	269	49	80	78	84	291	6
Morocco	750	37	106	40	15.0	108	17	31	31	41	120	25
Mauritania	551	12	142	..	4.0	65	11	0	10	15	36	36
Nepal	347	26	149	..	0.4	15	4	17	2	2	25	37
Pakistan	564	32	124	10	3.0	65	11	25	23	12	71	30
Panama	1 837	93	34	113	32.0	153	52	100	97	78	327	3
Paraguay	922	66	46	19	7.0	64	23	67	90	19	199	18
Peru	1 167	82	87	(45)	17.0	143	30	86	46	48	210	15
Philippines	683	87	54	19	8.0	43	15	93	78	19	205	16
Republic of Korea	1 128	82	43	108	2.0	402	29	86	98	68	281	7
Senegal	637	25	146	0.4	9.0	56	14	16	8	15	53	34
Sri Lanka	663	61	37	..	7.0	49	14	60	88	16	178	20
Sudan	431	32	123	6	2.0	74	7	25	19	11	62	33
Syrian Arab Republic	1 094	73	61	47	5.0	250	28	75	65	51	219	12
Thailand	643	62	54	17	5.0	131	14	62	81	25	182	19
Trinidad and Tobago	2 640	74	26	124	73.0	261	77	77	100	96	350	2
Tunisia	1 187	60	98	49	13.0	66	31	59	48	38	176	21
Venezuela	3 356	76	41	(120)	55.0	414	100	79	91	100	370	1
Yemen	342	19	160	0.0	..	18	4	9	0	2	15	38

Sources: For column (1), Kravis and others (1978); for column (2), United Nations Educational, Scientific and Cultural Organization (1981), pp. 111-128 ff.; for column (3), United Nations (1985); for columns (4)-(6), World Bank (1976), p. 524 ff.

NOTE: CARS = passenger motor cars per 1,000; ENROL = gross enrolment ratio; GDP = gross domestic product; ICOM = index of communication; IDEB = index of development; IENROL = index of gross enrolment ratio; IGDP = index of gross domestic product per capita; IMR = infant mortality rate; RADIOS = radios per 1,000; RANK = rank order of countries according to IDEV; TVS = television sets per 1,000.

[a] Formerly called the Ivory Coast.

The question arises whether estimates for one year, 1974, were appropriate for those WFS countries with relatively late survey dates. To answer this question it is important to know if there have been major changes in the relative positions of the countries with respect to GDP since 1974. An examination of more recent data for those countries whose survey occurred several years after the standard year, 1974, disclosed no important changes in their relative position *vis-à-vis* other countries with respect to GDP per capita. As the objective was only to order the countries and then sort them into four broad groups, it was felt that the advantage of using realistic GDP estimates for 1974 outweighed any gain from using nominal GDP per capita estimates for different years.

For the education component of the development index, two types of indicators are available.[7] One type is cumulative and measures the proportion of the population with certain characteristics relating to educational attainment, such as the percentage of the population literate or the percentage with primary schooling completed. The other type of measure is current and measures the proportion of the student-age population currently enrolled in school. Thus, the percentage literate is a measure of the stock of education embodied in the population at a moment in time while the enrolment ratio is a measure of the current input to that stock. Because the development process is dynamic and socio-economic change may be rapid in some countries, measures reflecting the current situation were considered preferable. Therefore, enrolment ratios were selected as being more representative of the current situation than literacy rates. The indicator selected was the gross enrolment ratio for males and females for the primary and secondary levels of schooling combined in 1975. This measure represents the total number of students enrolled at the primary and secondary levels, regardless of age, divided by population within the age groups normally attending these schooling levels. The net enrolment ratio, which includes only those enrolled students in the appropriate age group, would have been preferable but it was not available for all the countries. Enrolment ratios are shown in table 2, column (2); and the index of enrolment ratios, with values from 0 to 100, in column (8), with Mauritania having an index value of 0 and Panama a value of 100.

The selection of measures representing the level of health services was limited by the types of data available for all 38 WFS countries. The most widely available and perhaps most accurate information relating to service availability is the number of hospital beds. It is generally felt, however, that such a measure of the supply of health services is weak both because the distribution of services is not captured and because hospital care is only one component of the health care system. It was therefore decided to use the infant mortality rate (IMR) as an indirect measure of health-care accessibility, as suggested by the World Health Organization (1981). Although the infant mortality rate can be seen as reflecting the distribution of health services, it is obviously influenced by other factors as well, such as nutritional levels, general sanitation, access to transport and cultural practices. Estimates of infant mortality rates for 1975 or 1980 were used, depending upon when the survey was carried out (United Nations, 1985). The IMR values given in column (3) were transformed into an index (IIMR) in column (9) by using the highest observed value (Yemen, IMR = 170) and the lowest (Malaysia, and Trinidad and Tobago, IMR = 40) and subtracting the results from 100.

The final component of the development index relates to the extensiveness of the communications infrastructure and might be said also to measure the distribution of goods and services through the society. The role of such a component was to evaluate the degree of percolation throughout the community of those material goods which particularly relate to the communications network. Hence, it seemed worth while to examine ownership ratios of certain consumption items, such as passenger motor cars, television sets and radios, which are intimately involved in the development of transport and communications. A composite of three items was considered more reliable in the case of communications and consumption because each measure is liable to a fair amount of measurement error (e.g., the numbers of radios and television sets are only those officially registered in some countries but are all units in use in other countries). Also, no set of such data is universally available in all countries. The three specific measures used (columns (4)-(6) of table 2) were the number of passenger cars per 1,000 population in 1970; the number of television sets licensed and/or in use per 1,000 population in 1978; and the number of radio receivers licensed and/or in use per 1,000 population in 1978 (United Nations Educational, Scientific and Cultural Organization, 1981; World Bank, 1976). As can be seen, it was not possible to adhere to the standard year, 1975, in this case. The index measure derived, shown in column (10), was a composite of the two or three items for which data were available, with equal weight assigned to each.

The composite development index is presented in column (11) of table 2. Each of the four dimensions—production, education, health and communications—was given equal weight in the final index, which has a possible range of values from 0 to 400. The countries were then split into four groups based on this index (table 3).

TABLE 3. INDEX OF DEVELOPMENT AND RANK VALUES FOR 38 WORLD FERTILITY SURVEY COUNTRIES, AROUND 1975

	Index of development (1)	Rank value (2)
I. High level of development		
Venezuela	370	1
Trinidad and Tobago	350	2
Panama	327	3
Fiji	322	4
Jamaica	317	5
Mexico	291	6
Republic of Korea	281	7
Costa Rica	276	8
Malaysia	270	9
Guyana	269	10
Colombia	240	11
II. Middle-high level of development		
Syrian Arab Republic	219	12
Jordan	218	13
Ecuador	213	14
Peru	210	15
Philippines	205	16
Dominican Republic	202	17
Paraguay	199	18
Thailand	182	19
Sri Lanka	178	20
Tunisia	176	21
III. Middle-low level of development		
Egypt	133	22
Ghana	128	23
Kenya	126	24
Morocco	120	25
Lesotho	113	26
Indonesia	111	27
Cameroon	110	28
Côte d'Ivoire[a]	102	29
IV. Low level of development		
Pakistan	71	30
Haiti	67	31
Bangladesh	63	32
Sudan	62	33
Senegal	53	34
Benin	38	35
Mauritania	36	36
Nepal	25	37
Yemen	15	38

Source: Table 2.
[a] Formerly called the Ivory Coast.

Table 4 presents country ranks according to various indices of socio-economic development, including that derived here. The Mauldin and Berelson index (column (2)), which is unavailable for Benin and Guyana, is centred around 1970 and is made up of seven components: percentage of adults literate; percentage of those aged 5-19 enrolled in primary and secondary schools; life expectancy; infant mortality rate; percentage of males aged 15-64 in non-agricultural labour force; GNP per capita and percentage of the population in cities of 100,000 or more. The composite index developed by Fabri (column (3)), which is unavailable for seven of the 38 WFS countries included in this analysis, is also based on 1970. It includes 26 components drawn from three broad categories (demographic, economic and modernization factors) and includes a measure of fertility in the demographic category of variables—a component that would be inappropriate in this analysis. The quality-of-life index developed by Morris (column (4)) includes only infant mortality, life expectancy and literacy; thus, it is not fully comparable with those indices which give an important weight to economic development.

Although many alternative schemes could have been adopted, it is reassuring to note that the index developed from these components sorts the 38 countries into four broad groups which correspond almost exactly to the groups formed by other previously developed indices (see table 4). The few differences can be largely explained by the fact that this index has a more recent date and does not include any fertility component—a component that had been included in the Fabri index but that would be undesirable in this context because of the intention to link these groups to fertility differentials. The Spearman rank-order correlation coefficients between the index developed here and each of the successive indices shown in table 4 are 0.97, 0.85 and 0.89, respectively.

The high correlations between these four indices suggest that any cross-country findings based on these four broad groups of countries should be fairly robust. The main advantages of the index adopted for this report are its availability for all countries in the study and its timing in the mid-1970s.

Family planning programme effort

The measurement of strength of family planning programme effort is complex not only because many different factors contribute to the strength of a programme but because the measurements used must be comparable across countries. Given the difficulties entailed, it is not surprising that few have attempted to construct such a measure. It is very fortuitous for this project, however, that two very credible and thorough attempts have been made; one was centred on the year 1972 (Mauldin and Berelson, 1978) and one on 1983 (Lapham and Mauldin, 1984). In each case, all or almost all of the programmes of countries that participated in WFS were assessed. Since these years encompass all dates at which these surveys took place, it is possible to use these measures to construct for each country an index that applies to the year preceding the survey. It seemed advisable to make this adjustment because family planning programme strength is an instrument of government policy and therefore can change rapidly within the course of several years. Thus, it would not be advisable to choose either the 1972 or the 1983 index without making some interpolation to adjust for the timing of the actual survey date in each case. Table 5 presents the programme effort scores for both 1972 and 1983 as well as the interpolated index which was constructed for use in this study with the resulting grouping of countries into four categories of effort: strong; moderate; weak; very weak/none.

These groups corresponded to those listed in the 1984 *World Development Report* but the group labelled "strong" in table 5 includes the "strong" and "very strong" groups as defined by the World Bank. The methodology for constructing such an index was developed in 1972 (Lapham and Mauldin) and was further developed for the more recent rating (Lapham and Mauldin, 1984). Four major components of programme effort

TABLE 4. FOUR DEVELOPMENT INDICES AND RANK VALUES FOR 38 WORLD FERTILITY SURVEY COUNTRIES, AROUND 1975

Country	Rank N = 38 (1)	Mauldin and Berelson, 1970 N = 36 (2)	Composite Fabri index, 1970 N = 31 (3)	Physical quality-of-life index, 1970 N = 38 (4)
I. *High level of development*				
Venezuela	1	1	..	9
Trinidad and Tobago	2	3	..	1
Panama	3	3	1	7
Fiji	4	10	..	7
Jamaica	5	2	3	4
Mexico	6	6	7	11
Republic of Korea	7	7	2	5
Costa Rica	8	3	4	1
Malaysia	9	13	12	16
Guyana	10	..	5	1
Colombia	11	8	8	12
II. *Middle-high level of development*				
Syrian Arab Republic	12	16	14	19
Jordan	13	9	16	22
Ecuador	14	15	15	14
Peru	15	12	11	18
Philippines	16	13	17	12
Dominican Republic	17	16	18	17
Paraguay	18	10	10	10
Thailand	19	21	21	14
Sri Lanka	20	18	6	5
Tunisia	21	19	13	22
III. *Middle-low level of development*				
Egypt	22	20	9	24
Ghana	23	23	29	30
Kenya	24	26	24	26
Morocco	25	22	20	25
Lesotho	26	28	..	21
Indonesia	27	24	25	20
Cameroon	28	26	22	33
Côte d'Ivoire[a]	29	29	26	32
IV. *Low level of development*				
Pakistan	30	25	30	27
Haiti	31	30	19	28
Bangladesh	32	33	..	30
Sudan	33	32	27	28
Senegal	34	31	28	35
Benin	35	..	31	37
Mauritania	36	34	23	38
Nepal	37	36	..	35
Yemen	38	35	..	33

Sources: For column (1), table 3; for column (2), Mauldin and Berelson (1978), table 7; for column (3), Fabri (1978), table 1, column A; for column (4), Morris (1979), appendix A.

NOTE: When two or more countries have the same value, they are all assigned the same rank (i.e., the one that has the lowest value).

[a] Formerly called the Ivory Coast.

TABLE 5. FAMILY PLANNING PROGRAMME EFFORT SCORES AND GROUPING OF WORLD FERTILITY SURVEY COUNTRIES ACCORDING TO INTERPOLATED SCORES

Country	Elapsed years between 1972 and survey date (1)	Programme effort 1972 (2)	1983 (3)	Interpolated (4)
1. Strong effort: 60+				
Colombia	4	16	85.3	69.8
Costa Rica	4	21	39.8	71.9
Fiji	2	22	55.4	85.0
Indonesia	4	14	87.1	64.5
Jamaica	3	23	64.1	86.9
Malaysia	2	18	61.1	71.0
Panama	3	19	59.2	72.9
Philippines	6	16	63.6	63.8
Republic of Korea	2	24	96.9	96.1
2. Moderate effort: 40-59				
Dominican Republic	3	14	64.3	57.5
Egypt	8	8	45.7	40.7
Sri Lanka	3	12	81.6	54.1
Thailand	3	11	70.5	48.8
Trinidad and Tobago	5	15	55.0	58.2
Tunisia	6	12	69.8	57.9
3. Weak effort: 20-39				
Bangladesh	3	3	68.7	22.3
Ecuador	7	6	49.4	37.9
Guyana	3	..	29.9	29.9[a]
Haiti	5	3	43.8	23.6
Kenya	5	6	34.7	27.9
Mexico	4	4	78.6	33.1
Morocco	8	4	45.4	34.7
Nepal	4	6	46.3	30.1
Pakistan	3	8	48.5	35.0
Venezuela	5	7	37.5	31.5
4. Very weak/no effort: 0-19				
Benin	9	3	[b]	[b]
Cameroon	6	0	8.1	3.7
Côte d'Ivoire[c]	8	0	3.7	2.4
Ghana	7	3	20.5	16.6
Jordan	4	0	19.0	5.2
Lesotho	5	0	15.5	5.6
Mauritania	9	0	4.2	3.1
Paraguay	7	3	10.7	11.3
Peru	5	0	26.4	9.6
Senegal	6	0	22.9	10.4
Sudan	6	3	7.3	9.9
Syrian Arab Republic	6	0	7.3	3.3
Yemen	7	0	8.2	4.5

Sources: For column (2), Mauldin and Berelson (1978); for column (3), Lapham and Mauldin (1984), table 1, p. 112.

NOTES: In column (2), maximum score for 1972 = 30; in column (3), maximum score for 1983 = 120.

For column (4), the values were interpolated based on the assumption of a linear trend between 1972 and 1983 in programme effort scores. To get a value appropriate for the year before the survey, a weighted average of the 1972 and 1983 indices was calculated, giving the 1983 score a weight of one less than column (1) and the 1972 score a weight of 11 (the number of intervening years) minus the 1983 weight.

[a] It was not scored in 1972. Interpolated rating is based on 1983 scoring on the assumption that the programme effort remained constant.

[b] No information was available for 1983. It was therefore assumed that programme effort had not improved substantially, and thus Benin was included in group 4.

[c] Formerly called the Ivory Coast.

were evaluated: (*a*) policy and stage-setting activities; (*b*) service and service-related activities; (*c*) record-keeping and evaluation; and (*d*) availability and accessibility of fertility-control supplies and services. The strength of these components was measured by scaling the responses of knowledgeable informants in each country to a series of specific questions related to programme characteristics—a 15-item scale in 1972 and a 30-item scale in 1984. Many of these questions required subjective judgements on the part of the knowledgeable persons questioned, but given the lack of comparable objective data on many of the characteristics of the programme, this represented the only reasonable way to measure many of these characteristics systematically in as many countries as possible. When discrepancies occurred between informants in the rating of various items, the discrepant answers were not averaged; instead, the authors of the study tried to determine the most appropriate answers given information derived from other materials. Although the exact ranking of countries is doubtless subject to error because of the subjective nature of the questionnaire and variations between countries in the knowledgeability of informants, it is reasonable to expect that the broad groupings of countries by programme strength roughly captures the major differences between countries.

Although there is some overlap between these country-setting variables, each measures something quite different (table 6). All of the WFS countries in Latin America and the Caribbean fall in the upper half of the socio-economic scale, while all but one of the participating countries in Africa are in the lower development groups. Participating countries in Asia and Oceania, on the other hand, are found in all development groups. With respect to strength of the family planning programme effort, most of the countries in Africa (except for Egypt and Tunisia) have at best weak programmes, but participating countries in the other two regions can be found at all levels of programme strength. Therefore, a simple geographical grouping does not represent a measure of either development or programme strength because some regional diversity exists within each broad grouping of programme strength and socio-economic development. In fact, the examination of differences between regional groups within cells or groups of cells found in table 6 may suggest the independent importance of some socio-cultural characteristics of regions that are not captured by the economic and policy variables considered.

CHARACTERISTICS OF THE DATA

For purposes of this study, it is not necessary to discuss in detail all aspects of the selection of samples, the design of questionnaires and their respective implementation. These details are fully documented elsewhere (Scott and Harpham, 1984; Singh, 1984) and are outlined here when necessary for the discussion of individual topics in subsequent chapters. This section of the introduction focuses on those features of the survey design which are particularly relevant for proper interpretation of the comparative analysis of the World Fertility Survey data presented in this report, with respect both to comparisons between developed and developing countries and to comparisons within the developing countries.

The comparability of the WFS data is affected by a complex interaction between characteristics of the country setting which were discussed in the previous section and characteristics of the survey design which are outlined here (Lloyd, 1986). Figure I shows certain characteristics of the survey design and the country setting that have influenced the comparability of the WFS data. Only in

TABLE 6. CROSS-CLASSIFICATION OF COUNTRIES PARTICIPATING IN THE WORLD FERTILITY SURVEY, BY STRENGTH OF FAMILY PLANNING PROGRAMME EFFORT, LEVEL OF DEVELOPMENT AND REGION

Strength of family planning programme effort	I. High	II. Middle-high	III. Middle-low	IV. Low
1. Strong				
Latin America and the Caribbean	Colombia Costa Rica Jamaica Panama	—	—	—
Asia and Oceania	Fiji Malaysia Republic of Korea	Philippines	Indonesia	—
2. Moderate				
Africa	—	Tunisia	Egypt	—
Latin America and the Caribbean	Trinidad and Tobago	Dominican Republic	—	—
Asia and Oceania	—	Sri Lanka Thailand	—	—
3. Weak				
Africa	—	—	Kenya Morocco	—
Latin America and the Caribbean	Mexico Guyana Venezuela	Ecuador	—	Haiti
Asia and Oceania	—	—	—	Bangladesh Nepal Pakistan
4. Very weak/none				
Africa	—	—	Cameroon Côte d'Ivoire[a] Ghana Lesotho	Benin Mauritania Senegal Sudan
Latin America and the Caribbean		Paraguay Peru		
Asia and Oceania		Jordan Syrian Arab Republic	—	Yemen

Sources: Tables 3 and 5.
[a] Formerly called the Ivory Coast.

cases where the country settings are similar and the design and implementation of the surveys are identical can the resulting data be entirely comparable. Among these surveys, such comparability was achieved in certain groups of neighbouring countries with a similar historical and cultural tradition (e.g., the Caribbean countries and the Arab countries of Northern Africa and Western Asia). When all surveys are pooled, however, the picture is more complex.

Table 7 lists all the countries whose surveys were included in this study, by region and date of survey. While the dates of the surveys range from 1974 to 1982, within each region the dates cluster within a smaller range. In Europe, as is noted in chapter XIV, roughly 50 per cent of the surveys were conducted in 1975 and 1976 and roughly 50 per cent in 1977 and 1978. The distribution of the dates of the surveys in Latin America and the Caribbean is roughly similar. On the whole, the Asian countries were the earliest, with the large majority having been completed by 1976. Africa followed, building on previous experience. There the earliest surveys were in Kenya and Lesotho in 1977 but the majority took place in 1979 or later. Within the range of dates over which the surveys were conducted the ranking of country setting variables across countries has stayed sufficiently stable that comparative analysis can be based on meaningful groups of countries. While the data from many countries are already 10 years old, the value of these findings in the present context is based not so much on their timeliness as on their comparability across a range of demographic experiences and settings.

These surveys were intended to be nationally representative surveys of women currently in the reproductive ages who were exposed to the risks of childbearing. This goal was by and large realized. Table 8 presents details on the characteristics of the surveys from the developing countries in terms of population coverage, eligibility for interview and sample size. Similar information for the developed countries is given in chapter XIV (table 201). In the large majority of countries, the sample drawn was chosen to be national in scope, with all but five countries having more than 90 per cent of their resident population covered in the sampling design. In Indonesia, Jordan, Malaysia, Mauritania and the Sudan, however, coverage falls in the range of 67-85 per cent for several reasons, among which were anticipated sampling difficulties in remote areas or

Figure 1. Relationship between survey design, country setting and data comparability

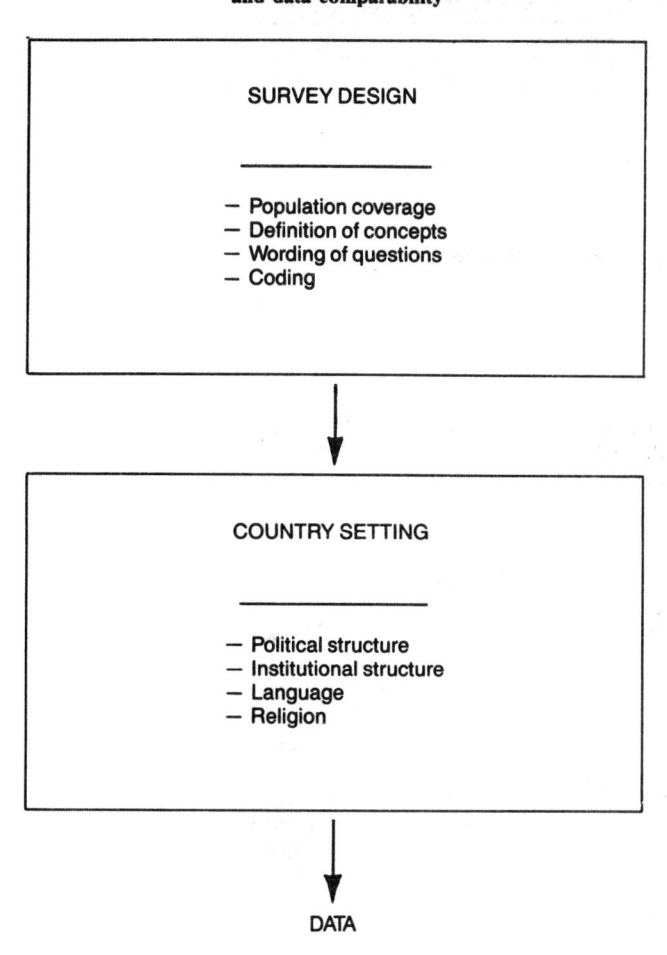

```
┌─────────────────────────────────┐
│         SURVEY DESIGN           │
│  ─────────────────────────────  │
│  — Population coverage          │
│  — Definition of concepts       │
│  — Wording of questions         │
│  — Coding                       │
└─────────────────────────────────┘
                │
                ▼
┌─────────────────────────────────┐
│        COUNTRY SETTING          │
│  ─────────────────────────────  │
│  — Political structure          │
│  — Institutional structure      │
│  — Language                     │
│  — Religion                     │
└─────────────────────────────────┘
                │
                ▼
              DATA
```

Source: Lloyd (1986).

TABLE 7. TIMING OF THE WORLD FERTILITY SURVEY IN COUNTRIES SELECTED FOR STUDY

Country	1974-1976	1977-1978	1979 onward
A. Developed countries			
Belgium	1975/76	—	—
Bulgaria	1976		
Czechoslovakia	—	1977	—
Denmark	1975	—	—
Finland	—	1977	
France	—	1977/78	—
Hungary	—	1977	—
Italy	—	—	1979
Netherlands	1975	—	—
Norway	—	1977/78	—
Poland	—	1977	—
Romania	—	1978	—
Spain	—	1977	—
United Kingdom[a]	1976	—	—
United States of America	1976	—	—
Yugoslavia	1976	—	—
TOTAL	7	8	1
B. Developing countries			
Africa			
Benin	—	—	1982
Cameroon	—	1978	—
Côte d'Ivoire[b]	—	—	1980
Egypt	—	—	1980
Ghana	—	—	1979/80
Kenya	—	1977/78	—

TABLE 7 (continued)

Country	1974-1976	1977-1978	1979 onward
Lesotho	—	1977	—
Mauritania	—	—	1981
Morocco	—	—	1979/80
Senegal	—	1978	—
Sudan	—	—	1978/79[c]
Tunisia	—	1978	—
TOTAL	0	5	7
Latin America and the Caribbean			
Colombia	1976	—	—
Costa Rica	1976	—	—
Dominican Republic	1975	—	—
Ecuador	—	—	1979
Guyana	—	1977	—
Haiti	—	1977	—
Jamaica	1975/76	—	—
Mexico	1976	—	—
Panama	1975/76	—	—
Paraguay	—	—	1979
Peru	—	1977/78	—
Trinidad and Tobago	—	1977	—
Venezuela	—	1977	—
TOTAL	6	5	2
Asia and Oceania			
Bangladesh	1975/76	—	—
Fiji	1974	—	—
Indonesia	1976	—	—
Jordan	1976	—	—
Malaysia	1974	—	—
Nepal	1976	—	—
Pakistan	1975	—	—
Philippines	—	1978	—
Republic of Korea	1974	—	—
Sri Lanka	1975	—	—
Syrian Arab Republic	—	1978	—
Thailand	1975	—	—
Yemen	—	—	1979
TOTAL	10	2	1

Source: World Fertility Survey (1984).
[a] Not including Northern Ireland.
[b] Formerly called the Ivory Coast.
[c] In the Sudan, most interviews were conducted during 1979.

among nomadic populations and political problems. The age range for interview was usually from 15 to 49 or 50 years. However, in two Latin American countries (Costa Rica and Panama), the youngest age of interview was 20 and in Venezuela the oldest age of interview was 44. While 19 of the surveys are based on interviews of all women in the requisite age groups, the other 19 are restricted to interviews with women who have ever been married. Usually, this choice was dictated by some knowledge of extra-marital fertility patterns in the country and by a concern to include most births without incurring unnecessary interviewing costs. Therefore, in Asia, where out-of-wedlock childbearing is thought to be relatively rare, only ever-married women were interviewed. At the other extreme, all women, regardless of marital status, were interviewed in all but one (Peru) of the Latin American surveys. The experience in Africa was mixed, but by and large, the sub-Saharan countries chose the all-women sample. For those countries excluding single women, fertility rates for all women have to be estimated using proportions married derived from the household survey, and such rates cannot be derived for certain sub-populations for which household data were not collected.

TABLE 8. CHARACTERISTICS OF POPULATION AND SAMPLE COVERED
BY THE WORLD FERTILITY SURVEY, BY REGION AND COUNTRY

Region and country	Population estimate, 1975 (millions) (1)	Sample domain target coverage (percentage) (2)	Sample size of the individual survey (3)	Age[a] (4)	Marital status (5)
Africa					
Benin	3.0	100	4 018	15-49	ALL
Cameroon	7.6	100	8 219	15-54	ALL
Egypt	36.3	100	8 788	-49	EM
Ghana	9.8	100	6 125	15-49	ALL
Côte d'Ivoire[b]	6.8	100	5 764	15-50	ALL
Kenya	13.7	95	8 100	15-50	ALL
Lesotho	1.2	100	3 603	15-49	EM
Mauritania	1.4	70	3 504	12-50	EM
Morocco	17.3	99	5 801	15-50	ALL
Senegal	4.8	100	3 985	15-49	ALL
Sudan	16.0	70	3 115	-50	EM
Tunisia	5.6	100	4 123	15-49	EM
Latin America and the Caribbean					
Colombia	23.2	99	5 378	15-49	ALL
Costa Rica	2.0	97	3 935	20-49	ALL
Dominican Republic	4.9	100	3 115	15-49	ALL
Ecuador	6.9	96	6 797	15-49	ALL
Guyana	0.8	92	4 642	15-49	ALL[c]
Haiti	5.2	100	3 365	15-49	ALL
Jamaica	2.0	100	3 096	15-49	ALL[c]
Mexico	60.2	100	7 310	15-49[d]	ALL
Panama	1.7	90	3 701	20-49	ALL
Paraguay	2.7	94	4 682	15-49	ALL
Peru	15.2	100	5 640	15-49	EM
Trinidad and Tobago	1.1	100	4 359	15-49	ALL[c]
Venezuela	13.1	98	4 361	15-44	ALL
Asia and Oceania					
Bangladesh	76.6	100	6 513	-49	EM
Fiji	0.6	96	4 298	15-49	EM
Indonesia	135.7	67	9 155	-50	EM
Jordan	1.7[e]	71	3 612	15-49	EM
Malaysia	12.4	85	6 316	-50	EM
Nepal	12.7	98	5 940	-49	EM
Pakistan	75.5	93	4 996	15-49	EM
Philippines	43.1	100	9 268	-49	EM
Republic of Korea	35.3	99	5 430	15-49	EM
Sri Lanka	13.6	100	6 812	-49	EM
Syrian Arab Republic	7.4	100	4 487	-49	EM
Thailand	41.9	100	3 778	-49	EM
Yemen	5.3	94	2 605	-50	EM

Sources: For column (1), United Nations (1985); for columns (2), (4) and (5), Scott and Harpham (1984); for column (3), Harpham and Scott (1984), table 7.

NOTE: EM = ever married; ALL = all women.

[a] When no lower age-limit is listed, it indicates that some women under age 15 were interviewed.
[b] Formerly called the Ivory Coast.
[c] Excluding full-time schoolgirls aged 15-19.
[d] At ages 15-19, including only women who had either had a baby or been in a union.
[e] Estimated by Population Division, United Nations, on basis of the 1979 census.

There was greater variability in the design of the surveys in developed countries in terms of the individual women interviewed. Many surveys limited the interview to women under age 45 and/or to only those women who were currently married or in the first marriage. These restrictions limited the topics selected for analysis by ECE in its comparative analysis project and also limited the comparison that can be drawn between the developed and developing countries, as is shown in chapter XV.

The high degree of comparability between the data from the different surveys in the developing countries is the result of a core questionnaire which was designed on the basis of certain essential concepts prior to the solicitation of country participation. Participating countries were not asked to follow the structure and wording of the core questionnaire exactly, but it was expected that all data specified in the core would be collected in such a way as to maintain comparability with other surveys in the WFS programme, as well as any earlier national fertility surveys. Countries were invited to pursue topics of special interest as supplements to the core through the use of special modules. Their use helped to minimize structural changes in the design of the individual country questionnaires as well as to preserve the integrity of the core elements of the survey. None the less, the wording of some questions was modified in some countries and these exceptions are discussed under individual topics in chapters I-IX.

Comparative analysis was further facilitated by the preparation of a standard recode tape for each survey, with a common format and naming conventions, which eliminated certain non-comparabilities from the analysts' concern, such as differences that existed between surveys in the sequence or wording of questions. For the developed countries, the comparative study required the creation of common files from non-standard surveys; and a large proportion of the resources for the ECE analysis had to be devoted to this recoding and file creation process.

Characteristics of the country settings are expected to affect not only actual demographic interrelationships (as discussed above) but the way in which the data themselves are measured or the way in which the questions posed are understood by those interviewed. Even when concepts are clear and questions are worded identically, non-comparabilities in the resulting data can arise if the completeness and accuracy of the responses are influenced by cultural traditions and education. Certain types of data-reporting problems occurred more frequently in some regions than in others. As a result, the quality of data on fertility levels and trends, as well as those on nuptiality and other topics, varies in ways that must be taken into account carefully before comparative conclusions can be drawn. Details relating the comparative quality of fertility estimates are presented in chapter I. The quality of other variables is discussed in the successive specific chapters devoted to those topics.

In some cases, where non-comparabilities in reporting were anticipated in advance, the questionnaire itself was adapted. Supplemented by method-specific probes, the inclusion of an open-ended question on knowledge of contraception would be one example (Vaessen, 1981). The result was greater comparability in the contraceptive prevalence estimates in countries with different method distributions. In the more complex case of marital unions, the definition of union status was allowed to vary from country to country in order to measure more comparably the dates and duration of each respondent's period of regular exposure to the risk of conception. This involved adapting the definition of union to the country setting while (in Latin America and the Caribbean) preserving the distinction between legal and other forms of union.

The background variables chosen for inclusion in the core questionnaire for the developing countries present special difficulties for comparative analysis because their definition is particularly tied to the political, administrative and institutional structures that are specific to each country. Urban and rural definitions are not at all consistent across countries and country definitions were applied in coding respondents' current residence status. The measurement of educational attainment is another variable that is bounded by country-specific definitions and institutions, with levels or degrees and content varying substantially across countries. To provide comparability with respect to at least one dimension of education, WFS measured years of schooling. This measurement was constructed out of the responses to two questions that were not asked in the same way in all countries: "What level of education did you attain?"; and "How many years did you achieve at that level?". Thus, the constructed variable representing years of schooling was based on local knowledge of WFS staff and country co-ordinators of the local educational systems. In some countries, such as Mauritania, there were two different educational tracks (Western style or Koranic), which added to the difficulty of arriving at a single measure of educational attainment.

One of the most challenging aspects of the core questionnaire for the developing countries was its work history for women. Unfortunately, despite considerable discussion and 17 core questions designed to probe many dimensions of the variable, this section of the interview was not successful in capturing a uniform concept of work across countries. The word "work", when translated into different languages, has subtly different meanings which proved hard to transcend in the absence of detailed guidelines and locally appropriate examples. Variations between countries in the concept of work occurred not only because of variations in the wording of the definition but because the definition itself left room for ambiguity. It is not known how interviewers resolved these ambiguities in the field but they are likely to have been heavily influenced by their own previous experience and their culture-bound views on women's work. Printed instructions to the interviewers did not clarify the concept as described in the core questionnaire. As a result of all these factors, the measured proportion of women currently working varies across countries in ways that are not always expected when such factors as level of development, religion (i.e., Muslim versus other) and percentage in agriculture are taken into account (see chapter IX). Thus, in the case of work, both the characteristics of the country setting and the design and implementation of the survey have contributed to non-comparabilities of the data.

Many of the non-comparabilities remaining in the data for the developing countries are unavoidable and can be attributed to differences between countries in culture, institutional settings and phase of development. The survey design went a long way towards enhancing the comparability of the data through the development of common concepts and wording as well as through the development of a uniform tool for further analysis—the standard recode tape. The foregoing discussion of remaining non-comparabilities is not meant to detract from the enormous achievement of the WFS programme, working as it did in such diverse settings with countries having a range of statistical needs and local institutional structures for the collection of data. The comparative analysis of these data presented in this report points to some of the factors influencing comparability, some of which may be accommodated more fully in the design of future surveys.

In the presentation of the findings from the developed countries given in chapter XIV, certain non-comparabilities are not immediately apparent because they affect the range of topics chosen for discussion. These countries, all of which have the infrastructure and experience to undertake surveys on their own, took a more individualistic approach in the design of their surveys. Although the quality of the data collected was undoubtedly high, their usefulness for comparative analysis is more limited, as can be seen in the concluding chapter (XV), where comparisons are drawn between the developing and developed countries.

PLAN OF ANALYSIS

The plan of analysis for this volume has been guided by the major subject areas designated for study by the World Fertility Survey and by the organizational structure of the United Nations system, which has been responsible for carrying out this comparative analysis project. The first three parts cover the World Fertility Survey findings from the developing countries and part four brings in the findings from the developed countries. The disproportionate attention given here to the findings in developing countries can be explained by the fact that a separate volume has been prepared to cover data from the developed countries (Economic Commission for Europe, forthcoming). Part four is therefore included in order to compare the broad conclusions from these two groups of countries and to provide a global overview on this important international survey programme.

Parts one and two, which present a comparative analysis of the findings from 38 surveys in developing countries, were prepared by the Population Division of the Department of International Economic and Social Affairs at United Nations Headquarters, using the conceptual framework described above. In part one (chapters I-VI), fertility, its major proximate determinants (i.e., nuptiality, contraception and breast-feeding) and fertility preferences are analysed in depth in successive chapters according to a country's level of development, region and, whenever appropriate, strength of the family planning programme effort. In chapter VI, estimates of the differential effect of each of the major proximate determinants on fertility are presented.

The theme of part two is socio-economic differentials and the topics chosen cover most of the major background variables systematically collected in the surveys in developing countries. In successive chapters on rural or urban residence, education and women's work, within-country differentials in fertility, fertility preferences and the major proximate determinants are compared across countries. Both bivariate and multivariate relationships are discussed. While the findings are drawn from cross-sectional data, demographic transition theories are re-explored in the light of the patterns in differentials observed among countries at different levels of development.

Part three provides regional perspectives on the WFS findings from the developing countries. Three of the four chapters in part three were prepared by the regional commission that participated actively in the United Nations Working Group on Comparative Analysis (Economic and Social Commission for Asia and the Pacific, Economic Commission for Latin America and the Caribbean and Economic Commission for Africa). A fourth chapter was prepared by a consultant on the data from the six participating Arab countries of Northern Africa and Western Asia, which were not covered by the work of the participating regional commissions mentioned above. In each of these four chapters, the perspective is regional, so topics of special importance for an understanding of reproductive behaviour in each region can be analysed in more depth. These chapters do not follow a standard format but reflect those regional issues.

The purpose of part four is to present some broad comparisons between the findings in developed and developing countries. In chapter XIV, ECE summarizes the findings from its comparative analysis project. Chapter XV provides conclusions for the entire study which compare the patterns observed for the developed countries as a group to the patterns observed across regions and development groups within the set of 38 WFS countries analysed in the first three parts of the volume. Not all topics covered in those parts could be compared in chapter XV because of differences both in survey coverage and in the design of the comparative analysis projects undertaken by the Population Division and by ECE. None the less, certain broad conclusions can be drawn which shed new light on the demographic changes currently occurring in the developing countries.

NOTES

[1] A survey was taken in the Islamic Republic of Iran in 1977, but the data have never been published.

[2] It should be noted, however, that the surveys in developed countries were not standardized. Although the participating countries recognized the desirability of international comparability, they also were concerned about comparability with previous surveys. Questionnaire guidelines for low-fertility countries developed by the World Fertility Survey and supplemented by the Economic Commission for Europe were drawn on by all countries and helped to assure a certain amount of common ground between them.

[3] For a full discussion of the strengths of World Fertility Survey data for multinational analysis, see Lloyd, 1986.

[4] Even the results from the testing of Easterlin's hybrid model (Easterlin and Crimmins, 1982; United Nations, 1984a) have been disappointing because of the lack of correspondence between actual variables and theoretical concepts.

[5] This measure, in any case, is highly correlated with nominal gross domestic product (GDP) per capita. For instance, the Spearman correlation coefficient between it and nominal GDP per capita for 1975 is 0.97 for the 40 developing countries participating in the World Fertility Survey.

[6] In a few cases, where 1974 data were unavailable, 1973 figures were used.

[7] Other indicators, such as government expenditure on education, pupil/teacher ratios and pupil/class-room ratios, are less adequate for a variety of reasons.

REFERENCES

Acsádi, George T. (1980). Research objectives, hypotheses and minimum tabulation plan (relevant to the United Nations Minimum Research Programme for Complete Analysis of World Fertility Survey Data). In *United Nations Programme for Comparative Analysis of World Fertility Survey Data*. New York: United Nations Fund for Population Activities, 63-90.

Adelman, Irma (1963). An econometric analysis of population growth. *American Economic Review*, 53(3):314-339.

Bongaarts, John (1978). A framework for analyzing the proximate determinants of fertility. *Population and Development Review* 4(1):105-132.

Boulier, Bryan L. (1985). Family planning programs and contraceptive availability: their effects on contraceptive use. In Nancy Birdsall, ed., *The Effects of Family Planning Programs on Fertility in the Developing World*. World Bank Staff Working Papers, No. 677; Population and Development Series, No. 2. Washington, D.C.: The World Bank, 41-115.

Caldwell, John C. (1982). *Theory of Fertility Decline*. London: Academic Press.

Casterline, John B., ed. (1985). *The Collection and Analysis of Community Data*. Voorburg, The Netherlands: International Statistical Institute.

_____ and others (1984). *The Proximate Determinants of Fertility*. World Fertility Survey Comparative Studies, No. 39. Voorburg, The Netherlands: International Statistical Institute.

Cleland, John (1985). Marital fertility decline in developing countries: theories and the evidence. In John Cleland and John Hobcraft, eds., in collaboration with Betzy Dinesen, *Reproductive Change in Developing Countries: Insights from the World Fertility Survey*. Oxford: Oxford University Press, 223-252.

Cutright, Phillips (1983). The ingredients of recent fertility decline in developing countries. *International Family Planning Perspectives* 9(4):101-109.

Demeny, Paul (1979). On the end of the population explosion. *Population and Development Review* 5(1):141-162.

Easterlin, Richard A. and Eileen M. Crimmins (1982). *An Exploratory Study of the 'Synthesis Framework' of Fertility Determination with World Fertility Survey Data*. World Fertility Survey Scientific Reports, No. 40. Voorburg, The Netherlands: International Statistical Institute.

Economic Commission for Europe (forthcoming). *Fertility and Family Planning in the ECE Region: A Comparative Analysis of WFS Surveys*.

Entwisle, Barbara and William Mason (1985). Multilevel effects of socio-economic development and family planning programs on children ever born. *American Journal of Sociology* 91(3).

Fabri, Marcel Y. (1978). The relationship between demographic and socio-economic factors in the context of development. In *Population Bulletin of the United Nations, No. 10—1977*. New York: United Nations, 1-13.
Sales No. E.78.XIII.6.

Friedlander, Stanley and Morris Silver (1967). A quantitative study of the determinants of fertility behaviour. *Demography* 4(I):30-70.

Grebenik, E. (1981). *The World Fertility Survey and its 1980 Conference*. Voorburg, The Netherlands: International Statistical Institute.

Harpham, Trudy and Chris S. Scott (1984). Implementation of sample designs. Background paper prepared for the World Fertility Survey Symposium, London, 24-27 April 1984.

Hermalin, Albert I. (1986). The multi-level approach: theory and concepts. In *Addendum, Manual IX. The Methodology of Measuring the Impact of Family Planning Programmes on Fertility*. New York: United Nations, 15-23.
Sales No. E.86.XIII.4.

_____ and William Mason (1980). A strategy for the comparative analysis of WFS data, with illustrative examples. In *The United Nations Programme for Comparative Analysis of World Fertility Survey Data*. New York: United Nations Fund for Population Activities, 90-168.

Hernandez, Donald J. (1981). A note on measuring the independent impact of family planning programs on fertility declines. *Demography* 18(4):627-634.

Hobcraft, John and J. B. Casterline (1983). *Speed of Reproduction*. World Fertility Survey Comparative Studies, No. 25. Voorburg, The Netherlands: International Statistical Institute.

Kravis, Irving and others (1975). *A System of International Comparisons of Gross Product and Purchasing Power*. Baltimore, Maryland: The Johns Hopkins University Press for the World Bank.

_____ and others (1978). Real GDP per capita for more than 100 countries. *The Economic Journal* 88(2):215-242.

Lapham, Robert J. and W. Parker Mauldin (1972). National family planning programs: review and evaluation. *Studies in Family Planning* 3(3):29-52.

_____ and W. Parker Mauldin (1984). Family planning program effort and birthrate decline in developing countries. *International Family Planning Perspectives* 10(4):109-118.

Lloyd, Cynthia B. (1974). An economic analysis of the impact of government on fertility: some examples from the developed countries. *Public Policy* 22(4):489-512.

_____ (1986). Multi-country analysis. In John Cleland and Chris Scott, eds., in collaboration with David Whitelegge, *World Fertility Survey: An Assessment of its Contribution*. London: Oxford University Press for the International Statistical Institute, 599-617.

McNicoll, Geoffrey (1980). Institutional determinants of fertility change, *Population and Development Review* 6(3):441-462.

Mason, William M. (1986). The multi-level approach: illustrative example. In *Addendum, Manual IX. The Methodology of Measuring the Impact of Family Planning Programmes on Fertility*. New York: United Nations, 24-31.
Sales No. E.86.XIII.4.

Mauldin, W. Parker and Bernard Berelson (1978). Conditions of fertility decline in developing countries, 1965-75. With section by Zenas Sykes. *Studies in Family Planning* 9(5):89-147.

Morris, Morris D. (1979). *Measuring the Condition of the World's Poor*. New York: Pergamon Press.

Rodríguez, Germán and John Cleland (1981). Socio-economic determinants of marital fertility in twenty countries: a multivariate analysis. In *World Fertility Survey Conference 1980: Record of Proceedings*. London, 7-11 July 1980. Voorburg, The Netherlands: International Statistical Institute, vol. 2, 337-414.

_____ and others (1984). *A Comparative Analysis of Determinants of Birth Intervals*. World Fertility Survey Comparative Studies, No. 30; Cross-National Summaries. Voorburg, The Netherlands: International Statistical Institute.

Russett, Bruce M. and others (1964). *World Handbook of Social and Political Indicators*. New Haven, Connecticut: Yale University Press.

Scott, Chris S. and Trudy Harpham (1984). Major issues of survey and sample design. Background paper prepared for the World Fertility Survey Symposium, London, 24-27 April 1984.

Singh, Susheela (1980). *Background Characteristics Used in WFS Surveys*. World Fertility Survey Comparative Studies, No. 4; Cross-National Summaries. Voorburg, The Netherlands: International Statistical Institute.

_____ (1984). *Comparability of Questionnaires: Forty-one WFS Countries*. World Fertility Survey Comparative Studies, No. 32; Cross-National Summaries. Voorburg, The Netherlands: International Statistical Institute.

United Nations (1969). Department of Economic and Social Affairs. Population Division. *Variables and Questionnaire for Comparative Studies*. Population Studies, No. 45. New York.
Sales No. E.69.XIII.4.

_____ (1975). *Report of the United Nations World Population Conference, 1974*. New York.
Sales No. E.75.XIII.3.

_____ (1981). Department of International Economic and Social Affairs. Population Division. *Variations in the Incidence of Knowledge and Use of Contraception: A Comparative Analysis of World Fertility Survey Results for Twenty Developing Countries*. Non-sales publication E/ESA/SER.R/40. New York.

_____ (1981a). *Selected Factors Affecting Fertility and Fertility Preferences in Developing Countries*. Non-sales publication E/ESA/SER.R/37. New York.

_____ (1982). *The Impact of Population Structure on Crude Fertility Measures: A Comparative Analysis of World Fertility Survey Results for Twenty-one Developing Countries*. Non-sales publication ST/ESA/SER.R/49. New York.

_____ (1982a). Some demographic characteristics of women's work patterns and rates in ten World Fertility Survey countries. In *World Population Trends and Policies, 1981 Monitoring Report*, vol. I, *Population Trends*. Population Studies, No. 79. New York, 207-215.
Sales No. E.82.XIII.2.

_____ (1983). *Fertility Levels and Trends as Assessed from Twenty World Fertility Surveys*. Non-sales publication ST/ESA/SER.R/50. New York.

_____ (1983a). *Marital Status and Fertility: A Comparative Analysis of World Fertility Survey Data for Twenty-one Countries*. Non-sales publication ST/ESA/SER.R/52. New York.

_____ (1983b). *Relationships Between Fertility and Education: A Comparative Analysis of World Fertility Survey Data for Twenty-two Developing Countries*. Non-sales publication ST/ESA/SER.R/48. New York.

_____ (1984). *Some Relationships Between Nuptiality and Fertility in Countries of the West Indies*. Non-sales publication ST/ESA/SER.R/46. New York.

_____ (1984a). Socio-economic development and fertility decline: an application of the Easterlin synthesis approach to World Fertility Survey. Working paper ESA/P/WP/88. New York.

_____ (1985). *World Population Prospects: Estimates and Projections as Assessed in 1982*. Population Studies, No. 86. New York.
Sales No. E.83.XIII.5.

_____ (1986). *Review and Appraisal of the World Population Plan of Action*. Population Studies, No. 99. New York.
Sales No. E.86.XIII.2.

United Nations Educational, Scientific and Cultural Organization (1981). *UNESCO Statistical Yearbook 1981*. Paris.

Vaessen, Martin (1981). Knowledge of contraceptives: an assessment of World Fertility Survey data collection procedures. *Population Studies* 35(3):357-374.

_____ (1984). *Childlessness and Infecundity*. World Fertility Survey Comparative Studies, No. 31; Cross-National Summaries. Voorburg, The Netherlands: International Statistical Institute.

World Bank (1976). *World Tables 1976*. Baltimore, Maryland: The Johns Hopkins University Press.

_____(1980). *World Tables*. 2nd ed. Baltimore, Maryland: The Johns Hopkins University Press.

_____(1984). *World Development Report*. New York: Oxford University Press.

World Fertility Survey (1984). *Major Findings and Implications*. Voorburg, The Netherlands: International Statistical Institute.

World Health Organization (1981). *Global Strategy for Health for All by the Year 2000*. "Health for All" Series, No. 3. Geneva.

PART ONE. FERTILITY AND ITS PROXIMATE DETERMINANTS IN THE DEVELOPING COUNTRIES

I. LEVELS AND TRENDS IN FERTILITY

ABSTRACT

This chapter describes levels and trends in fertility as assessed from data for 38 World Fertility Survey countries and includes a comparative assessment of the quality of estimates of fertility levels and trends. Fertility in the adolescent years and the extent of childlessness are also discussed.

A systematic scrutiny of the data from the birth and marriage histories and the household survey reveal that 27 of these countries had estimates of fertility for the five-year period preceding the survey that were at least reasonably reliable and 19 had at least reasonably reliable estimates of fertility trends (periods from 0-4 to 10-14 years prior to the survey). Of the countries with less reliable recent estimates, 6 were in Africa and 5 in Asia and Oceania, while in the case of trend estimates, 10 countries were in Africa, 6 in Asia and Oceania and 3 in Latin America and the Caribbean. A strong relationship between a country's level of development and the quality of its survey estimates of fertility was observed.

Fertility rates for the five-year period before the survey ranged from fewer than four children per woman in Costa Rica, Sri Lanka, and Trinidad and Tobago to more than eight children in Kenya and Yemen. Fertility among African women was estimated to be the highest—6.5 children, on average—while that of Latin American and Caribbean women was estimated at 4.9 children, on average. Within-region variation was particularly large in Africa, where fertility among the Northern African countries was lower than that of countries in the sub-Saharan region. Similar regional variation exists in Asia and Oceania, where countries in Southern and Western Asia had relatively high fertility. Fertility was strongly related to level of development and family planning programme effort. Substantial declines in total fertility rates, ranging from 16 to 46 per cent, occurred over the 10-year period before the survey. The declines were positively related to level of development and family planning programme strength. While declines occurred in all age groups, the largest declines were among women aged 15-19 and among older women aged 35-49. Marital fertility showed particularly large declines among older women. In some countries, a slight increase in marital fertility was observed among young women, but this was more than offset by large declines among older women.

Childbearing among adolescents, defined as women aged 15-19, made up about 10 per cent of the total fertility rate, although except for several African countries and Bangladesh and Mexico, fertility among women aged 15 and 16 years was low. For most countries, the proportion of childless women was not large—between 3 and 4 per cent.

One of the primary outcomes of the World Fertility Survey (WFS) was information on fertility levels and trends. For populations that have not had a tradition of population surveys or censuses and where vital registration systems are deficient, the WFS data have made an especially valuable contribution to establishing the level and trends in fertility. Even among populations that have conducted censuses and fertility surveys, fertility levels estimated from the World Fertility Survey add to the picture which has developed with data from other sources; and in countries that have relatively good vital registration, these data act, in addition, as a check on the registration system.

The WFS estimates of fertility for 38 countries (12 in Africa, 13 in Latin America and the Caribbean and 13 in Asia and Oceania) are presented in this chapter. Of these countries, only 11 (Costa Rica, Egypt, Fiji, Guyana, Jamaica, Malaysia, Panama, Sri Lanka, Trinidad and Tobago, Tunisia and Venezuela) have "complete"[1] birth registration data which were available for comparison with the WFS estimates for comparable time periods. For most of the remaining countries, fertility estimates were available from censuses or surveys for periods comparable to the survey date or for some period during the 15 years prior to the survey. Only Benin, Ghana and Senegal did not have any data from external sources for comparison. The lack of demographic data from other sources for these three countries means that the WFS data are invaluable for establishment of levels and trends in fertility at the national level, but it also means that estimates derived from the World Fertility Survey cannot yet be checked against an independent data source.

An assessment of the quality of estimates is necessary in any analysis of fertility levels and trends, whether the estimates are derived from censuses, surveys or birth registration. A critical scrutiny of the data from detailed birth histories can reveal the usefulness of fertility estimates derived from them and indicate the degree of uncertainty surrounding these estimates. Reasonably accurate date reporting in the birth and marriage histories, as well as accurate reporting of the respondent's age, is necessary if reliable age-specific and marital age-specific fertility rates are to be derived from a maternity history survey, not only for the period immediately preceding the survey but for a period of from 15 to 20 years prior to the survey. Owing to the scarcity of reliable fertility estimates for most developing countries, estimates from the World Fertility Survey represent an important addition to demographic knowledge but their interpretation requires some concept of data quality.

The WFS programme has provided a unique opportunity for data quality to be examined in a comparative context because an assessment of the quality of any one country's fertility estimates can be made in relation to that of all other countries. This assessment is possible because of the uniformity of the household and individual questionnaires. Such an investigation of data quality was carried out by the United Nations for the first 20 WFS countries and is being done for another 18 countries (United Nations, 1983 and forthcoming). The age distribution and the reporting of births and marriages were scrutinized systematically for each country. Using a specified set of measures, data quality was compared across countries for the age, marriage and birth distributions, all of which are direct or indirect inputs in the computation of fertility rates. The results of this assessment are utilized in this chapter to indicate the degree of uncertainty surrounding the estimates of fertility levels and trends that can be derived from the WFS data. A brief description of the steps leading to assessment of the quality is presented below in section A.

This chapter presents a descriptive and demographic picture of childbearing that has emerged from the WFS data. Detailed analysis and explanations of the fertility patterns are not dealt with here but are discussed in subsequent chapters. Section A includes an overview of the quality of WFS fertility estimates and a brief summary of how the quality assessment was undertaken. This is followed by a presentation of fertility estimates and cumulative fertility. Trends in fertility are given next for those countries whose data are judged to be at least reasonably reliable. The age pattern of fertility and trends therein are also studied. Lastly, two special aspects of fertility—adolescent fertility and childlessness—are discussed. All of the information is summarized for groups of countries according to region, level of development and strength of family planning programme effort.

A. THE DATA

The fertility measures presented in this chapter are the crude birth rate, the total fertility rate (TFR), the fertility rate among ever-married women and the mean number of children ever born. The total fertility rate is a synthetic-cohort measure or period rate. It is the sum of all age-specific rates and is interpreted as the total number of children a women would bear by the end of her reproductive period if the prevailing fertility rates were to apply to her from age 15 to age 49 years. In the case of the WFS data, it is obtained by dividing the number of births to women at a given age over a specified period (five years) by the number of women-years of exposure in that age over the same period. Summed over all ages, the total fertility rate is obtained:

$$TFR = \sum_{i=15}^{49} b_i/w_i$$

where b_i is births to women aged i and w_i is the woman-years in age group i. The mean number of children ever born to a birth cohort of women gives a similar summary measure but because the fertility experience of the younger birth cohorts is truncated by the survey, it is only for the cohort aged 45-49 years at the time of the survey that fertility is essentially complete.[2]

Under certain conditions or assumptions, a comparison of the number of children born to women aged 45-49, a cohort rate, and the total fertility rate, a period rate, can give an indication of the extent of fertility change over an extensive period prior to the survey. This is only possible, however, if the data are reasonably accurate. Timing errors in the dating of births and omission of births can be especially serious among the older cohorts; and if they are present, any interpretation of fertility change based on such a comparison would be misleading. Alternatively, the comparison of cumulative fertility of the oldest cohort (P) with the cumulated period measure (F) can be used to evaluate the quality of data in a survey in the absence of notable trends; this is known as the P/F procedure. In practice, it is difficult to distinguish errors in data from actual trends using this comparison when both are suspected to be present. A detailed discussion of this comparison and its drawbacks is presented in Goldman and Hobcraft (1982) and in United Nations (1983a). Patterns of rates in the birth history can also be examined graphically, as was done in the United Nations studies (United Nations, forthcoming) in conjunction with the other checks described below. While the most accurate estimation of trends in fertility for any country in the absence of complete vital registration data would be from a series of surveys with overlapping birth histories, the intent of this chapter is to focus primarily on the WFS results. Indeed, in only a few of the WFS countries are there multiple surveys with full birth histories to allow such a comparison.

Data for the compilation of fertility rates presented in this chapter come from the birth and marriage history in the individual questionnaire and from the age and marital status distribution derived from the household questionnaire. Details of the calculation of the rates from birth history data are given in Verma (1980). For the 20 countries that administered the individual questionnaire only to ever-married women, the denominator of the fertility estimate (the woman-years of exposure) was inflated to include all women, using estimates of proportions ever married from the household schedule.[3] In order to arrive at estimates of the crude birth rate for all countries, one further step was necessary. Age-specific rates were multiplied by age-specific proportions female from the household questionnaire and summed over the age groups from 15 to 49 years.

Age-specific rates and other rates presented in this paper are averaged over five-year periods before the survey date and refer to the mid-point of the period. Annual rates would be ideal to discern changes within five-year periods but sampling errors for single-year rates are estimated to be rather high (Little, 1982). The sampling error decreases considerably for rates averaged over three years (Hanenberg, 1980) and decreases further for rates averaged over five years. Five-year averages were chosen for presentation here because an examination of single-year rates revealed underreporting of births in the one- to two-year period before the survey for some countries, with corresponding heaping on zero and three or four years, leading to the possibility that estimates based on a three-year average might underestimate recent fertility (United Nations, 1983).

Detailed country evaluations of the WFS data were undertaken by country personnel with the assistance of the World Fertility Survey.[4] These evaluations were subsequently used along with other sources of data in United Nations studies (United Nations, 1983 and forthcoming) to evaluate the data in a cross-country comparative context. In the United Nations study, fertility estimates of different countries were sorted into one of three crude categories with respect to data quality so that users would have a rough idea of the reliability of the estimates. These categories are used in this chapter whenever fertility estimates are presented. A summary of the procedures applied to arrive at these crude categories and the categories themselves are presented below.

The most common errors that occur in the data involve recall problems, age misreporting and dating of events, which can affect not only the estimation of trends in fertility but recent fertility estimates. Internal and external checks were used to evaluate each aspect of data quality with respect to women's age, their union status at the time of the survey and their union and birth histories, as each of these is an important input in the calculation of fertility rates. A summary of the results of these checks is presented in the annex (tables 23-28); a technical introduction and detailed footnotes provide unambiguous definitions of each of the measures applied. A full rationale for and discussion of the approach can be found in United Nations (1983 and forthcoming).

Age reporting was examined for digit preference, completeness of reporting of birth dates and distortions in five-year female age distribution (annex, table 23). The female age distribution from the household data was also compared with an external source, usually a recent census (United Nations, forthcoming). Next, the quality of the marriage history was assessed by studying, first, the completeness of reporting of dates of marriages. In addition, the single-year distribution of marriage duration was examined for suggestions of preference for particular durations, and trends in proportions married were compared with marital status distributions from other censuses or surveys (annex, table 24).

The assessment of the quality of the birth history was done in two steps: recent birth reporting was assessed and then reporting over the period 0-14 years prior to the survey was assessed, so that separate ratings could be given to first recent fertility estimates and to the trends implied by comparisons with earlier fertility estimates (annex, tables 23-28). The period 0-14 years was chosen for two reasons. First, as the oldest women interviewed were 49, data are progressively truncated, reducing the age range over which fertility estimates can be derived. For example, in the 15-19 years before the survey, information in the birth history was available for ages 15-34 only. The second reason for choosing the period 0-14 years is that reporting errors in the birth history become more problematical and numerous the further back into the past one goes.

Steps that were taken in assessing the enumeration of recent births included comparisons of the parity distribution with that from an external source in order to discern omissions of births, an examination of the completeness of reporting of birth dates, a comparison of recent fertility levels from the World Fertility Survey with those estimated from external sources and the extent of irregularity in annual rates in the period 0-4 years before the survey. In addition, annual rates for the five-year period before the survey were examined for any shifting of births out of the period from one to two years before the survey into the adjacent periods (annex, table 25). The quality of trends in births over the period 0-14 years prior to the survey was assessed not only through a comparison of WFS estimates with trends implied by external sources but through direct comparisons between cohorts in age profiles of fertility and in parity at the older ages for evidence of omissions and date misplacements. An index of irregularity in annual rates was also used. If differences between sources in the level and age pattern appeared, these are noted, as in table 27 (see annex) and are considered a possible indication of uncertainty surrounding the rates.

Using the tests described above, age reporting, marriage-date reporting and birth-date reporting were successively rated for quality and categorized into three broad groups with respect to reliability. These ratings in turn were used to arrive at an assessment of the quality of recent fertility estimates for all women and ever-married women and of fertility trends (annex, tables 26 and 28). A three-way rating scheme was adopted. Countries with data that ranked relatively high with respect to most or all of the criteria outlined above were rated "A" and were considered to have fertility rates of good quality. A rating of "B" was given to those countries with data that ranked at least moderately on a fair number of the criteria used. For these countries, the estimated rates are considered to be of acceptable quality, but uncertainty about the estimates exists. The third group, rated "C", is composed of countries with data that ranked poorly with respect to some of the more crucial criteria established so that estimates of fertility from these data are problematical in the absence of additional evidence to the contrary.

Of the 38 countries for which data were examined, recent fertility rates were considered to be of good quality in 13 while recent rates of another 14 countries were thought to be generally acceptable. Fertility rates of the remaining 11 countries were thought to be less reliable under the criteria used. Recent fertility estimates for all the countries in Latin America and the Caribbean were of at least acceptable quality, whereas in Africa and in Asia and Oceania, six and five countries, respectively, had recent estimates that were classified as less reliable (table 9, panel A). All of these 11 countries were in development groups III and IV (table 9, panel B), while all 13 countries with "good" recent fertility estimates were in development groups I and II. This association between level of development and the reliability of fertility estimates probably reflects the existence of better survey mechanisms in the more developed of these countries as well as better knowledge on the part of the respondents of the dates of their vital events. It also highlights the fact that in the very countries where good demographic estimates are more sought after and greatly needed, such estimates are difficult to provide. In many instances, however, the WFS data have provided estimates that represent a substantial improvement over previous national data. In addition, given the incompleteness of vital registration, reliable survey and census data for many countries at the lower development levels, the WFS estimates are occasionally the only ones available.

TABLE 9. NUMBER OF COUNTRIES CLASSIFIED BY ASSESSMENT OF QUALITY OF RECENT FERTILITY ESTIMATES AND FERTILITY TRENDS, BY REGION AND LEVEL OF DEVELOPMENT

	Fertility rates assessed as being:		
	Of good quality	Of acceptable quality	Less reliable
A. Assessment of recent rates			
Region			
Africa	1	5	6
Latin America and the Caribbean	7	6	—
Asia and Oceania	5	3	5
Level of development			
I. High	9	2	—
II. Middle-high	4	6	—
III. Middle-low	—	5	3
IV. Low	—	1	8
B. Assessment of trends			
Region			
Africa	1	1	10
Latin America and the Caribbean	4	6	3
Asia and Oceania	4	3	6
Level of development			
I. High	6	4	1
II. Middle-high	3	5	2
III. Middle-low	—	1	7
IV. Low	—	—	9

Sources: Tables 26 and 28, in annex to this chapter.

The results of the assessment of the quality of estimates of fertility trends over the period 0-14 years prior to the survey are much the same. Because of chronic problems of misreporting of dates in most of the African countries, only two—Morocco and Tunisia—were assessed as having acceptable trend information. In Latin America and the Caribbean and in Asia and Oceania, on the other hand, in only three and six countries, respectively, was information on fertility trends considered less reliable (table 9). When classified by level of socio-economic development, a strong positive relationship is seen between that level and the quality of trend estimates, as was the case for recent fertility estimates. Indeed, all of the countries in the low development group (IV) had unreliable estimates of trends in fertility from birth history information. In addition, it was mostly these countries where a lack of data from other sources made it most difficult to verify the trend estimates from the World Fertility Survey. In development group IV, data from other sources for comparison with the WFS estimates were available in only two out of nine countries, whereas in development group I, all 11 countries had data from other sources for comparison.

B. RECENT FERTILITY

Crude birth rates and total fertility rates

Crude birth rates for the five-year period preceding the survey date show a wide range for the 38 countries included here (table 10). While Costa Rica, Sri Lanka, and Trinidad and Tobago had birth rates below 30 per 1,000 population, Benin, Côte d'Ivoire,[5] Senegal and Yemen had extremely high rates, over 50 births per 1,000 population. African countries in general had higher rates than the countries in Latin America and the Caribbean and in Asia and Oceania, the average rate for Africa being 45 births per 1,000 population, compared with 35 and 39 births per 1,000 population in the other two regions, respectively.[6] Even within regions, birth rates had a wide range, especially in Asia. Among the Asian countries, those of Southern and Western Asia generally had higher rates than those of East Asia, while in Africa, the Northern African countries generally had lower rates than the sub-Saharan countries.

The crude birth rate is a measure that can be influenced by the age and sex structure of a population, whereas the total fertility rate is not influenced by age distribution. Total fertility rates for the five years preceding the survey are included in table 10. Except for a few countries, the relative positions of countries with respect to fertility levels is the same for the two measures.[7] Total fertility rates for the 38 countries range from fewer than four children per woman in Costa Rica, Sri Lanka, and Trinidad and Tobago to more than eight children in Kenya and Yemen. At the prevailing fertility rates for the five-year period before the survey, African women are estimated to bear, on average, 6.5 children, while women in Asia and Oceania are estimated to bear about one child less, 5.7 children; and Latin American and Caribbean women will bear, on average, 4.9 children. As was the case for crude birth rates, these regional averages mask considerable variation within regions, especially in Asia and Oceania, where the difference between the highest and lowest rate was more than four births. Within the regions of Africa and of Asia and Oceania, subregional patterns emerge. The Northern African countries generally have lower fertility than the sub-Saharan countries, while the other countries in Asia and Oceania generally have lower fertility than those in Southern or Western Asia.

Unfortunately, countries with the highest fertility rates are those with less reliable rates. Of the 13 countries that had fertility rates of more than six children, only two—Mexico and the Syrian Arab Republic—had fertility estimates that were assessed as being of good quality. For three countries, Cameroon, Jordan and Kenya, recent fertility rates were considered acceptable, while for the remaining eight countries, recent rates were considered unreliable (table 10). By contrast, of the 12 countries where total fertility rates were below five children, only one—Indonesia—had recent rates that were assessed as being less reliable.

When averaged by level of development and strength of family planning programme effort, a strong relationship is seen between the level of recent fertility and development level and programme effort (table 11). Women in countries in the high development group (I) are estimated to have, on average, two children fewer than women in countries in the low development group (IV).

TABLE 10. POPULATION ESTIMATES, CRUDE BIRTH RATES AND TOTAL FERTILITY RATES FOR THE FIVE YEARS PRECEDING THE SURVEY DATE, BY REGION AND COUNTRY

Region and country	Population estimates, 1975[a] (millions) (1)	Year of survey (2)	Crude birth rate (3)	Total fertility rate (4)	Assessment of rates (5)
Africa					
Benin	3.5	1982	54.0	7.1	C
Cameroon	8.6	1978	45.5	6.4	B
Côte d'Ivoire[b]	8.2	1980	52.6	7.4	C
Egypt	41.2	1980	39.4	5.3	B
Ghana	11.5	1979/80	43.5	6.5	C
Kenya	13.7	1977/78	48.4	8.3	B
Lesotho	1.2	1977	40.2	5.8	B
Mauritania	1.6	1981	45.5	6.2	C
Morocco	20.0	1979/80	41.5	5.9	B
Senegal	5.7	1978	51.9	7.2	C
Sudan	18.7	1978/79	40.6	5.9	C
Tunisia	6.4	1978	37.1	5.8	A
AVERAGE[c]	—	—	45.0	6.5	—
Latin America and the Caribbean					
Colombia	23.2	1976	34.8	4.7	A
Costa Rica	2.0	1976	29.6	3.8	A
Dominican Republic	4.9	1975	41.4	5.7	B
Ecuador	8.0	1979	38.2	5.3	B
Guyana	0.8	1975	35.3	4.9	A
Haiti	5.2	1977	37.6	5.5	B
Jamaica	2.0	1975/76	31.1	5.0	A
Mexico	60.1	1976	41.4	6.2	A
Panama	1.7	1975/76	30.4	4.5	B
Paraguay	3.2	1979	35.3	5.0	B
Peru	15.2	1977/78	37.5	5.6	A
Trinidad and Tobago	1.1	1977	26.5	3.4	A
Venezuela	13.1	1977	35.4[d]	4.6[d]	B
AVERAGE[c]	—	—	35.0	4.9	—
Asia and Oceania					
Bangladesh	76.6	1975/76	42.9	6.1	C
Fiji	0.6	1974	31.9	4.2	A
Indonesia	135.7	1976	35.8	4.7	C
Jordan	2.6	1976	47.7	7.6	B
Malaysia	12.3	1974	33.2	4.7	A
Nepal	13.0	1976	44.1	6.0	C
Pakistan	75.2	1975	42.2	6.3	C
Philippines	48.3	1978	35.4	5.3	A
Republic of Korea	35.3	1974	30.7	4.3	A
Sri Lanka	13.6	1975	28.3	3.8	B
Syrian Arab Republic	8.8	1978	45.7	7.5	A
Thailand	41.4	1975	32.9	4.6	B
Yemen	5.8	1979	58.0	8.5	C
AVERAGE[c]	—	—	39.1	5.7	—

Sources: For column (1), United Nations (1985); for columns (2) and (4), World Fertility Survey standard recode tapes; for column (5), table 26, in annex to this chapter.

NOTES: Rates assessed as: A = good quality; B = acceptable quality; C = less reliable.

[a] For surveys conducted in 1978 or more recently, the estimates are for 1980.
[b] Formerly called the Ivory Coast.
[c] Averages are not weighted.
[d] The fertility rate for age group 45-49 is the same as that from the birth registration data for the period 1972-1976. Women aged 45-49 were not included in the individual questionnaire for Venezuela.

Similarly, women in countries with a strong family planning programme are estimated to have, on average, two fewer children than women in countries that had no programme or a very weak one.

Age-specific fertility rates

Differences that were seen in the levels of recent fertility between regions also occur in the age pattern of recent fertility (table 12 and figure 2). Average rates for African countries are higher in all age groups than those for Latin America and the Caribbean and for Asia and Oceania, particularly in age groups 25-29 and 30-34, where the differences between the average for Africa and that for Latin America and the Caribbean were 64 and 58 births per 1,000 women, respectively. The age patterns of fertility for Asia and Oceania and for Africa are similar except that rates for the former are lower than those for the latter in all age groups. There is considerable variation in the age pattern of fertility within regions also. The average pattern for the three Western Asian countries—Jordan, the Syrian Arab Republic and Yemen—shown in figure 2 have the highest rates in all age groups compared with other subregions of Asia. Large differences

TABLE 11. CRUDE BIRTH RATES AND TOTAL FERTILITY RATES, BY LEVEL OF DEVELOPMENT AND STRENGTH OF FAMILY PLANNING PROGRAMME EFFORT

	Crude birth rate	Total fertility rate
Level of development		
I. High	32.8	4.6
II. Middle-high	38.0	5.6
III. Middle-low	43.4	6.3
IV. Low	46.3	6.5
Strength of family planning programme effort		
1. Strong	32.5	4.6
2. Moderate	34.3	4.8
3. Weak	40.7	5.9
4. Very weak/none	46.0	6.7

Source: Table 10.

are seen especially among women aged 25-29, 30-34 and 35-39 years. By contrast, age-specific rates for Fiji, Indonesia, Malaysia, the Philippines, the Republic of Korea and Thailand (East and South Eastern Asia and Oceania in figure 2) are more concentrated in the age groups from 20 to 34 years and are significantly lower than those for Southern and Western Asia. In Africa, age-specific rates among age groups 15-19 and 20-24 were distinctly lower for Northern African countries (Egypt, Morocco and Tunisia).

Age-specific rates were averaged by level of development and strength of family planning programme effort (figure 3). Countries in the high development group (I) had lower fertility in all age groups, compared with countries in the low development group (IV), while the age-specific rates for development groups II and III fell in between. Age-specific rates by strength of family

TABLE 12. AGE-SPECIFIC FERTILITY RATES AND TOTAL FERTILITY RATES FOR FIVE YEARS PRECEDING THE SURVEY DATE, BY REGION AND COUNTRY

Region and country	15-19	20-24	25-29	30-34	35-39	40-44	45-49	Total fertility rate	Assessment of rates
Africa									
Benin	0.151	0.314	0.329	0.278	0.193	0.099	0.051	7.10	C
Cameroon	0.187	0.295	0.277	0.220	0.155	0.106	0.041	6.40	B
Côte d'Ivoire[a]	0.216	0.314	0.299	0.246	0.207	0.129	0.060	7.40	C
Egypt	0.099	0.256	0.286	0.217	0.130	0.048	0.016	5.26	B
Ghana	0.136	0.255	0.276	0.245	0.188	0.132	0.061	6.46	C
Kenya	0.178	0.346	0.356	0.298	0.244	0.164	0.066	8.26	B
Lesotho	0.102	0.268	0.258	0.233	0.173	0.094	0.030	5.79	B
Mauritania	0.154	0.264	0.290	0.242	0.168	0.086	0.044	6.20	C
Morocco	0.093	0.265	0.296	0.222	0.178	0.098	0.029	5.90	B
Senegal	0.188	0.304	0.331	0.270	0.197	0.106	0.036	7.16	C
Sudan	0.108	0.260	0.282	0.251	0.146	0.107	0.035	5.94	C
Tunisia	0.034	0.225	0.304	0.260	0.199	0.112	0.035	5.85	A
AVERAGE	0.137	0.281	0.299	0.249	0.182	0.107	0.042	6.48	—
Latin America and the Caribbean									
Colombia	0.101	0.230	0.221	0.172	0.130	0.062	0.023	4.70	A
Costa Rica	0.103[b]	0.193	0.178	0.137	0.093	0.053	0.010	3.84	A
Dominican Republic	0.123	0.286	0.265	0.233	0.166	0.054	0.015	5.71	B
Ecuador	0.103	0.237	0.262	0.200	0.161	0.083	0.017	5.32	B
Guyana	0.114	0.283	0.242	0.184	0.112	0.042	0.006	4.92	A
Haiti	0.057	0.204	0.266	0.226	0.178	0.116	0.054	5.50	B
Jamaica	0.147	0.262	0.227	0.178	0.114	0.058	0.013	5.00	A
Mexico	0.114	0.290	0.294	0.254	0.178	0.084	0.021	6.18	A
Panama	0.127[c]	0.237	0.214	0.153	0.111	0.039	0.008	4.44	B
Paraguay	0.086	0.221	0.239	0.207	0.150	0.074	0.016	4.96	B
Peru	0.084	0.237	0.262	0.242	0.171	0.092	0.026	5.57	A
Trinidad and Tobago	0.078	0.188	0.171	0.118	0.081	0.029	0.010	3.38	A
Venezuela	0.097	0.234	0.216	0.178	0.120	0.060	0.012[d]	4.59	B
AVERAGE	0.103	0.239	0.235	0.191	0.136	0.065	0.018	4.93	—
Asia and Oceania									
Bangladesh	0.219	0.304	0.260	0.214	0.142	0.064	0.012	6.08	C
Fiji	0.061	0.247	0.225	0.165	0.092	0.045	0.009	4.22	A
Indonesia	0.124	0.249	0.226	0.167	0.112	0.050	0.018	4.73	C
Jordan	0.124	0.343	0.365	0.332	0.240	0.103	0.019	7.63	B
Malaysia	0.063	0.232	0.252	0.201	0.132	0.041	0.011	4.66	A
Nepal	0.131	0.283	0.287	0.236	0.159	0.079	0.027	6.01	C
Pakistan	0.152	0.283	0.312	0.252	0.180	0.064	0.010	6.26	C
Philippines	0.054	0.214	0.253	0.239	0.179	0.089	0.022	5.25	A
Republic of Korea	0.012	0.188	0.319	0.196	0.094	0.040	0.006	4.28	A
Sri Lanka	0.038	0.151	0.207	0.181	0.116	0.045	0.012	3.75	B
Syrian Arab Republic	0.123	0.297	0.339	0.312	0.245	0.136	0.044	7.48	B
Thailand	0.069	0.213	0.220	0.179	0.154	0.071	0.020	4.63	B
Yemen	0.175	0.346	0.346	0.334	0.229	0.197	0.075	8.51	C
AVERAGE	0.104	0.258	0.278	0.231	0.160	0.079	0.022	5.66	—

Source: World Fertility Survey standard recode tapes.
NOTES: Rates assessed as: A = good quality; B = acceptable quality; C = less reliable.
[a] Formerly called the Ivory Coast.
[b] Estimate based on vital registration data for age group 15-19 averaged from 1970 to 1976, from Costa Rica (1978), p. 74.
[c] Estimate based on vital registration data for age group 15-19 averaged from 1971 to 1975, from United Nations (1979), table 6.
[d] Estimate based on vital registration data for age group 45-49 averaged from 1972 to 1976, from Vielma (1982).

Figure 2. Age-specific fertility rates, by region

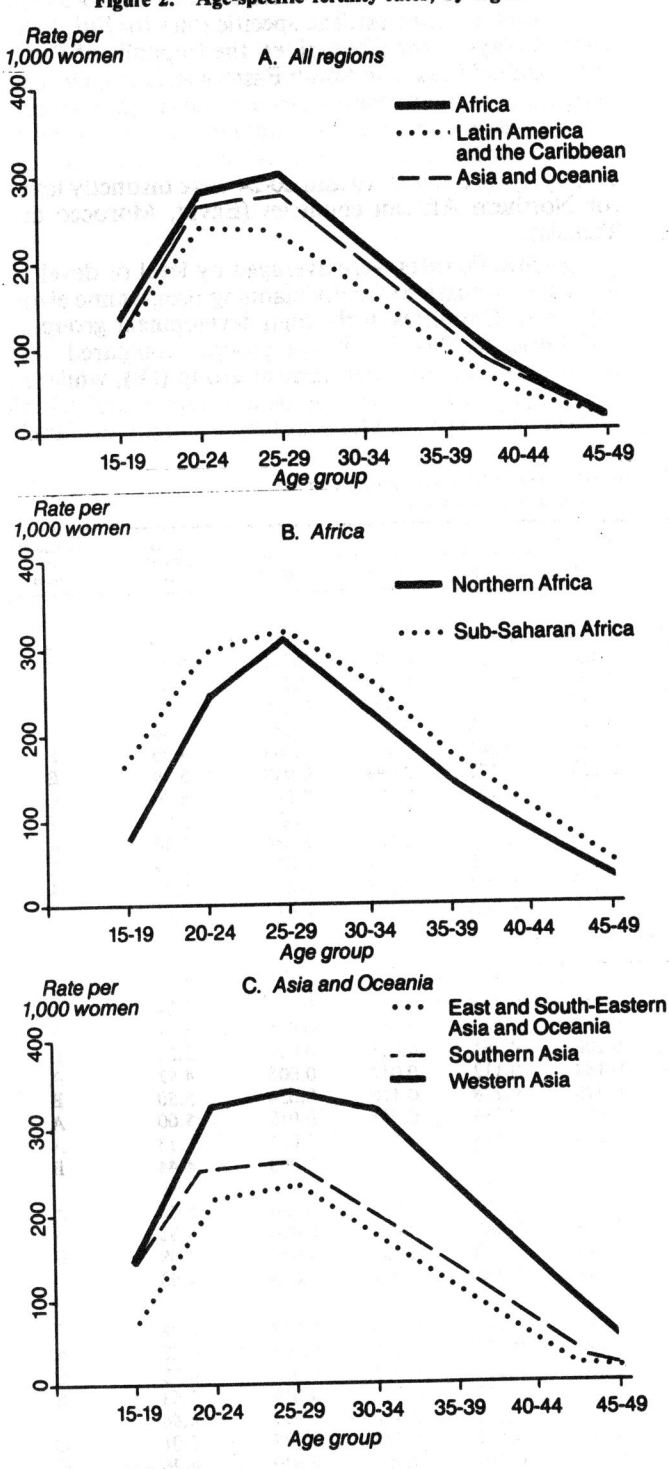

A. All regions
B. Africa
C. Asia and Oceania

Source: Table 12.

Figure 3. Age-specific fertility rates, by level of development and strength of family planning programme effort

A. Level of development
B. Family planning programme effort

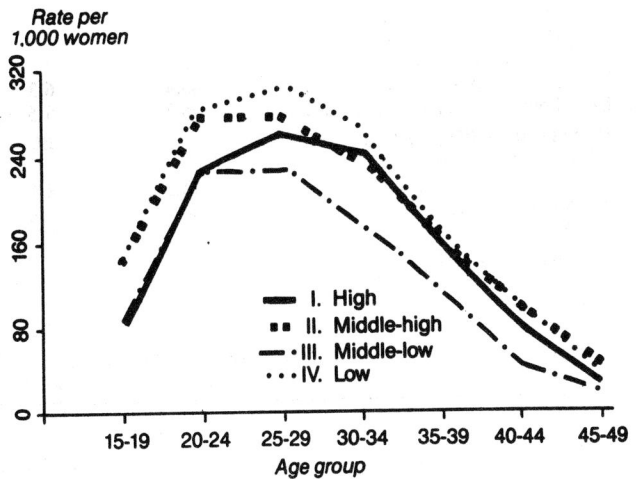

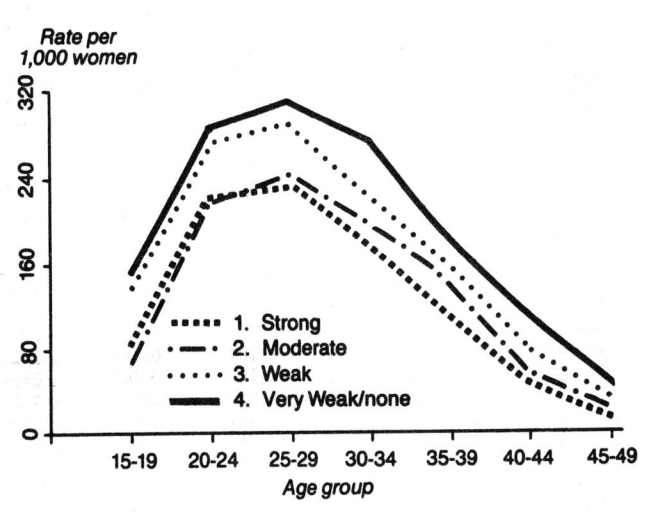

Source: Table 12.

planning programme effort reflect the same type of differences as were found for development levels. Fertility rates for countries with a strong programme were lower at all ages than those of countries with a very weak or no programme. At the older ages, fertility rates become progressively higher as one moves from the strong to the very weak category. Differences in the age pattern of fertility among countries at various levels of development and levels of programme strength reflect differences in proportions married or proportions sexually active in the younger age groups, while in the older age groups, differences probably reflect differences in contraceptive use. Of course, in every age group, differences in fecundability could also account for some of the differences in observed levels. All of these points are discussed in greater detail in chapters III and VI.

Marital age-specific fertility rates

The measurement of marital fertility is restricted to women ever exposed to risk of conception through the formation of unions; and when tabulated by age, the differences between marital age-specific rates and age-specific rates reflect differences in proportions ever married.[8] With marital fertility, variation due to differences in marital patterns between countries is eliminated although marital dissolution and remarriage could still affect rates. None the less, variation due to other factors, such as the extent of breast-feeding, post-partum abstinence and most importantly, contraceptive use, can be observed. The effect of these factors on marital fertility is discussed in detail in succeeding chapters. In this chapter, the level and pattern of age-specific rates among women ever in a union are described.

The World Fertility Survey guidelines included in their definition of unions all socially recognized unions, not just legal unions. Thus, in a number of countries, especially those in Latin America and the Caribbean, consensual and non-cohabiting sexual unions were also included (Singh, 1984). A full discussion of the various types of unions is presented in chapter III. As in the case of age-specific rates, marital age-specific fertility rates were also evaluated and the quality assessments are presented in table 28 (see annex).

Despite the fact that marital fertility rates are controlled for variations in proportions ever married, there still is considerable variation in rates between countries. In age group 15-19, for example, marital fertility ranges from 0.229 and 0.213 in Haiti and Nepal, respectively, to double that (0.479) in Jordan (table 13). Ever-married women aged 20-24 years in Trinidad and Tobago had 0.256 birth per woman, while those in Jordan and the Syrian Arab Republic had 0.482 and 0.454 birth per woman, respectively.

TABLE 13. AGE-SPECIFIC MARITAL FERTILITY RATES FOR THE FIVE YEARS PRECEDING THE SURVEY DATE, BY REGION AND COUNTRY

Region and country	15-19	20-24	25-29	30-34	35-39	40-44	45-49	Assessment of rate
Africa								
Benin	0.336	0.351	0.334	0.280	0.193	0.099	0.051	C
Cameroon	0.294	0.313	0.280	0.222	0.156	0.107	0.042	B
Côte d'Ivoire[a]	0.326	0.330	0.305	0.247	0.207	0.130	0.060	C
Egypt	0.346	0.378	0.318	0.224	0.134	0.049	0.016	B
Ghana	0.330	0.292	0.281	0.246	0.190	0.132	0.062	C
Kenya	0.404	0.389	0.364	0.299	0.244	0.165	0.066	B
Lesotho	0.310	0.322	0.276	0.244	0.177	0.095	0.031	B
Mauritania	0.300	0.320	0.307	0.253	0.171	0.088	0.045	C
Morocco	0.340	0.366	0.322	0.226	0.178	0.098	0.029	B
Senegal	0.310	0.344	0.336	0.270	0.198	0.106	0.037	C
Sudan	0.346	0.350	0.308	0.259	0.152	0.109	0.036	C
Tunisia	0.385	0.434	0.358	0.271	0.203	0.113	0.037	A
AVERAGE	0.336	0.349	0.316	0.253	0.184	0.108	0.043	—
Latin America and the Caribbean								
Colombia	0.429	0.366	0.265	0.194	0.145	0.066	0.023	A
Costa Rica	0.368[b]	0.311	0.213	0.152	0.106	0.058	0.011	A
Dominican Republic	0.368	0.373	0.288	0.241	0.170	0.055	0.015	B
Ecuador	0.404	0.361	0.311	0.218	0.174	0.089	0.017	B
Guyana	0.362	0.357	0.255	0.190	0.115	0.043	0.006	B
Haiti	0.229	0.311	0.300	0.235	0.181	0.119	0.056	B
Jamaica	0.310	0.300	0.232	0.183	0.117	0.058	0.013	B
Mexico	0.443	0.422	0.339	0.274	0.187	0.088	0.022	A
Panama	0.392[b]	0.346	0.238	0.164	0.116	0.040	0.008	B
Paraguay	0.376	0.354	0.286	0.225	0.156	0.077	0.017	B
Peru	0.451	0.414	0.323	0.268	0.184	0.097	0.028	B
Trinidad and Tobago	0.251	0.256	0.187	0.123	0.083	0.030	0.010	A
Venezuela	0.429	0.369	0.256	0.189	0.125	0.062	0.010[c]	B
AVERAGE	0.370	0.349	0.269	0.204	0.143	0.068	0.018	—
Asia and Oceania								
Bangladesh	0.275	0.315	0.261	0.215	0.142	0.065	0.012	C
Fiji	0.344	0.344	0.242	0.172	0.094	0.046	0.009	A
Indonesia	0.274	0.293	0.235	0.170	0.114	0.051	0.018	C
Jordan	0.479	0.482	0.407	0.346	0.247	0.106	0.020	B
Malaysia	0.432	0.402	0.296	0.213	0.135	0.041	0.011	A
Nepal	0.213	0.310	0.303	0.254	0.180	0.099	0.035	C
Pakistan	0.313	0.344	0.331	0.260	0.182	0.064	0.010	C
Philippines	0.429	0.432	0.330	0.267	0.194	0.094	0.024	B
Republic of Korea	0.364	0.403	0.347	0.198	0.094	0.040	0.006	A
Sri Lanka	0.363	0.348	0.284	0.201	0.123	0.047	0.012	B
Syrian Arab Republic	0.447	0.454	0.394	0.332	0.256	0.140	0.044	A
Thailand	0.377	0.348	0.264	0.197	0.162	0.074	0.021	B
Yemen	0.274	0.382	0.357	0.340	0.233	0.199	0.075	C
AVERAGE	0.353	0.374	0.312	0.243	0.166	0.082	0.023	—

Source: World Fertility Survey standard recode tapes.

NOTES: Rates assessed as: A = good quality; B = acceptable quality; C = less reliable.

[a] Formerly called the Ivory Coast.
[b] Obtained by multiplying the rate for age group 15-19 by the reciprocal of the proportion married at ages 15-19. This proportion is obtained from the marriage history for the period 0-4 years prior to the survey in the individual questionnaire and is 0.280 for Costa Rica and 0.324 for Panama.
[c] Obtained by multiplying the rate for age group 45-49 by the reciprocal of the proportion married at ages 45-49 from the 1971 census.

The age pattern of marital fertility varies between regions. Among the countries of Africa and of Asia and Oceania, marital fertility peaks at ages 20-24 and then declines at older ages, whereas among the Latin American and Caribbean countries, the highest rates were found among those aged 15-19 years. These differences are even more pronounced when the rates are averaged according to levels of development and strength of family planning programme effort (figure 4). At ages 20-24, the level of marital fertility among all development groups (except middle-high) and at all levels of programme effort were similar. Below this age group (i.e., ages 15-19), the countries in the upper development groups and those with stronger family planning programmes had higher rates, while the reverse was true among older women. Indeed, differences in marital fertility rates between the high and low development groups are most pronounced in age groups 15-19 (positive relationship) and 25-39 (negative relationship). When averaged by programme strength, marital fertility rates are progressively higher among women aged 25-39 as one moves from the strong to the very weak effort categories (figure 4).

C. CUMULATIVE FERTILITY

The large differences earlier observed in the level of recent fertility between countries are not reflected in the data on children ever born to women aged 40-49 years at the time of the survey (table 14). This is mainly because the fertility measure, children ever born, represents the cumulative experience for the oldest cohort and most of the births to women in this cohort took place a long time ago while other measures of fertility are current. Completed family size ranged from 5.1 children in Lesotho to 8.5 children in Jordan. Only Cameroon, Indonesia, Lesotho and the Republic of Korea have completed family sizes of fewer than 5.5 children, while Jordan, Kenya, Morocco and the Syrian Arab Republic had an average completed family size of more than seven children. In 23 countries, family size was in the range from 5.5 to 6.5 children. Averaged by level of development (figure 5) and strength of family planning programme effort (not shown), the mean number of children ever born increases monotonically with age at all levels of development and programme strength. However, differences among women aged 40-49 years are not large. While women aged 40-49 in countries in the high development group and in countries with a strong programme had about 6.1 children, those in countries in the low development group and in countries with a very weak programme had about 0.5 child more at the end of their childbearing period. These small differences are not surprising, as births to women aged 40-49 years occurred over a period in the past while the ranking of countries according to levels of development and family planning programme strength is based on current indicators.

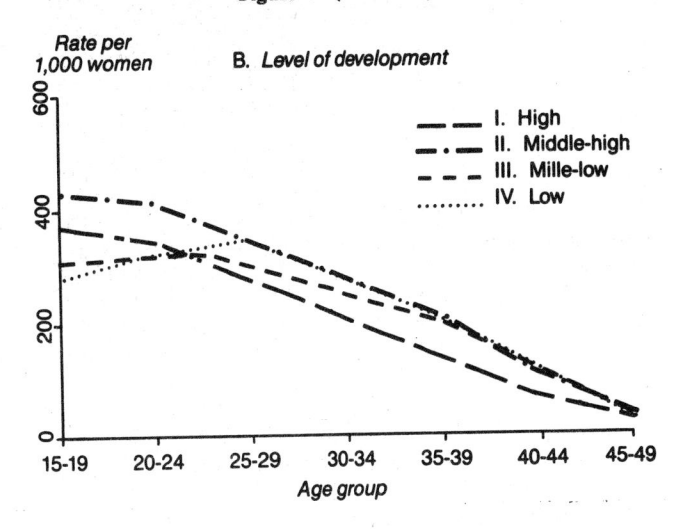

When countries are classed according to level of development, patterns differ for number of children born and number surviving (table 15 and figure 5). At ages 35 and older, the number of living children is lowest in development groups III and IV. For women aged 40-49, the difference between the high level (I) and the two lower groups (III and IV) amounts to roughly 0.8 child, and the difference between group II and the lower groups is about one child. At the lower ages, differential mortality has largely cancelled the effect of higher rates of childbearing in development groups III and IV. At ages 20-24, for instance, the average number of children born is 0.5 child greater in development group IV than in group I,

Figure 4. Marital age-specific fertility rates, by region, level of development and strength of family planning program effort

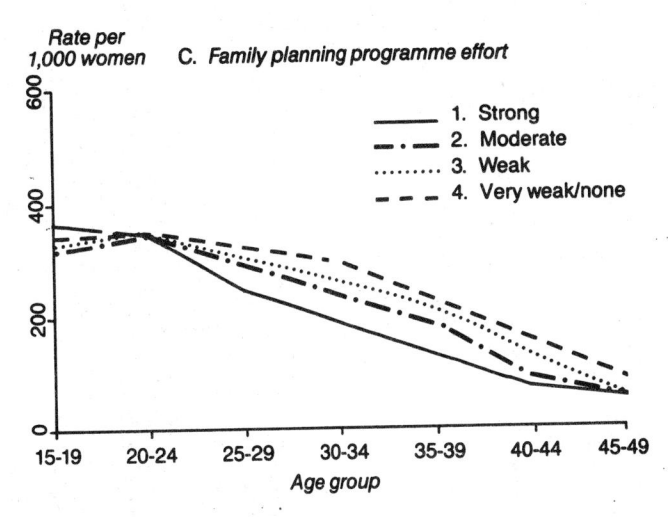

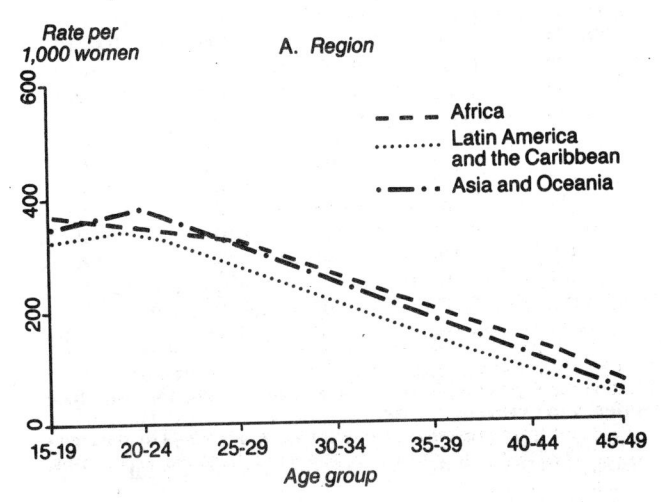

TABLE 14. MEAN NUMBERS OF CHILDREN EVER BORN, BY AGE OF WOMAN AND BY REGION AND COUNTRY

Region and country	15-19	20-24	25-29	30-34	35-39	40-44	45-49	40-49
Africa								
Benin	0.3	1.5	3.1	4.7	5.7	6.1	6.3	6.2
Cameroon	0.4	1.6	3.0	4.2	4.9	5.2	5.2	5.2
Côte d'Ivoire[a]	0.5	1.9	3.3	4.7	5.9	6.7	6.9	6.8
Egypt	0.1	1.2	2.6	4.4	5.7	6.3	6.8	6.3
Ghana	0.2	1.4	2.7	4.0	5.4	6.1	6.7	6.4
Kenya	0.3	1.8	3.8	5.6	6.8	7.6	7.9	7.7
Lesotho	0.2	1.2	2.4	3.8	4.6	5.0	5.2	5.1
Mauritania	0.4	1.6	3.4	4.8	5.7	5.9	5.9	5.9
Morocco	0.2	1.2	2.9	4.8	5.7	5.9	5.9	5.9
Senegal	0.4	1.7	3.4	5.3	5.9	7.1	7.1	7.1
Sudan	0.2	1.4	3.0	4.8	5.8	6.8	7.2	6.9
Tunisia	0.0	0.6	2.3	4.3	5.7	6.5	7.0	6.7
AVERAGE	0.3	1.4	3.0	4.6	5.7	6.3	6.5	6.4
Latin America and the Caribbean								
Colombia	0.2	1.1	2.4	4.0	5.0	6.1	6.7	6.4
Costa Rica	..	1.0	2.0	3.5	4.8	6.1	6.7	6.4
Dominican Republic	0.2	1.3	3.0	4.6	6.3	6.4	6.5	6.5
Ecuador	0.2	1.2	2.5	4.0	5.5	6.4	6.8	6.6
Guyana	0.2	1.3	2.8	4.8	5.7	6.3	6.4	6.3
Haiti	0.1	0.8	2.0	3.4	4.5	5.6	5.9	5.8
Jamaica	0.3	1.6	2.8	4.1	5.1	5.4	5.5	5.5
Mexico	0.2	1.3	2.9	4.6	6.0	6.6	6.8	6.7
Panama	..	1.2	2.6	3.8	4.9	5.6	5.8	5.7
Paraguay	0.1	1.0	2.2	3.5	4.6	5.8	6.3	6.0
Peru	0.1	1.0	2.5	4.0	5.4	6.3	6.6	6.4
Trinidad and Tobago	0.1	0.9	2.0	3.2	4.3	5.2	5.8	5.5
Venezuela	0.2	1.1	2.4	3.9	5.0	6.1	..	6.1[b]
AVERAGE	0.2[c]	1.1	2.5	4.0	5.2	6.0	6.3[d]	6.2[d]
Asia and Oceania								
Bangladesh	0.6	2.3	4.2	5.6	6.7	7.1	6.8	6.9
Fiji	0.1	1.0	2.5	4.1	5.0	6.0	6.5	6.2
Indonesia	0.2	1.3	2.7	3.9	4.8	5.3	5.2	5.2
Jordan	0.2	1.6	3.7	5.6	7.1	8.4	8.6	8.5
Malaysia	0.1	0.9	2.3	4.0	5.3	6.0	6.1	6.1
Nepal	0.2	1.3	2.8	4.1	5.1	5.5	5.8	5.6
Pakistan	0.2	1.5	3.1	4.8	5.9	6.9	6.8	6.9
Philippines	0.1	0.8	2.1	3.7	5.2	6.4	6.6	6.5
Republic of Korea	0.0	0.4	1.8	3.3	4.4	5.1	5.7	5.4
Sri Lanka	0.0	0.6	1.7	3.3	4.6	5.3	5.9	5.6
Syrian Arab Republic	0.2	1.3	3.1	4.8	6.3	7.3	7.7	7.5
Thailand	0.1	0.9	2.1	3.5	4.6	5.8	6.5	6.1
Yemen	0.4	1.7	3.2	5.0	6.0	6.4	7.2	6.8
AVERAGE	0.2	1.2	2.7	4.3	5.5	6.3	6.6	6.4

Sources: Goldman and Hobcraft (1982); and Singh (1984).
[a] Formerly called the Ivory Coast.
[b] Mean for age group 40-44 only.
[c] Excluding Costa Rica and Panama.
[d] Excluding Venezuela.

while the contrast in number living is 0.2 child. Contrasts between the number born and the number surviving are much smaller by region and family planning effort than by development level—not surprisingly, because the current level of infant mortality is a component of the development index. Higher overall mortality in Africa, however, means that the older women in that region have an average number of living children about 0.5 child lower than in Latin America and the Caribbean, even though the number of children ever born is slightly higher in Africa.

D. FERTILITY TRENDS

Trends in age-specific fertility rates

Fertility trends estimated from the birth histories were assessed as being of good or acceptable quality for 19 of the 38 countries (see annex, table 28). For these 19 countries, trends in age-specific fertility rates over the 14-year period preceding the survey are discussed in the text.[9] Table 16 shows the age-specific rates averaged over three five-year periods prior to the survey: 0-4; 5-9; and 10-14 years.

All of the 19 countries recorded substantial declines in total fertility rates from the period 10-14 years before the survey to the period 0-4 years prior to the survey (table 16).[10] Declines range from 17 and 16 per cent in Mexico and Morocco, respectively, to 46 per cent in Costa Rica. With only a few exceptions, declines were greater in the more recent period than in the earlier period. The average decline for all countries over the 10-year period (from 12.5 years to 2.5 years before the survey) was 26 per cent, with an 11 per cent decline during the earlier period and a 17 per cent decline for the more recent period. There does not appear to be a strong relationship

TABLE 15. MEAN NUMBERS OF LIVING CHILDREN, BY AGE OF WOMAN AND BY REGION AND COUNTRY

Region and country	15-19	20-24	25-29	30-34	35-39	40-44	45-49	40-49
Africa								
Benin	0.3	1.3	2.5	3.6	4.3	4.2	4.3	4.2
Cameroon	0.3	1.4	2.5	3.3	3.7	3.9	3.7	3.8
Côte d'Ivoire[a]	0.4	1.6	2.7	3.7	4.5	4.9	4.7	4.8
Egypt	0.1	1.0	2.1	3.5	4.3	4.6	4.7	4.6
Ghana	0.2	1.2	2.4	3.5	4.6	5.1	5.4	5.2
Kenya	0.3	1.6	3.2	4.7	5.6	6.1	6.0	6.1
Lesotho	0.1	1.0	2.1	3.1	3.7	4.0	4.1	4.0
Mauritania	0.3	1.4	2.8	3.9	4.6	4.4	4.4	4.4
Morocco	0.1	1.1	2.4	4.1	5.0	5.6	5.5	5.6
Senegal	0.4	1.4	2.5	3.9	4.2	4.6	4.9	4.7
Sudan	0.1	1.2	2.7	4.1	4.9	5.0	5.0	5.0
Tunisia	0.0	0.6	2.1	3.7	4.9	5.3	5.6	5.4
MEAN	0.2	1.2	2.5	3.8	4.5	4.8	4.8	4.8
Latin America and the Caribbean								
Colombia	0.1	1.0	2.2	3.6	4.4	5.2	5.6	5.4
Costa Rica	..	0.9	1.8	3.2	4.3	5.5	5.8	5.6
Dominican Republic	0.2	1.2	2.7	4.0	5.4	5.4	5.5	5.5
Ecuador	0.2	1.0	2.2	3.5	4.7	5.3	5.5	5.3
Guyana	0.3	1.2	2.6	4.5	5.1	5.6	5.5	5.6
Haiti	0.1	0.6	1.6	2.8	3.4	4.3	4.5	4.4
Jamaica	0.5	1.5	2.7	3.9	4.7	4.9	5.0	4.9
Mexico	0.9	1.2	2.6	4.0	5.3	5.7	5.6	5.6
Panama	..	1.1	2.5	3.5	4.5	5.2	5.1	5.2
Paraguay	.1	0.9	2.0	3.3	4.3	5.3	5.7	5.5
Peru	0.1	0.9	2.1	3.4	4.3	4.9	4.9	4.9
Trinidad and Tobago	0.1	0.8	1.9	3.0	4.0	4.8	5.3	5.1
Venezuela	0.2	1.1	2.3	3.6	4.7	5.6	..	5.6[b]
MEAN	0.3	1.0	2.3	3.6	4.5	5.2	5.3	5.3
Asia and Oceania								
Bangladesh	0.5	1.8	3.2	4.3	5.0	5.1	4.7	4.9
Fiji	0.1	0.9	2.4	3.8	4.6	5.5	5.8	5.6
Indonesia	0.2	1.1	2.3	3.2	3.8	4.1	3.8	4.0
Jordan	0.2	1.4	3.4	5.1	6.4	7.0	7.2	7.1
Malaysia	0.1	0.8	2.2	3.7	4.9	5.4	5.3	5.4
Nepal	0.2	1.1	2.2	3.0	3.7	3.8	3.9	3.9
Pakistan	0.2	1.2	2.5	3.8	4.7	4.9	4.9	4.9
Philippines	0.1	0.7	1.9	3.4	4.7	5.7	5.7	5.7
Republic of Korea	0.0	0.4	1.7	3.1	4.0	4.5	4.7	4.6
Sri Lanka	0.0	0.6	1.6	3.0	4.2	4.7	5.1	4.9
Syrian Arab Republic	0.2	1.2	2.8	4.4	5.6	6.3	6.6	6.5
Thailand	0.1	0.8	1.9	3.1	4.1	4.9	5.4	5.1
Yemen	0.3	1.3	2.5	3.6	4.3	4.3	4.6	4.5
MEAN	0.2	1.0	2.4	3.7	4.6	5.1	5.2	5.1
TOTAL MEAN	0.2	1.1	2.4	3.7	4.6	5.0	5.1	5.1

Source: World Fertility Survey standard recode tapes.
[a] Formerly called the Ivory Coast.
[b] For age group 40-44.

between initial fertility levels and the amount of decline over the period. In general, however, countries that had total fertility rates of seven children in the earlier period had fertility declines of about two children, while those which began with fertility rates of about five or six children had declines of about 1.5 children over the 10-year period.

The 19 countries for which data are presented here are not evenly distributed across the three regions. Only 2 (Morocco and Tunisia) are in Africa, 7 in Asia and Oceania and 10 in Latin America and the Caribbean. Regional averages are not presented in table 16 but an inspection of the percentage declines in fertility rates shows that the declines for the two Northern African countries were smaller than that for Asia and Oceania, where the decline was in turn slightly smaller than in Latin America and the Caribbean.

Table 17 shows fertility trends for two levels of development (high and medium-high) and of family planning programme effort. Unfortunately, the 19 countries were concentrated in development groups I and II, so the trend information is averaged over only those two levels. Countries in the high development group recorded larger decreases in fertility than those in the medium-high group, 30 per cent versus 22 per cent, declines being larger in both groups in the more recent period. When averaged by strength of programme effort, it is seen that the stronger the programme, the larger the decline in fertility.

Figure 5. **Age-specific fertility rates for the periods 10-14 and 0-4 years prior to the survey date, by level of development and strength of family planning programme effort, 19 countries**

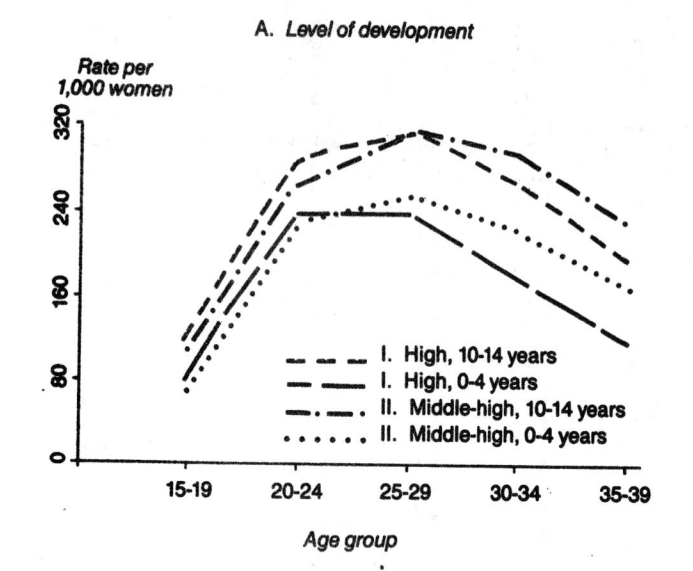

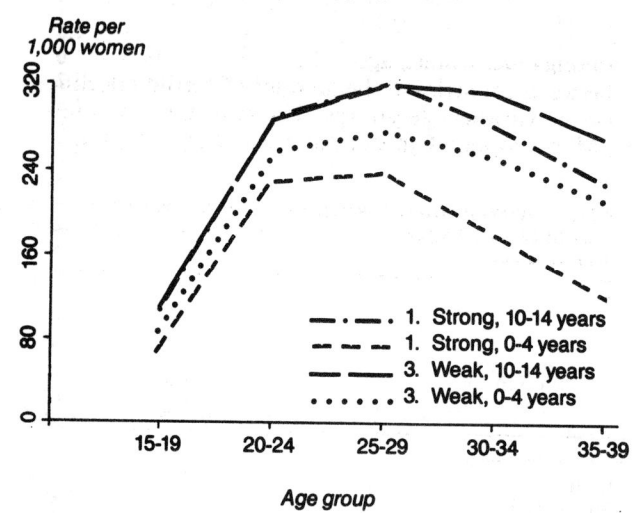

A. *Level of development*

- — — — I. High, 10-14 years
- — — — I. High, 0-4 years
- —·—·— II. Middle-high, 10-14 years
- ······· II. Middle-high, 0-4 years

B. *Family planning programme effort*

- —·—·— 1. Strong, 10-14 years
- — — — 1. Strong, 0-4 years
- ——— 3. Weak, 10-14 years
- ······· 3. Weak, 0-4 years

Source: World Fertility Survey standard recode tapes.

TABLE 16. TOTAL FERTILITY RATES FOR WOMEN AGED 15-44 AND PERCENTAGE CHANGE IN TOTAL FERTILITY RATES FOR THE PERIODS FROM 10-14 TO 0-4 YEARS PRIOR TO THE SURVEY DATE, BY REGION, 19 COUNTRIES[a]

Region and country	10-14	5-9 (years)	0-4	From 10-14 to 5-9 years	From 5-9 to 0-4 years	From 10-14 to 0-4 years
Africa						
Morocco	6.9	6.7	5.8	−3	−13	−16
Tunisia	7.0	6.1	5.7	−13	−7	−19
Latin America and the Caribbean						
Colombia	7.2	6.1	4.6	−14	−25	−36
Costa Rica	7.1	5.5	3.8	−23	−31	−46
Ecuador	6.8	6.2	5.2	−9	−16	−24
Guyana	7.0	6.1	4.9	−12	−20	−30
Jamaica	6.5	5.9	4.9	−10	−16	−25
Mexico	7.3	6.9	6.1	−6	−12	−17
Paraguay	6.1	5.6	4.9	−8	−13	−20
Peru	6.7	6.3	5.4	−5	−14	−18
Trinidad and Tobago	5.3	4.0	3.3	−25	−18	−38
Venezuela	6.0	5.6	4.5	−7	−20	−25
Asia and Oceania						
Fiji	6.8	5.4	4.2	−20	−23	−38
Malaysia	6.1	5.4	4.6	−12	−15	−25
Philippines	6.7	6.3	5.1	−5	−19	−23
Republic of Korea	5.5	4.7	4.2	−15	−10	−23
Sri Lanka	5.5	4.7	3.7	−15	−22	−33
Syrian Arab Republic	8.3	7.6	7.3	−8	−4	−12
Thailand	6.6	5.9	4.5	−10	−24	−31

Source: World Fertility Survey standard recode tapes.

[a] These 19 countries were assessed as having trend information of more reliable quality. See table 28, in annex to this chapter.

The average decline for countries with a very weak programme or no programme was 16 per cent, while that for countries with a strong programme was twice as great.

Percentage changes in age-specific rates from 10-14 to 0-4 years prior to the survey are presented in table 18. The average change by age group for the 19 countries shows that greater declines occurred in age group 15-19 and among older women aged 35-39. There is some variation between countries in the amount of fertility decline among the various age groups. The two African countries, Morocco and Tunisia, recorded relatively greater declines in fertility among younger women than older ones, whereas fertility declines among Latin American and the Caribbean countries were larger among older women. In all regions, however, substantial declines in fertility rates were recorded for every age group. The 19 countries when grouped by level of development (only two levels had enough countries—the high and the middle-high) showed similar amounts of decline among younger women but declines among older women were substantially larger in countries in development group I (see figure 6). For strength of programme effort, classification by four levels was possible. Percentage declines in fertility were higher in all age groups in the strong category, compared with countries in the very weak/none category. As can be seen quite clearly in figure 6, the decline in fertility among older women was substantially higher in countries with a strong family planning programme than in those with a very weak programme or no programme, although differences in the decline are also large among women in age group 15-19.

TABLE 17. TRENDS IN TOTAL FERTILITY RATES FOR WOMEN AGED 15-44 AND PERCENTAGE CHANGE IN TOTAL FERTILITY RATES FOR THE PERIODS FROM 10-14 TO 0-4 YEARS PRIOR TO THE SURVEY DATE, BY LEVEL OF DEVELOPMENT AND STRENGTH OF FAMILY PLANNING PROGRAMME EFFORT, 19 COUNTRIES[a]

	Number of countries	Total fertility rate in periods prior to the survey			Percentage change		
		10-14	5-9 (years)	0-4	From 10-14 to 5-9 years	From 5-9 to 0-4 years	From 10-14 to 0-4 years
Level of development							
I. High	10	6.4	5.6	4.5	−13	−20	−30
II. Middle-high	8	6.7	6.1	5.2	−9	−15	−22
Strength of family planning programme effort							
1. Strong	7	6.6	5.6	4.5	−15	−20	−32
2. Moderate	4	6.1	5.2	4.3	−15	−17	−30
3. Weak	5	6.8	6.3	5.3	−7	−16	−22
4. Very weak/none	3	7.0	6.5	5.9	−7	−9	−16

Source: Table 16.

[a] These 19 countries were assessed as having trend information of more reliable quality. See table 28, in annex to this chapter. However, as only one country was at the middle-low level of development, this level was omitted in the upper panel of this table.

TABLE 18. PERCENTAGE CHANGE IN AGE-SPECIFIC FERTILITY RATES FOR WOMEN AGED 15-39 FROM 10-14 TO 0-4 YEARS PRIOR TO THE SURVEY DATE, BY REGION, FOR 19 COUNTRIES[a]

Region and country	Age group				
	15-19	20-24	25-29	30-34	35-39
Africa					
Morocco	−42	−18	−10	−16	−15
Tunisia	−65	−27	−11	−17	−15
Latin America and the Caribbean					
Colombia	−24	−23	−33	−40	−50
Costa Rica	..	−38	−45	−56	−61
Ecuador	−20	−22	−15	−30	−27
Guyana	−28	−23	−25	−30	−42
Jamaica	−23	−9	−24	−33	−42
Mexico	−24	−8	−14	−13	−26
Paraguay	−12	−9	−9	−21	−32
Peru	−25	−16	−15	−17	−21
Trinidad and Tobago	−32	−34	−38	−44	−41
Venezuela	−26	−18	−29	−32	..
Asia and Oceania					
Fiji	−57	−24	−27	−39	−55
Malaysia	−48	−22	−18	−19	−27
Philippines	−26	−18	−23	−22	−26
Republic of Korea	−25	−20	−4	−26	−50
Sri Lanka	−59	−38	−27	−24	−38
Syrian Arab Republic	−17	−12	−9	−12	−15
Thailand	−19	−20	−29	−39	−36
AVERAGE	−32	−21	−21	−28	−34

Source: United Nations (1985), table 29.

[a] These 19 countries were assessed as having information of more reliable quality. See table 28, in annex to this chapter.

Trends in marital age-specific fertility rates

The data used in compiling trends in marital fertility rates were assessed as being reliable for 16 of the 38 countries for the period from 12.5 to 2.5 years prior to the survey. There were considerable reductions in marital fertility among older women in all 16 countries (table 19). In Costa Rica and Fiji, the declines in marital fertility were as much as 59 and 55 per cent, respectively, among women aged 35-39 years. The amount of decline increases with age for all countries. Among the younger age groups, however, increases in marital fertility were recorded for some countries. For the two Northern African countries and most of the Asian countries, marital fertility increased among younger women, although this was not the case among the Latin American and Caribbean countries, except for Venezuela. Increases are not large, however, except for age group 15-19 in Malaysia, the Philippines, the Republic of Korea and the Syrian Arab Republic. The small sample size probably accounts in part

Figure 6. Mean number of children ever born and living, by age group of woman and level of development

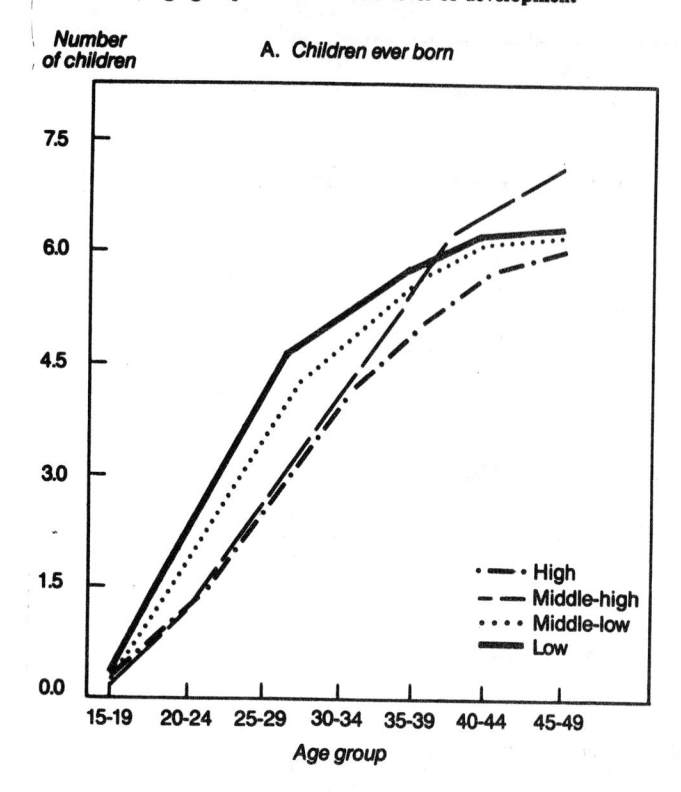

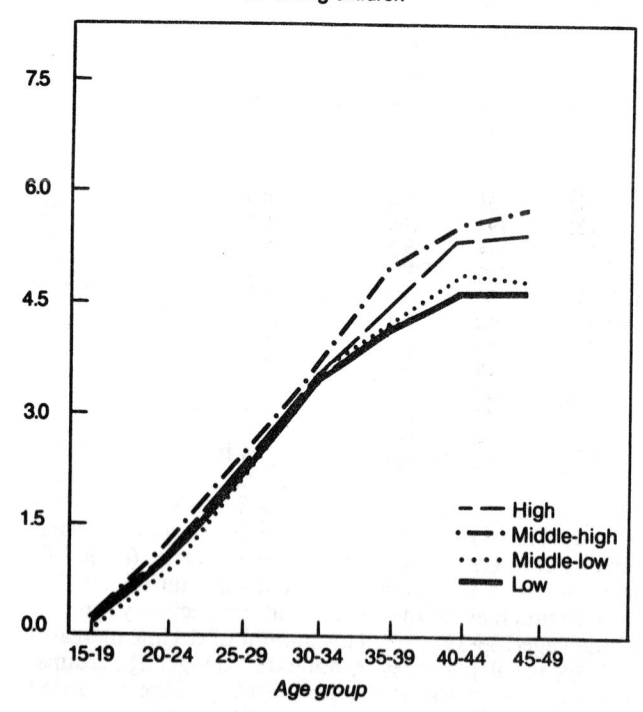

A. Children ever born

B. Living children

Sources: Tables 14 and 15.
NOTE: Based on all women, regardless of marital status.

for the 56 per cent increase observed among women aged 15-19 years in the Republic of Korea because so few women were married in this age group. The large declines among older women offset the small increases among young women, so that for all countries, the overall marital fertility rate had declined over the 14-year period.

TABLE 19. PERCENTAGE CHANGE IN MARITAL AGE-SPECIFIC FERTILITY RATES FOR WOMEN AGED 15-39 FROM 10-14 TO 0-4 YEARS PRIOR TO THE SURVEY DATE, BY REGION, 16 COUNTRIES[a]

Region and country	15-19	20-24	25-29	30-34	35-39
Africa					
Morocco	+ 4	+ 3	− 4	− 15	− 16
Tunisia	+ 4	+ 9	− 2	− 16	− 15
Latin America and the Caribbean					
Colombia	− 7	− 18	− 34	− 39	− 49
Costa Rica	..	− 37	− 48	− 57	− 59
Ecuador	− 4	− 16	− 13	− 29	− 25
Mexico	− 1	− 3	− 11	− 13	− 26
Paraguay	− 5	− 5	− 6	− 21	− 34
Trinidad and Tobago	− 27	− 31	− 37	− 44	− 41
Venezuela	+ 4	− 9	− 26	− 33	..
Asia and Oceania					
Fiji	− 10	− 13	− 26	− 38	− 55
Malaysia	+ 12	− 3	− 12	− 17	− 26
Philippines	+ 10	+ 1	− 15	− 21	− 26
Rep. of Korea	+56[b]	+ 3	+ 2	− 26	− 50
Sri Lanka	0	− 7	− 15	− 20	− 36
Syrian Arab Republic	+ 14	0	− 7	− 11	− 13
Thailand	+ 9	− 8	− 24	− 37	− 36
AVERAGE	+ 4	− 8	− 17	− 27	− 34

Source: World Fertility Survey standard recode tapes.
[a] These 16 countries were assessed as having information of more reliable quality. See table 28, in annex to this chapter.
[b] Large decline caused by unstable rates due to small sample size.

Increases in marital fertility among young women have been previously recorded in a number of countries, the Republic of Korea (Donaldson and Nichols, 1978); India (Srinivasan, Reddy and Raju, 1978); Kuwait (Hill, 1979); Latin America (Collver, 1965); and rural central Asia (Coale, Anderson and Härm, 1979). Declines in primary infertility and a possible rise in fecundability through changing practices associated with breast-feeding and abstinence all contribute to an increase in marital fertility. Such increases however are believed to be short-lived (Singh, Casterline and Cleland, 1985). A more likely explanation is that proportions of women married at ages under 20 have declined substantially due to rising age at marriage in many countries; and women who continue to marry at young ages are likely to be self-selected on a number of characteristics related to high fertility (Knodel, 1977).

Both level of development and strength of family planning programme effort have a strong positive relationship with the amount of decline in marital fertility rates among older women. It should be borne in mind, however, that these groups only have data for a subset of countries (16 in all) for which marital fertility trend data were assessed as being of more reliable or adequate quality. In the high and middle-high development groups, the difference in amount of decline between groups increases with age (table 20). In other words, among those aged 15-19 years, there was little or no difference in the amount of change in rates but among women aged 35-39 years, the difference is largest. The same is true of the different levels of programme strength.

TABLE 20. PERCENTAGE CHANGE IN MARITAL AGE-SPECIFIC FERTILITY RATES FOR WOMEN AGED 15-39 FROM 10-14 TO 0-4 YEARS PRIOR TO THE SURVEY DATE, BY LEVEL OF DEVELOPMENT AND STRENGTH OF FAMILY PLANNING PROGRAMME EFFORT, 16 COUNTRIES[a]

	Number of countries	15-19	20-24	25-29	30-34	35-39
Level of development						
I. High	8	+ 4	−14	−24	−33	−44
II. Middle-high	6	+ 4	− 6	−13	−23	−28
Strength of family planning programme effort						
1. Strong	5	+12	−10	−21	−34	−47
2. Moderate	4	− 4	− 9	−19	−29	−32
3. Weak	4	+ 1	− 6	−13	−23	−22
4. Very weak/none	2	+ 5	− 2	− 6	−16	−24

Source: Table 19.

[a] These 16 countries were assessed as having information of more reliable quality. See table 28, in annex to this chapter.

TABLE 21. AGE-SPECIFIC FERTILITY RATES FOR WOMEN AGED 15-19 FOR THE PERIOD 0-4 YEARS PRIOR TO THE SURVEY DATE, BY REGION AND COUNTRY
(PER 1,000 WOMEN)

Region and country	15	16	17	18	19	Age group 15-19 as percentage of total fertility rate
Africa						
Benin	45	69	128	190	286	10.6
Cameroon	102	134	183	244	274	14.6
Côte d'Ivoire[a]	104	172	226	277	311	14.6
Egypt	23	52	105	142	196	9.4
Ghana	39	76	148	203	227	10.5
Kenya	48	129	207	243	284	10.8
Lesotho	13	51	102	154	226	8.8
Mauritania	90	112	175	184	233	12.4
Morocco	14	55	96	142	181	7.9
Senegal	78	162	187	268	266	13.1
Sudan	29	89	106	152	188	9.1
Tunisia	3	4	21	48	109	2.9
AVERAGE	49	92	140	187	232	10.4
Latin America and the Caribbean[b]						
Colombia	22	59	95	161	194	10.7
Dominican Republic	34	76	122	194	206	10.8
Ecuador	21	60	113	154	183	9.7
Guyana	32	72	122	189	220	11.6
Haiti	13	24	50	97	107	5.2
Jamaica	54	110	170	200	248	14.7
Mexico	109	146	199	196	247	9.2
Paraguay	25	49	94	128	147	8.7
Peru	23	52	78	127	159	7.5
Trinidad and Tobago	23	38	75	117	149	11.5
Venezuela	39	50	111	139	168	10.6
AVERAGE	36	67	112	155	184	10.0
Asia and Oceania						
Bangladesh	140	211	230	272	259	18.0
Fiji	3	15	44	110	157	7.2
Indonesia	50	83	130	171	215	13.1
Jordan	29	80	125	216	256	8.1
Malaysia	11	25	59	94	145	6.8
Nepal	29	76	130	181	220	10.9
Pakistan	39	104	147	172	229	12.1
Philippines	8	17	53	82	122	5.1
Republic of Korea	0	2	8	22	40	1.4
Sri Lanka	4	17	30	65	82	5.1
Syrian Arab Republic	49	85	122	174	218	8.2
Thailand	13	35	68	105	142	7.4
Yemen	70	134	188	244	270	10.3
AVERAGE	34	68	103	147	181	8.7

Source: World Fertility Survey standard recode tapes.

[a] Formerly called the Ivory Coast.
[b] Not including Costa Rica and Panama because women aged 15-19 were not included in the individual interviews.

E. ADOLESCENT FERTILITY

Recently, there has been a growing concern over the fertility of women under age 20—adolescent fertility. High adolescent fertility is seen to have adverse effects on the health of teen-age mothers and their infants, whether childbearing is within or outside marriage. An early start to childbearing may mean an interruption in education, resulting in low future income through lesser labour force options and larger completed family size. Data for developing countries show that levels of adolescent fertility are high compared with developed countries, although fertility among women aged 15-19 years appears to be declining in some countries. In a majority of countries, especially in Africa and in Latin America and the Caribbean, more than 10 per cent of the total fertility rate is contributed by women aged 15-19; thus, women below age 20 are important contributors to total childbearing among all women (Senderowitz and Paxman, 1985).

Fertility rates among adolescents, who are defined in this study as women aged 15-19 years, rise steeply across the age range (table 21). Adolescent fertility rates among African women were, on average, higher than among those in Latin America and the Caribbean and in Asia and Oceania. However, as in the case of fertility rates in other age groups, there is much variation within regions. Cameroon and Côte d'Ivoire had exceptional high fertility among women aged 15 and 16 years; and in these two countries, fertility rates were as high as 274 and 311 per 1,000 women, respectively, by age 19. In Latin America and the Caribbean and in Asia and Oceania, only Bangladesh, Jamaica, Jordan, Mexico and Yemen had comparable high rates among women aged 15 and 16 years.

Childbearing among adolescents (ages 15-19) contributes a sizeable percentage of childbearing, on average, about 10 per cent of the fertility rate. In Bangladesh, Cameroon, Côte d'Ivoire and Jamaica, about 15 per cent of the total fertility is contributed by adolescents. In contrast, in the Philippines and the Republic of Korea, only 5.1 and 1.4 per cent, respectively, of the total fertility is contributed by that group.

A strong dichotomy in the relationship with levels of development and programme strength is seen when adolescent rates are grouped by these two variables. The low and middle-low groups have similar rates and are higher at every age than the high and middle-high groups. The same is true for categories of family planning programme strength (figure 7).

F. CHILDLESSNESS

Childlessness or infecundity is the "inability to conceive after several years of exposure to the risk of pregnancy" (Vaessen, 1984, p. 7).[11] Disease is considered a principal cause of subfecundity; and such diseases as tuberculosis, malaria, African sleeping sickness, leprosy, venereal disease, chagas disease, smallpox and filariasis are especially influential (Poston and others, 1982). Unfortunately, infecundity is a difficult condition to measure. Two aspects of infecundity can be distinguished: (a) "primary" infertility, which is the inability to bear any children as a result of an inability either to conceive or to carry a pregnancy to term; and (b) "secondary" infertility, which relates to the inability to have a child subsequent to an earlier birth after a reasonably long period of exposure.[12]

As a measure of primary infertility, the proportion of women who have never experienced any fertile pregnancy is used. Fertile pregnancies are children ever born plus current pregnancies. Since miscarriages usually occur within the first three or four months of pregnancy and most of the pregnancies reported in WFS were of longer durations, the proportion of pregnant women who will not have a live birth will be small (Vaessen, 1984).

Figure 7. **Adolescent fertility rates, by age of woman and by region, level of development and strength of family planning programme effort**

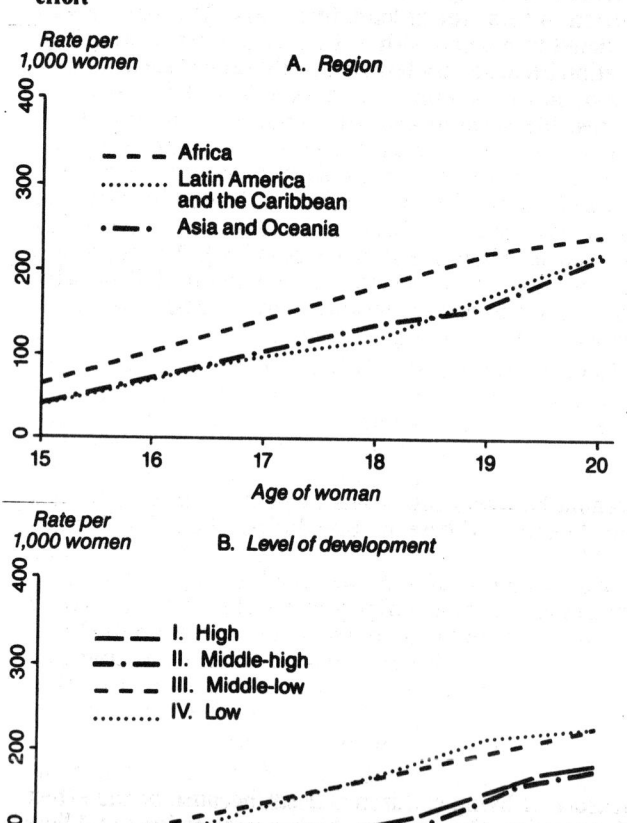

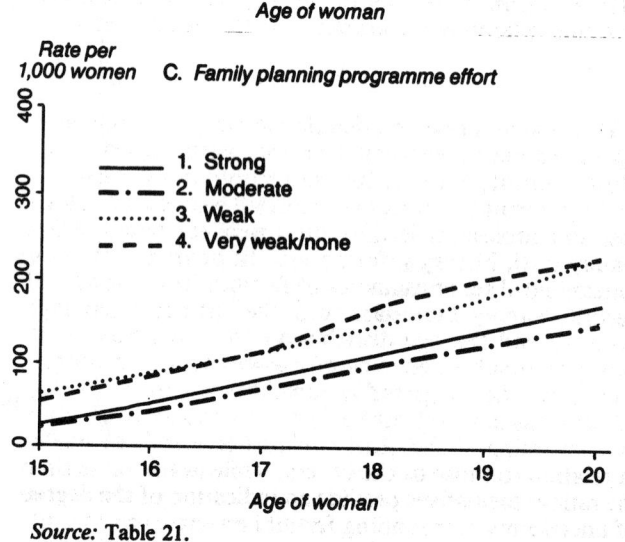

Source: Table 21.

Another measure of childlessness is the proportion of women with no living children. This measure is influenced by both fecundity and the levels of mortality to which children are subject throughout their lifetime. Although this indicator is not, strictly speaking, a measure of primary infertility, it is of importance for economic and social reasons as well.

Table 22 shows the proportion of women without any living children or fertile pregnancies, based on currently married women aged from 30 to 44 years who had been married in total for at least five years. The sample was restricted to women with at least five years of marriage duration because very few first births take place after that period, so that a woman who experienced five years of married life without bearing a child is very unlikely to have one after that period (Vaessen, 1984). The lower age-limit of 30 was chosen because if younger women were included, some of whom might be infecund in their first few years of marriage because of adolescent infecundity (in countries where age at marriage is low), the proportion childless might be overestimated. Women aged 45 or older were excluded because reporting may have been of poorer quality than for younger women.

Table 22 (column (1)) shows that, for most countries, the proportion of women with no fertile pregnancies was not large; and in only one country, Cameroon, was the percentage rather high—10.4 per cent. Many countries in Latin America and the Caribbean and in Asia and Oceania had very low levels of primary infertility, less than 2 per cent. These are Bangladesh, Ecuador, Malaysia, Mexico, Panama, Peru, the Philippines, the Republic of Korea and Thailand. Regional averages show that African countries had higher levels of primary infertility than did those in the other two regions. Within the Latin American and Caribbean region, the Caribbean countries and Guyana had higher primary infertility than the other countries—an average of 4.0 per cent compared with 1.9 per cent for the rest of the region.

Higher proportions childless are recorded when the measure of living children is used, because of the effect of mortality. On average, higher proportions childless were recorded among women in Africa (5.3 per cent) than among those in Latin America and the Caribbean (3.4 per cent) and those in Asia and Oceania (3.2 per cent). The measures of primary infertility and childlessness show little relationship to level of development and strength of family planning programme effort (not shown).

G. CONCLUSION

This chapter presents a descriptive picture of childbearing for 38 developing countries that participated in the World Fertility Survey. Recent fertility rates, trends in fertility, fertility among ever-married women, childlessness and adolescent fertility rates were estimated, using mainly birth history information. In order to arrive at a meaningful set of estimates of fertility from the World Fertility Survey data, data from the birth and marriage histories and the age distribution from the household survey were subjected to careful assessment on a systematic basis. The comparative context in which the quality of data was assessed makes it possible to provide some kind of rating of the quality of one country's estimates in relation to those of the others, while at the same time the ratings themselves provide an indication of the degree of uncertainty surrounding fertility estimates and trends and the amount of confidence that can be placed on them.

TABLE 22. PERCENTAGE OF WOMEN WITH NO LIVING CHILDREN AND PERCENTAGE WITH NO FERTILE PREGNANCIES AMONG CURRENTLY MARRIED WOMEN AGED 30-44 AND MARRIED FOR AT LEAST A TOTAL OF FIVE YEARS, BY REGION AND COUNTRY

Region and country	No fertile pregnancies (1)	No living children (2)
Africa		
Benin	2.4	3.8
Cameroon	10.4	14.4
Côte d'Ivoire[a]	3.2	5.4
Egypt	2.8	3.7
Ghana	2.2	3.2
Kenya	2.2	3.2
Lesotho	3.8	5.6
Mauritania	2.5	3.1
Morocco	4.5	5.5
Senegal	3.4	6.3
Sudan	4.3	5.6
Tunisia	2.9	3.4
AVERAGE	3.7	5.3
Latin America and the Caribbean		
Colombia	2.1	2.6
Costa Rica	2.2	2.6
Dominican Republic	3.7	4.3
Ecuador	1.4	1.6
Guyana	3.7	4.8
Haiti	3.3	5.9
Jamaica	4.2	5.5
Mexico	1.9	2.3
Panama	1.2	1.7
Paraguay	3.3	3.4
Peru	1.2	1.7
Trinidad and Tobago	4.9	5.9
Venezuela	2.1	2.1
AVERAGE	2.7	3.4
Asia and Oceania		
Bangladesh	1.7	2.5
Fiji	4.0	4.7
Indonesia	4.5	6.7
Jordan	2.0	2.4
Malaysia	1.6	1.9
Nepal	3.1	5.0
Pakistan	3.2	4.0
Philippines	1.7	1.9
Republic of Korea	1.1	1.2
Sri Lanka	2.8	3.2
Syrian Arab Republic	2.6	2.8
Thailand	1.4	1.9
Yemen	2.3	3.2
AVERAGE	2.5	3.2

Source: World Fertility Survey standard recode tapes.
[a] Formerly called the Ivory Coast.

Using a threefold ranking system for the quality of rates with the first two categories representing reliable estimates and the third, less reliable, 11 countries were assessed as having recent fertility estimates that were less reliable. All of these countries were in the middle-low and low development groups and were in Africa and Asia. For trend information, 19 countries were assessed as having less reliable rates and a strong positive correlation also was observed between level of development and quality of the estimates. These findings suggest that both respondents' knowledge of the dates of their vital events and better survey mechanisms tend to improve with development. They also highlight the fact that where good demographic estimates are most needed, such estimates are most difficult to provide. In the case of information on fertility trends, all of the countries in the low development group had less reliable trend information. Although this categorization paints a rather gloomy picture of the reliability of estimates derived from surveys conducted in countries at the lower development levels, it should be borne in mind that for a number of countries, the WFS estimates are the only estimates available for a comparable period; and in many instances, WFS was successful in providing estimates that represent a substantial improvement in quality and coverage over those from other sources. Indeed, in six of the least developed countries, WFS was successful in providing what were assessed as being reliable estimates of recent fertility. While more remains to be done, it must be emphasized that WFS has made an important contribution to improving national survey capability and the development of standardized questionnaires (Scott and Chidambaram, 1985; Verma, 1985).

Recent fertility rates were presented for all 38 countries, although trends in fertility were discussed only for those countries with reasonably reliable information. Fertility rates for the five-year period before the survey ranged from fewer than four children per woman in Costa Rica, Sri Lanka, and Trinidad and Tobago to more than eight children in Kenya and Yemen. Fertility among African women was the highest—6.5 children, on average—while in Latin America and the Caribbean, the estimate is 4.9 children per woman. Total fertility rates among women in Asia and Oceania averaged 5.7 children. There is considerable variation within regions. Northern African countries generally had lower fertility than the sub-Saharan countries, while the East Asian countries usually had considerably lower fertility than Southern or Western Asian countries. The average rate for the three Western Asian countries, Jordan, the Syrian Arab Republic and Yemen, was extremely high—7.8 births per woman.

A strong relationship was observed between countries' recent fertility and the level of development and strength of family planning programme effort. Women in countries in the high development group were estimated to have two fewer children than women in countries in the low development group. A similar differential was observed when groups of countries were compared according to family planning programme effort.

All of the 20 countries recorded substantial declines in total fertility rates, ranging from 16 to 46 per cent between the period 10-14 years prior to the survey and the period 0-4 years before the survey. The higher the level of development and the greater the programme strength, the larger the decline in total fertility rates over the 10-year period preceding the survey. The Northern African countries, Morocco and Tunisia, recorded relatively larger declines among younger women, whereas fertility declines were larger among older women in the Latin American and Caribbean countries.

Very high marital fertility rates were recorded among ever-married women in the Western Asian countries and in some sub-Saharan African countries. Age-specific rates at ages above 25 years were found to be negatively related to levels of development and strength of programme effort. Over time, marital fertility showed large declines among older women. The amount of decline increased with age among women older than 25. Among young women, a slight increase in marital fertility was observed in certain countries but this was more than offset by the large declines among older women.

Childbearing among adolescents, defined as women aged 15-19 years, makes up about 10 per cent of the total fertility rate. In general, fertility was found to be low among women aged 15 and 16 although several African countries and Bangladesh and Mexico recorded high fertility rates at these two ages.

The proportion of childless women was not large for most countries, ranging between 3 and 4 per cent. In only one country, Cameroon, was the proportion rather high —10.4 per cent.

NOTES

[1] Birth registration is regarded as "complete" if it is at least 90 per cent complete as reported by the countries to the United Nations Statistical Office.

[2] Strictly speaking, the cohort aged 45-49 years at the time of the survey is still in the reproductive process for five more years. However, the number of children born to women aged 45-49 is not large and the mean number of children ever born to these women can be considered to approximate completed family size.

[3] In Guyana, Jamaica, and Trinidad and Tobago, women aged 15-19 years who were attending school full time were excluded; in Mexico, those aged 15-19 who had never been in a union and who were childless were excluded (Singh, 1984).

[4] Workshops were conducted in the London office of the World Fertility Survey for personnel from the different countries. Evaluations were subsequently published in the WFS Scientific Reports series.

[5] Formerly called the Ivory Coast.

[6] All averages by region, level of development and strength of family planning programme effort presented in this chapter are unweighted.

[7] Kenya is an example of a country where the age distribution did influence the level of the crude birth rate. The total fertility rate for Kenya was 8.3, one of the highest among the 38 countries, but the crude birth rate of Kenya was 48, which does not top the list. A United Nations study (1982) that standardized crude birth rates of 21 World Fertility Survey countries for age and sex structure found that the crude birth rate for Kenya would be higher than 48.7 if it had not been for its young age/sex population distribution. Another factor that has to be taken into account is that the age/sex distribution from the household surveys is used to convert total fertility rates into crude birth rates, and any anomalies in the age/sex distribution will affect the crude birth rates. The assessment of the household age distribution (see annex, table 23) should therefore be kept in mind when interpreting crude birth rates.

[8] All those ever married are included in the calculations regardless of their union status at the time of the survey. The definition used in this chapter differs from that in chapter III, on marital status, in that in this chapter, exposure is counted from the first union whereas in chapter III only exposure within unions is included in the denominator.

[9] Estimates of trends for all 38 countries are given in United Nations (forthcoming).

[10] Total fertility rates were computed for the ages from 15 to 44 years only, because birth history information is available only up to 44 years for the period 5-9 years prior to the survey. For the period 10-14 years prior to the survey, information is available only up to age group 35-39. For this period, in computing the total fertility rates, the rate for age group 40-44 was assumed to be the same as that in the period 5-9 years prior to the survey.

[11] The definition used by the World Health Organization (1975) is inability to conceive within two years.

[12] In medical terminology, primary infertility is defined as never having conceived and secondary infertility as not being able to conceive after one or more conceptions have occurred earlier in a woman's life.

REFERENCES

Chidambaram, V. C. and Zeba A. Sathar (1984). *Age and Date Reporting*. World Fertility Survey Comparative Studies, No. 5; Cross-National Summaries. Voorburg, The Netherlands: International Statistical Institute.

Coale, Ansley J., Barbara A. Anderson and Erna Härm (1979). *Human Fertility in Russia since the Nineteenth Century*. Princeton, New Jersey: Princeton University Press.

Collver, O. Andrew (1965). *Birth Rates in Latin America: New Estimates of Historical Trends and Fluctuations*. Institute of International Studies Research Series, No. 7. Berkeley: University of California.

Costa Rica (1978). Dirección General de Estadística y Censos. *Encuesta Nacional de Fecundidad de 1976*. San José.

Donaldson, Peter J. and Douglas J. Nichols (1978). The changing tempo of fertility in Korea. *Population Studies* 32(2):231-249. The data in this article refer to the Republic of Korea.

Goldman, Noreen and John Hobcraft (1982). *Birth Histories*. World Fertility Survey Comparative Studies, No. 17: Cross-National Summaries. Voorburg, The Netherlands, International Statistical Institute.

Hanenberg, Robert (1980). *Current Fertility*. World Fertility Survey Comparative Studies, No. 11: Cross-National Summaries. Voorburg, The Netherlands: International Statistical Institute.

Hill, G. (1979). Levels and trends of fertility and mortality in Kuwait. In Kornel Abu Jabar, ed., *Levels and Trends of Fertility and Mortality in Selected Arab Countries of West Asia*. Amman: Population Studies Programme of the University of Jordan, 75-81.

Hobcraft, J. N., Noreen Goldman and V. C. Chidambaram (1982). Advances in the P/F ratio method for analysis of birth histories. *Population Studies* 36(2):291-316.

Knodel, J. (1977). Family limitation and the fertility transition: evidence from the age pattern of fertility in Europe and Asia. *Population Studies* 31(2):219-249.

Little, Roderick J. A. (1982). *Sampling Errors of Fertility Rates from the WFS*. World Fertility Survey Technical Bulletin, No. 10. Voorburg, The Netherlands: International Statistical Institute.

Poston, Dudley L., Jr. and others (1982). *Estimating Voluntary and Involuntary Childlessness in the Developing Countries of the World*. Texas Population Research Center Papers, Series 4, paper No. 4.003. Austin, Texas: University of Texas.

Rutstein, Shea (1984). An assessment of the quality of WFS data for direct estimate of childhood mortality. Paper submitted to the World Fertility Survey Symposium, London, 24-27 April 1984.

Santow, G. and A. Bioumla (1983). An Evaluation of the Cameroon Fertility Survey, 1976. World Fertility Survey Technical Papers, Tech. 2173. Voorburg, The Netherlands, International Statistical Institute.

Scott, Chris and V. C. Chidambaram (1985). World Fertility Survey: origins and achievements. In John Cleland and John Hobcraft, eds., in collaboration with Betzy Dinesen, *Reproductive Change in Developing Countries: Insights from the World Fertility Survey*. Oxford: Oxford University Press, 7-26.

Senderowitz, Judith and John M. Paxman (1985). *Adolescent Fertility: Worldwide Concerns*, Population Bulletin, vol. 40, No. 2. Washington, D.C.: Population Reference Bureau.

Singh, Susheela (1984). *Comparability of Questionnaires: Forty-one WFS Countries*. World Fertility Survey Comparative Studies, No. 32; Cross-National Summaries. Voorburg, The Netherlands: International Statistical Institute.

_____(1984a). Birth histories: levels and trends in fertility in 41 WFS countries. Additional tables for World Fertility Survey Comparative Studies; Cross-National Summaries. Voorburg, The Netherlands, International Statistical Institute, unpublished.

_____J. B. Casterline and J. G. Cleland (1985). The proximate determinants of fertility: Sub-national variations, *Population Studies* 39(1):113-135.

Srinivasan, K., P. H. Reddy and K. N. M. Raju (1978). From one generation to the next: changes in fertility, family size preferences and family planning in an Indian state between 1951 and 1975. *Studies in Family Planning* 9(10/11):258-271.

United Nations (1979). Department of International Economic and Social Affairs, Statistical Office. *Demographic Yearbook—Special Issue: Historical Supplement*. New York.
Sales No. E/F.79.XIII.8.

_____(1982). Department of International Economic and Social Affairs. Population Division. *The Impact of Population Structure on Crude Fertility Measures: A Comparative Analysis of World Fertility Survey Results for Twenty-One Developing Countries*. Non-sales publication ST/ESA/SER.R/49. New York.

_____(1983). *Fertility Levels and Trends as Assessed from Twenty World Fertility Surveys*. Non-sales publication ST/ESA/SER.R/50. New York.

_____(1983a). *Manual X. Indirect Techniques for Demographic Estimation*. Population Studies, No. 81. New York.
Sales No. E.83.XIII.2.

_____(1985). Levels and trends in fertility: selected findings from the World Fertility Survey data. Working paper IESA/P/WP.91. New York.

_____(1985a). *World Population Prospects: Estimates and Projections as Assessed in 1982*. Population Studies, No. 86. New York.
Sales No. E.83.XIII.5.

_____(1986). *A Comparative Evaluation of Data Quality in Thirty-eight World Fertility Surveys*. Non-sales publication ST/ESA/SER.R/50/Rev.1. New York.

Vaessen, Martin (1984). *Childlessness and Infecundity*. World Fertility Survey Comparative Studies, No. 31; Cross-National Summaries. Voorburg, The Netherlands: International Statistical Institute.

Verma, Vijay (1980). *Basic Fertility Measures from Retrospective Birth Histories*. World Fertility Survey Technical Bulletins, No. 4. Voorburg, The Netherlands: International Statistical Institute.

_____(1985). WFS survey methods. In John Cleland and John Hobcraft, eds., in collaboration with Betzy Dinesen, *Reproductive Change in Developing Countries: Insights from the World Fertility Survey*. Oxford: Oxford University Press, 27-44.

Vielma, Gilberto (1982). *Evaluation of the Venezuela Fertility Survey 1977*. World Fertility Survey Scientific Reports, No. 35. Voorburg, The Netherlands: International Statistical Institute.

World Health Organization, (1975). Scientific Group on the Epidemiology of Infertility. *The Epidemiology of Infertility*. Technical Report Series, No. 582. Geneva.

Annex

COMPARATIVE ASSESSMENT OF DATA QUALITY

TECHNICAL INTRODUCTION

This technical introduction is intended as a detailed guide to tables 23-28, which present material used to assess the quality of the World Fertility Survey (WFS) fertility estimates. For each table, there is a detailed explanation of the rationale behind the measures and comparisons selected to be applied in every country. For each of the 38 countries, a more detailed discussion of these measures is presented elsewhere in the form of country chapters (United Nations, forthcoming).

Age data: table 23

Two general indices of the overall quality of age reporting were chosen: (a) the percentage of respondents who supplied a month and calendar year for their date of birth from the individual interview (column (1)); and (b) Myers' index of digital preference based on the single-year age distribution from the household survey (column (2)). The first statistic measures the degree to which women have accurate knowledge of calendar dates in the past and the second measures the degree of heaping on preferred digits. It can be interpreted as an estimate of the minimum proportion of persons in the population for whom an age with an incorrect final digit is reported (Shryock, Siegel and others). Although the household age distribution is not always used directly in estimation of age-specific fertility rates,[a] it can be used as an index of data quality if it is assumed that the relative ranking of countries with respect to the degree of digit preference in the household schedule is similar to their ranking in the individual schedule.

The household age distribution of females was examined carefully for evidence of possible shifting of women out of the eligible ages and also for evidence of possible overrepresentation of certain age groups within the eligible (that is, reproductive) age range. Measures of the existence and extent of possible shifting and overrepresentation of the eligible age groups are presented in columns (3)-(6).

TABLE 23. INDICATORS OF THE QUALITY OF WORLD FERTILITY SURVEY AGE DATA

Region and country	Month and year reported by women interviewed (percentage) (1)	Myers' index household data estimates for females ranging from 0 to 90 years (2)	Shifting-out of eligible ages To younger[a] (3)	To older[b] (4)	Eligible age groups overrepresented (5)	Extent of overrepresentation[c] (6)	Overall quality (7)
Africa							
Benin	9	17.5	d	Some	20-24, 25-29	A lot, a lot	C
Cameroon	28	15.4	d	A lot	30-34, 40-44	Some, a lot	C
Côte d'Ivoire[e]	20	7.1	d	A lot	20-24, 40-44	Some, some	C
Egypt	26	17.5	d	d	d	d	B
Ghana	52	16.7	d	A lot	d	d	B
Kenya	34	7.6	Some	d	25-29, 35-39	A lot, some	C
Lesotho	72	6.2	d	d	40-44	A lot	B
Mauritania	4	25.5	d	A lot	d	d	C
Morocco	22	17.8	d	Some	d	d	B
Senegal	38	3.7	d	Some	30-34[f]	Some	B
Sudan	22	28.5	d	d	25-29, 35-39, 45-49	A lot, a lot, A lot	C
Tunisia	88	6.8	d	A lot	d	d	A
Latin America and the Caribbean							
Colombia	97	5.7	d	d	35-39	A lot	B
Costa Rica	..	2.8	Some[g]	Some	d	d	A
Dominican Republic	86	8.5	d	d	35-39	A lot	B
Ecuador	100	6.0	d	Some	d	d	A
Guyana	98[h]	4.8[i]	..	..	d	d	A
Haiti	92	9.9	d	A lot	30-34[f], 20-24, 40-44[f, j]	Some, some, some	B
Jamaica	95	4.7	d	A lot	d	d	A
Mexico	95	6.6	d	d	35-39	A lot	B
Panama	99	3.7	Some[g]	A lot	30-34	Some	A
Paraguay	100	..	d	Some	35-39	Some	A
Peru	95	6.5	d	d	35-39	Some	B
Trinidad and Tobago	98	2.1	d	A lot	15-19, 25-29[f], 40-44[j]	Some, a lot, a lot	B
Venezuela	..	4.7	d	Some[k]	35-39	Some	A
Asia and Oceania							
Bangladesh	1	7.8	Some	d	25-29, 45-49	Some, some	C
Fiji	68	5.1	d	A lot	d	d	B
Indonesia	22	11.6	d	A lot	35-39	Some	C
Jordan	30	24.3	d	Some	35-39	Some	C
Malaysia	57	8.5	d	d	d	d	B
Nepal	13	16.3	Some	A lot	20-29, 40-44	Some, a lot	C
Pakistan	7	12.1	d	d	25-34, 40-44	Some, a lot	C
Philippines	97	2.4	d	Some	35-39	Some	A
Republic of Korea	100	1.9	d	d	d	d	A
Sri Lanka	67	8.8	d	d	35-39, 45-49	Some, a lot	B
Syrian Arab Republic	57	9.2	d	A lot	20-24[f], 25-29[f], 30-34[f, j]	Some, a lot, some	B

38

TABLE 23 (continued)

Region and country	Month and year reported by women interviewed (percentage) (1)	Myers' index household data estimates for females ranging from 0 to 90 years (2)	Shifting-out of eligible ages To younger[a] (3)	Shifting-out of eligible ages To older[b] (4)	Eligible age groups overrepresented (5)	Extent of overrepresentation[c] (6)	Overall quality (7)
Thailand	85	2.5	d	d	d	d	A
Yemen	0	41.8	d	A lot	25-29	A lot	C

Sources: Table 13 and country chapters in United Nations (forthcoming); for column (1), Chidambaram and Sathar (1984), except for Colombia and Mexico; for column (2), Myers' index from Rutstein (1984).

NOTE: Age data assessed as: A = good quality; B = acceptable quality; C = less reliable.

[a] If $2P_{15-19}/(P_{10-14} + P_{20-24})$ is less than 0.90 and greater than 0.75, "Some" evidence of shifting to younger ages is said to exist. If the ratio is less than 0.75, then "A lot" of shifting to younger ages is said to exist.

[b] If $2P_{50-54}/(P_{45-49} + P_{55-59})$ is greater than 1.10 and less than 1.30, then "Some" evidence of shifting to older ages is said to exist. If the ratio is greater than 1.30 then "A lot" of shifting to older ages is said to exist.

[c] If the ratio of two times the overrepresented age group to the sum of the adjacent age groups is greater than 1.05 and less than 1.15 "Some" overrepresentation is said to exist. If the ratio is greater than 1.15, "A lot" of overrepresentation is said to exist. A stricter criteria than for [a] and [b] is used as these age groups are within childbearing ages and therefore a greater impact on fertility rates is expected.

[d] The characteristic referred to does not exist to a significant degree according to the criteria mentioned above.

[e] Formerly called the Ivory Coast.

[f] Underrepresented.

[g] Ages 15-19.

[h] Women in the individual questionnaire only.

[i] Based on ages 20-49.

[j] Migration distorts the age distribution.

[k] The oldest eligible age group was 40-44 years.

An assumption of linearity is made in the criteria used to measure shifting and overrepresentation of age groups. For example, to measure the degree of overrepresentation of an age group within the eligible age range, the ratio of two times the overrepresented age group to the sum of the adjacent age groups is examined. If this ratio is greater than 1.05 and less than 1.15 then "some" overrepresentation is said to exist. If the ratio is greater than 1.15 then "a lot" of overrepresentation is said to exist. In each of the detailed country chapters (United Nations, forthcoming), the female age distribution by five-year age groups is compared to the male age distribution and the female age distribution from a recent external source. Any country peculiarities were noted and taken into account in making the quality assessments.

Marriage history data: table 24

Again, the percentage of first unions reported with a month and year was used as a crude index of the quality of date reporting (column (1)). An index measuring the degree of annual fluctuation in marital duration provides one summary measure of the quality of marriage-date reporting (column (2)). This index is based on the annual marital duration distribution for the period 0-14 years prior to the survey. It is similar in concept to the age-ratio score and is derived from the ratio of the actual number of marriages in the period x years from the survey to the average number of marriages in the period $x - 1$, x and $x + 1$ years prior to the survey. The index is the average over 15 years of the absolute deviation of the ratio from one.

TABLE 24. INDICATORS OF THE QUALITY OF WORLD FERTILITY SURVEY MARITAL HISTORY DATA
(*Period 0-14 years prior to the survey*)

Region and country	Percentage of first unions reported by month and year (1)	Duration index[a] (2)	Deficit of unions 0-4 years prior to survey[b] (3)	Cohort proportion overestimated[c] (4)	Age group for which trend inconsistent with external sources (5)	Overall quality rating (6)
Africa						
Benin	5	0.169	d	(25-29) (35-39)[e]	..	C
Cameroon	21	0.103	d	d	..	C
Côte d'Ivoire[f]	12	0.075	d	(25-29)[g] (35-39)	(15-29)	C
Egypt	37	0.076	d	(25-29)[g]	d	B
Ghana	40	0.071	d	(20-24) (35-39)	..	C
Kenya	69	0.102	d	(30-34)	d	B
Lesotho	88	0.080	d	d	(15-19)	A
Mauritania	7	0.105	Yes	(25-29) (35-39)	(15-29)	C
Morocco	35	0.071	d	(35-39)	d	B
Senegal	69	0.119	d	(30-34)	(15-29)	C
Sudan	41	0.146	Yes	(35-39)	..	C
Tunisia	53	0.086[h]	d	d	d	A
Latin America and the Caribbean						
Colombia	97[i]	0.060	d	(30-34)	(15-19)	B
Costa Rica	..	0.060	j	(30-34)	(15-29)	B
Dominican Republic	73	0.142	d	(35-39)	(15-19)	C
Ecuador	67	0.078	d	(25-29)[g]	(15-29)	B
Guyana	79[k]	0.153	d	(30-34)	d	C
Haiti	93	0.105	Yes	d	..	C
Jamaica	53[k]	0.163	Yes	d	d	C
Mexico	94	0.077	d	(40-44)	(15-19)	A
Panama	100	0.114	j	d	(15-24)	B
Paraguay	98	0.125	d	(40-44)	(15-29)	B
Peru	81	0.109	Yes	(40-44)	(15-29)	C

TABLE 24 (continued)

Region and country	Percentage of first unions reported by month and year (1)	Distribution by years since first union		Trend in proportions ever married		Overall quality rating (6)
		Duration index[a] (2)	Deficit of unions 0-4 years prior to survey[b] (3)	Cohort proportion overestimated[c] (4)	Age group for which trend inconsistent with external sources (5)	
Trinidad and Tobago	100	0.094	Yes	d	..	B
Venezuela	..	0.099	d	(35-39)	(25-29)	B
Asia and Oceania						
Bangladesh	11[k]	0.080	d	d	(15-19)	C
Fiji	85	0.064	d	d	(15-24)	A
Indonesia	46[k]	0.048	d	d	(15-19)	C
Jordan	58[k]	0.101	d	(35-39)	(15-29)	C
Malaysia	62	0.064	d	d	d	A
Nepal	27	0.169	Yes	d	(15-24)	C
Pakistan	73	0.117	d	d	(15-24)	C
Philippines	96	0.084	Yes	(40-44)	(20-29)	B
Republic of Korea	100	0.077	d	d	d	A
Sri Lanka	70	0.094	d	d	(15-24)	B
Syrian Arab Republic	79	0.062	d	(30-34)	(15-19)	B
Thailand	75	0.102	d	(40-44)	(15-29)	B
Yemen	8	0.140	d	(25-29)[g]	(30-34)[e]	..	C

Sources: Table 14 and figures 3 and 4 of country chapters in United Nations (forthcoming); for column (1), Chidambaram and Sathar (1984).

NOTES: Marriage data assessed as: A = good quality; B = acceptable quality; C = less reliable.

[a] This index is based on the period 0-14 years prior to the survey and is designed to measure fluctuations in annual rates. The index is similar in concept to the age ratio score and is derived from the ratio of the actual number of marriages in year x to the average number of marriages in year $x - 1$, x and $x + 1$. The index is the average over 15 years of the absolute deviations of the ratio from one.

[b] There was considered to be a deficit of unions reported in the recent period if the number of marriages taking place 0-4 years prior to the survey was less than or equal to the number occurring 5-9 years before the survey.

[c] The cohort named in this column showed a proportion married at each age (see United Nations, forthcoming, figure 4 in each country chapter) which was too high in relationship to the observed trend for that age.

[d] The characteristic referred to does not exist to a significant degree.
[e] Excess in most recent period among all cohorts.
[f] Formerly called the Ivory Coast.
[g] Underestimated.
[h] Fluctuations in Tunisia caused by changes in marriage laws.
[i] Based on current marriages. The percentage reporting month and year of former marriage was 80 per cent for Costa Rica.
[j] The deficit observed in the case of Costa Rica and Panama can be explained by the fact that only women aged 20 years and older were eligible for interview.
[k] Some responses were given in the form of age at union: Guyana, 15 per cent; Jamaica, 47 per cent; Bangladesh, 67 per cent; Indonesia, 41 per cent; Jordan, 21 per cent.

Possible backdating of recent unions was checked by comparing the numbers of unions taking place 0-4 years prior to the survey with those 5-9 years before the survey (column (3)). If the number of marriages during the period 0-4 years was less than or equal to the number of occurring during the period 5-9 years prior to the survey, then under-reporting of unions in the recent period is considered to have occurred.

Information on trends in proportions ever married at five-year intervals before the survey, as implied by the WFS data, was compared with other census or survey information for dates in the past. Systematic misreporting of age, resulting in the overrepresentation of one age group in the eligible age range, sometimes has the effect of distorting the trend in proportions married by age with the distortion occurring further back in time the younger the age group for which trends are being measured (column (4)). This can easily be detected by examining trends in proportions married by age group as reconstructed from the WFS marriage history. A figure of these trends is presented for each country in another United Nations study (forthcoming) and is not shown here. In addition, any discrepancies in trends between the World Fertility Survey and other sources are noted (column (5)). Trends in the WFS data may be distorted due to either the omission of early unions or the misdating of first unions; but, on the other hand, trends in proportions ever married from the census data may be affected by changes in the quality of age misreporting over time as well as, in the case of Latin America and the Caribbean, changing definitions of consensual unions. Thus, the possible conclusions to be drawn from this comparison of trends in proportions ever married depend very much upon the country context and the quality of other data sources.

Recent birth history data: table 25

As before, the first index of the quality of birth reporting is the percentage of all live births recorded that were reported with a month and a year (column (1)). The relative completeness of birth enumeration from WFS was evaluated by comparing parity at the time of the survey with parity from a recent census or survey (columns (2)-(4)). If the most recent external data for comparison do not fall within three years of the WFS data, then the WFS parity is estimated for the date for which the external data are available. It was not possible to measure parity on a comparable basis (that is, per woman or per ever-married woman) for all countries but the comparisons are always consistent within countries.

Age-specific fertility rates from vital registration or from other sources if registration is not complete, for dates within the 0-4 years prior to the WFS date are compared with rates obtained from WFS. Total fertility rates from this comparison are presented in columns (5)-(9). For purposes of comparison, the WFS data are always based on an average of a minimum of three calendar years (because of sampling errors) and whenever possible are centred on the same dates as the outside data sources chosen for comparison.

In order to assess the possibility of a deficit in births from one to two years preceding the survey, which, if serious enough, could indicate a displacement of births out of the most recent period (0-4 years prior to the survey), the ratio of the sum of the number of births in years 1-2 before the survey to the sum of the number of births in years 0 and 3 before the survey (column (10)). If this ratio was less than 0.90, the deficit is considered to be "a lot"; and if it is less than 0.95 and greater than or equal to 0.90, then there is "some" deficit of births. In cases that fall into the category, "a lot", backward shifting of births from 0-4 to 5-9 years prior to the survey is strongly suspected.

An index measuring the degree of annual fluctuations in fertility rates in the period 0-4 years before the survey was computed. Fluctuations in annual age-specific rates are examined for each age group in the country chapters of the forthcoming United Nations publication, but the

TABLE 25. OVERALL QUALITY OF ENUMERATION OF RECENT BIRTHS FROM THE WORLD FERTILITY SURVEY
(Period 0-4 years prior to the survey)

Region and country	Percentage of live births reported by month and year (1)	Parity comparison Year of WFS (2)	Parity comparison Other source date (3)	WFS higher than other source for age groups (4)	WFS Date (5)	WFS Level (6)	Other source Date (7)	Other source Type of data[a] (8)	Other source Level (9)	Deficit in births in years 1-2 before survey[a] (10)	Index of irregularity in recent annual average fertility rates[b] (11)	Overall quality (12)
Africa												
Benin	12[c]	...	...	...	...	...	...	...	...	A lot	0.038	C
Cameroon	41	...	...	...	1975-1977	6.4	1976	C	6.0	[d]	0.012	B
Côte d'Ivoire[e]	28[c]	1980/81	1978/79	35-49	1977-1979	7.5	1978-1979	S	6.8	A lot	0.054	C
Egypt	41[c]	1976	1976	15-49	1975-1977	5.5	1975-1977	BR	5.4	A lot	0.035	B
Ghana	64[c]	1970	1970	Lower	...	...	...	...	...	A lot	0.045	C
Kenya	75[c]	1977/78	1977	35-49	1976-1978	8.0	1977/78	S	8.1	Some	0.016	B
Lesotho	90	1977	1976	15-49	1975-1977	5.9	1976	C	5.9	[d]	0.065	B
Mauritania	12[c]	...	...	...	1975-1977	6.9	1976	C	6.6	A lot	0.067	C
Morocco	60[c]	1972/73	1972/73	15-39	...	...	...	...	...	[d]	0.023	B
Senegal	99[c]	...	...	...	...	...	...	...	...	Some	0.054	C
Sudan	63[c]	1973	1973	15-44	1972-1974	6.8	1973	C	5.3	A lot	0.054	C
Tunisia	70	1978	1975	Lower	1974-1978	5.9	1974-1978	BR	5.6	[d]	0.025	A
Latin America and the Caribbean												
Colombia	91	1976	1973	40-49[f]	1970-1974	4.9	1972-1973	C	4.4	[d]	0.035	A
Costa Rica	...	1976	1973	Lower	1970-1974	4.3	1970-1974	BR	4.3	[d]	0.018	A
Dominican Republic	91	1975	1970	35-49	1971-1975	5.7	...	...	...[g]	Some	0.025	B
Ecuador	78	1974	1974	25-44	1976-1979	5.3	1976-1979	S	5.7	[d]	0.026	B
Guyana	91	1975	1970	40-49	1970-1974	5.1	1970-1974	BR	4.5	Some	0.029	A
Haiti	94[c]	1971	1971	30-34	1972-1974	5.5	1973	S	5.1	[d]	0.025	B
Jamaica	91	1975-1976	1970	35-49	1971-1975	5.0	...	[h]	...	Some	0.037	A
Mexico	99	1976	1970	35-49	1971-1972	6.5	1971-1972	BR	6.3	[d]	0.010	A
Panama	98	1975/76	1971	40-49	1971-1975	4.5	1971-1975	BR	4.6	Some	0.064	B
Paraguay	100	1979	1977	20-24	1975-1978	4.9	1976-1977	S	4.7	Some	0.033	B
Peru	93	1975/76	1975/76	35-49	1974-1976	5.5	1975	S	5.3	[d]	0.014	A
Trinidad and Tobago	94	1970	1970	15-44	1972-1976	3.4	1972-1976	BR	3.3	Some	0.025	B
Venezuela	...	1977	1981	25-44	1972-1976	4.7	1972-1976	BR	5.0	Some	0.024	B
Asia and Oceania												
Bangladesh	12	1975	1974	15-49	1971-1975	6.3	1974	S	7.2	A lot[i]	0.031	C
Fiji	86	1974	1976	20-49	1970-1974	4.1	1970-1974	BR	3.6	[d]	0.036	A
Indonesia	46[c]	1976	1976	Lower	1971-1975	4.7	1971-1975	S	4.9	A lot	0.042	C
Jordan	66	1976	1972	40-49	1971-1976	7.8	1972-1976	S	7.8[j]	[d]	0.036	B
Malaysia	86[c]	1974	1970	40-49	1970-1974	4.7	1970-1974	BR	4.5	[d]	0.013	A
Nepal	...[k]	1976	1971	20-49	1971-1974	6.0	1974-1976	S	6.3[l]	[d]	0.036	B
Pakistan	80	1975	1971	20-49	1971-1975	6.2	...	...	...	A lot	0.040	C
Philippines	96	1975	1975	20-49	1974-1978	5.1	...	C	...	[d]	0.022	A
Republic of Korea	100[c]	1974	1975	30-49	1972-1974	4.0	1972-1974	BR	3.9	[d]	0.014	C
Sri Lanka	73	1975	1971	40-49	1972-1974	3.6	1972-1974	BR	3.7	Some	0.034	B
Syria	83[c]	1978	1976	20-34	1975-1977	7.4	1977-1978	S	7.4	[m]	0.006	A

TABLE 25 (continued)

	Percentage of live births reported by month and year (1)	Parity comparison			Recent fertility (total fertility rate) comparison						Deficit in births in years 1-2 before survey[a] (10)	Index of irregularity in recent annual average fertility rates[b] (11)	Overall quality (12)
		Year of WFS (2)	Other source date (3)	WFS higher than other source for age groups (4)	WFS		Other source						
Region and country					Date (5)	Level (6)	Date (7)	Type of data[a] (8)	Level (9)				
Thailand	84	1975	1970	45-49	1970-1974	4.8	1970-1974	S	4.9		A lot	0.032	B
Yemen	11[c]	1979	1981	45-49	1976-1978	8.1	1981	S	7.9		A lot	0.041	C

Sources: Table 15 and country chapters in United Nations (forthcoming); for column (1), Chidambaram and Sathar (1984).

NOTES: Recent birth data assessed as: A = good quality; B = acceptable quality; C = less reliable.

WFS = World Fertility Survey.

For type of data: S = estimated from result of survey; BR = based on birth registration data; C = estimated from population census data.

[a] Deficit in births in years 1-2 before the survey is measured as "A lot" if $(P_1 + P_2)/(P_0 + P_1)$ is less than 0.90 and "Some" if this ratio is less than 0.95 and greater than or equal to 0.90. In cases coded "A lot", backward shifting of births from 0-4 to 5-9 years before the survey is strongly suspected.

[b] This index is based on the average fertility rate. P_i (defined as births to women of all ages divided by total exposure) for the period 0-4 years prior to the survey. The index is defined as the average absolute deviation from 1.0 of the ratio of average fertility rate to a three-year moving average centred on the rate:

$$\frac{1}{4} \sum_{i=1}^{4} \left| 1 - 3P_i / (P_{i-1} + P_i + P_{i+1}) \right|$$

[c] Used event chart.
[d] Index greater than 0.95.
[e] Formerly called the Ivory Coast.
[f] However, parity at ages 45-49 is shown to be higher in the 1978 Contraceptive Prevalence Survey.
[g] Cohort-period rates from a subsequent survey in 1980 allowed a comparison of recent rates in the country chapter.
[h] Registered vital statistics have not been published since 1964.
[i] Although the index of Bangladesh is greater than 0.95, backdating of births from 0-4 to 5-9 years before the survey is strongly suspected, as shown in the country chapter in United Nations (forthcoming).
[j] This is not really an independent estimate, because it is based on the parity changes between the 1972 survey and World Fertility Survey, to permit a comparison with the period 0-4 years prior to the survey.
[k] The birth history automatically imputes only calendar year for all births.
[l] An average of estimates from 1974/75 survey and the 1976 survey.
[m] There is a deficit for the period 4-5 years prior to the survey.

42

index given in column (11) of table 25 is based on the average annual fertility rate, which is total births in each year divided by total woman-years of exposure. This index is a useful tool for detecting any evidence of digit or year preferences or other evidence of irregular patterns. It is computed by taking the average absolute deviation from 1.0 of the ratio of the average fertility rate to a three-year moving average centred on the rate.

Quality of recent rates: table 26

The ratings on the quality of recent births, age distribution and current marital status distribution are combined in table 26 for a rating on the overall quality of recent age-specific fertility rates (column (3)) and recent marital age-specific rates (column (5)).

TABLE 26. OVERALL QUALITY OF RECENT AGE-SPECIFIC FERTILITY RATES AND RECENT MARITAL AGE-SPECIFIC FERTILITY RATES

Region and country	Quality of recent births (1)	Quality of age distribution (2)	Quality of recent age-specific rates (3)	Quality of marital history [a] (4)	Quality of recent marital age-specific rates (5)
Africa					
Benin	C	C	C	C	C
Cameroon	B	C	B	C	B
Côte d'Ivoire [b]	C	C	C	C	C
Egypt	B	B	B	B	B
Ghana	C	B	C	C	C
Kenya	B	C	B	B	B
Lesotho	B	B	B	A	B
Mauritania	C	C	C	C	C
Morocco	B	B	B	B	B
Senegal	C	B	C	C	C
Sudan	C	C	C	C	C
Tunisia	A	A	A	A	A
Latin America and the Caribbean					
Colombia	A	B	A	B	A
Costa Rica	A	A	A	B	A
Dominican Republic	B	B	B	C	B
Ecuador	B	A	B	B	B
Guyana	A	A	A	C	B [c]
Haiti	B	B	B	C	B
Jamaica	A	A	A	C	B [c]
Mexico	A	B	A	A	A
Panama	B	A	B	B	B
Paraguay	B	A	B	B	B
Peru	A	B	A	C	B [c]
Trinidad and Tobago	A	B	A	B	A
Venezuela	B	A	B	B	B
Asia and Oceania					
Bangladesh	C	C	C	C	C
Fiji	A	B	A	A	A
Indonesia	C	C	C	C	C
Jordan	B	C	B	C	B
Malaysia	A	B	A	A	A
Nepal	B	C	C [d]	C	C
Pakistan	C	C	C	C	C
Philippines	A	A	A	B	B [c]
Republic of Korea	A	A	A	A	A
Sri Lanka	B	B	B	B	B
Syrian Arab Republic	A	B	A	B	A
Thailand	B	A	B	B	B
Yemen	C	C	C	C	C

Source: United Nations (forthcoming), table 8.
NOTES: Rates assessed as: A = good quality; B = acceptable quality; C = less reliable.
[a] Current marital status consistent except for Pakistan, age group 15-19; and Thailand, age group 15-24.
[b] Formerly called the Ivory Coast.
[c] Change from column (4).
[d] Change from column (1).

Trends in births: table 27

An index that measures the extent of annual fluctuations in average fertility rates over the 14-year period prior to the survey is presented in column (2) of table 27. This index is similar to the one in column (11) of table 25 but covers the period 0-14 years prior to the survey.

The possibility of omissions of births among older women was examined by looking at cumulative cohort-period fertility rates among the 40-44 and 45-49 cohorts; first, at the time of the survey (column (3)), then at ages 40-44 for both cohorts (column (4)). If cumulative fertility of the 45-49 cohort is less than that of the 40-44 cohort at the time of the survey and/or ages 40-44, then evidence of omission of births is said to be present.

Cohort fertility profiles were examined for evidence of shifting of dates of births forward from the distant past. The effect of this type of misstatement of birth dates can be seen in the cohort fertility profiles.

TABLE 27. OVERALL QUALITY OF TRENDS IN BIRTHS FROM THE WORLD FERTILITY SURVEY
(From 0-4 to 10-14 years prior to the survey)

			Omissions			Recent trend comparison (total fertility rate)							
			P40-44 more than P45-49			World Fertility Survey		Other source					Overall quality trends (from 0-4 to 10-14 years) (12)
Region and country	Quality of birth data[a] (0-4 years) (1)	Index of irregularity in average fertility rate[a] (2)	At survey (3)	At age 40-44[b] (4)	Displacement in age profile of cohort fertility[c] (5)	Dates (6)	Percentage change (7)	Dates (8)	Percentage change (9)	Type of data (10)	Trends consistent by age of mother[d] (11)	
Africa													
Benin	C	0.053	e	Yes	A lot	67/71-77/81	+1	...	...	...	...	C
Cameroon	B	0.024	Yes	Yes	e	64/68-74/78	-5	...	...	...	...	B
Côte d'Ivoire[f]	C	0.030	e	Yes	Some	66/70-76/80	-1	...	...	...	...	C
Egypt	B	0.047	e	e	e	65/67-75/77	-26	66-75/77	-13	S/BR	e	C
Ghana	C	0.043	e	e	e	65/69-75/79	-6	...	...	...	...	C
Kenya	A	0.035	e	Yes	A lot	68/70-76/78	-11	69-77/78	+7	C/S	e	C
Lesotho	B	0.056	e	Yes	e	71/73-75/77	+7	71/73-76	+4	S/C	e	C
Mauritania	C	0.047	e	Yes	A lot	67/71-77/81	-4	...	...	...	...	C
Morocco	B	0.027	Same	e	e	61/63-71/73	-7	61/63-72	0	S/S	e	B
Senegal	C	0.039	e	e	A lot	64/68-74/78	-4	...	...	...	...	C
Sudan	C	0.037	e	Yes	A lot	64/68-74/78	-14	...	...	...	...	C
Tunisia	A	0.021	e	e	Some	65/67-74/78	-19	66-74/78	-21	BR	Yes	A
Latin America and the Caribbean													
Colombia	A	0.024	e	g	Some	66/69-71/74	-21	67/68-72/73	-27	S/C	e	A
Costa Rica	A	0.026	e	e	e	60/64-70/74	-39	60/64-70/74	-39	BR	Yes	A
Dominican Republic	B	0.021	e	Yes	A lot[h]	61/65-71/75	-24	...	...	...	e	C
Ecuador	B	0.020	e	e	Some	67/70-76/79	-22	67/70-76/79	-21	S/S	Yes[i]	B
Guyana	A	0.026	e	Same	Some	60/64-70/74	-23	60/64-70/74	-26	BR	Yes	B
Haiti	B	0.050	e	Yes	A lot	53/66-73/76	-12	...	...	...	...	C
Jamaica	A	0.032	e	Same	A lot	60/64-69/71	-8	60/64-70	-4	BR/C	e	B
Mexico	A	0.021	e	Yes	Some	66/70-74/76	-15	66/70-78	-18	BR/C	j	A
Panama	B	0.044	e	Same	e	59/61-71/75	-20	59/61-71/75	-14	BR	e	C
Paraguay	B	0.031	e	e	Some	65/69-75/79	-17	...	...	...	...	B
Peru	A	0.024	e	e	e	67/69-74/76	-18	67/68-75	-20	S	Yes	A
Trinidad and Tobago	A	0.034	e	e	e	62/66-72/76	-38	62/66-72/76	-30	BR	Yes	A
Venezuela	B	0.046	e	k	e	67/71-72/76	-19	67/71-72/76	-12	BR	Yes	B
Asia and Oceania													
Bangladesh	C	0.029	Yes	Yes	A lot	63/65-71/75	-21	63/65-74	+3	S	e	C
Fiji	A	0.023	e	e	Some	60/64-70/74	-38	60/64-70/74	-33	BR	Yes	A
Indonesia	C	0.064	Yes	Yes	A lot	67/70-71/76	-16	67/70-71/75	-6	S	e	C
Jordan	B	0.030	e	e	Some	60/62-71/76	-7	61-72/76	+5	C/S	e	C
Malaysia	A	0.020	e	Same	Some	66/69-70/74	-10	66/69-70/74	-10	BR	Yes	A
Nepal	B	0.038	e	Same	e	62/66-72/76	9	...	...	...	...	C
Pakistan	C	0.051	Yes	Yes	A lot	63/65-68/71	-1	63/65-68/71	-14	S	e	C
Philippines	A	0.017	e	Yes	Some	64/66-69/71	-2	63/67-60/72	-6	S	e	A
Republic of Korea	A	0.020	e	e	Some	59/61-72/74	-35	60-72/74	-35	C	e	A
Sri Lanka	B	0.026	e	e	Some	64/66-72/74	-27	65-72/74	-23	BR	e	B
Syrian Arab Republic	A	0.014	e	Same	Some	69/71-75/77	-5	70-77/78	-8	C/S	Yes	A
Thailand	B	0.031	e	e	e	60/64-70/74	-27	60/64-70/74	-25	C/S	Yes	B
Yemen	C	0.064	e	Yes	A lot	65/69-75/79	+12	...	...	...	...	C

44

Source: United Nations (forthcoming), table 9.

NOTES: Trend data assessed as: A = good quality; B = acceptable quality; C = less reliable.

For type of data: S = estimated from results of survey; BR = based on birth registration data; C = estimated from population census data.

For dates, 63/65-71/75, for example, indicates the period 1963-1965 – 1971-1975.

[a] This index is defined in the same manner as that for the period 0-4 years prior to the survey (table 25) but includes the period 0-14 years prior to the survey.

[b] P_{40-44} is the parity of the 40-44 cohort and P_{45-49}, the parity of the 45-49 cohort.

[c] "A lot" of displacement occurred if the age profile of cohort fertility (figure 5 of country chapters of United Nations (forthcoming)) became progressively older for the older cohorts, that is, the age group at which fertility peaks moved from younger to older age groups as the cohorts got older. "Some" displacement occurred if only the oldest cohort (45-49) showed an older pattern of fertility. The displacement in the age pattern indicates the extent to which forward-dating of births from the distant past occurred (the Potter type of effect).

[d] Trends by age are available in each country chapter in United Nations (forthcoming, table 3). Trends were rated as consistent and given a "yes" if all age groups showed similar trends or if all age groups but the 15-19 group showed similar trends.

[e] The characteristic referred to does not exist to a significant degree according to the criteria mentioned above.

[f] Formerly called the Ivory Coast.

[g] Comparisons with a 1978 Contraceptive Prevalence Survey suggest the possibility of some omissions among women aged 45-49.

[h] The 35-39 cohort shows unusually high fertility at ages 25 and 30, which somewhat masks the effect of displacement using the criteria given above.

[i] Not for age groups 15-19 and 25-29.

[j] Time periods are not the same.

[k] Parity compared is that of the 40-44 and 35-39 cohorts.

The older cohorts reported older age patterns of fertility in relation to the younger cohorts. Fertility profiles for the 30-34, 35-39, 40-44 and 45-49 cohorts were examined to see if there was a trend towards older pattern of childbearing from the younger to the older cohorts (column (5)). "A lot" of displacement occurred if the age profile of cohort fertility was older progressively from the younger to older cohorts. "Some" displacement occurred if only the oldest cohort (45-49) showed an older pattern of fertility.

Trends in total fertility from WFS data are compared with trends from outside sources where available (columns (6)-(11)). Unfortunately, the quality of rates from other sources is not always known so that inconsistency between two sources cannot be considered necessarily a sign that the data are of poor quality; in fact, the opposite may be true.

Overall quality of trends in fertility rates: table 28

The quality of trends in births (column (1)) and the age distribution (column (2)) were combined for a rating of the quality of overall trends in age-specific rates over a 15-year period. Trends in marital age-specific rates also were assessed, based on the rating of the quality of the marriage history (column (4)).

TABLE 28. OVERALL QUALITY OF 15-YEAR TRENDS IN AGE-SPECIFIC FERTILITY RATES AND MARITAL AGE-SPECIFIC FERTILITY RATES

Region and country	Quality of birth trends (1)	Quality of age distribution (2)	Quality of trends in age-specific rates (3)	Quality of marital history (4)	Quality of trends in marital age-specific rates (5)
Africa					
Benin	C	C	C	C	C
Cameroon	B	C	C[a]	C	C
Côte d'Ivoire[b]	C	C	C	C	C
Egypt	C	B	C	B	C
Ghana	C	B	C	C	C
Kenya	C	C	C	B	C
Lesotho	C	B	C	A	C
Mauritania	C	C	C	C	C
Morocco	B	B	B	B	B
Senegal	C	B	C	C	C
Sudan	C	C	C	C	C
Tunisia	A	A	A	A	A
Latin America and the Caribbean					
Colombia	A	B	A	B	B[c]
Costa Rica	A	A	A	B	B[c]
Dominican Republic	C	C	C	C	C
Ecuador	B	A	B	C	B
Guyana	B	A	B	C	C[c]
Haiti	C	B	C	C	C
Jamaica	B	A	B	C	C[c]
Mexico	A	B	A	A	A
Panama	C	A	C	B	C
Paraguay	B	A	B	B	B
Peru	A	B	A	C	C[c]
Trinidad and Tobago	A	B	B[a]	B	B
Venezuela	B	A	B	B	B
Asia and Oceania					
Bangladesh	C	C	C	C	C
Fiji	A	B	A	A	A
Indonesia	C	C	C	C	C
Jordan	C	C	C	C	C
Malaysia	A	B	A	A	A
Nepal	C	C	C	C	C
Pakistan	C	C	C	C	C
Philippines	A	A	A	B	B[c]
Republic of Korea	A	A	A	A	A
Sri Lanka	B	C	B	B	B
Syrian Arab Republic	A	B	B[a]	B	B
Thailand	B	A	B	B	B
Yemen	C	C	C	C	C

Source: United Nations (forthcoming), table 10.
NOTES: Rates assessed as: A = good quality; B = acceptable quality; C = less reliable.
[a] Change from column (1).
[b] Formerly called the Ivory Coast.
[c] Change from column (3).

Note

[a] The distribution according to age by marital status, however, does enter into the calculation of age-specific fertility rates for surveys that sampled ever-married women for the individual interview.

References

Chidambaram, V. C. and Zeba A. Sathar (1984). *Age and Date Reporting*. World Fertility Survey Comparative Studies, No. 5; Cross-National Summaries. Voorburg, The Netherlands: International Statistical Institute.

Rutstein, Shea (1984). An assessment of the quality of WFS data for direct estimate of childhood mortality. Paper submitted to the World Fertility Survey Symposium, London, 24-27 April 1984.

Shryock, Henry S., Jacob Siegel and others (1973). *The Methods and Materials of Demography*. Washington, D.C.: United States Department of Commerce, Bureau of the Census, vol. 1.

II. FERTILITY PREFERENCES

ABSTRACT

This chapter gives an overview of women's answers to questions about desired family size, current desire for more children and unwanted fertility. Problems of measurement are discussed. Differentials in preferences according to demographic characteristics, particularly family size and sex composition, are also examined.

The average number of children desired, according to a direct question, lies between three and five in most countries, but is from five to six in Western Asia and from six to nine in sub-Saharan Africa. Women in sub-Saharan Africa were also likely to give non-numerical answers to this question. An average of 11 per cent of married and fecund women in the sub-Saharan countries said they currently wanted no more children, as compared with 46-48 per cent in the rest of Africa and in Asia and Oceania, and 53 per cent in Latin America and the Caribbean. Very few women reported wanting no children or only one child, and in only two countries did over half the women with two children want no more. Among women with three children, however, over 50 per cent in nearly half the countries wanted to stop. Women generally preferred at least one child of each sex, but in most of Asia, and some countries elsewhere, a strong preference for sons coexists with a weaker desire for at least one daughter.

The data imply rather large declines in fertility in many countries if women were to avoid unwanted births, the projected decline depending upon the type of measure employed. Using a conservative criterion, "unwanted fertility" averaged 21 per cent of the total fertility rate in Latin America and the Caribbean and 16 per cent in Asia and Oceania, but only 8 per cent in Africa. Estimates of unwanted fertility are roughly 80 per cent higher using another measure.

Regardless of the preference indicator, regional (or cultural) differences in fertility preferences are more pronounced than those associated with development level. Indeed, development shows no relation to desired family size if sub-Saharan countries are considered separately. Other indicators do show that women in the more developed countries are more interested in limiting family size. Notably, "wanted fertility" (a different measure from desired family size) is relatively low in the upper development groups, but unwanted fertility is not—even though the level of contraceptive use is much higher than average in these countries. Reasons for this probably include high rates of childbearing in the past, which, coupled with relatively favourable mortality conditions, have left older women in the more economically advanced countries with large families; this elevates their levels of current exposure to the risk of unwanted fertility.

Preferences for the size of family or for the sex of child reflect the values attributed to children by both society and the individual. Such preferences indicate the demand for children. In theory, the concept of demand for children is intended to capture views on alternate family-building outcomes, abstracting from attitudes towards intercourse, abortion, contraception, breast-feeding and other fertility-related behaviour included in the family-building process (Lee and Bulatao, 1983). In empirical research, however, data on fertility preferences are derived from responses to sample survey questions in which such qualifications are rarely articulated and in which usually only one response is solicited.

Research has shown that family size preferences, as expressed in survey responses, can be strong predictors of future fertility levels, at least in the developed countries. Based on data for the United States of America obtained from a sample of urban women interviewed first in 1957 and again three years later, it was found that the strongest predictor of fertility at the second interview was the number of additional children desired at the initial interview (Westoff, Potter and Sagi, 1963). A similar result was obtained by Coombs (1974) in her study of the relation between family size preferences and subsequent fertility. Using data from a panel study conducted in a United States city from 1962 to 1965, Coombs (1974) found that women with preferences for large families subsequently had more pregnancies and births than those with preferences for smaller families.

Studies linking size preferences to subsequent fertility in developing countries are limited. On the basis of data from a longitudinal study in Taiwan, Province of China, it was found that, among women who said they wanted no more children in 1967, 14 per cent had a live birth within the next three years, compared with 75 per cent among those who wanted more (Freedman, Hermalin and Chang, 1975). Similar results for the period from 1973 to 1977 in Taiwan, Province of China, were obtained by Coombs (1979), using different measures of preferences. Rodgers (1976), using longitudinal data from Thailand, found a positive relationship between expressed desires for additional children in 1969 and subsequent fertility four years later. Without question, further longitudinal studies in other developing countries are necessary in order to examine whether these relationships are universal and to assess their strength.

It has generally been hypothesized that sex preferences (i.e., preferences for children of a particular sex or for a particular combination of sons and daughters) may influence family size as well. This may happen when women go on to have more children than they had originally desired in order to achieve their preferred family compositions. Empirical studies have found a relationship at the individual level between the sex composition of the family and subsequent childbearing. Studies based on United States data show that couples with both sons and daughters are less likely to have an additional child than those with all sons or all daughters (Williamson, 1976). Studies by Freedman and Takeshita (1969) and by Williamson (1976) found that strong son preference has resulted in higher prospective fertility in Taiwan, Province of China, while Coombs (1979) found, at the individual level, that women with a stronger son preference varied in their reproductive behaviour, depending upon their parity. In India, however, mixed results were obtained. Williamson (1976) reports that, in one study based on the National Sample Survey of 1961-1962, a larger proportion of couples of parity 2 had a third child within the following three years if both their children were girls than did couples with other sex compositions. On the other hand, Repetto (1972) found no evidence of this effect in his samples from India. Neither was this effect found in Bangladesh or Morocco (where son preferences are assumed to be strong). In her review of sex preference studies, Williamson (1976) concludes that even strong sex preferences cannot be expected to affect family size in the presence of one or more of the following conditions: high infant/child mortality; low use of contraception; and desire for large families.

Recently, attention in the literature has shifted to the question of the impact of preferences for the sex of children on the overall level of fertility. Based on a comparative analysis of fertility survey data from 27 countries, Arnold (1986) concludes that in most cases sex preference has only a weak effect on overall fertility rates. The reason for this is that simple laws of probability assure that the majority of families will achieve their desired sex distribution by chance and only a small percentage of families will be in the position of going on to a higher parity to achieve a desired sex distribution. Even in countries where strong son preference exists, estimated fertility effects were only moderate. Similar conclusions were also reached by Park (1986) and Feeney (1986) in the case of China. For this reason, although data on sex preferences are presented, the discussion of the fertility implications of preferences focuses on the more important effects of family size preferences.

Unwanted fertility is another topic of policy interest. Simple comparisons of the average level of desired and actual fertility underestimate the number of unwanted births, because the averages reflect a degree of counter-balancing between couples who have more children than desired and those who have fewer. For instance, in many industrialized countries recent surveys show the persistence of substantial levels of unwanted fertility, even though the average preferred or ideal family size is in some countries slightly lower than the average number of children women expect to have (see chapter XIV). To study the achievement of fertility goals, individuals' fertility can be divided into "wanted" and "unwanted" components.

Measures of fertility preferences have long been controversial. On the one hand, if they can be taken at face value, the data have clear implications for social policy. Evidence of unwanted fertility may lead to a strengthening of family planning programmes. Indications of a desire for longer birth-spacing may bring about a reorientation of programmes to strengthen the provision of reversible contraceptive methods and methods suited for use by nursing mothers. Data suggesting a preference for large families or a preference for sons over daughters may, depending upon national social and demographic goals, spur a reorientation of development programmes in ways thought to alter these preferences.

On the other hand, the use of such data to guide policy is complicated by the considerations that fertility preferences are imperfectly measured and that the social forces determining these preferences are not well understood. It is always necessary to consider in what ways the answers to preference questions may be biased. Furthermore, there is usually little basis for saying whether the preferences are strongly held, or whether, on the contrary, they are easily overridden by competing circumstances and easily changed.

At the same time, it is possible to over-emphasize the drawbacks of preference measures. Although preference questions generally score lower on conventional tests of reliability than do measures of social and demographic characteristics, such as number of children or education, preference questions usually rank well by comparison with other attitudinal items (McClelland, 1983). The longitudinal studies mentioned earlier provide some reassurance that individuals' preferences are sufficiently stable to have a large effect on subsequent fertility, in societies where contraception is widely practised. Lastly, it must be recognized that, despite their shortcomings, survey data on fertility preferences usually provide the only direct information available on couples' fertility goals, and as such the data deserve serious consideration.

This chapter examines the extent of size and sex preferences and the levels of unwanted fertility found in the 38 developing countries included in this study. Further, in order to facilitate comparisons among countries, these preferences (and unwanted fertility) are examined for countries grouped by level of socio-economic development and strength of family planning programme effort. Socio-economic correlates of these preferences and unwanted fertility are not included here but are discussed in later chapters. The next section describes the data in general terms with respect to both their characteristics and their quality. Section B discusses size preferences as indicated by responses to the questions on desired family size and whether more children were wanted. Where necessary, demographic controls for age and family size are introduced. Section C discusses the prevalence of preferences for sons or daughters or both in these countries. The basic source of information for these preferences are responses to questions on the desired sex of the next child and whether more children were wanted. Section D presents estimates of levels of unwanted fertility, together with the levels of fertility that would occur if women were to implement their desires. The chapter concludes with a summary and discussion of the findings.

A. THE DATA

The World Fertility Survey (WFS) questionnaire contains a series of questions designed to measure respondents' preferences concerning fertility. Women who were currently married and fecund were asked whether they wanted to have another child sometime. Women who responded "Yes" were then asked how many additional children they would like to have. These women were also asked whether they would prefer their next child to be a girl or a boy. Pregnant women were asked instead whether they wanted another child in addition to the one they were expecting. If the response was "Yes", they were then asked the number of additional children they would like to have. They were also asked the preferred sex of the child they were expecting (not the preferred sex of the next child). Lastly, all women, regardless of their fecundity, pregnancy and current marital status, were asked about their desired family size. In addition, in 20 WFS countries, all women with one or more children were asked whether they had wanted any more children before the last child was conceived.

The quality of WFS preference data can be ascertained to some extent through test-retest reliability studies (which examine the stability of responses over time) and through inter-item consistency tests (which examine the extent to which responses to different questions in the same survey are consistent with one another). Unfortunately, the available evidence on the test-retest reliability of the WFS preference questions is limited. Published results from reinterviews of subsamples of the original WFS samples are available from just six countries: Costa Rica; Dominican Republic; Fiji; Indonesia; Peru; and Sri Lanka.[1] Test-retest data on the variable "whether more children are wanted" were available for only three countries, Fiji, the Dominican Republic and Sri Lanka. Identical responses in both the interviews to this question were given by 81 per cent of respondents in Fiji, 86 per cent in the Dominican Republic and 91 per cent in Sri Lanka. Available summary data (Lightbourne, 1984b) on the test-retest reliability of desired family size indicate that the proportions of respondents giving identical responses in both the initial and subsequent surveys were 48 per cent in the Dominican Republic, 44 per cent in Costa Rica, 54 per cent in Indonesia and 43 per cent in Sri Lanka. However, much larger proportions of respondents (70 per cent in the Dominican Republic, 71 per cent in Costa Rica, 81 per cent in Indonesia and 77 per cent in Sri Lanka) differed by not more than one child in the number of children they said they desired. Two reasons for this pattern have been suggested. First, it is unreasonable to think that all respondents have a fixed desire for a single number. It is more plausible that many respondents think in terms of a range (three or four children, say) so that a discrepancy of one child is not surprising (Lightbourne and MacDonald, 1982). Secondly, there may be a tendency for respondents to report their current family size as desired family size. The surveys from Costa Rica and Sri Lanka showed evidence that women who originally had not wanted any more children, but had had a subsequent birth, tended to revise upward their stated desired family size (Lightbourne, 1984b).

Inter-item consistency analyses for the WFS preference data were also conducted (Lightbourne, 1984b). With respect to the variable "whether more children are wanted", women were regarded as consistent either if they wanted more children and their actual family size was less than their desired family size, or if they did not want more children and their actual family size was greater than their desired size. Using this definition, inconsistency was found to be very low among women who wanted additional children, but was much higher among women who did not want more. Discrepancies of this type are substantial in most countries of Latin America and the Caribbean but tend to be much smaller elsewhere (Lightbourne, 1985a). There are two interpretations for the inconsistency among women who did not want any more children. First, it could be that in the abstract such women would have liked to have more children, but in reality felt they should not have any because of age, marital problems or economic problems (Palmore and Concepción, 1981; Pullum, 1980; Lightbourne and MacDonald, 1982). Alternatively, it could be that respondents misunderstood the question to mean whether they wanted another child in the near future, rather than whether they wanted to stop childbearing altogether (United Nations, 1981). Additional analyses reported in Lightbourne (1984b) provide some evidence in support of the latter interpretation.

With respect to the variable "whether last birth was wanted", women were considered consistent either if they had wanted their last birth and their actual family size was less than their desired size or if they had not wanted their last birth and their actual family size was greater than their desired size. Among women who had not wanted their last birth, the proportion of responses that were consistent ranged from 82 per cent in Fiji to 33 per cent in Guyana. According to Lightbourne (1984b), some of this inconsistency probably reflected births that were mistimed rather than unwanted.

Two further points about the data used in this analysis can be noted here. First, the data pertain to only one point in a woman's life cycle, and inferences about fertility are based on these one-time measured preferences. It is generally believed, however, that preferences do not remain constant over the childbearing years (Morgan, 1982). Preferences may change at different points in the family cycle: at marriage; or after the birth of the first child, the second child etc. Furthermore, preferences may also change independently of life-cycle changes. Shifts in the economic situation, for example, may result in a revision of family preferences. Thus, fertility levels calculated on the basis of stated preferences should be viewed with some caution. While there is no evidence from developing countries as yet, evidence of a downward revision of preferences for additional children over a woman's life cycle was obtained in a longitudinal study in the United States (Morgan, 1982). If this finding holds in developing countries (where it may not), then estimates of wanted fertility based on WFS preference data may be overestimates.

Secondly, the data analysed here pertain to women only. However, husbands and wives may have very different preferences, and these differences may have important implications for future fertility levels. In surveys that have asked both sexes about preferences, the mean number of children desired by men has frequently been higher, but usually only slightly so, than the number desired by wives (Mauldin, 1965). The level of disagreement tends to be greater for individual couples. These points are well illustrated by WFS results for two countries that interviewed husbands as well as wives. In Egypt and Thailand, the aggregate proportion who wanted no more children differed by one or two percentage points for husbands and for wives, but in roughly 20 per cent of couples, one spouse wanted more children while the other did not (Lightbourne, 1985a). In one study in Malaysia, Coombs and Fernandez (1978) found high overall aggregate agreement of men and women for size preferences, somewhat lower agreement for sex preferences and much lower agreement between individual marital partners. With respect to sex preferences, wives were more likely to prefer girls or equal numbers of boys and girls; husbands were more likely to prefer sons. This has also been observed in other countries (see Knodel and Prachuabmoh (1976) for Thailand; Williamson (1976) mentions other cases).

The effect of such disagreement on contraceptive use and fertility has been studied in very few societies. In some cases, the wife's preferences have been found to be more influential than those of the husband: in Thailand and Egypt, with respect to contraceptive use (Lightbourne, 1985a; Hallouda and others, 1983); and in Taiwan, Province of China, with respect to subsequent fertility, as measured in a longitudinal study (Coombs and Chang, 1981). Also, in the United States of America, the wife's preferred timing for the next birth appeared to affect contraceptive practice more than the husband's, given that both wanted another child eventually (Thomson, 1984). This does not mean that the husband's preference carries no weight. In Egypt, for instance, among exposed couples interviewed in the World Fertility Survey, the proportion who were using contraception was 52 per cent if both partners wanted no more children, 41 per cent if the husband wanted more but the wife did not, 26 per cent if the wife wanted more but the husband did not and 13 per cent if both wanted more (Hallouda and others, 1983).[2] This pattern suggests that in Egypt disagreement often results in the birth of more children, although this occurs less frequently than when partners agree that they want more. By contrast, in the United States of America, "marital conflict in desires for another child is apparently resolved in favour of contraception and therefore no births" (Thomson, 1984, p. 10).

These studies indicate that understanding of fertility behaviour could be improved if both partners' preferences were routinely obtained in surveys. However, the limited evidence does not suggest that the husband's fertility desires are usually more influential than those of the wife. It has also been argued that in traditional societies other family members (grandparents, for example) may have a large role in fertility decision-making for the couple (Caldwell, 1983). Again, little research exists to confirm this.

The reader should keep in mind first that the preferences in this study refer to one point in the life cycle of women; and secondly, that the preferences pertain to wives only. It should be emphasized, however, that the amount of bias introduced due to these limitations is not known. Other issues of measurement and bias are discussed below in more detail for each of the preference measures, in connection with the substantive findings.

B. SIZE PREFERENCES

The measurement of preferences in sample surveys has always been problematical, with little agreement on how best to measure them. As a result, many different types of questions or series of questions have been asked in various surveys. McClelland (1983) provides a classification of these questions which have attempted to capture the preferences of women concerning their family size. Four basic categories of questions are identified, namely: "how many more"; "over again"; ordering; and projective. The WFS data derived from the surveys in the developing countries relate primarily to the first two categories.

In the first category, the respondent is asked how many more children are wanted in addition to the children already in the family. Then, wanted family size is calculated by adding this number to the respondent's number of living children. Also included in this category is a question whether more children are desired in the future. Both these questions were asked in the World Fertility Survey programme and are included in the analysis.

The "over again" category includes asking the respondent to state the number of children that would be desired if it were possible to begin childbearing all over again. The questions on desired family size included in WFS fall in this category. In some other surveys, a set of conditions was given which the respondent had to consider before stating her desired family size.

In the ordering category, respondents are generally asked to rank a series of family sizes, beginning with the most desired family size. Based on the order of these rankings, an index is then calculated. The most frequently used measure of this type is the Coombs scale. Such questions were not included in most WFS questionnaires. The final category includes questions about the ideal or typical family size rather than about the respondent's personal desires. For example, the Pakistan Fertility Survey asked its respondents, "In your opinion, how many children should a married couple have?". When such questions are used as measures of individual family-size desires, it is assumed that the respondent's desires bias her judgement about the typical family size, so that the typical family size reported by her is assumed to approximate her own desires (McClelland, 1983). Such an assumption may or may not be true.

Desired family size

The question recommended for measuring desired family size was, "If you could choose exactly the number of children to have in your whole life, how many would that be?". All but four countries asked the question exactly as recommended for ever-married women. The exceptions were Cameroon, Fiji, Malaysia and Pakistan. Malaysia retained the meaning of the standard question but changed the wording slightly.[3] Pakistan, however, used a completely different question, which measured "ideal" rather than "desired" family size.[4] In Fiji, the measure of desired family size was obtained in different ways for different groups of women. Furthermore, this measure was restricted to currently married women who were fecund. Although Cameroon used the recommended question, it restricted it to particular parity and age groups of women (which consisted of 55 per cent of the total sample). Because of these deviations from the standard, the data on desired family size for Cameroon, Fiji and Pakistan are considered to be non-comparable with other countries. Results for these three countries are therefore not discussed in this section although they are available for reference in the accompanying tables.

Before presenting the WFS data, certain limitations of this measure should be noted. The question on desired family size did not make clear whether the respondent should respond in terms of the desired number of births or the desired number of surviving children. According to Lightbourne and MacDonald (1982), this could have important implications for estimating desired fertility levels, especially in countries with high infant/child mortality, because it is generally assumed that respondents answer in terms of surviving children. In addition, a measure such as desired family size does not consider the intensity of desires concerning family size or what family size would be preferred if stated desires are not achieved. Thus, it is not known how hard a woman would try in order to achieve her desired family size or whether her second or third choice would be higher or lower fertility. This measure also mixes up size and sex preferences. For example, a woman may say she wants three children, but in reality she would choose to stop with three children only if she had at least two sons. Thus, in cases where size preferences are strongly contingent on sex preferences, measures like desired family size may not be accurate predictors of subsequent fertility levels.[5]

Lastly, questions on the meaningfulness of the concept of desired family size in developing countries have often been raised (for example, Knodel and Prachuabmoh, 1973;

and Ware, 1974). It has been suggested that these concepts make little sense to respondents so that the answers they provide have basically no meaning (Mauldin, 1965; Hauser, 1967). As a result, it has been argued that respondents often answer the question on family size preferences by giving the number of children they already have or are unable to give any numerical response at all, further limiting the usability of measures like desired family size. Evidence to the contrary, however, has slowly accumulated (Knodel and Prachuabmoh, 1973; Coombs, 1976). Both non-response and rationalization effects are examined here. In spite of these criticisms, important information on the preferences of respondents can still be obtained from the question on desired family size.

Table 29 shows for each country the percentage of ever-married women who gave a non-numerical response to the question on desired family size. There were low rates (below 5 per cent) of non-numerical responses in over 60 per cent of the countries, including all those in Latin America and the Caribbean, and most of those in Asia and Oceania. The exceptions are Bangladesh in Southern Asia, where 30 per cent did not give a numerical answer; and the Syrian Arab Republic and Yemen in Western Asia, with 7 and 44 per cent, respectively. In sharp contrast to the generally low rates in Latin America and the Caribbean and in Asia and Oceania, nearly all countries in Africa had high rates of non-response, varying from about 11 per cent in Ghana and Morocco to 31 per cent in Mauritania. Low rates are found in only two countries: Egypt (1.4 per cent); and Lesotho (2.1 per cent). Not surprisingly, the regional averages show that Africa, as a whole, had the highest non-numerical response rate (16.0 per cent), while Latin America and the Caribbean had the lowest (0.4 per cent).

TABLE 29. PERCENTAGE OF NON-NUMERICAL RESPONSES, MEAN DESIRED FAMILY SIZE AND PROPORTIONS WHO DESIRED EXACTLY i[a] CHILDREN AMONG EVER-MARRIED WOMEN AGED 15-49[b]

Region and country	Non-numerical responses (percentage)	Mean desired family size	Percentage who desired i[a] children							
			None	One	Two	Three	Four	Five	Six	Seven or more
Africa										
Benin	21.9	7.4	0.0	0.3	1.2	2.9	10.1	10.6	19.6	55.3
Cameroon[c]	25.9	8.1	0.0	1.4	6.9	5.7	7.1	12.6	8.4	57.9
Côte d'Ivoire[d]	24.9	8.4	0.2	0.2	1.1	2.0	6.5	9.5	12.9	67.5
Egypt	1.4	4.1	0.2	2.0	28.2	23.2	19.3	8.1	6.3	12.9
Ghana	10.8	6.0	0.0	0.2	1.5	4.2	26.0	12.0	24.6	31.6
Kenya	19.2	7.2	0.0	0.2	1.2	2.4	13.4	12.7	20.5	49.5
Lesotho	2.1	6.0	0.0	0.7	2.9	6.8	23.3	14.1	21.7	30.5
Mauritania	30.6	8.7	0.8	1.9	5.1	5.9	8.2	9.2	9.8	59.3
Morocco	11.1	4.9	0.5	1.1	10.9	11.3	29.1	11.9	17.5	17.6
Senegal	28.6	8.3	0.0	0.5	1.9	2.8	7.0	10.4	11.3	66.0
Sudan	18.2	6.3	0.4	1.2	4.6	7.1	18.1	13.2	13.8	41.6
Tunisia	5.5	4.1	0.4	1.3	11.1	17.8	43.5	11.8	7.4	6.8
SUB-AVERAGE	16.0	6.5	0.2	0.9	6.3	7.9	18.6	11.2	15.0	39.9
Latin America and the Caribbean										
Colombia	0.6	4.1	0.6	3.3	22.8	25.6	19.3	9.5	6.6	12.4
Costa Rica	0.0	4.7	0.6	2.3	16.9	23.8	20.7	9.8	9.2	16.8
Dominican Republic	0.0	4.6	1.2	1.0	12.3	24.7	25.6	12.2	8.3	14.6
Ecuador	0.1	4.1	0.7	3.4	20.8	24.2	22.1	8.5	8.9	11.4
Guyana	0.0	4.6	0.8	1.3	14.4	18.9	26.8	12.3	11.2	14.4
Haiti	0.3	3.5	0.2	3.9	25.6	26.1	25.8	8.1	5.2	5.1
Jamaica	0.2	4.0	1.6	3.6	21.7	18.2	28.7	6.6	9.3	10.3
Mexico	0.0	4.5	0.9	2.0	19.3	21.8	21.8	9.8	9.6	14.8
Panama	0.1	4.2	0.7	1.5	15.6	27.2	24.6	10.0	9.6	11.0
Paraguay	0.7	5.1	0.1	2.4	10.3	18.7	20.0	14.3	11.2	23.1
Peru	1.8	3.8	1.2	4.0	23.4	22.6	24.8	7.9	9.0	7.0
Trinidad and Tobago	0.0	3.8	0.9	2.0	23.3	17.7	36.2	6.7	7.7	5.5
Venezuela	1.1	4.2	0.4	2.6	19.3	23.4	25.4	8.7	9.7	10.5
SUB-AVERAGE	0.4	4.2	0.8	2.6	18.9	22.5	24.8	9.6	8.9	12.1

TABLE 29 (continued)

| Region and country | Non-numerical responses (percentage) | Mean desired family size | \multicolumn{8}{c}{Percentage who desired i[a] children} |
			None	One	Two	Three	Four	Five	Six	Seven or more
Asia and Oceania										
Bangladesh	30.0	4.1	0.5	1.4	12.9	24.7	32.5	13.8	7.1	7.1
Fiji[c]	..	4.2	0.3	1.7	17.5	22.3	22.9	15.0	9.5	11.0
Indonesia	4.4	4.2	0.3	3.9	15.4	22.0	23.2	15.7	8.9	10.7
Jordan	0.0	6.3	0.1	0.5	5.6	8.1	20.7	12.3	15.1	37.7
Malaysia	0.8	4.4	0.2	0.6	8.9	11.3	46.3	14.3	11.1	7.3
Nepal	0.2	3.9	0.2	1.2	14.0	29.8	28.5	13.9	6.7	5.9
Pakistan[c]	2.9	4.2	0.0	0.4	10.3	18.5	40.9	16.1	8.8	5.0
Philippines	0.0	4.4	0.0	1.5	12.9	23.6	25.5	13.2	9.3	14.0
Republic of Korea	1.0	3.2	0.4	1.8	24.6	41.2	19.0	10.9	1.3	0.8
Sri Lanka	0.2	3.8	0.1	3.4	22.0	27.7	19.0	12.7	6.3	8.9
Syrian Arab Republic	7.2	6.1	0.0	0.3	6.6	10.9	22.9	12.4	13.4	33.5
Thailand	2.9	3.7	0.0	3.2	20.6	25.0	27.1	12.8	6.8	4.6
Yemen	43.8	5.4	0.7	2.8	9.9	9.2	20.0	18.3	14.8	24.4
SUB-AVERAGE	8.2	4.5	0.2	1.9	13.9	21.2	25.9	13.7	9.2	14.1
TOTAL	7.7	5.0	0.4	1.8	13.4	17.5	23.2	11.4	10.9	21.5

Source: World Fertility Survey standard recode tapes.
[a] i = 1, 2, ..., 7+ children.
[b] Excluding Costa Rica and Panama (20-49) and Venezuela (15-44).
[c] Data not considered comparable and not included in calculation of sub-averages.
[d] Formerly called the Ivory Coast.

Non-numerical responses do not necessarily imply that women have no preferences as to the number of children they would like to have. Non-response may occur when women who are indifferent among several possible family sizes are forced to give only one response, as in the question used here (Coombs, 1976).[6] Alternatively, women may not respond to the question on desired family size because they believe that their family size is decided by God or fate (Ware, 1974). Such women, however, often provide a numerical response when asked the number of children they hope God will send them. Therefore, the evidence seems to indicate that many women who do not answer questions about their desired family size have family size preferences but often cannot respond to questions worded in a certain way.

In many of the countries with high non-numerical rates, controlling the supply of children may be impossible or very costly (McClelland, 1983). Thus, many people may not have thought about how many children they would like to have. As means for controlling fertility become more widely available, however, couples will be able to make decisions about family size. For example, it has been reported that, in countries where contraception has become increasingly available and acceptable, respondents think about their family size (Bulatao and Arnold, 1977). Table 30 provides a crude way of testing this relationship by comparing average non-numerical response rates in groups of countries classified according to level of socio-economic development and strength of family planning programme effort.

The percentage of non-numerical responses can be seen to decline monotonically with either increasing development or increasing family planning programme strength. In both cases, the largest absolute differences are found for comparisons between the low category (IV, 4) and the next one (III, 3). For example, while slightly over a fifth of the respondents in development group IV gave non-numerical responses, this proportion falls to about 11 per cent in group III.

The question whether the large percentages of non-numerical responses observed in several countries bias the

TABLE 30. MEAN PERCENTAGE OF NON-NUMERICAL RESPONSES,[a] BY LEVEL OF DEVELOPMENT AND STRENGTH OF FAMILY PLANNING PROGRAMME EFFORT

Level of development	Non-numerical responses (percentage)	Strength of family planning programme effort	Non-numerical responses (percentage)
I. High	0.4	1. Strong	0.9
II. Middle-high	1.8	2. Moderate	1.7
III. Middle-low	10.6	3. Weak	6.9
IV. Low	21.7	4. Very weak/none	15.9

Source: Table 29.
[a] Not including Cameroon, Fiji and Pakistan in calculation of means.

mean numbers of children desired has been investigated (Lightbourne and MacDonald, 1982; Lightbourne, 1984b). Based on the evidence that, at each family size, women who gave non-numerical responses and those who gave numerical answers had very similar proportions of women who had not wanted the last birth, while at the same time the likelihood of providing a non-numerical response was the same at all family sizes, it was concluded that the high rates of non-response for Bangladesh did not bias the mean number of children desired (Lightbourne and MacDonald, 1982). Jensen (1985) used a different technique but reached a similar conclusion for surveys (non-WFS) in Guatemala and India. For the countries of Africa, Lightbourne (1984b) found that synthetic-cohort estimates of desired family size were usually similar to the means obtained from the direct question on desired family size, suggesting that the estimates were not seriously affected by the high rates of non-numerical response.[7]

Table 29 and figure 8 present the mean number of children desired for each country. The means range from a low of 3.2 in the Republic of Korea to a high of 8.7 in Mauritania. Regional averages show that Africa, as a whole, has the highest mean number of children desired (6.5), followed by Asia and Oceania (4.5) and Latin America and the Caribbean (4.2). The range is narrowest in Latin America and the Caribbean (1.6 children), where the lowest mean is 3.5 (Haiti) and the highest is 5.1

Figure 8. Mean desired family size, by region, level of development and strength of family planning programme effort

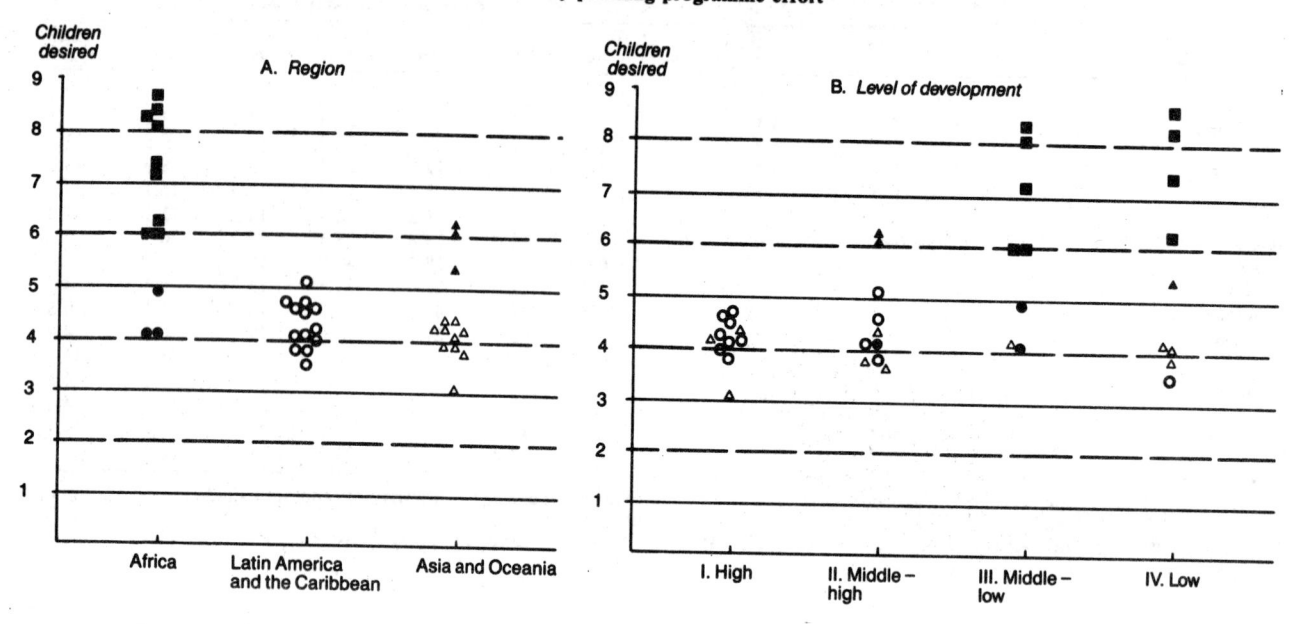

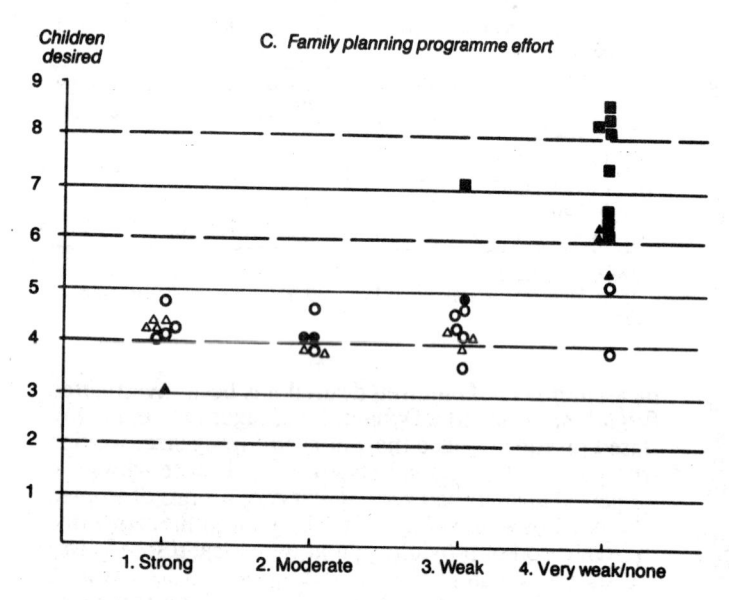

A. Region

B. Level of development

C. Family planning programme effort

Legend:
- ■ Sub-Saharan Africa[a]
- ● Other Africa
- ○ Latin America and the Caribbean
- ▲ Western Asia
- △ Other Asia and Oceania

Source: Table 29.

[a] Including the Sudan.

(Paraguay). In Asia and Oceania, the range is wider, a bit more than three children. Relatively higher averages are found in the three Western Asian countries, Jordan, the Syrian Arab Republic and Yemen; and lower means in the rest of Asia, varying between 3.2 and 4.4. The largest range in average desired family size is found in Africa. Several countries stand out as having very high means, such as Côte d'Ivoire,[8] Mauritania and Senegal, with over eight; and Benin and Kenya, with over seven. Although a wide range of values is seen in sub-Saharan Africa, all the sub-Saharan countries have means of at least six children desired. This level is reached elsewhere only in Jordan and the Syrian Arab Republic. Apart from the distinctive subregions of Western Asia and sub-Saharan Africa, average desired family size falls in the roughly two-child range of from 3.2 to 5.1 children.

It is reasonable to expect the mean desired family size in the relatively more developed of the developing countries to be lower than in the least developed ones. This is because socio-economic development, among other things, generally increases the costs of children, while at the same time reducing their economic benefits. As can be seen from table 31, mean desired family size is indeed higher in development group IV than in group I, by 1.7 children. However, as table 31 and figure 8 also show, the overall relationship is entirely due to the sub-Saharan countries; when the latter are removed from the averages, there is no difference in mean desired family size between groups I and IV. Even with the sub-Saharan countries included, the development index accounts for only about one quarter of the variance in desired family size, as compared with roughly one half of the variance in current fertility levels.[9]

TABLE 31. MEAN DESIRED FAMILY SIZE,[a] BY LEVEL OF DEVELOPMENT AND STRENGTH OF FAMILY PLANNING PROGRAMME EFFORT

	All regions	Excluding sub-Saharan Africa
Level of development		
I. High	4.2	4.2
II. Middle-high	4.6	4.6
III. Middle-low	5.8	4.4
IV. Low	5.9	4.2
Strength of family planning programme effort		
1. Strong	4.1	4.1
2. Moderate	4.0	4.0
3. Weak	4.5	4.2
4. Very weak/none	6.2	5.3

Source: Table 29.

[a] Not including Cameroon, Fiji and Pakistan in calculation of means.

Thus, low levels of development appear compatible with a wide range of fertility desires, depending upon regional (presumably cultural) factors that are not closely associated with socio-economic indicators. Mean desired family size in development group IV ranges from 3.5 to 8.7, and in group III from 4.1 to 8.4 (see figure 8). A much smaller range is evident in group I, though the average desired family size of roughly four children is still approximately double the level seen in most of the highly industrialized countries of Europe (see chapter XIV). While these data provide no reason to doubt that very high levels of development are incompatible with very high levels of desired family size, it is plain that development factors do not distinguish well between societies with high, as opposed to moderate, fertility desires.

Desired family size can also be expected to vary with strength of family planning effort, in part because programme effort is correlated with development. In addition, the family planning programme itself may be successful in lowering preferences for large families, and/or countries with low preferences may be more successful in developing programmes. Whatever the reason for the association—and this, unfortunately, cannot be established here—nearly all the countries with a very weak programme or no programme exhibit preferences for very large families (table 31 and figure 8). Only one country in this group, Peru, has a mean desired family size under five children. All but one of the sub-Saharan countries (Kenya) and all three of the Western Asian countries with high preferences have family planning effort scores classed as "very weak/none". There is little variation in desired family size among the other three family planning groups.

Table 29 also presents, for each country, the percentage distribution of women according to desired family size. Very few women wished to remain childless—the proportion of women who expressed a desire for no children never exceeds 2 per cent. Only in Jamaica and Peru did more than 5 per cent of the women say that they wanted at most one child, and it is notable that in no country did more than 35 per cent of the women prefer at most two children. In most countries, over half the women desired from two to four children. This is true for all the countries in Latin America and the Caribbean and most of the countries in Asia and Oceania, but only two (Egypt and Tunisia) in Africa. At the other extreme, in 12 countries (including Cameroon), over 20 per cent of the women desired at least seven children. Eight of those countries are in Africa; in Benin, Côte d'Ivoire, Mauritania and Senegal, over half the women desired seven or more children. The other countries are Jordan, the Syrian Arab Republic and Yemen in Western Asia, and Paraguay in Latin America.

Below-average national values of desired family size come about almost entirely through a concentration of responses in ranges of from two to four or from two to five children, and not through a greater popularity of families with no children or one child. In the country with the lowest mean, the Republic of Korea, only 2 per cent preferred no children or one child, while 85 per cent gave answers in the range from two to four and 96 per cent in the range from two to five. In no other country were responses so heavily concentrated in a narrow span, but in roughly one quarter of the cases, a three-child range (either from two to four or from two to five children) accounts for at least 70 per cent of the answers.

In contrast to these countries, where there is something approaching a social consensus in favour of moderate-sized families, the countries with very high mean values of desired family size tended to have responses distributed over a wide range of numbers of children, with even numbers given most often. In four of the sub-Saharan countries, 10 children was the most common single answer, attracting 22-33 per cent of the numerical answers in Cameroon, Côte d'Ivoire, Mauritania and Senegal. Responses of 12, 15 and even 20 children were also fairly common in these countries. Because few women will have so many children, such answers are tantamount to saying "as many as possible". Unrealistically large (or unachievable) family sizes were given much less frequently in some of the other sub-Saharan countries. In Ghana and Lesotho, about one quarter of women reported four children as the desired number and about 60 per cent of numerical answers were in the range of from four to six children.

Regional averages highlight the differences among geographical areas. As table 29 shows, Latin America and the Caribbean and Asia and Oceania have roughly similar distributions: 12-14 per cent desired large families of seven or more children while 16-22 per cent preferred small families of at most two children. In contrast, in Africa almost 40 per cent of the respondents expressed a desire for seven or more children while only 8 per cent wanted at most two. These differences are illustrated in figure 9, which uses the data from table 29 to plot the proportion of ever-married women against the distribution of number of children desired for the three regional groups.

Recent research has found that desired family size is positively associated with both age and parity (for example, Lightbourne and MacDonald, 1982). Thus, older women and women with more children generally expressed a desire for larger families, compared with younger women and women with fewer children. When women of the same parity are compared across age groups, differences in fertility desires are negligible (Lightbourne and MacDonald, 1982). Standardization for family size tends to remove the association between age and desired family size not just in countries where birth control is widely practised, and where the correlation of desired and actual fertility could conceivably be due to successful birth planning, but in societies where there is little evidence of deliberate fertility control. This indicates that

Figure 9. Percentage of ever-married women by number of children desired, regional groups

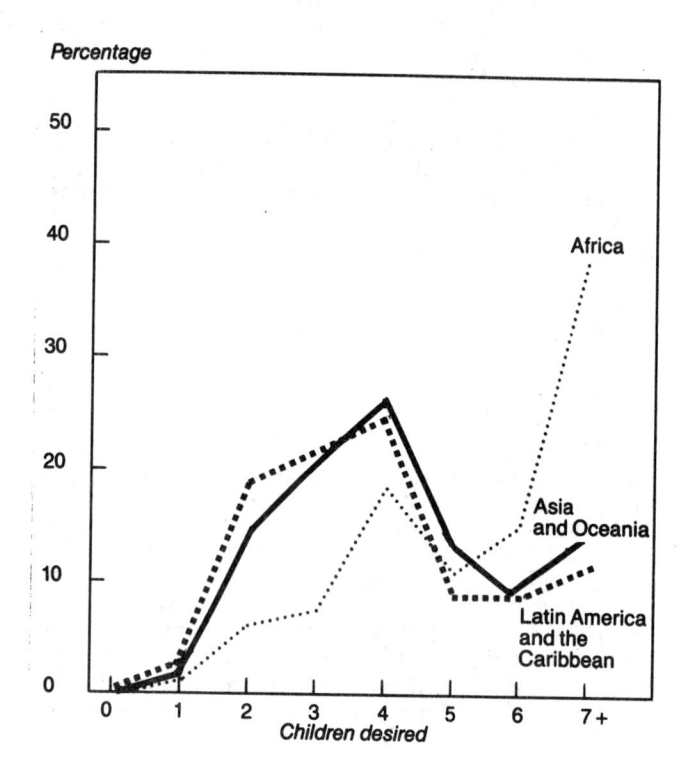

Source: Table 29.

age differences in mean desired family size cannot be interpreted as indicating a trend towards lower desired family size among women born more recently. Whether such a trend exists, either within birth cohorts or between successive cohorts, can be assessed only through a series of surveys. Age differences in mean desired family size are not presented here.

Women who had large families tended to report relatively large desired family sizes, whether age is held constant or not (Lightbourne and MacDonald, 1982). Table 32 shows that mean desired family size, averaged over all countries, increases from 4.0-4.1 children for women with from none to two living children to 6.8 for women with seven or more living children. The increments in desired family size are not similar across countries. Paraguay and Indonesia, for example, have large increments in desired family size, while Egypt, Malaysia, Peru, the Republic of Korea, Thailand and Tunisia have relatively small increments. Senegal also has small increments, but women with no children began at a very high desired family size of 7.5.

The literature provides several possible reasons for the strong association observed between the number of living children and mean desired family size (for example, Knodel and Prachuabmoh, 1973; Lightbourne and MacDonald, 1982). First, it is logical that women who have smaller desired family sizes would try to restrict their fertility once they achieve their preferred size, while women who want larger families would continue childbearing. This should be the case particularly in populations where methods of fertility limitation are widely used and where women have an idea of how many children

TABLE 32. MEAN DESIRED FAMILY SIZE, BY NUMBER OF LIVING CHILDREN, INCLUDING CURRENT PREGNANCY, AMONG EVER-MARRIED WOMEN AGED 15-49[a]

Region and country	None	One	Two	Three	Four	Five	Six	Seven or more	Overall mean
Africa									
Benin	6.85	6.82	7.03	7.03	7.55	8.05	8.60	9.45	7.42
Cameroon[c]	7.39	7.03	7.72	8.08	8.57	8.63	8.54	9.52	8.08
Côte d'Ivoire[d]	7.39	7.51	7.82	8.14	8.84	9.20	9.65	10.34	8.35
Egypt	3.65	3.46	3.68	3.87	4.20	4.58	4.71	5.33	4.08
Ghana	5.29	4.95	5.22	5.63	6.20	6.88	7.41	8.65	6.03
Kenya	6.29	6.27	6.39	6.69	6.78	7.24	8.01	8.75	7.17
Lesotho	5.54	5.30	5.52	5.80	6.23	6.73	7.45	8.17	5.96
Mauritania	9.14	7.93	8.20	8.22	8.85	9.04	9.16	10.54	8.69
Morocco	4.01	4.02	4.13	4.48	5.06	5.16	5.65	6.37	4.90
Senegal	7.51	7.95	8.25	8.54	8.34	8.64	9.10	8.89	8.29
Sudan	5.39	5.40	5.44	5.99	6.24	7.05	7.22	7.94	6.32
Tunisia	3.63	3.40	3.58	3.83	4.27	4.63	4.68	4.75	4.13
SUB-AVERAGE	5.88	5.73	5.93	6.20	6.60	7.02	7.42	8.10	6.49
Latin America and the Caribbean									
Colombia	2.67	2.75	3.17	3.84	4.25	4.72	4.87	6.14	4.08
Costa Rica	2.85	3.04	3.49	4.30	4.81	5.47	6.08	7.53	4.72
Dominican Republic	3.47	3.48	3.79	4.39	4.84	5.27	5.53	6.48	4.61
Ecuador	2.87	2.72	3.04	3.74	4.44	4.79	5.33	6.13	4.08
Guyana	3.44	3.44	3.56	4.05	4.65	5.18	5.64	6.90	4.60
Haiti	2.87	2.81	3.05	3.89	4.13	4.10	4.48	4.90	3.52
Jamaica	3.14	2.97	3.36	3.83	4.32	4.78	5.17	5.79	4.01
Mexico	3.26	3.29	3.43	4.11	4.56	5.03	5.38	5.87	4.45
Panama	3.09	3.01	3.37	3.75	4.44	4.88	5.48	5.90	4.22
Paraguay	3.29	3.41	3.81	4.63	5.25	6.11	6.93	8.77	5.13
Peru	3.23	2.78	3.09	3.66	4.10	4.25	4.56	4.85	3.78
Trinidad and Tobago	3.14	3.08	3.41	3.75	4.14	4.54	4.59	5.17	3.77
Venezuela	2.81	2.86	3.31	3.79	4.58	5.00	5.38	6.85	4.15
SUB-AVERAGE	3.09	3.05	3.38	3.98	4.50	4.93	5.34	6.25	4.24

TABLE 32 (continued)

Region and country	Number of living children[b]								Overall mean
	None	One	Two	Three	Four	Five	Six	Seven or more	
Asia and Oceania									
Bangladesh	3.44	3.50	3.72	3.90	4.21	4.66	4.90	5.53	4.08
Fiji[c]	2.57	2.69	2.98	3.54	4.14	4.91	5.75	7.10	4.16
Indonesia	2.88	3.04	3.42	4.02	4.75	5.57	6.04	7.04	4.14
Jordan	4.42	4.70	4.71	5.58	5.60	6.44	6.80	8.00	6.31
Malaysia	3.64	3.71	3.83	4.22	4.62	4.81	4.80	5.02	4.36
Nepal	3.42	3.47	3.51	3.81	4.37	4.75	5.13	5.78	3.91
Pakistan[c]	3.83	3.82	3.93	4.05	4.24	4.45	4.40	4.72	4.15
Philippines	2.81	2.81	3.15	3.59	4.30	4.94	5.53	6.44	4.42
Republic of Korea	2.55	2.62	2.79	3.11	3.42	3.65	3.96	4.08	3.19
Sri Lanka	2.50	2.29	2.65	3.31	3.95	4.69	5.24	6.28	3.79
Syrian Arab Republic	4.61	4.81	5.29	5.53	5.64	6.05	6.80	7.80	6.10
Thailand	2.99	2.82	3.18	3.57	4.00	4.32	4.73	4.81	3.71
Yemen	4.44	4.66	4.51	5.19	5.66	6.06	6.36	8.19	5.35
SUB-AVERAGE	3.42	3.50	3.71	4.17	4.59	5.08	5.48	6.26	4.49
TOTAL	4.07	4.03	4.09	4.74	5.19	5.63	6.04	6.83	5.03

Source: World Fertility Survey standard recode tapes.
[a] For Costa Rica and Panama, 20-49; for Venezuela, 15-44.
[b] A current pregnancy is counted as a living child.
[c] Data not considered comparable and not included in calculation of sub-averages.
[d] Formerly called the Ivory Coast.

they prefer, so that fertility preferences influence fertility behaviour. Secondly, the reverse relationship could hold, with actual fertility behaviour influencing fertility preferences. This is generally called the "rationalization effect", where women have more children than they had originally desired and yet report their actual family size as their desired family size so as to avoid implying that some of their children are unwanted. The rationalization of unwanted fertility should not affect the answers of women who have recently begun childbearing, since they generally have not had time to reach the desired family size. Their responses, however, could give a misleadingly low impression of the number of children these women will eventually want to have, if the target family size tends to be revised upward once the original goal is approached. Lightbourne and MacDonald (1982) found that the proportion of women who desired more than a particular number of children, N, was greater for women who already had N than for women who had fewer children. For example, in 19 countries, among women who currently had four children, an average of 33 per cent desired more than four, compared with 12 per cent among women who currently had none or one. This pattern of response could reflect either trends between age cohorts or effects of deliberate fertility control (causing women who wanted very small families to be clustered at lower parities), as well as upward revision of targets once several children are born. In any case, the responses of low-parity women are likely to underestimate the "true" average desired family size for the society as a whole. The responses of low-parity and high-parity women should thus represent lower and upper bounds, respectively, to the number of children women would have if they could freely choose and were not affected by infecundity or other circumstances that may cause family size to fall below the expressed desire.

Figure 10 plots the mean total number of children desired against the number of living children for regions. The diagonal indicates the points at which actual family size equalled desired family size. Women to the left of the diagonal had not yet reached their desired parity, while women to the right of the diagonal had exceeded their average desired parity. As figure 10 shows, the distributions for Latin America and the Caribbean and Asia and Oceania are very similar. In each region desired family size rises from just over three for women with no children to over six for women with seven or more children. In sharp contrast, women in Africa had much greater desired family sizes, from over five and a half for women with no children to nearly eight for women with seven or more children. Further, at no parity was their desired size less than the actual number of children living whereas, in most countries of Latin America and the Caribbean and of Asia and Oceania, women with more than five children had more children than they desired. Control for number of living children does not alter the conclusions reached earlier about associations between desired family size and level of development or family planning effort.

Proportions wanting no more children

With only two exceptions, all countries asked the question, "Do you want to have another child sometime?", of women who were currently married and fecund.[10] The wording of the question varied slightly, depending upon whether the respondent had no birth, had at least one birth or was pregnant at the time of the interview. In addition to respondents who answered "No" to this question, respondents who were sterilized for contraceptive reasons were also coded as wanting no more children in most countries.[11] Data on this variable are available for all countries included in this project. The results for Bangladesh, Cameroon and Senegal, however, are not considered to be comparable;[12] therefore, although data for these three countries are presented in the tables, they are not included in this discussion.

As mentioned earlier, consistency tests have led researchers of WFS data to speculate about the accuracy of the responses to the question on "desire for more children". There is the possibility that some of the women who responded "No" to this question may, in fact, wish to postpone births rather than stop childbearing entirely (Lightbourne, 1984b). Thus, results based on this question may overestimate the actual extent of the desire to stop childbearing. On the other hand, it has also been

Figure 10. **Mean number of children desired, by number of living children, for regions**

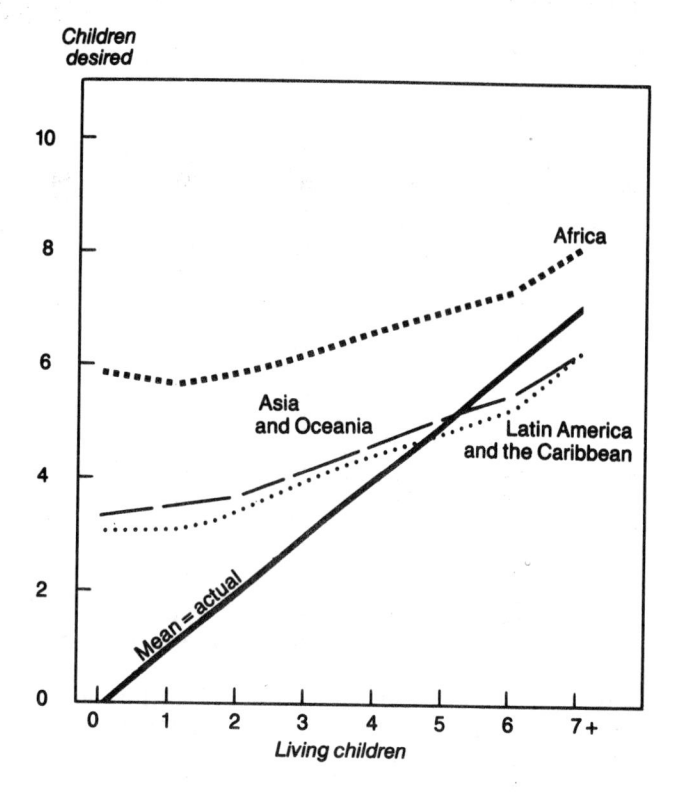

[Chart showing children desired (y-axis, 0-10) vs living children (x-axis, 0-7+). Curves shown for Africa (rising from ~6 to ~8), Asia and Oceania (rising from ~3 to ~6), Latin America and the Caribbean (rising from ~3 to ~6), and a diagonal line labeled "Mean = actual".]

Source: Table 32.

suggested that many of the women who said they wanted more children or were undecided are potential "permanent postponers". That is, there may be many women who wish to postpone the next birth for an extended period and who, if they succeed at delaying the birth for several years, will eventually decide to have no more children at all (Lightbourne, 1985a).

Table 33 gives the overall proportions of women who did not want any more children for each country. These range from a minimum of 3 per cent in Cameroon to a maximum of 72 per cent in the Republic of Korea. Countries in Africa, except for Egypt, Morocco and Tunisia in Northern Africa, stand out as having relatively low proportions (under 20 per cent) of women who did not want more children. The only country outside Africa with a similarly low proportion is Yemen. In all other countries covered, substantial proportions of women reported that they wanted to stop childbearing, in ranges from 32 to 63 per cent in Latin America and the Caribbean and from 30 to 72 per cent in Asia and Oceania.

However, such comparisons of proportions who wanted no more children can be misleading. Two populations with identical distributions of desired family size could have very different proportions who did not want more children if they had very different tempos of childbearing, which depend upon such factors as breast-feeding patterns, contraceptive use and post-partum abstinence (Lightbourne and MacDonald, 1982). This is because the population with a slower tempo of childbearing (due, for example, to longer breast-feeding intervals or more use of contraception for spacing purposes) will take longer to achieve its desired family size and so will generally produce a lower proportion wanting to stop childbearing when observed in a cross-sectional survey. Consider, for example, Peru, and Trinidad and Tobago. Both have similar desired family sizes of about 3.8. Yet, while 61 per cent of the women in Peru did not want any more children, only 47 per cent in Trinidad and Tobago had the same desire. In part, the lower percentage in Trinidad and Tobago may be explained by its slower speed of reproduction due to more widespread use of contraception to space births.

Table 33 also presents the proportions who wanted no more children categorized by number of living children. In general, in most countries, the proportion increases rapidly with increasing numbers of living children between families with no children and those with five children; it then either remains stable at the higher parities or increases more slowly. Several countries in Africa, however, do not exhibit this pattern. Instead, they have relatively small increases with increasing family size (Ghana, Kenya and the Sudan, for example).

In most countries, sharp increases in the proportions who did not want any more children generally occurred after two or three children, although a few countries show a rapid increase only after four children. After three or fewer children, over half the women in all the countries of Latin America and the Caribbean (except Peru) wanted no more children. In Asia and Oceania, however, there were only four countries—the Philippines, the Republic of Korea, Sri Lanka and Thailand—in which over 50 per cent wanted no more children after having had three (or fewer), while in Africa only Egypt has this characteristic. In general, the family size at which over 50 per cent wanted no more children is three in Latin America and the Caribbean, four in Asia and Oceania, and seven or more in sub-Saharan Africa.

Table 33 further indicates that the proportion of childless women who stated that they did not want any children varies from almost zero in several countries to over 12 per cent in the Republic of Korea. In several countries (nearly all of them in Latin America and the Caribbean), over 5 per cent of childless women did not want any children. This proportion implies that a rather large number of women wanted to remain childless and is not entirely consistent with earlier findings based on the question about desired family size, where the proportion of women who desired no children never exceeded 2 per cent (table 29).[13]

The proportion of women with two children who did not want any more children is of interest. In only two countries, Colombia and the Republic of Korea, did over half the women with two children desire to cease childbearing. There are several countries (mostly in Latin America and the Caribbean) where 40-49 per cent wanted no more children. Lower proportions (20-30 per cent) are generally found in Asia and Oceania, while the lowest proportions are found in Africa.

Even after controlling for number of children, as in table 33, however, the problems of drawing conclusions about inter-country differences in family size preferences from comparisons of proportions who did not want more children remain, because differential use of contraception can produce major differences in such proportions. Consider, for example, two countries, A and B, with identical distributions of desired family size. Assume for the

TABLE 33. PERCENTAGE OF CURRENTLY MARRIED, FECUND WOMEN WHO WANTED NO MORE CHILDREN,
BY NUMBER OF LIVING CHILDREN, INCLUDING CURRENT PREGNANCY

Region and country	None	One	Two	Three	Four	Five	Six	Seven or more	Total
Africa									
Benin	0	1	3	6	10	12	20	29	8
Cameroon[b]	1	2	4	4	3	8	9	27	3
Côte d'Ivoire[c]	0	1	2	3	3	6	11	19	4
Egypt	0	7	43	64	76	81	90	90	54
Ghana	1	1	3	6	15	19	35	49	12
Kenya	2	1	4	7	16	18	25	45	17
Lesotho	0	3	8	15	26	42	45	57	15
Mauritania	3	4	7	11	13	16	15	23	11
Morocco	3	7	18	34	45	66	69	84	42
Senegal[b]	0	2	1	1	5	8	18	40	8
Sudan	1	4	8	11	17	22	32	41	17
Tunisia	1	5	25	43	62	73	81	88	49
SUB-AVERAGE	1	3	12	20	28	36	42	52	23
Latin America and the Caribbean									
Colombia	9	19	52	65	79	78	85	91	61
Costa Rica	5	13	35	59	68	75	78	84	52
Dominican Republic	5	11	39	62	70	78	74	79	52
Ecuador	4	14	46	61	68	77	80	82	56
Guyana	9	17	42	57	64	84	90	92	55
Haiti	3	16	42	59	69	77	79	87	46
Jamaica	4	23	41	53	64	77	79	91	51
Mexico	10	10	42	54	69	77	82	89	57
Panama	8	12	42	73	82	85	87	87	63
Paraguay	1	5	21	31	41	46	53	66	32
Peru	6	20	48	62	74	80	81	89	61
Trinidad and Tobago	5	13	39	60	75	79	86	90	47
Venezuela	9	10	41	64	74	85	85	88	55
SUB-AVERAGE	6	14	41	58	69	77	80	86	53
Asia and Oceania									
Bangladesh[b]	12	43	56	66	77	84	90	93	63
Fiji	2	7	34	48	67	76	80	90	50
Indonesia	4	9	29	45	57	69	78	88	39
Jordan	4	5	15	25	38	47	54	73	42
Malaysia	0	4	22	32	54	65	79	91	45
Nepal	2	5	24	41	59	66	81	90	30
Pakistan	0	3	23	39	61	71	87	90	43
Philippines	1	7	33	51	69	73	76	85	54
Republic of Korea	12	13	66	86	92	95	96	99	72
Sri Lanka	2	14	49	73	87	89	94	94	61
Syrian Arab Republic	1	2	13	28	45	52	54	66	37
Thailand	6	19	49	70	85	92	92	96	61
Yemen	6	5	11	20	25	35	48	52	19
SUB-AVERAGE	3	7	31	47	62	69	77	84	46
TOTAL	4	8	29	43	55	63	68	76	42

Source: World Fertility Survey standard recode tapes.
[a] A current pregnancy is counted as a living child.
[b] Data not considered comparable and not included in calculation of sub-averages.
[c] Formerly called the Ivory Coast.

moment that women in the two countries do not use contraception, so that the women progress from parity to parity at the same tempo, regardless of whether they want additional children. Then, the two countries will have identical parity distributions and identical proportions wanting no more children at each parity. Now assume that the women in country A successfully adopt contraception for stopping purposes. Then, the women of country A will be concentrated at their desired family sizes, and at each desired parity they will want no more children. As a result, at each parity the proportions of women wanting no more children will be higher than those in country B. In other words, extensive contraceptive use for stopping purposes can increase parity-specific proportions wanting no more children.[14]

The reverse effect can theoretically occur, however, with the widespread use of contraception for spacing purposes or, alternatively, with the use of traditional birth-spacing practices, such as breast-feeding and postpartum abstinence. Again, assume that in country A women use contraception for spacing purposes at a given parity. In a cross-sectional survey, women will be more concentrated at that parity than in country B but will want more children. Thus, the proportion wanting no more children at that parity will be lower than that in country B. If such contraceptive use is widespread enough and women wait long enough at a given parity, then this depressing effect on the proportion not wanting additional children will be sufficient to offset any increasing effect due to contraceptive use for stopping purposes.

Thus, countries with identical desired family size distributions may have very different proportions wanting no more children at each parity, if they differ with respect to the extent of contraceptive use for stopping or spacing purposes. These effects should be kept in mind when making international comparisons of parity-specific proportions not wanting additional children.

Figure 11 summarizes the regional differences in mean proportions who wanted no more children by graphing those mean percentages by the number of living children. Women in Latin America and the Caribbean and in Asia and Oceania had very similar distributions, with slightly larger proportions of women who wanted to stop childbearing at each family size in the former region. Women in Africa had much lower proportions who wanted to cease childbearing at each family size.

Figure 11. Percentage who wanted no more children, by number of living children, for regions

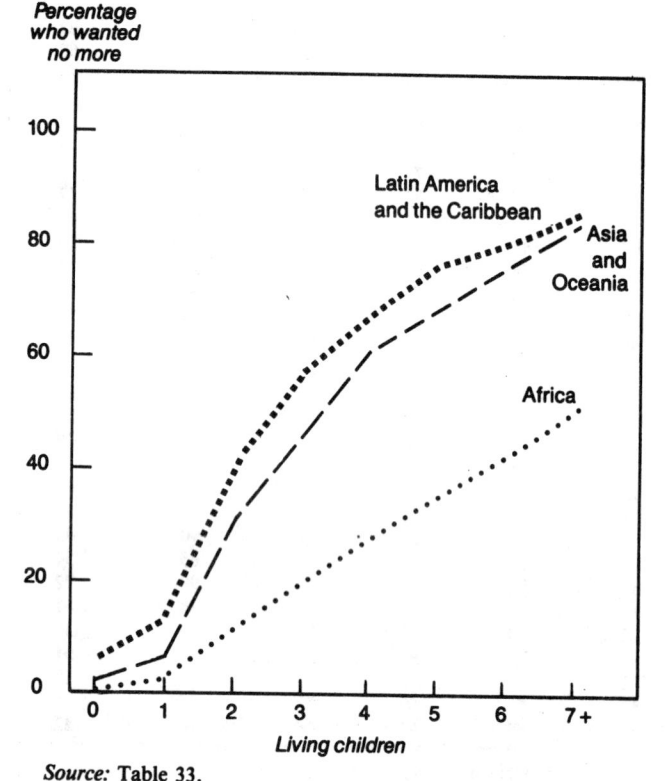

Source: Table 33.

When the countries are grouped by level of development and strength of family planning programme effort, the overall percentage of women who wanted no more children increases steadily from 25 to 55 with increasing levels of development, and from 23 to 54 with increasing family planning programme activity (table 34). Even when the sub-Saharan countries are removed from the averages, there remains a difference of 15 percentage points between development groups I and IV and a 17-point difference between the extreme family planning groups. Most of the overall contrast is due to differing proportions of women who wanted to stop childbearing at each family size rather than to differing underlying distributions of children ever born (figures 12 and 13, table 34). These results offer support for a link between socio-economic development and the desire for smaller

Figure 12. Percentage who wanted no more children, by number of living children, various levels of development

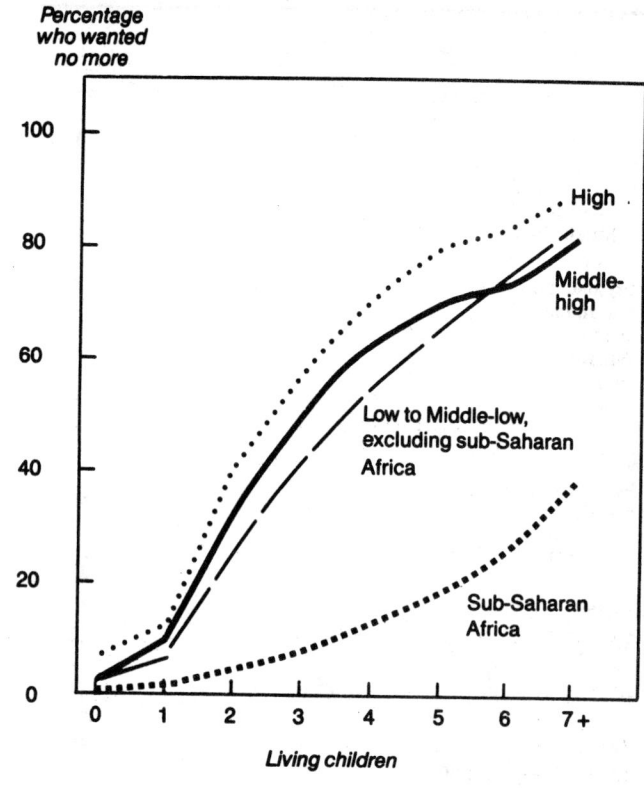

Source: Table 33.

Figure 13. Percentage who wanted no more children, by number of living children, for strength of family planning programme effort

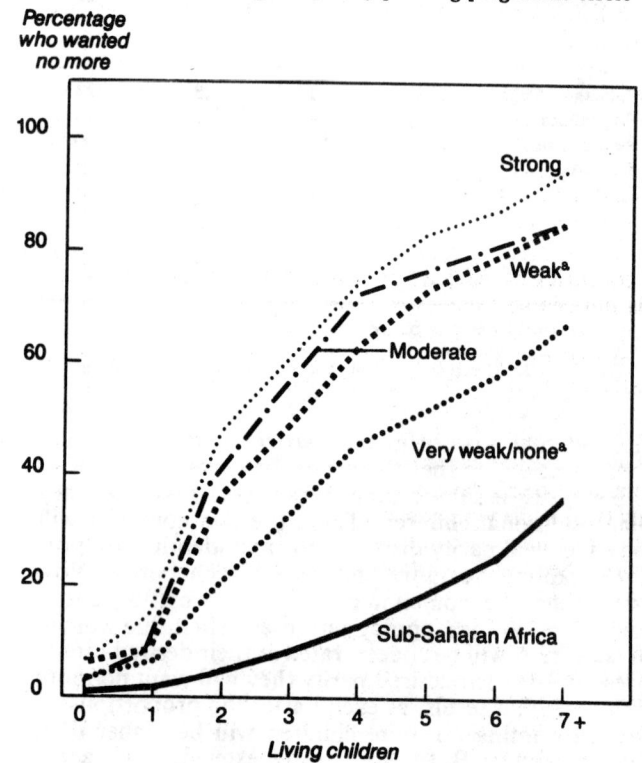

Source: Table 33.
[a] Excluding sub-Saharan Africa.

TABLE 34. OBSERVED AND STANDARDIZED PERCENTAGES OF CURRENTLY MARRIED, FECUND WOMEN WHO WANTED NO MORE CHILDREN: AVERAGES BY LEVEL OF DEVELOPMENT AND STRENGTH OF FAMILY PLANNING PROGRAMME EFFORT

	All countries		Excluding sub-Saharan Africa	
	Observed	Standardized[a]	Observed	Standardized[a]
Level of development				
I. High	55	54	55	54
II. Middle-high	50	47	50	47
III. Middle-low	26	30	45	46
IV. Low	25	28	40	41
Family planning programme effort				
1. Strong	54	57	54	57
2. Moderate	54	52	54	52
3. Weak	45	47	48	49
4. Very weak/none	23	25	38	35

Source: Table 33.

NOTES: Averages excluding data for Bangladesh, Cameroon and Senegal. For sub-Saharan Africa, average proportion who wanted no more children is 12 per cent before and 13 per cent after standardization.

[a] Standardized for number of living children using a standard distribution approximating the average for all countries.

families. It remains true, however, that the most impressive contrast in proportion wanting to stop childbearing is not that between the highest and lowest development groups, but that between sub-Saharan countries and all others.

Besides the number of children already born to a woman, there are other factors which may affect her decision to cease childbearing. Age is one such factor. Table 35 presents the percentage of women who wanted no more children for family sizes two, four and six, classified by age groups 15-24, 25-34 and 35-49. In general, at each of the family sizes considered, older women were much more likely than younger women to want to stop childbearing. This tendency is particularly noticeable at family sizes two and four, when comparing women aged 35-49 years with those aged 15-24 years. Consider Malaysia, for example. For two-child families, only 12 per cent of the women aged 15-24 years and 21 per cent of those aged 25-34 years wanted no more children. However, among women aged 35-49 years, 50 per cent wanted no more. A similar pattern, though not always as vivid, is observed in most other countries. In a majority of countries of Africa for which data can be obtained, it is noticeable that, even for women with six children, the proportion who wanted to stop childbearing did not exceed 40 per cent, even for the oldest women. Several reasons can be offered to explain this finding of higher proportions of older women not wanting more children after controlling for family size. The first is the selection effect discussed earlier—that is, by age 35 most of the women who still have only two children may have wanted only two, while younger women with only two may prefer more but have not yet had time fully to achieve their desires. Secondly, it may be that older women want to avoid births once they have children old enough to marry and bear children themselves. This has often been called the "grand maternal effect". Lastly, it could be that women who have fewer children by a given age are more likely to be aware of childbearing costs as they become older, and so wish to cease childbearing. This may imply that women who postpone births may ultimately not have these births, so that in the long run they have fewer children then they had originally desired.

Alternative estimates of mean desired family size can be derived from the question on the desire for more children and the additional number desired and compared with the directly reported desired family size. Two such approaches are briefly described below. The first type of estimate is called the "stopping-point approach" and is based on a synthetic-cohort measure. In brief, this procedure estimates the average number of children a synthetic cohort of women would have at the end of their reproductive life if they progressed to each parity at the same rate as observed from the actual data and stopped childbearing according to the actual reported proportion of women who wanted no more children at each parity. Several methods of estimation using this approach have been proposed, including those by Udry, Bauman and Chase (1973), Pullum (1979), Rodríguez and Trussell (1981), Lightbourne (1977) and Nour (1983).

Based on extensive simulations, it was concluded that for many countries "reasonably good" measures of preferred family size could be obtained through combining the Rodríguez and Trussell estimates with those of Lightbourne.[15] The Lightbourne measure is based on information on the number of living children and whether the respondent wanted more children. The Rodríguez and Trussell measure, in addition to this, also used information on whether the last birth was wanted[16] (Lightbourne, 1985a). However, when actual birth intervals were particularly long, either because of effective use of contraception for postponing the next birth or because of traditional birth-spacing practices, both measures were found to be overestimates of the actual mean desired family size. With the exceptions noted above, it can be said that the mean desired family size, as reported directly, generally does offer a reasonably good approximation to the mean number of living children women would have if they stopped childbearing when they wanted no more children (Lightbourne, 1985a).

Family size preferences can also be measured by the "wanted family size" variable, which is constructed by adding the number of living children (counting a current pregnancy as a living child) to the number of additional children wanted. This latter variable is defined for respondents who replied "Yes" or "No" to the question whether more children were wanted, but the variable is undefined for respondents who were undecided about whether to cease childbearing because those women were not asked about the number of additional children desired.[17] Several criticisms of the "wanted family size" variable have been noted (Ryder, 1973). First, this variable is indeterminate in meaning because it combines a varying factual component (number of living children) with a varying attitudinal component (number of additional children wanted). Thus, a woman with a wanted family size of three may have had zero children and wanted three, or she may have had three and wanted no more, etc. Secondly, as mentioned earlier, this variable is not defined for women who were undecided about their desire to cease childbearing. Thirdly, this variable has some inherent upward bias, because no adjustment is made for unwanted children already born to women who indicated a current desire to cease childbearing.

C. SEX PREFERENCES

As with size preferences, various questions have been asked in surveys to measure sex preferences. These questions can also be conveniently grouped into the four basic

TABLE 35. PERCENTAGE WHO WANTED NO MORE CHILDREN AT PARITIES 2, 4 AND 6 FOR AGE GROUPS 15-24, 25-34 AND 35-39[a]

	Parity 2			Parity 4			Parity 6[b]	
	15-24	25-34	35-39	15-24	25-34	35-39	25-34	35-39
Africa								
Benin	1	2	12	8	4	23	14	23
Cameroon[c]	4	2	d	d	5	d	10	d
Côte d'Ivoire[e]	3	1	1	3	2	6	7	14
Egypt	30	49	61	65	76	79	87	91
Ghana	3	2	10	19	13	18	27	38
Kenya	3	2	12	14	15	22	22	30
Lesotho	9	6	13	d	27	23	d	45
Mauritania	7	8	6	16	10	16	12	21
Morocco	17	17	29	49	46	39	65	72
Senegal[c]	0	3	d	0	0	d	d	d
Sudan	8	4	17	11	17	21	32	32
Tunisia	19	26	47	d	57	72	71	85
Latin America and the Caribbean								
Colombia	52	49	63	69	78	86	90	81
Costa Rica	28	34	54	d	66	75	73	83
Dominican Republic	39	31	d	69	72	66	79	69
Ecuador	42	44	68	58	67	73	82	78
Guyana	47	28	61	66	60	74	87	94
Haiti	45	39	49	d	76	62	86	76
Jamaica	36	39	62	59	59	77	79	81
Mexico	39	45	55	61	70	75	78	85
Panama	27	42	72	70	80	88	84	89
Paraguay	21	11	45	d	29	59	47	56
Peru	49	46	52	70	73	78	82	80
Trinidad and Tobago	33	34	61	58	69	86	83	87
Venezuela	39	37	65	69	69	84	80	89
Asia and Oceania								
Bangladesh[c]	56	54	73	74	74	88	85	95
Fiji	30	33	53	59	62	80	76	82
Indonesia	20	31	51	43	53	68	72	82
Jordan	7	20	d	33	36	56	48	65
Malaysia	12	21	50	39	51	64	74	83
Nepal	21	22	40	56	57	63	71	85
Pakistan	18	21	58	69	54	74	81	92
Philippines	26	33	50	60	67	73	70	80
Republic of Korea	53	65	85	d	87	97	d	97
Sri Lanka	42	45	67	79	84	93	89	97
Syrian Arab Republic	9	16	41	39	42	56	47	61
Thailand	45	51	56	d	81	93	89	94
Yemen	11	10	22	30	21	31	48	48

Source: World Fertility Survey standard recode tapes.
[a] The age range for Costa Rica and Panama is 20-49; for Venezuela, 15-44; and for all other countries, 15-49.
[b] Age group 15-24 for parity 6 was omitted because the sample size was fewer than 10 for most countries.
[c] Data not considered comparable.
[d] Sample size is fewer than 10.
[e] Formerly called the Ivory Coast.

categories proposed by McClelland (1983) for classifying size preference questions. The parallel to the "how many more" category for size preferences can be called the "sex of next child" category, where the desired sex of the next birth is ascertained for women who say that they want more children. The "over again" category includes questions that ask the respondents to state their desired sex compositions if life could be lived over again. As in the case of desired family size, this measure is subject to rationalization effects based on the existing sex composition of the respondent's family. In the "ordering" category, respondents are generally asked to rank-order a series of family compositions.[18] Lastly, in the projective category, respondents are asked to state their ideal family compositions for their ideal family size.

In the absence of such data, sex preferences have often been inferred from comparisons of behavioural responses to various compositions of families. Examples include whether baby boys were more likely to be breast-fed or were breast-fed longer than baby girls (Millman, 1981); whether contraceptive use was more likely among women with sons than among women with no sons (Lee, 1977); or whether parents had another child sooner following the death of an infant son than that of an infant daughter (Rukanuddin, 1982). As indicated previously, these types of analyses are not included in this chapter.

A related method of measuring sex preferences (and the effect of sex preferences on fertility) is through an examination of parity progression ratios as a function of the existing sex composition of the family, assuming that women with undesirable sex compositions are more likely to proceed to the next higher parity than women with desirable sex compositions. There are two major problems in using parity progression ratios to indicate sex preferences. First, in order to calculate these ratios, the data have to be aggregated over many women. This requirement of aggregation means that any pattern of progression from parity to parity can be observed only if a large majority of the sample population has the same sex preference. Secondly, this assumption ignores the possibility that some women may not have additional children because if the next child is not of the desired sex the resulting family composition may be even less desirable. Further details concerning these problems can be found in McClelland (1979). These limitations can also be applied to other behavioural response studies and may explain why many parity progression ratio studies (and other studies based on behavioural responses) failed to find any consistent effect of sex preferences on fertility.

The WFS questionnaires included only one specific question to ascertain the sex preferences of respondents, namely, the desired sex of the respondent's next child. Additional information on sex preferences can also be obtained from the data based on responses to the question on the desire for more children. Even though the absence of any other questions to elicit the sex preferences of respondents limits the understanding of these preferences, the information derived from these data can be useful, especially because a large number of countries are being compared. Results based on these two questions are discussed next. Since sex preferences are not expected to be affected by strength of family planning programme effort, averages for programme strength are not presented.

Preferred sex of next child

The question asked to obtain the respondent's preferences for the sex of her next child was, "Would you prefer your next child to be a boy or a girl?". Slight modifications in the wording were made if the respondent had no children or was pregnant at the time of the interview. In all countries, this question was limited to currently married women who considered themselves fecund and who had expressed a desire for more children. Thus, women who did not want any more children were not asked about their preferences as to family composition. This exclusion should be kept in mind, particularly because in many countries close to half the sample did not want any more children.[19] The findings with respect to this question are presented in table 36. Responses to this question were grouped into three categories: "Prefer boy"; "Prefer girl"; and "Undecided". Included in this last category are women who said either sex was equally acceptable and women who could not (or did not) state a preference.

Son preference, as indicated by the much larger proportion of women who preferred sons over daughters, was found to be strongest in the Southern Asian countries of Bangladesh, Nepal and Pakistan (in each country over 50 per cent of the women preferred a son, compared with under 10 per cent who preferred a daughter); and in Jordan, Mauritania, the Republic of Korea and the Syrian Arab Republic. Daughter preference is evident only in Jamaica, where over 52 per cent expressed a desire for a daughter, compared with 31 per cent who wanted a son. Roughly equal preferences for sons and daughters can be found in several countries, most of which are in the Latin America and the Caribbean region. These countries include Colombia, Costa Rica, Panama, Paraguay and Ghana. From the regional point of view, son preference seems strongest in Asia and Oceania, where close to 50 per cent preferred a son, compared with just 20 per cent who wanted a daughter.

TABLE 36. PREFERENCES FOR SEX OF NEXT CHILD AND PREFERENCE RATIO AMONG CURRENTLY MARRIED, FECUND WOMEN WHO WANTED ANOTHER CHILD

Region and country	Preference Boy (percentage) (1)	Girl (percentage)	Undecided (percentage) (2)	Preference ratio[a] (3)
Africa				
Benin	18.9	11.6	69.4	1.2
Cameroon[b]	23.0	14.8	62.2	1.2
Côte d'Ivoire[c]	23.6	17.2	59.2	1.1
Egypt	40.5	20.6	38.9	1.5
Ghana	32.9	34.4	32.7	1.0
Kenya	25.0	20.8	54.2	1.1
Lesotho	51.1	31.3	17.6	1.5
Mauritania	44.1	9.8	46.0	2.1
Morocco	26.1	17.7	56.1	1.2
Senegal	42.1	22.9	34.9	1.5
Sudan	41.8	22.3	35.9	1.5
Tunisia	29.0	17.5	53.5	1.3
SUB-AVERAGE	34.1	20.6	45.3	1.4
Latin America and the Caribbean				
Colombia	42.1	40.5	17.4	1.0
Costa Rica	31.6	32.5	35.8	1.0
Dominican Republic	46.8	39.4	13.8	1.2
Ecuador	41.9	32.8	25.2	1.2
Guyana	39.1	35.8	25.1	1.1
Haiti	24.8	28.8	46.3	0.9
Jamaica	31.1	52.2	16.6	0.7
Mexico	37.2	28.3	34.5	1.2
Panama	39.4	40.7	19.9	1.0
Paraguay	35.5	37.3	27.2	1.0
Peru	38.9	33.8	27.2	1.1
Trinidad and Tobago	42.4	35.5	22.1	1.1
Venezuela	33.0	42.8	24.2	0.8
SUB-AVERAGE	36.7	37.5	25.8	1.0
Asia and Oceania				
Bangladesh	59.9	8.3	31.8	3.3
Fiji	43.3	30.5	26.1	1.3
Indonesia	34.5	29.2	36.3	1.1
Jordan	40.8	12.0	47.2	1.9
Malaysia	36.1	28.5	35.4	1.2
Nepal	67.2	7.5	25.3	4.0
Pakistan	71.6	5.0	23.4	4.9
Philippines	33.7	36.9	29.4	0.9
Republic of Korea	67.1	13.7	19.3	3.3
Sri Lanka	52.2	30.6	17.2	1.5
Syrian Arab Republic	49.6	11.0	39.4	2.3
Thailand	49.0	34.5	16.5	1.4
Yemen	20.5	9.1	70.4	1.3
SUB-AVERAGE	48.1	19.8	32.1	2.2
TOTAL	39.9	26.3	33.8	1.5

Source: World Fertility Survey standard recode tapes.
[a] Ratio of the number of women who preferred a son to those who preferred a daughter, after allocating the "undecideds" equally between the "preferred boy" and "preferred girl" groups.
[b] Data not considered comparable and not included in calculation of sub-averages.
[c] Formerly called the Ivory Coast.

A noticeable feature of table 36 is the substantial proportions of women who did not state a specific preference for the sex of their next child and were coded as "undecided". This proportion ranges from 14 per cent in the Dominican Republic to over 70 per cent in Yemen. For most countries, the range is from 15 to 40 per cent. Six countries in Africa recorded proportions higher than 40 per cent (Benin, Côte d'Ivoire, Kenya, Mauritania, Morocco and Tunisia) as well as Haiti in the Caribbean, and Jordan and Yemen in Western Asia. Considering the regions as a whole, 45 per cent in Africa had no preference, followed by Asia and Oceania, with 32 per cent, and Latin America and the Caribbean, with 26 per cent.

The response "Undecided" to the sex preference question captures very different aspects of sex preference. A woman may be undecided and express no preference for a particular sex because she really does not care whether her next child is a boy or girl. This could be because either she genuinely has no preferences about the sex composition of her family or she has already achieved her desired sex composition (say, at least one child of each sex). Again, she may be undecided because it is against the cultural norm to express a desire for a specific sex of a future child, since basically the sex of one's child is not amenable to choice. These various explanations about the "undecided" category make it difficult to interpret the differences in proportions undecided among the countries.

Further, the large proportions of women who are coded as "undecided" create a problem of interpretation in the case of proportions who expressed a clear preference for either boys or girls. To take an extreme example, consider Yemen, where 70 per cent were undecided. At the same time, 21 per cent of the respondents wanted a son, 9 per cent a daughter. Does this mean that women in Yemen have no preferences as to the sex composition of their families? Or does it mean that son preference is strong because the ratio of women who preferred sons to those who preferred daughters is greater than two to one?

Two strategies are followed to help answer such questions. First, inferences about sex preferences based on the responses "Prefer boy" and "Prefer girl" are made only for those countries where fewer than 50 per cent are reported as undecided. Secondly, a "preference ratio" is calculated, based on the assumption that on average the "undecideds" are more or less evenly split between their desire for a son or daughter (Cleland, Verrall and Vaessen, 1983). These ratios are given in column (3) of table 36. Values of 0.8 or less are considered to indicate daughter preference; values between 0.9 and 1.1, equal preferences for sons and daughters; values between 1.2 and 1.5, moderate son preference; and values greater than 1.6, strong son preference (Cleland, Verrall and Vaessen, 1983). Using this classification, daughter preference is found in Jamaica and Venezuela, and very strong son preferences are found in Bangladesh, Jordan, Mauritania, Nepal, Pakistan, the Republic of Korea and the Syrian Arab Republic. Most countries fall in the "moderate son" or "equal" preference group. Regional averages indicate a strong son preference in Asia and Oceania, a moderate son preference in Africa and an equal preference for sons and daughters in Latin America and the Caribbean.

Table 37 shows the average proportion of women who wanted a son, a daughter or either, and the average "preference ratio" for the countries grouped according to level of development. The general expectation is that, as development increases, preferences for a particular sex become less strong. The data seem to indicate this tendency. The preference ratio indicates a strong son preference in the low development group and a moderate son preference in the other groups. It is, once again, difficult to isolate the regional/cultural component of this relationship from the effects of socio-economic development. The example of the Republic of Korea (high development)

TABLE 37. PREFERENCES FOR SEX OF NEXT CHILD AND PREFERENCE RATIO AMONG CURRENTLY MARRIED, FECUND WOMEN WHO WANTED ANOTHER CHILD, BY LEVEL OF DEVELOPMENT

Level of development	Boy (percentage)	Girl (percentage)	Undecided (percentage)	Preference ratio
I. High	40.0	34.6	25.1	1.2
II. Middle-high	41.0	29.0	29.7	1.4
III. Middle-low	34.5	25.2	40.3	1.2
IV. Low	46.5	14.2	39.2	2.4

Source: Table 36.

shows that a high degree of son preference can persist after considerable socio-economic progress has occurred.

The proportion indifferent or undecided about the sex of the next child is lowest in the upper development groups. It is unclear whether this represents a genuine difference in underlying preferences or simply a greater willingness to express an opinion. Women in the relatively developed countries tend, among other things, to be more educated than their counterparts in the least developed countries, a factor that may increase respondents' confidence and willingness to speak out. Whatever the reason, the proportion undecided or indifferent about the sex of the next child tended to be high in the same countries where many women gave non-numerical answers to the question about desired family size: in countries where under 5 per cent of women did not report a desired size, roughly one quarter, on average, were undecided or indifferent about the sex of the next child, compared with roughly 50 per cent where the level of non-numerical responses to the question on family size was higher than 5 per cent.

Sex preference for the next child is strongly influenced by the existing sex composition of the family. To examine this, table 38 presents the sex preferences for five types of family composition: all sons; more sons than daughters; equal numbers of sons and daughters; more daughters than sons; and all daughters. The evidence from this table overwhelmingly points to a preference for a two-sex family, though, at the same time, there is evidence of strong son preference in a few countries, including Bangladesh, Nepal, Pakistan and the Republic of Korea. Among families with only sons, the general tendency is for women to want a daughter. This tendency is especially prevalent in countries of the Latin America and the Caribbean region, where, in each country, at least about 70 per cent of the women with all sons desired a daughter for their next child, compared with fewer than 10 per cent who desired yet another son. A strong preference for at least one daughter is also generally found in the countries of Africa and of Asia and Oceania, but this pattern is not prevalent in all countries. In Mauritania, Nepal and Pakistan, women are more likely to want another son than a daughter even if their existing children are all boys. At least 20 per cent of women with all-boy families wanted another son in these three countries, plus Bangladesh, the Republic of Korea and the Syrian Arab Republic. By contrast, among women with all-girl families, the proportion who wanted another daughter never exceeds 12 per cent (in Jamaica) and does not exceed 5 per cent in Africa or in Asia and Oceania.

A similar picture emerges when considering families with either more sons than daughters or the reverse. In

TABLE 38. PREFERENCES FOR SEX OF NEXT CHILD, BY FAMILY COMPOSITION AMONG CURRENTLY MARRIED, FECUND WOMEN WHO WANTED ANOTHER CHILD
(Percentage)

Region and country	All boys Preference Boy	All boys Preference Girl	All boys Undecided	More boys Preference Boy	More boys Preference Girl	More boys Undecided	Balance Preference Boy	Balance Preference Girl	Balance Undecided	More girls Preference Boy	More girls Preference Girl	More girls Undecided	All girls Preference Boy	All girls Preference Girl	All girls Undecided
Africa															
Benin	4.4	30.7	64.9	8.9	15.9	75.2	15.2	5.5	79.2	30.4	3.3	66.3	37.3	2.0	60.7
Cameroon[a]	7.3	27.0	65.7	16.4	14.8	68.9	21.3	16.0	62.7	17.1	1.4	81.4	40.6	0.7	58.7
Côte d'Ivoire[b]	5.6	41.8	52.6	8.2	28.9	62.9	17.7	9.6	72.7	41.9	2.3	55.8	47.1	2.1	50.8
Egypt	13.8	58.2	28.1	30.7	20.1	49.2	39.1	8.2	52.7	60.9	2.3	36.8	72.1	2.2	25.7
Ghana	4.3	70.0	25.7	7.7	58.5	33.8	33.4	27.3	39.3	56.9	8.6	34.5	69.7	4.1	26.2
Kenya	6.5	40.3	53.2	6.6	36.3	57.1	17.3	19.2	63.5	38.2	4.8	57.1	54.9	3.1	42.0
Lesotho	11.5	71.4	17.1	16.7	64.7	18.7	52.1	20.3	27.6	78.1	6.5	15.4	87.4	1.8	10.8
Mauritania	34.3	22.2	43.5	32.7	18.0	49.3	46.8	5.2	48.0	52.8	3.0	44.2	51.6	3.2	45.2
Morocco	3.2	51.4	45.4	6.9	34.4	58.8	22.9	4.3	72.9	42.2	2.6	55.2	58.1	3.1	38.8
Senegal	13.9	59.5	26.6	20.6	32.9	46.6	50.0	10.0	40.0	53.5	2.3	44.2	66.1	1.8	32.1
Sudan	15.4	54.9	29.7	27.4	35.8	36.9	41.4	13.6	45.1	58.1	6.4	35.5	70.3	3.1	26.6
Tunisia	3.8	52.9	43.3	9.4	30.9	59.7	18.7	4.4	76.9	61.5	0.6	37.9	67.8	1.1	31.1
SUB-AVERAGE	10.6	50.3	39.1	16.0	34.2	49.8	32.2	11.6	56.2	52.2	3.9	43.9	62.1	2.5	35.4
Latin America and the Caribbean															
Colombia	4.6	84.3	11.1	16.7	61.7	21.7	34.9	41.9	23.3	75.8	8.8	15.4	78.5	6.5	15.0
Costa Rica	8.5	69.4	22.1	11.8	52.0	36.2	20.4	18.9	60.7	54.8	7.9	37.3	72.5	7.8	19.7
Dominican Republic	6.9	88.9	4.2	13.2	64.7	22.1	20.2	28.1	51.7	67.1	14.8	18.2	86.2	8.0	5.8
Ecuador	7.4	76.4	16.2	17.8	49.6	32.6	36.6	25.0	38.4	63.3	11.5	25.2	79.4	5.6	15.0
Guyana	4.4	81.4	14.3	13.8	68.8	17.5	32.2	25.2	42.7	65.0	8.8	26.3	81.2	4.4	14.4
Haiti	1.2	69.7	29.1	2.4	31.0	66.7	22.9	14.3	62.9	26.2	11.9	61.9	62.4	0.6	36.9
Jamaica	3.9	87.7	8.4	13.9	69.6	16.5	23.1	57.0	19.8	62.7	18.6	18.6	74.1	12.1	13.9
Mexico	8.9	69.6	21.5	14.0	47.1	38.9	32.7	18.7	48.6	61.1	5.9	33.0	72.1	6.4	21.6
Panama	6.1	83.8	10.1	18.1	60.2	21.7	30.2	41.9	27.9	64.9	13.2	21.9	80.2	6.4	13.4
Paraguay	8.0	78.5	13.5	10.9	61.5	27.6	24.2	30.1	45.8	59.6	9.1	31.4	77.7	6.3	16.0
Peru	8.4	75.2	16.4	13.7	61.4	24.8	40.9	20.0	39.1	57.1	5.1	37.9	76.6	4.0	19.4
Trinidad and Tobago	6.7	81.3	12.0	18.3	67.6	14.1	26.2	31.6	42.3	79.0	11.6	9.5	80.7	5.2	14.1
Venezuela	3.0	83.0	14.0	5.3	71.1	23.7	20.8	40.8	38.3	56.5	13.0	30.4	75.2	8.3	16.5
SUB-AVERAGE	6.0	79.2	14.8	13.1	58.9	28.0	28.1	30.0	41.9	61.0	10.8	28.2	76.7	6.3	17.0
Asia and Oceania															
Bangladesh	26.7	38.2	35.1	47.3	5.5	47.3	60.9	1.5	37.7	64.8	0.0	35.2	85.3	0.9	13.8
Fiji	6.3	80.3	13.4	9.5	67.1	23.4	37.6	18.6	43.8	71.1	4.7	24.2	87.5	2.4	10.1
Indonesia	3.8	72.1	24.1	9.5	52.3	38.3	25.8	19.9	54.3	54.2	6.5	39.2	71.0	2.1	26.8
Jordan	14.1	43.8	42.2	23.1	15.5	61.4	35.6	3.6	60.7	62.9	0.3	36.8	63.8	1.5	34.8
Malaysia	3.5	73.4	23.1	9.6	55.9	34.5	33.7	16.4	50.0	67.6	3.9	28.5	76.0	0.9	23.2
Nepal	34.6	29.2	36.2	44.2	15.8	40.0	67.9	2.4	29.6	86.2	0.5	13.3	88.4	0.7	10.8
Pakistan	41.2	19.4	39.4	55.0	6.0	38.9	71.4	0.4	28.2	87.4	0.7	11.9	93.2	0.2	6.6
Philippines	2.4	82.8	14.8	5.0	63.2	31.9	24.4	30.9	44.7	59.3	4.9	35.7	79.0	2.6	18.4
Republic of Korea	24.5	47.2	28.3	31.3	31.3	37.5	80.0	0.9	19.1	100.0	0.0	...	95.9	0.0	4.1
Sri Lanka	5.9	83.6	10.6	32.2	32.2	35.6	59.0	7.6	33.3	84.3	2.3	13.5	92.3	1.5	6.2
Syrian Arab Republic	22.0	37.0	41.0	37.2	13.8	49.0	43.8	2.4	53.8	71.8	1.2	26.9	72.6	1.2	26.2
Thailand	3.8	87.2	9.0	18.2	63.6	18.2	48.5	21.6	29.9	74.4	6.1	19.5	90.2	2.9	6.9
Yemen	9.9	23.1	67.0	14.6	10.2	75.2	17.9	6.6	75.5	27.4	4.3	68.3	38.3	1.6	60.2
SUB-AVERAGE	15.3	55.2	29.6	25.9	33.3	40.9	46.7	10.2	43.1	70.1	2.7	29.4	79.5	1.4	19.1

Source: World Fertility Survey standard recode tapes.
[a] Data not considered comparable and not used in calculation of sub-averages.
[b] Formerly called the Ivory Coast.

each case, the preference is generally in the direction of a balance in the sex composition of the family. Thus, in families with more sons than daughters, women tend to want another daughter, while their preference is for a son if they have more daughters. For example, in Costa Rica, among families with more sons than daughters, 52 per cent of the respondents preferred a daughter, compared with 12 per cent who preferred a son. On the other hand, among families with more daughters than sons, 55 per cent preferred a son, and 8 per cent, a daughter. There are, however, a number of exceptions to this pattern. Among families with more sons, larger proportions of women wanted an additional son rather than a daughter in Bangladesh, Egypt, Jordan, Mauritania, Nepal, Pakistan, the Syrian Arab Republic and Yemen. This preference was particularly strong in Bangladesh, Nepal and Pakistan. In the last country, for instance, 55 per cent wanted another son, compared with just 6 per cent who wanted another daughter. In all countries in Latin America and the Caribbean, however, more women preferred a daughter.

Among families with more daughters, women tended to prefer a son. As in all-daughter families, this pattern appears universal. No more than 10 per cent in any country in Africa or Asia and Oceania desired another daughter. In several Latin American and Caribbean countries, the proportion is a bit higher, reaching a maximum of 19 per cent in Jamaica.

In spite of the evidence pointing to a desire for a balanced family, in most countries a large proportion of women in each category of the sex composition variable remained undecided. Among women with only sons in the family, over 50 per cent were undecided in Benin, Côte d'Ivoire, Kenya and Yemen, and over 40 per cent in Jordan, Mauritania, Morocco, the Syrian Arab Republic and Tunisia. Among women with all daughters, over 50 per cent were undecided in Benin, Côte d'Ivoire and Yemen. High proportions are also found in Kenya and Mauritania. In a number of countries, the proportion of undecided is much greater in all-son families than in all-daughter families. Countries with this characteristic include Bangladesh (35 versus 14 per cent), Nepal (36 versus 11 per cent), Pakistan (39 versus 7 per cent) and the Republic of Korea (28 versus 4 per cent). One interpretation of this may be that in these countries women with all sons are likely to be unconcerned about the sex of their next child. Having yet another son would be acceptable to them. However, women with only daughters may have a stronger desire for a child of the other sex. Thus, a much lower proportion of these women are undecided. Such an explanation seems particularly appropriate for those countries where strong son preferences have been established by other studies.

In general, the proportions of women who were undecided are higher in the two-sex families than in the one-sex families. For example, in Haiti, from 29 to 37 per cent of women with one-sex families were undecided, in comparison with over 60 per cent of women with two-sex families, adding to the evidence that women desire children of both sexes.

Table 39 presents the sex preferences for each type of family composition by level of development. Two patterns are evident. In general, for each type of composition, the proportion of women coded as "undecided" declines with increasing levels of development, as noted earlier. Among families with all boys, for example, the

TABLE 39. PREFERENCES FOR SEX OF NEXT CHILD, BY LEVEL OF DEVELOPMENT AND FAMILY COMPOSITION
(*Percentage*)

Level of development and sex composition	Boy	Girl	Undecided
I. High			
All boys	7	76	16
More boys	15	59	26
Balance	34	28	38
More girls	69	9	22
All girls	79	6	15
II. Middle-high			
All boys	8	69	23
More boys	19	43	38
Balance	35	19	46
More girls	66	5	29
All girls	78	3	19
III. Middle-low			
All boys	7	54	39
More boys	13	39	48
Balance	29	16	56
More girls	49	4	47
All girls	63	2	35
IV. Low			
All boys	20	39	41
More boys	28	19	53
Balance	44	7	50
More girls	54	4	42
All girls	66	2	33

Source: Table 38.

proportion undecided declines from 41 per cent in development group IV to 16 per cent in development group I. At the same time, there is evidence that, with development, respondents are more likely to desire for their next child that sex which will help to balance the family.

Proportions wanting no more children

In this section, inferences about the sex preferences of women are made based on information on whether more children were wanted. Table 40 presents the proportion of currently married, fecund women who did not want any more children, controlling for current family size and sex composition. This sex composition variable was described above. Only proportions for family sizes two, three and four are shown because sample sizes for larger families are extremely small.

Regional averages show that very few African women wish to stop childbearing at any of the family sizes shown, resulting in very little variation across the sex composition variable. Only in Egypt, Morocco and Tunisia can some inferences about sex preferences be made. In each of these countries, some son preference is implied because, for women with three or four children, larger proportions wanted to stop childbearing if they had at least two sons. This pattern is also prevalent in Asia and Oceania, where the differences are more pronounced than in either Africa or Latin America and the Caribbean. For example, in Asia and Oceania, among women with four children, an average of 66-67 per cent desired no more children if they had two or three sons, compared with 35 per cent if they had no sons and 55 per cent if they had no daughters. No comparable range exists for Latin America and the Caribbean. For each type of sex composition, the proportion who did not want more children averages 64-70 per cent for women who had four children. Thus, in Asia

TABLE 40. PERCENTAGE WHO WANTED NO MORE CHILDREN, BY FAMILY COMPOSITION AMONG CURRENTLY MARRIED, FECUND AND NON-PREGNANT WOMEN WITH FROM TWO TO FOUR LIVING CHILDREN

Region and country	Two children				Three children				Four children			
	All boys	Both	All girls	All boys	More boys	More girls	All girls	All boys	More boys	Equal	More girls	All girls
Africa												
Benin	4	3	2	9	9	7	2	0[a]	13	13	9	0
Cameroon[b]	5	5	1	10	10	7	15	20	14	9	11	7
Côte d'Ivoire[c]	3	3	2	3	3	3	6	8[a]	5	4	1	0[a]
Egypt	42	45	34	63	70	63	38	79	83	82	62	47
Ghana	1	4	3	13	5	5	9	9[a]	15	17	14	7
Kenya	4	3	6	8	7	9	2	18[a]	17	16	12	15
Lesotho	9	8	5	14	14	14	13	20[a]	24	24	28	25[a]
Mauritania	8	8	9	7	11	9	10	13[a]	10	15	16	0[a]
Morocco	17	18	24	27	45	33	21	57[a]	49	44	34	31[a]
Sudan	8	8	6	7	7	11	6	5[a]	17	13	16	0[a]
Tunisia	18	30	18	49	47	39	14	54	64	66	48	40[a]
SUB-AVERAGE	11	13	11	20	22	19	12	26	30	29	24	16
Latin America and the Caribbean												
Colombia	49	53	45	52	68	61	53	73[a]	73	81	81	85[a]
Costa Rica	32	35	38	55	58	59	48	71[a]	68	65	74	67[a]
Dominican Republic	37	28	39	68[a]	62	63	42[a]	90[a]	62	74	70	60[a]
Ecuador	46	45	41	45	71	61	43	60	64	69	67	68[a]
Guyana	33	39	39	46	60	59	36	46[a]	63	64	65	60[a]
Haiti	35	36	37	51	53	63	57[a]	57[d]	78	66	68	79[a]
Jamaica	38	37	42	52[a]	48	52	50	47[a]	57	62	61	88[d]
Mexico	37	41	32	48	61	47	47	55	68	74	64	56
Panama	34	49	34	71	77	70	59	80[a]	85	84	72	77
Paraguay	20	22	19	26	35	31	27	53[a]	36	37	41	60[a]
Peru	42	49	47	57	67	63	56	75	72	76	68	74
Trinidad and Tobago	36	40	34	52	68	55	51	58	76	80	76	49[a]
Venezuela	32	48	26	40	73	61	57	71[a]	75	71	76	77[a]
SUB-AVERAGE	36	40	36	51	62	57	48	64	67	70	68	70
Asia and Oceania												
Bangladesh[b]	69	66	49	71	80	67	56	75	91	82	81	61
Fiji	29	36	23	35	56	51	28	56	67	77	64	30[a]
Indonesia	18	35	32	31	50	51	35	39	54	63	64	46
Jordan	17	20	5	30	33	15	22	45[a]	41	38	28	18[a]
Malaysia	17	26	16	24	42	29	15	41	58	66	41	8[a]
Nepal	33	28	10	43	55	36	10	61	76	65	52	7
Pakistan	35	26	4	54	60	21	5	59	83	67	37	20[a]
Philippines	23	44	22	40	58	53	35	55	65	71	69	51
Republic of Korea	77	71	35	93	97	82	47	100	99	97	81	55
Sri Lanka	42	60	37	64	81	75	43	71	92	91	86	69
Syrian Arab Republic	15	17	3	29	35	23	17[a]	37	52	50	41	23[a]
Thailand	49	54	38	60	78	66	62	75[a]	90	87	81	88[a]
Yemen	10	16	9	24	20	23	11	23[a]	29	26	25	0[d]
SUB-AVERAGE	30	36	20	44	55	44	28	55	67	66	56	35
TOTAL AVERAGE	27	31	23	40	48	42	31	50	57	57	51	42

Source: World Fertility Survey standard recode data.
NOTE: Excluding Senegal because of lack of data. For Cameroon, percentages refer to women who either stated that they wanted no more children or reported a desired family size smaller than or equal to the current family size.
[a] From 10 to 24 cases.
[b] Data not considered comparable and not included in calculation of sub-average.
[c] Formerly called the Ivory Coast.
[d] Fewer than 10 cases.

and Oceania, women tended to be more responsive to the sex composition of the family when deciding whether to have more children.

The most extreme examples of son preference are a few countries of Asia and Northern Africa, where women with one or two sons are much more likely to want no more children than those who have only daughters, whereas the absence of a daughter has, in itself, almost no effect on proportions wanting to stop. For example, in the Republic of Korea, among women with four children, 97-100 per cent wanted to stop if they had two or more sons, as opposed to 55 per cent of those who had only daughters. In Jordan, the proportion of women with four children who wanted to stop is much lower, but it ranges from 45 per cent among women with four boys to 18 per cent among those with four girls. Egypt also shows a pattern indicating a strong preference for sons, though there is some sign that absence of a daughter may slightly decrease the proportion who wanted to stop, compared with women who had at least two sons and a daughter.

More often, a pronounced demand for at least one daughter coexists with a strong preference for sons. For example, in Nepal and Pakistan, 55-83 per cent of those with a daughter and at least two sons were willing to stop, compared with 43-61 per cent of those with three or four sons and no daughter and only 5-20 per cent of those with no sons. In several other countries, the contrasts are of the same general type but are smaller: Fiji; Malaysia; Sri Lanka; the Syrian Arab Republic; Tunisia; and Yemen. In some of these countries, the most satisfactory combination for women with four children is two sons and two daughters; and in others, it is three sons and one daughter. In all these cases, however, women with no daughters are substantially more likely to want no more children than are women with no sons. Bangladesh probably also belongs in this group, although the information is not strictly comparable to that obtained elsewhere.

Still other Asian societies show the highest levels of satisfaction with a balanced family (or, at least, a two-sex family), with all-boy and all-girl combinations viewed as adequate by roughly equal percentages of women in Indonesia, the Philippines and Thailand. A weak pattern of this type also appears in much of Latin America and the Caribbean, where it tends to be most evident for women with three children.

D. UNWANTED FERTILITY

An important objective in obtaining preference data is to estimate the levels of unwanted fertility, defined as the differences between actual fertility levels and wanted fertility levels. Measures of unwanted fertility provide one type of indicator of the potential demand for services provided by family planning programmes. While the more common method of obtaining such measures of potential demand is through measurement of the "unmet need" for contraception (covered in chapter V), this section is concerned with the measurement of the demographic significance of unmet need.

Estimates of unmet contraceptive need based on the WFS data consider the proportion of women at risk of unwanted fertility but not using contraception. Such estimates vary widely, depending upon the criteria used to select the respondents to whom the estimates apply. The study by Westoff and Pebley (1981) demonstrates this quite effectively. In their study of 18 WFS countries, they derive 11 estimates of unmet need, ranging from 7 to 40 per cent of married women of reproductive ages. The broadest measure of unmet need (which yielded the estimate of 40 per cent) was the proportion of married women who did not want any more children and were not using an effective method of contraception. The most stringent measure (which yielded the estimate of 7 per cent) was the proportion of married women who did not want any more children, who desired no more children than they had (i.e., whose desired family size was not more than current family size); who were fecund, not pregnant and not breast-feeding; and who were not using any method of contraception but intended to do so in the future. Intermediate estimates were produced by different combinations of these criteria defining exposure status and desire for additional children.

Using an intermediate measure of unmet need (the proportion of married women who wanted no more children; and who were fecund, not pregnant and not using any method of contraception), Westoff and Pebley (1981) calculated the percentage declines in fertility if all such unmet need were met. Their fertility measure was the average annual number of births per 1,000 currently married women in the previous two years. A number of assumptions were made to obtain an estimate of the hypothetical fertility applicable to a condition of no unmet need, namely: (a) that the fertility of women in the "unmet need" category (if they were to practise contraception) would be equal to the observed fertility of women who wanted no more children and were using some contraception; (b) that contraception had been used during the previous two years by women in the "met need" category and that their desire to have no more children preceded the two-year period; and (c) that women in the "unmet need" category would use the same contraceptive methods with the same regularity and effectiveness as those in the "met need" category. A comparison of actual and hypothetical fertility led to estimates of potential declines in fertility ranging from about 5 per cent in Costa Rica and Kenya, to about 15 per cent in Colombia, Nepal, Pakistan and Panama, and to just over 25 per cent in the Republic of Korea, as well as to indirect measures of unwanted fertility.

A variety of indicators of unwanted fertility can be calculated from the WFS data, based either on comparisons of actual fertility with desired family size (from the "over again" question) or on a direct question about whether, at the time the last birth was conceived, the woman had wanted any more children. The latter question was asked in only 20 of the developing countries, and none of the sub-Saharan countries included it.

For women nearing the end of the childbearing period, the cumulative incidence of unwanted fertility is shown in columns (1) and (2) of table 41. According to the direct question, column (1), between 16 per cent (in Paraguay) and 66 per cent (in the Republic of Korea) of last births had been unwanted. The mean for all 20 countries is 47 per cent. The comparison between desired and actual fertility, column (2), produces an impression of somewhat lower levels of unwanted fertility,[20] although at least 25 per cent of older women had more children than desired in 23 of 38 countries. In Yemen and most sub-Saharan countries, fewer than 10 per cent had more than the desired number of children; Kenya and the Sudan had slightly higher proportions, 10-16 per cent. Thus, regardless of which indicator is used, the proportion of women

TABLE 41. MEASURES OF UNWANTED AND WANTED FERTILITY

Region and country	For ever-married women aged 40-49 Percentage whose last birth was not wanted[a] (1)	Percentage with more children than the desired number[b] (2)	Total fertility rate[c] (3)	Wanted total fertility rate[d] (4)	Unwanted fertility rate (3) − (4) (5)	Percentage of fertility that is unwanted (5)/(3) (6)
Africa						
Benin	..	2	7.3	7.3	0.0	0
Cameroon[e]	..	6	6.4	6.1	0.3	5
Côte d'Ivoire[f]	..	0.5	7.2	7.2	0.0	0
Egypt	49	43	5.0	3.6	1.4	28
Ghana	..	3	6.1	6.0	0.1	2
Kenya	..	10	7.9	7.6	0.3	4
Lesotho	..	7	6.0	5.6	0.4	7
Mauritania	..	7	7.5	7.1	0.4	5
Morocco	41	28	5.5	4.4	1.1	20
Senegal	..	6	7.1	6.9	0.2	3
Sudan	..	16	5.6	5.0	0.6	11
Tunisia	..	48	5.5	4.1	1.4	25
SUB-AVERAGE	..	16	6.4	5.9	0.5	8
Latin America and the Caribbean						
Colombia	56	42	4.6	3.4	1.2	26
Costa Rica	44	33	3.5	3.0	0.5	17
Dominican Republic	41	39	5.2	3.8	1.4	27
Ecuador	58	39	5.2	4.1	1.1	21
Guyana	61	30	4.4	3.8	0.6	14
Haiti	..	36	5.6	4.3	1.3	23
Jamaica	61	32	4.4	3.4	1.0	23
Mexico	..	41	5.7	4.5	1.2	21
Panama	46	34	4.2	3.9	0.3	7
Paraguay	16	13	5.0	4.5	0.5	10
Peru	60	44	5.3	3.5	1.8	34
Trinidad and Tobago	38	42	3.2	2.5	0.7	22
Venezuela	48	29	4.3	3.6	0.7	16
SUB-AVERAGE	..	35	4.7	3.7	1.0	21
Asia and Oceania						
Bangladesh	58	21	5.4	4.6	0.8	15
Fiji[e]	25	18	4.0	3.6	0.4	10
Indonesia	29	11	4.3	4.0	0.3	7
Jordan	44	29	7.0	6.0	1.0	14
Malaysia	..	47	4.5	3.3	1.2	27
Nepal	..	22	6.1	5.4	0.7	11
Pakistan[e]	..	46	6.0	4.3	1.7	28
Philippines	43	35	5.1	4.1	1.0	20
Republic of Korea	66	57	3.9	2.8	1.1	28
Sri Lanka	51	28	3.4	2.9	0.5	15
Syrian Arab Republic	..	28	7.4	6.3	1.1	15
Thailand	..	46	4.3	3.2	1.1	26
Yemen	..	5	8.9	8.2	0.7	8
SUB-AVERAGE	..	30	5.5	4.6	0.9	16

Sources: For columns (1) and (2), World Fertility Survey standard recode tapes; for columns (3)-(6), Lightbourne (1985).

[a] In response to a direct question about whether more children were wanted before the last child was conceived; including current pregnancy, if any.

[b] Based on a comparison of desired family size with the current number of living children.

[c] Total fertility rate for the two years preceding each survey.

[d] Births in excess of respondent's desired family size are deleted.

[e] Data not considered comparable for wanted fertility estimates and therefore not included in calculation of sub-averages.

[f] Formerly called the Ivory Coast.

who experienced unwanted fertility appears substantial in most countries outside sub-Saharan Africa.

Another type of indicator concerns the impact of unwanted birth on level of current fertility. Table 41 presents, in columns (3)-(5), the total fertility rates and the wanted and unwanted total fertility rates, calculated by Lightbourne (1985a) from age-specific birth rates for the two years preceding the survey. The wanted rate is calculated exactly like the conventional rate, except that births in excess of the respondent's desired family size are not counted. "The wanted TFR thus reflects the number of wanted births the average woman will have over her lifetime, if she has only wanted births, and if there is no change in reproductive motivation or in the proximate determinants of fertility (e.g., fecundity, breastfeeding or proportions married)" (Lightbourne,

1985, p. 34). This measure implicitly takes account of the toll of child mortality, since the count of wanted births rests on a comparison of desired family size with the number of surviving children rather than with the cumulative number of live births. The unwanted total fertility rate is the difference between the total and wanted rates. Column (6) of the table shows the estimated percentage decline in total fertility should all unwanted births be prevented.

As columns (4) and (5) show, there is a wide variation among the countries in the amount (and proportion) of unwanted fertility. It is practically non-existent in Benin and Côte d'Ivoire, while in Peru it amounts to 1.8 children per woman. In other words, in Benin and Côte d'Ivoire there would be virtually no change in fertility levels, while in Peru fertility would decline by 34 per cent if unwanted births were prevented. Africa, as a whole, stands out as having a very small percentage of unwanted fertility—about 8 per cent—with unwanted fertility representing roughly 0.5 child per woman. Within Africa, however, a regional pattern is observed. The Northern African countries have the highest proportions of unwanted fertility. In the Sudan, this proportion is 11 per cent; in Egypt, Morocco and Tunisia, it is 20 per cent or more. In sharp contrast, all of the remaining countries of Africa have less than 10 per cent unwanted fertility. In Latin America and the Caribbean and in Asia and Oceania, the unwanted fertility rate is roughly one child per woman, but because of the slightly lower average fertility in Latin America and the Caribbean, this represents a larger proportion of fertility in that region. In most of the countries of East and South-eastern Asia (specifically in Malaysia, the Philippines, the Republic of Korea and Thailand), there is more than 20 per cent unwanted fertility.

Other estimates of the unwanted fertility rate can be calculated from the direct question about whether the last birth had been wanted. The average unwanted fertility rate is about 80 per cent higher than shown in table 41, on average, when births reported to be unwanted at the time of the conception are included in the unwanted fertility rate (Lightbourne, 1985a). Lightbourne argues that these higher estimates more nearly reflect the true situation and may even underestimate the amount of unwanted fertility, because there are signs that these retrospective estimates are influenced by rationalization (Lightbourne, 1985). Employing an indirect technique for countries where the direct question about the last birth was not asked, Lightbourne estimates that the average unwanted total fertility rate is roughly one third of the average total fertility rate, or 1.6 children per woman, in countries outside sub-Saharan Africa. (The comparable figure from table 41 is 0.9 child per woman.) For sub-Saharan Africa, Lightbourne's alternative estimates imply an average unwanted total fertility rate of 0.6 child per woman, compared with 0.3 in table 41.

There are conflicting hypotheses about the direction of the relationship between "unwanted" fertility and the level of socio-economic development or family planning programme strength. It may be argued that with development (and increasing family planning activity) unwanted fertility should decrease due to the availability of contraception. It can also be argued that development (and increased programme activity) may increase the awareness of respondents that births can be postponed or prevented and reduce fertility preferences, thus increasing at least at first the levels of unwanted fertility. In addition, variations in the pace of childbearing and child mortality mean that countries differ in the proportion of women at risk of unwanted fertility, even if desired family size does not vary.

In this connection, it is important to note that the countries where current fertility rates were lowest (development group I and Latin America and the Caribbean) did not therefore have the lowest numbers of living children. At ages 40-49, women in the low development group (IV) averaged about 0.8 less living child than did those in group I and about one child less than those in group II. This is mainly the result of differential child mortality, since the lower two development groups had mean numbers of children ever born that are close to the average for all countries (chapter I). These differences in current family size are confined to older women, but these are, of course, the women who are most likely to be at risk of unwanted fertility. As a result, even though there is little variation in desired family size according to development level, for countries outside sub-Saharan Africa, older women in development groups I and II are more likely to have reached or exceeded the desired family size (not shown).

Table 42 presents the average total wanted and unwanted fertility rates (from table 41), and the proportion of fertility that is unwanted, for countries grouped by level of development and strength of family planning programme effort. The wanted fertility rate declines monotonically with each increase in development level and family planning programme effort. The difference from the low to the high level is close to three children per woman, from 6.1 to 3.4 both for development and for family planning programme effort. The relationship is weakened but not eliminated if attention is confined to countries outside sub-Saharan Africa. For instance, the difference in wanted total fertility rate between development groups I and IV is 2.0 children, rather than 2.7, for countries outside sub-Saharan Africa.

Unwanted fertility levels do not show as regular a pattern. Unwanted fertility is about half a child (0.5-0.6) per woman for development groups III and IV, and about one child (0.8-1.0) per woman for groups I and II. In the case of strength of family planning programme effort, unwanted fertility varies from 0.6 in countries with little or no effort to 0.9-1.0 in countries with a more active family planning programme. In general, then, the unwanted fertility rate appears to be greater at higher levels of development or with the presence of some family planning activity. The proportion of fertility that is unwanted is more strongly positively related to both development and programme strength, primarily because of the significantly lower levels of wanted fertility at higher levels of development and programme effort. In development groups III and IV, unwanted fertility is estimated to be 8-9 per cent of total fertility, as compared with 19 per cent in groups I and II. With each increment in strength of family planning programme effort, the proportion of total fertility that is unwanted increases, from 9 per cent of countries with a very weak or no programme to 21-23 per cent in countries with moderate or strong programmes. If only the countries outside sub-Saharan Africa are considered, however, there is essentially no relation between the unwanted fertility rate and either development or family planning strength.

TABLE 42. TOTAL FERTILITY RATE, WANTED AND UNWANTED TOTAL FERTILITY RATE AND PROPORTION OF UNWANTED FERTILITY, BY LEVEL OF DEVELOPMENT AND STRENGTH OF FAMILY PLANNING PROGRAMME EFFORT

	Total fertility rate (1)	Wanted total fertility rate (2)	Unwanted total fertility rate (3) = (1) − (2)	Unwanted fertility as a percentage of total rate (4) = (3)/(1)
Level of development				
I. High	4.2	3.4	0.8	19
II. Middle-high	5.3	4.3	1.0	19
III. Middle-low	6.0	5.5	0.5	8
IV. Low	6.7	6.1	0.6	9
Excluding sub-Saharan Africa				
III. Middle-low	4.9	4.0	0.9	19
IV. Low	6.4	5.4	1.0	16
Strength of family planning programme effort				
1. Strong	4.3	3.4	0.9	21
2. Moderate	4.4	3.4	1.0	23
3. Weak	5.6	4.7	0.9	16
4. Very weak/none	6.7	6.1	0.6	9
Excluding sub-Saharan Africa				
3. Weak	5.4	4.3	1.0	19
4. Very weak/none	6.7	5.7	1.0	16

Source: Table 41.
NOTE: Not including Cameroon, Fiji and Pakistan in calculation of means.

The higher proportions of women at risk of unwanted fertility, mentioned earlier, are probably responsible for the failure of unwanted fertility rates to decline with level of development or family planning effort, as might otherwise be expected from the higher levels of contraceptive use in these groups of countries. The marked relation between the wanted fertility rate and the index of development is, however, somewhat surprising, when it is considered that the classification of births into "unwanted" and "wanted" components rests, in table 42, on a comparison of desired with actual family size, and that desired family size, outside of sub-Saharan Africa, shows no relationship with development (see section B above).

It is also notable that the wanted fertility rate is usually lower than the mean number of children desired (compare tables 29 and 41). In sub-Saharan Africa, this probably reflects physiological limits on fertility, but fecundity impairments are unlikely to account for all of the difference of 1.1-1.7 children between desired family size and the wanted fertility rate in Costa Rica, Malaysia, and Trinidad and Tobago, where the mean desired family size of 3.8-4.7 children is within the physical capacity of most women. Substantial differences of this type are particularly characteristic of the high development group; on average, the wanted fertility rate for countries in this group is 0.8 child lower than the desired family size, and an even larger difference is implied by Lightbourne's alternative estimates (1985).

Various factors other than infecundity might cause the wanted fertility rate to diverge from desired family size. It may be that in some cases the difference is temporary or spurious, for instance if the total fertility rate immediately before the survey was atypically high or low, or merely appeared to be so because of problems with dating of events (see chapter I).[21] However, there could also be more enduring factors. The implicit adjustment of the wanted total fertility rate for effects of child mortality, mentioned earlier, may contribute to the existence of a stronger relation between development and the wanted rate than between development and desired family size. This does not explain, though, why the wanted rate tends to fall so far below desired family size in the countries where contraceptive practice is widespread.

A possible explanation draws upon the observation that many births, while not definitely unwanted, occurred to women who were uncertain whether they wanted more children or who wanted more, but later. In societies where contraception is widely practised, many of these births will be postponed (though "timing failures" remain common even in industrialized countries (Berent, 1982)). Lightbourne (1985a) suggests that many deliberately postponed births may never occur, because of intervening sterility or marital disruption, or because economic hardship or simply advancing maternal age makes the prospect of another infant less attractive. Some empirical support for this idea comes from responses to a question about whether women wanted another child soon. In some countries, over half the women said they wanted to delay the next birth further even when it had already been from five to seven years since their last child was born. This was true, for instance, in Ecuador, Paraguay and Portugal (but not in Egypt or Ghana) (Lightbourne, 1985a). If there are indeed many "permanent postponers", wanted fertility, as measured here, will tend persistently to fall below desired family size, possibly by a substantial amount, in countries where contraceptive practice is widespread. This line of argument also suggests that the potential for additional fertility decline through adoption of birth control may be larger than indicated by measurements of unwanted fertility alone.

Results in some respects parallel to those discussed above were obtained by Westoff (1981) and Blanc (1982), who analysed trends in wanted and unwanted marital fertility in 11 WFS countries by comparing rates for marriage cohorts whose childbearing was near completion to synthetic-cohort rates for the period immediately preceding the survey. Just as, in table 42, most of the difference in current fertility is due to lower rates of wanted fertility in groups of countries with higher levels of contraceptive practice, Westoff and Blanc found that most of the within-country fertility decline was attributable to lower wanted, rather than unwanted, fertility rates. Bias in reporting of unwanted fertility may have influenced these apparent trends.[22] With this reservation, however, it can be concluded that both trend indicators and cross-national comparisons strongly suggest that wanted fertility rates tend to drop as contraception is adopted in developing countries. It is an open question whether changes in wanted fertility rates, which combine demographic and attitudinal information, can be fully explained by concurrent trends in purely attitudinal measures, such as desired family size. Decreases in desired family size have been documented for some developing countries (Lightbourne, 1984b; McClelland, 1983), but usually only after fertility had already appreciably declined (Cleland, 1985).

In summary, rather large declines in fertility could be expected in many countries if women were to implement successfully their stated preferences. The exceptions are

Yemen and the African countries (excluding the countries in Northern Africa), where the high wanted fertility rates imply very little prospect for fertility decline. Furthermore, when the countries were grouped by level of development and strength of family planning programme effort, a general increase in the amount of potential fertility decline was observed with greater development and stronger programmes. It should be emphasized, however, that these conclusions are based on estimates that are possibly very rough, particularly in cases where a large percentage of women did not express any numerical preference. Studies that clearly establish desired spacing intervals and desired stopping parities may yield different results. The unwanted fertility rates shown here are a conservative measure of the amount of fertility decline that would occur if women completely implemented their preferences.

E. Conclusion

In this chapter, the extent of size and sex preferences was investigated for the 38 WFS countries included in the United Nations comparative project. The evidence indicates that the mean total number of children desired lies between three and five children in most countries. However, a number of countries (most in sub-Saharan Africa) have preferences for much larger families, on average. Strong son preferences were observed in a few countries, mostly in Asia. The most common pattern was a preference for children of both sexes. In certain of the least developed countries, however, high levels of non-numerical responses raise some doubts about the interpretation of the mean size preferences for those countries, while high levels of uncertainty with respect to the sex preferred for the next birth reflect the fact that preferences for sex may be less clearly formulated than size preferences.

One striking finding is the extent to which most aspects of fertility preferences vary along regional or cultural lines. For several indicators, the contrasts according to the index of socio-economic development are modest by comparison with the regional differences. It is notable that desired family size is more weakly related to development level than is the current level of fertility, although an indicator that contains a component of actual fertility, the "wanted fertility rate", shows a stronger association with development than does desired family size alone. These results are reviewed in more detail below.

Mean desired family size was found to be highest in Africa (6.5), followed by Asia and Oceania (4.5) and by Latin America and the Caribbean (4.2). High mean desired family sizes—over five and, in most cases, over six children—were found in sub-Saharan Africa and in Western Asia. Nearly all the remaining countries have average desired family sizes somewhere between three and five children.

Very few women wished either to remain childless or to have an only child. Nor had the two-child family become popular among these women. In no country did more than about a third of the respondents desire two children.

It is widely believed, and these data provide no reason to doubt, that high levels of socio-economic development eventually erode traditional cultural supports for high fertility. Yet it is easy to overstate the extent to which low levels of development are currently linked to the desire for large families. Low levels of development appear compatible with a wide range of preferred family sizes—in the least developed groups of WFS countries mean desired family size ranges from 3.5 to 8.7 children. Within development groups, the values vary according to cultural divisions represented by geographical region; and if the sub-Saharan region is removed, there is no remaining relationship between level of development and mean desired family size: women in poor Asian countries, such as Nepal, did not express a desire to have larger families than women in more economically advanced Asian and Latin American countries, such as Malaysia or Mexico.

A second indicator of desired family size shows a more robust relationship to development: the proportion of women who wanted to stop childbearing, standardized for current family size, is 13 percentage points higher in development group I than in group IV, even if the sub-Saharan countries are excluded. (Including the sub-Saharan countries, this contrast is 26 points.) Even so, the contrast between the sub-Saharan countries and all others is much larger than the differences according to the development index. The overall proportion of married and fecund women who wanted no more children averages 12 per cent in sub-Saharan Africa, 46-48 per cent in Asia and Oceania and in Northern Africa, and 53 per cent in Latin America and the Caribbean. Within countries, the proportion who wanted to stop childbearing varies strongly with number of children living and, controlling for family size, the proportion increases with age.

Differentials in number preferences were also examined for countries classed by strength of family planning programme effort. Women in countries with a very weak family planning programme, or no programme, tended to prefer much-larger-than-average families, while the contrast between countries with weak, moderate and strong programmes is small. The "very weak" group consists of all but one of the sub-Saharan countries (Kenya), the three Western Asian countries, and Paraguay and Peru—only in Peru is the mean desired family size below five children. It is not possible to say from this finding whether the association between family planning strength and family size preferences reflects an effect of such programmes or whether a lack of official attention to family planning merely reflects a lack of strong demand from the populace.

The most notable finding for sex preferences was that women desire at least one child of each sex. Strong son preferences were generally found in the Western Asian and Southern Asian countries as well as in the Republic of Korea. Even in these countries, however, a desire for at least one daughter was generally found.

Regional differences in sex preferences were also established in this chapter. Although Northern African women showed a preference for sons, in sub-Saharan Africa no consistent evidence of either son or daughter preference was found in general. It should be noted, however, that, on average, about 40 per cent of the women were undecided. Only Mauritania showed consistent evidence of some son preference. Preferences for families of both sexes were widespread in all countries in Latin America and the Caribbean, but in this region the sex composition of the current family usually did not have a large effect on willingness to stop childbearing. A tendency towards daughter preference was observed in Jamaica. More variations in the strength and patterns of sex preferences were found in Asia and Oceania, though most populations in this region exhibited some degree of son preference. Especially strong son preferences were evident in Bangladesh, Nepal, Pakistan and the Republic of Korea. In Indonesia and the Philippines, women preferred an equally balanced family. When countries were classified by level of development, there was some evidence of a decline in son preference with development. This was particularly noticeable when comparing the middle-low level with the low level of development.

Indicators of unwanted fertility imply very little prospect for fertility decline in sub-Saharan Africa, but a substantial potential for decline in most other countries. Two criteria for assessing unwanted fertility were discussed: a direct question about whether any more children were wanted before the last child was conceived; and a comparison of current family size with the total number of children desired. According to the first criterion, the proportion of last births that had not been wanted averages nearly 50 per cent for women aged 40-49. The amount of unwanted fertility appears lower but is still quite large in most cases, according to the second criterion; in countries outside sub-Saharan Africa, an average of 33 per cent had more children than desired. This figure is under 10 per cent in most sub-Saharan countries. Using the more conservative (second) criterion, unwanted fertility averages 17 per cent of recent fertility (TFR) in Asia and Oceania and 21 per cent in Latin America and the Caribbean, but only 8 per cent in Africa.

When current fertility (TFR) is disaggregated into "wanted" and "unwanted" components, it is apparent that differences in the wanted fertility rate are responsible for the inverse relationship between level of development and the total fertility rate. The unwanted fertility rate is in fact higher in the upper development groups, even though the level of contraceptive use is also greater there. Greater exposure to risk of unwanted fertility is probably the reason for this. The association between the wanted fertility rate and development is stronger than might be expected from the earlier examination of fertility preference measures. Especially in the more developed countries, wanted birth rates would, if continued over women's lifetimes, produce completed family sizes well below the average desired family size reported by ever-married women. This may not in fact occur, particularly if desired family size declines. Indeed, where declines in stated desired family size have been observed, they have usually occurred only after fertility rates had already fallen substantially (Cleland, 1985). It should be noted, however, that in highly industrialized societies where birth control is well established, it is not uncommon for stated fertility desired to remain slightly above the level of fertility (and more substantially above the level of wanted fertility; see chapter XIV).

In summary, although the preference measures suggest that family size desires do not present a serious obstacle to lower fertility in most developing countries, they indicate that there is as yet little interest in limiting fertility in the sub-Saharan countries included in this report. And, while unwanted fertility is common in most countries of other regions, even the lowest mean desired family sizes reported in the World Fertility Survey are substantially above the level required for long-term population replacement. The value of these indicators for prediction over the coming decades is, however, very uncertain. In addition to the possibility that desired family size may decline, there are signs that, in some circumstances, couples may deliberately restrict fertility well below the level suggested by responses to questions about desired size. Thus, although it is unclear how far fertility might fall given current preferences, the current fertility desires reported in these surveys cannot be assumed to represent a solid floor that will halt the fertility declines.

NOTES

[1] Not all preference questions were asked in the reinterviews. The reinterviews in the Dominican Republic, Fiji, Indonesia and Peru took place from several weeks to several months after the initial interview; in Costa Rica, about 18 months later; and in Sri Lanka, about four years later.

[2] The figures mentioned in the text refer to the wife's report of current contraceptive use and the direct question about whether more children were wanted. If the husband's report of current use is employed, the husband's desire for more children appears to affect use nearly as much as does the wife's desire for more children. However, most husband-wife discrepancies with respect to current contraceptive use involved use of the pill—a method practised by women (Hallouda and others, 1983, pp. 88, 92).

[3] "If you were just married and could have just the number of children you want, how many would you want by the time you were 50?"

[4] "In your opinion, how many children should a married couple have?"

[5] In general, this influence of sex preference on the average number of children chosen is probably not very great; of women whose actual family size is at least as large as the number reported as desired, few stated that they wanted to have another child (Lightbourne and MacDonald, 1982).

[6] In a Bangladesh study on size and sex preferences, Ahmed (1981) reports that 96 per cent of the respondents successfully completed the Coombs scale procedure for measuring preferences. This is in sharp contrast to the 30 per cent non-response rate obtained by the World Fertility Survey in Bangladesh. Evidently, many women found it easier to order an array of choices rather than choose a single most preferred number.

[7] Lightbourne (1984b), however, warns against using the data for the countries of Africa for analysis of group differences in fertility preferences, particularly if there is a tendency for certain social groups to answer non-numerically.

[8] Formerly called the Ivory Coast.

[9] Based on correlations between the development index scores shown in the Introduction to this volume and the mean desired family size and total fertility rate values shown, respectively, in tables 29 and 10.

[10] Benin asked all fecund women regardless of marital status and Cameroon asked only specific age or parity groups.

[11] Couples who were sterilized for contraceptive reasons could not be identified in Côte d'Ivoire and Senegal. Additional details can be found in Singh (1984).

[12] Bangladesh asked non-pregnant women with at least one child, "Do you want to have another child soon?". Childless and pregnant women were asked the usual question. Again, in Cameroon, the question was limited to specific groups, depending upon age or parity. The results for Senegal should be viewed with caution, because for a very large proportion (about 85 per cent) of women, the data on those who wanted no more children were missing.

[13] However, following extensive consistency tests, Lightbourne and MacDonald (1982) concluded that there were no countries in which the data consistently indicated a widespread desire to remain childless.

[14] Extensive simulations by Lightbourne (reported in Lightbourne and MacDonald, 1982) confirm these effects.

[15] As Lightbourne (1985, p. 181) states:
"Simulation is based on a reverse logic: the analyst begins with a known desired family size distribution, then generates from this a set of parity-specific percentages wanting more children and percentages wanting the last birth, under various assumptions about contraception for spacing and stopping purposes. The analyst then applies each procedure to the generated data to see how well the procedure recovers the true mean."

[16] It should be noted that the main reason for the absence of the question on desire for the last birth in many countries was that such a question was meaningless in populations where the notion that fertility could be controlled had not yet emerged.

[17] Respondents who said they wanted no more children were coded as wanting zero additional children. Respondents who wanted more children were asked, "How many more children do you want?", with suitable modifications in the wording if the respondent was childless or pregnant.

[18] The most frequently used measure of this type is the Coombs scale for sex preferences, which ranges from a strong daughter preference, to a preference for equal numbers of sons and daughters, to a strong son preference. This scale can be developed from the same information obtained for the construction of the size preference scale.

[19] In addition to the criteria mentioned above, Cameroon further limited this question to specific parity and age groups of women. Results for Cameroon are therefore not considered comparable with other countries. Further details about the comparability of these questions can be found in Cleland, Verrall and Vaessen (1983) and in Singh (1984).

[20] The proportions in column (1) of table 41 are based on women with at least one birth (or current pregnancy) while those in column (2) are based on all ever-married women. Although this difference in base populations contributes to the higher proportions in column (1), the main reason for the difference is that many women who reported that the last birth was not wanted, in answer to the direct question, also reported a total desired family size at least as large as the current family size (Lightbourne, 1985a; Lightbourne and MacDonald, 1982).

[21] In addition, if the timing of fertility as well as its quantity has been altered in those countries (primarily in development groups I and II) which have experienced large declines in fertility, this could affect the wanted fertility rates. Pronounced increases in age at marriage or increases in the interval between wanted births could temporarily depress period fertility rates, while shorter birth-spacing would have the opposite effect. It is difficult to tell from World Fertility Survey data alone how much change in timing of births has occurred (Hobcraft and McDonald, 1984, pp. 16-17) and still more so to measure the effect of such change on the wanted fertility rates shown here.

[22] It is possible that fertility intentions are better recalled, and less often rationalized, for recent than for more remote events; and, therefore, that the responses of women with nearly completed childbearing may understate the number of births that were unwanted at conception to a greater degree than the responses of women who had recently given birth. There are few before-and-after comparisons that might indicate the amount of rationalization. One reinterview survey of women in the United States of America suggests that retrospective reports may lead to an appreciable underestimate of unwanted fertility, even for recent births (Westoff and Ryder, 1977).

REFERENCES

Ahmed, Nilufer R. (1981). Family size and sex preferences among women in rural Bangladesh. *Studies in Family Planning* 12(3):100-109.

Anderson, John E. and Leo Morris (1981). Fertility differences and the need for family planning services in five Latin American countries. *International Family Planning Perspectives* 7(1):16-21.

Arnold, Fred (1986). The effect of sex preference on fertility and family planning: empirical evidence. Paper prepared for the Annual Meeting of the Population Association of America, San Francisco, California, 3-5 April 1986.

Berent, Jerzy (1982). *Family Planning in Europe and USA in the 1970s*. World Fertility Survey Comparative Studies, No. 20; ECE Analyses of WFS Surveys in Europe and USA. Voorburg, The Netherlands: International Statistical Institute.

Blanc, Ann K. (1982). Unwanted fertility in Latin America and the Caribbean. *International Family Planning Perspectives* 8(4):156-162.

Bulatao, Rodolfo A. and F. Arnold (1977). Relationships between the value and cost of children and fertility: cross-cultural evidence. In *International Population Conference, Mexico 1977*. Liège: International Union for the Scientific Study of Population, vol. 1, 141-156.

Caldwell, John C. (1983). Direct economic costs and benefits of children. In Rodolfo A. Bulatao and Ronald D. Lee, eds., with Paula E. Hollerbach and John Bongaarts, *Determinants of Fertility in Developing Countries*, vol. 1, *Supply and Demand for Children*. Report of the National Research Council Committee on Population and Demography, Panel on Fertility Determinants. New York: Academic Press, 458-493.

Cleland, John (1985). Marital fertility decline in developing countries: theories and the evidence. In John Cleland and John Hobcraft, eds., in collaboration with Betzy Dinesen, *Reproductive Change in Developing Countries: Insights from the World Fertility Survey*. Oxford: Oxford University Press, 223-252.

_____, Jane Verrall and Martin Vaessen (1983). *Preferences for the Sex of Children and Their Influence on Reproductive Behaviour*. World Fertility Survey Comparative Studies, No. 27; Cross-National Summaries. Voorburg, The Netherlands: International Statistical Institute.

Coombs, Lolagene C. (1974). The measurement of family size preferences and subsequent fertility. *Demography* 11(4):587-611.

_____ (1976). *Are Cross-cultural Preference Comparisons Possible? —A Measurement-Theoretic Approach*. International Union for the Scientific Study of Population Paper, No. 5. Liège.

_____ (1979). Prospective fertility and underlying preferences: a longitudinal study in Taiwan. *Population Studies* 33(3):447-455. The data in this article refer to Taiwan, Province of China.

_____ and Ming-cheng Chang (1981). Do husbands and wives agree? Fertility attitudes and later behavior. *Population and Environment* 4(2):109-127.

_____ and Dorothy Fernandez (1978). Husband-wife agreement about reproductive goals. *Demography* 15(1):57-73.

Feeney, Griffith M. (1986). The effect of son preference on fertility in China and its provinces. Paper submitted to the Annual Meeting of the Population Association of America, San Francisco, California, 3-5 April 1986.

Freedman, Ronald and John Y. Takeshita (1969). *Family Planning in Taiwan: An Experiment in Social Change*. Princeton, New Jersey: Princeton University Press. The data in this book refer to Taiwan, Province of China.

_____, Albert I. Hermalin and Ming-cheng Chang (1975). Do statements about desired family size predict fertility? The case of Taiwan, 1967-1970. *Demography* 12(3):407-416. The data in this article refer to Taiwan, Province of China.

Hallouda, Awad M. and others, eds. (1983). *The Egyptian Fertility Survey 1980*, vol. III, *Socio-economic Differentials and Comparative Data from Husbands and Wives*. Cairo: Central Agency for Public Mobilisation and Statistics.

Hauser, Philip M. (1967). "Family planning and population programs" —A book review article. *Demography* 4(1):397-414.

Hobcraft, John and John McDonald (1984). *Birth Intervals*. World Fertility Survey Comparative Studies, No. 28; Cross-National Summaries. Voorburg, The Netherlands: International Statistical Institute.

Jensen, Eric (1985). Desired fertility, the "up to God" response, and sample selection bias. *Demography* 22(3):445-454.

Knodel, John and Visid Prachuabmoh (1973). Desired family size in Thailand: are the responses meaningful? *Demography* 10(4):619-637.

_____ and Visid Prachuabmoh (1976). Preferences for sex of children in Thailand: a comparison of husbands' and wives' attitudes. *Studies in Family Planning* 7(5):137-143.

Lee, Ronald D. and Rodolfo A. Bulatao (1983). The demand for children: a critical essay. In Rodolfo A. Bulatao and Ronald D. Lee, eds., with Paula E. Hollerbach and John Bongaarts, *Determinants of Fertility in Developing Countries*, vol. 1, *Supply and Demand for Children*. Report of the National Research Council Committee on Population and Demography, Panel on Fertility Determinants. New York: Academic Press, 233-287.

Lee, S. B. (1977). System effects on family planning behaviour. Unpublished doctoral dissertation, University of Michigan, Ann Arbor.

Lightbourne, Robert E. (1977). Family size desires and the birth rates they imply. Doctoral dissertation, University of California, Berkeley.

_____ (1980). *Urban-Rural Differentials in Contraceptive Use*. World Fertility Survey Comparative Studies, No. 10; Cross-National Summaries. Voorburg, The Netherlands: International Statistical Institute.

_____ (1981). Some improved measures of desired family size: an application to developing countries. Paper presented at the Annual Meeting of the Population Association of America, Washington, D.C., 26-28 March 1981.

_____ (1984). *Fertility Preferences in Guyana, Jamaica and Trinidad and Tobago, from World Fertility Survey 1975-77—A Multiple Indicator Approach*. World Fertility Survey Scientific Reports, No. 68. Voorburg, The Netherlands: International Statistical Institute.

_____ (1984a). Comparing old and new approaches to forecasting fertility change in developing countries. Paper submitted to the Annual Meeting of the Population Association of America, Minneapolis, Minnesota, 3-5 May 1984.

_____ (1984b). Quality of the WFS fertility preference data. Background paper submitted to the World Fertility Survey Symposium, London, 24-27 April 1984.

_____ (1985). Desired number of births and prospects for fertility decline in 40 countries. *International Family Planning Perspectives* 11(2):34-39.

_____ (1985a). Individual preferences and fertility behaviour. In John Cleland and John Hobcraft, eds., in collaboration with Betzy Dinesen, *Reproductive Change in Developing Countries: Insights from the World Fertility Survey*. Oxford: Oxford University Press, 165-198.

_____ and Alphonse L. MacDonald (1982). *Family Size Preferences*. World Fertility Survey Comparative Studies, No. 14; Cross-National Summaries. Voorburg, The Netherlands: International Statistical Institute.

McClelland, Gary H. (1979). Determining the impact of sex preferences on fertility: a consideration of parity progression ratio, dominance, and stopping rule measures. *Demography* 16(3):377-388.

_____ (1983). Family-size desires as measures of demand. In Rodolfo A. Bulatao and Ronald D. Lee, eds., with Paula E. Hollerbach and John Bongaarts, *Determinants of Fertility in Developing Countries*, vol. 1, *Supply and Demand for Children*. Report of the National Research Council Committee on Population and Demography, Panel on Fertility Determinants. New York: Academic Press, 288-343.

Mauldin, W. Parker (1965). Fertility studies: knowledge, attitude and practice. *Studies in Family Planning* 7:1-10.

_____ and Bernard Berelson (1978). Conditions of fertility decline in developing countries, 1965-75. With section by Zenas Sykes. *Studies in Family Planning* 9(5):89-147.

Millman, Sara (1981). Breastfeeding in Taiwan: trends and differentials. Unpublished doctoral dissertation. University of Michigan, Ann Arbor. The data in this dissertation refer to Taiwan, Province of China.

Morgan, S. Philip (1982). Parity-specific fertility intentions and uncertainty: the United States, 1970 to 1976. *Demography* 19(3):315-334.

Nour, El-Sayed (1983). On the estimation of the distribution of desired family size for a synthetic cohort. *Population Studies* 37(2):315-322.

Palmore, James A. and Mercedes B. Concepción (1981). Desired family size and contraceptive use: an 11-country comparison. *International Family Planning Perspectives* 7(1):37-40.

Park, Chai Bin (1986). How many births are attributable to preference for sex of children? Paper submitted to the Annual Meeting of the Population Association of America, San Francisco, California, 3-5 April 1986.

Pullum, Thomas W. (1979). Adjusting stated fertility preferences for the effect of actual family size with applications to World Fertility Survey data. Paper submitted to the Annual Meeting of the Population Association of America, Philadelphia, Pennsylvania, 26-28 April 1979.

_____ (1980). *Illustrative Analysis: Fertility Preferences in Sri Lanka*. World Fertility Survey Scientific Reports, No. 9. Voorburg, The Netherlands: International Statistical Institute.

Repetto, Robert (1972). Son preference and fertility behaviour in developing countries. *Studies in Family Planning* 3(4):70-76.

Rodgers, G. B. (1976). Fertility and desired fertility: longitudinal evidence from Thailand. *Population Studies* 30(3):511-526.

Rodríguez, Germán and T. J. Trussell (1981). A note on synthetic cohort estimates of average desired family size. *Population Studies* 35(2):321-328.

Rukanuddin, Abdul R. (1982). Infant child mortality and son preference as factors influencing fertility in Pakistan. *The Pakistan Development Review* 21(4):297-328.

Ryder, Norman B. (1973). A critique of the national fertility survey. *Demography* 10(4):495-506.

_____ (1979). Consistency of reporting fertility planning status. *Studies in Family Planning* 10(4):115-128.

Singh, Susheela (1984). *Comparability of Questionnaires: Forty-one WFS Countries*. World Fertility Survey Comparative Studies, No. 32; Cross-National Summaries. Voorburg, The Netherlands: International Statistical Institute.

Thomson, Elizabeth (1984). Marital conflict and contraceptive choice. Paper submitted to the Annual Meeting of the Population Association of America. Minneapolis, Minnesota, 3-5 May 1985. Revised.

Udry, J. Richard, Karl E. Bauman and Charles L. Chase (1973). Population growth in perfect contraceptive populations. *Population Studies* 27(2):365-371.

United Nations (1981). Department of International Economic and Social Affairs. Population Division. Selected factors affecting fertility and fertility preferences in developing countries: evidence from the first fifteen World Fertility Survey country reports. In *World Fertility Survey Conference 1980: Record of Proceedings*. London, 7-11 July 1980. Voorburg, The Netherlands: International Statistical Institute, 147-227.

Ware, Helen (1974). *Ideal Family Size*. World Fertility Survey Occasional Papers, No. 13. Voorburg, The Netherlands: International Statistical Institute.

Westoff, Charles F. (1981). Unwanted fertility in six developing countries. *International Family Planning Perspectives* 7(2):43-52.

_____ and Anne R. Pebley (1981). Alternative measures of unmet need for family planning in developing countries. *International Family Planning Perspectives* 7(4):126-136.

_____ and Norman B. Ryder (1977). The predictive value of reproductive intentions. *Demography* 14(4):431-453.

_____, Robert G. Potter and Philip C. Sagi (1963). *The Third Child: A Study in the Prediction of Fertility*. Princeton, New Jersey: Princeton University Press.

Williamson, Nancy E. (1976). *Sons or Daughters: A Cross-Cultural Survey of Parental Preferences*. Beverly Hills, California: Sage publications.

III. NUPTIALITY

ABSTRACT

This chapter describes country differences in women's age at marriage, the proportion ever marrying, marital disruption and remarriage, and several types of relationships between marriage and fertility.

With few exceptions, over 95 per cent of women eventually marry, but the average age at first marriage ranges from 16 years in Bangladesh to 25 years in Sri Lanka. Overall marriage age is currently higher and shows greater increase over time in more economically advanced developing countries. Increases in marriage age are more pronounced in Asia and Oceania but the average age at entry into unions is still somewhat later in Latin America and the Caribbean (and earliest in Africa). Averaged over all countries, nearly three quarters of the typical woman's reproductive years (ages 15-49) are spent within marriage, 18 per cent before first marriage, 5 per cent divorced or separated and only 3 per cent in widowhood.

Africa, and Latin America and the Caribbean have the highest levels of marital disruption, proportions in informal unions and rates of childbearing outside marriage. These aspects of marriage and reproduction are determined by societal norms and customs and therefore are more closely related to geographical region than to level of development. Countries where marital disruption is common tend to have high remarriage rates, so that the impact of disruption on aggregate fertility levels is usually not large.

Within each country, later age at marriage is associated with lower completed family size. On average, among women aged 40-49, those who first married under age 17 had borne 0.8 child more than those marrying at ages 17-20 years, 1.7 children more than those marrying at 21-24 and 3.2 more than those marrying at 25 or over. However, elimination of early marriages would not itself produce low levels of fertility; even women who married after age 25 usually averaged at least four children. Many Governments regard early marriage with concern, not simply because it is associated with high fertility but because of health risks to adolescent mothers and their children and because early marriage and childbearing may foreclose opportunities for women's education, employment and involvement in the wider society. Despite recent increases in marriage age, the World Fertility Survey data show that large proportions of adolescent women in developing countries still marry and bear children. Of all women currently in their early twenties, an average of 22 per cent had entered a union before age 16, some 40 per cent before age 18 and 57 per cent before age 20. Twenty-two per cent had borne a child before the age of 18. In the least developed countries, roughly one third had become mothers by this age.

Although marital unions form the predominant context for childbearing and child-rearing throughout the world, the structure and associated customs, as well as the initial timing, prevalence and stability of unions, vary widely. The date of entry into first union is an important milestone in a woman's life; it represents not only a major change in the composition of her family but usually the beginning of regular exposure to the risk of childbearing. Thus, any study of cross-country differentials in fertility must examine closely the role that the timing of first union plays in explaining these differentials and how these patterns relate to various characteristics of the countries' settings. Other aspects of nuptiality that can affect the length and timing of regular sexual exposure and that have implications for fertility include the incidence of divorce and widowhood and the prevalence and timing of remarriage.

A trend towards delay of first marriage has been documented in recent decades in countries with widely different economic, social and cultural configurations (Henry and Piotrow, 1979; Smith, 1984). These increases in the age of entry into unions (except where the changes have occurred primarily in the early teen-age years) have been credited with a large share of the observed fertility decline. When marriage behaviour is viewed as a proximate determinant of fertility, this interpretation is, strictly speaking, correct. However, a broader view must consider that social and economic changes, such as increased schooling for women, lead both to delays in marriage and to declines in marital fertility. This complicates the interpretation of relationships between the timing of entry into regular sexual exposure and completed fertility, particularly when such findings are to be adapted for policy application. Furthermore, while a rise in age at first marriage may be a sufficient condition for fertility decline, it is not a necessary one. In many Latin American and Caribbean countries, for instance, little of the fertility decline has been attributed to rising age at first union.

When comparing women within a country at a single point in time, differences between them in age at entry into union can be related to differences in timing of first births, spacing of births and termination of childbearing (McDonald, 1984). In the absence of comparable trend data for a wide range of countries, a comparative analysis of such country patterns can reveal not only the range of nuptiality patterns across countries but the possible links between marriage timing and fertility. Knowledge of these patterns and interrelationships has important policy relevance, with respect to the susceptibility of marriage timing to available policy measures, the likely relationship between changes in marriage timing and fertility, and the extent of extra-marital fertility and childbearing among the very young.[1] Family planning policy-makers can use this information to direct programmes and services to all those in need. In this area of policy-making, information on marital-status distribution by age can help in deciding from what age contraceptive information and services are needed.

This chapter provides basic information on marital status distributions and on the age at first marriage for 38 countries participating in the World Fertility Survey (WFS). In addition, childbearing among unmarried and married women is compared, and the effect of marriage on fertility is examined. Variations in fertility and in childlessness according to age at first marriage and marital status are also analysed. Several reports analysing nuptiality or nuptiality and fertility in a comparative context have appeared in recent years.[2]

More than any other factor affecting fertility, marriage forms and practices vary according to culture. These variations in customs have important implications for understanding the obligations and rights of men and women and the control of property and children. Such variations, however, are often relatively unimportant in an analysis of fertility, which depends instead upon knowledge of variations in sexual exposure. The focus of WFS was on measurement of sexual exposure within the context of socially recognized unions, rather than on obtaining information about the customs surrounding particular forms of unions and marriages.

In order to achieve some degree of comparability across different cultures, a wide definition of marriage was used in all surveys (Singh, 1984). Where types of unions other than legal marriage were known to exist, "marriage" was defined to include unions sanctioned legally or by religious or customary ceremonies as well as unions where the couple lived together, but the union had not been formally sanctioned. In a few countries where legal marriage considerably precedes the consummation of marriage, the age at which the consummation ceremony occurred was obtained and this was used as the age at first marriage instead of the age at the official (betrothal) ceremony. The chief exception to this generalization occurred in the Caribbean, where four countries (Guyana,[3] Haiti, Jamaica, and Trinidad and Tobago) also recorded "visiting" unions, in which a regular sexual relationship existed but the couple did not live together. In this report, marriage, common-law or consensual unions and visiting unions are all considered to be "marriages" or unions in which sexual exposure does not differ substantially. The adoption of such a wide definition of marriage resulted in fairly complete coverage of exposure within unions in all countries, possibly excluding those in which "free" unions were not explicitly included in the definition of marital unions. Such an omission could be especially important in the present context if it involved unions preceding that recorded as the first (Jemai and Singh, 1984). The analysis of nuptiality and fertility implicitly assumes that the frequency of intercourse within unions is the same regardless of the type of union (i.e., legal, religious or customary marriage and various types of informal union) or the country setting. No direct information is available on this point.

The terms "union" and "marriage" were used interchangeably here to denote all of the above-mentioned types of sexual relationships as recorded in WFS. It is interesting to note that even this liberal definition of marriage did not eliminate all "extra-marital" fertility. Although there may be ambiguity about the exact time of beginning and end of unions when these events are not marked by a legal or social ceremony, the survey respondents plainly did not report all periods of sexual activity as time spent in a union.

This chapter begins with a discussion of proportions ever married and the mean age at first marriage. Trends in the age at first marriage are then estimated and the experience of older women is compared with that of younger women. The distribution of time spent in the different marital statuses and the status of the first marriage are also described. Section B discusses the overall relationship between fertility and marital exposure (that is, time spent in a union), including the age pattern of fertility, childbearing outside marriage and the effect of standardizing for proportions married on the level of fertility. The levels of recent fertility within periods spent single, not currently married and currently married are also compared, to estimate the amount of fertility occurring outside unions. In addition, the mean number of children ever born to women aged 40-49 is compared for subgroups according to the status of the first marriage in order to estimate the effect of dissolution of marriages on cumulative fertility.

Section C also addresses the relationship between marriage and fertility, but it focuses on age at first marriage. Differences in the duration of the first birth interval and in marital fertility rates between two large age-at-marriage subgroups are analysed, and cumulative fertility and the percentage childless among women aged 40-49 are compared across age-at-marriage subgroups. This section also considers the interrelated factors of age, duration of marriage and age at first marriage, and their effect on fertility.

The final section looks at early childbearing and marriage among a recent cohort of women with the aim of estimating the current prevalence of teen-age childbearing and sexual activity within unions.

A. Marital status of women

In this section, inter-country variations in women's marriage patterns are examined. Given the cultural diversity in marriage patterns, regional differences in the prevalence of informal unions and in marital dissolution and remarriage are expected. In addition, the level of socio-economic development is expected to be related to the age of marriage and proportions married, since greater economic development is likely to result in better opportunities for women, thus leading to later ages at first marriage. Proportions ever married and a synthetic summary of these proportions, the singulate mean age at first marriage (Hajnal, 1953), are described first. Then, trends over time in the proportions ever married and in the mean age at marriage are estimated from cohort differences. Lastly, variations in the prevalence of marital dissulution and remarriage are discussed.

Proportions single and the singulate mean age at marriage

Of the three major regional groups, the highest proportions remaining single at each age are found in Latin America and the Caribbean, on average (table 43). The African region shows the greatest propensity for early marriage, with as many as 35 per cent of women aged 15-19, on average, having entered their first marriage at the time of the surveys. Asia and Oceania occupies the

TABLE 43. PERCENTAGE OF WOMEN NEVER MARRIED IN FIVE-YEAR CURRENT AGE GROUPS AND SINGULATE MEAN AGE AT MARRIAGE, BY REGION, COUNTRY AND LEVEL OF DEVELOPMENT

	15-19	20-24	25-29	30-34	35-39	40-44	45-49	Singulate mean age at marriage
Africa								
Benin	56	10	1	0	0	0	0	18.2
Cameroon	47	10	4	2	1	1	2	17.5
Côte d'Ivoire[a]	44	10	5	2	1	0	0	17.8
Egypt	78	36	14	4	2	2	2	21.3
Ghana	69	15	3	1	1	1	0	19.3
Kenya	72	21	4	2	1	1	1	19.9
Lesotho	68	16	7	5	3	2	2	19.6
Mauritania	61	24	9	5	2	2	2	19.2
Morocco	79	36	12	3	1	1	0	21.3
Senegal	41	14	4	0	0	0	0	17.7
Sudan	78	36	11	4	2	1	1	21.3
Tunisia	94	57	20	6	2	2	1	23.9
AVERAGE	65	24	7	3	1	1	1	19.8
Latin America and the Caribbean								
Colombia	85	44	22	11	12	9	9	22.1
Costa Rica	85	45	25	12	13	11	10	22.7
Dominican Republic	72	27	10	5	2	3	3	20.5
Ecuador	82	43	20	11	7	8	6	22.1
Guyana	72	26	7	2	3	2	2	20.0
Haiti	84	41	14	4	3	2	1	21.8
Jamaica	70	12	4	1	3	1	2	19.2
Mexico	81	34	15	9	6	6	5	21.7
Panama	80	35	12	7	5	3	2	21.2
Paraguay	83	43	19	11	6	5	5	22.1
Peru	86	49	23	11	9	5	6	23.2
Trinidad and Tobago	80	32	10	5	3	2	2	20.9
Venezuela	80	41	18	8	4	3	3	21.8
AVERAGE	80	36	15	7	6	5	4	21.5
Asia and Oceania								
Bangladesh	30	5	1	0	1	0	0	16.3
Fiji	88	34	9	4	3	2	1	21.8
Indonesia	63	20	5	2	2	1	1	19.4
Jordan	81	37	12	4	2	3	2	21.6
Malaysia	89	47	17	7	4	2	1	23.1
Nepal	42	7	2	1	1	1	1	17.1
Pakistan	62	22	9	3	3	1	1	19.8
Philippines	92	58	29	14	9	5	6	24.5
Republic of Korea	97	60	11	1	1	0	0	23.2
Sri Lanka	93	61	32	13	6	5	2	25.1
Syrian Arab Republic	77	40	17	8	6	3	2	22.1
Thailand	85	42	19	10	6	4	3	22.5
Yemen	39	7	3	2	0	2	1	16.9
AVERAGE	72	34	12	5	3	2	1	21.0
Level of development								
I. High	82	37	13	6	5	3	3	21.6
II. Middle-high	84	45	20	9	6	4	4	22.7
III. Middle-low	64	20	6	2	1	1	1	19.5
IV. Low	55	18	6	2	1	1	1	18.7
ALL COUNTRIES	73	32	12	5	3	3	2	20.8

Sources: Smith (1980), and Ebanks and Singh (1984).   [a] Formerly called the Ivory Coast.

middle position between these two extremes. While almost universal marriage is found in all three regions, with only 3-7 per cent remaining single by ages 30-34, moderate regional differences persist at ages 20-29. Only in Latin America and the Caribbean does celibacy remain significant, at 4-5 per cent, on average, at ages over 40. These regional differences are reflected in the summary measure, singulate mean age at marriage (SMAM), which is based on marital status distribution and can be interpreted as the average number of years lived before the first marriage, by women who eventually marry.[4] These results show that a very young age at marriage characterizes the African region, which has an average SMAM of 19.8 years, compared with 21.0 in Asia and Oceania and 21.5 in Latin America and the Caribbean.

As might be expected, these regional averages conceal large differences between countries (see figure 14 and table 43). Within Africa, for example, the Northern African countries (Egypt, Morocco, the Sudan and Tunisia) have much higher proportions remaining single up to age 30, compared with the sub-Saharan countries, where marriage is almost universal over age 25, and where in several countries, only 40-60 per cent of teenagers (ages 15-19) are still single. Most of the Caribbean countries (the Dominican Republic, Guyana, Jamaica, and Trinidad and Tobago) have lower proportions remaining single under age 25 than other countries in the region. The Asia and Oceania region contains two highly contrasting groups which do not, however, form distinct geographical clusters—Bangladesh, Nepal and Yemen, with extremely low proportions single at each age; and Malaysia, the Philippines, the Republic of Korea and Sri Lanka, with very high proportions delaying the first marriage until the late twenties or the early thirties. Over all, Asia displays the greatest range of mean ages at marriage; Africa also has a large range and the countries of Latin America and the Caribbean a narrower one.

The expected pattern of larger delays in first marriage and a higher mean age among relatively highly developed countries is partially supported. Interestingly, the high development group (I) has a noticeably earlier marriage pattern, on average, than the middle-high group (SMAMs of 21.6 and 22.7 years, respectively) suggesting that factors other than socio-economic development affect the average age of marriage in these societies. The inclusion of three Caribbean countries in group I is partially responsible for this result. The two lower groups (III and IV) do have substantially earlier patterns of marriage, however, supporting the hypotheses of a relationship between the level of development and the timing of the first marriage. It can also be seen from figure 14 that the level of development in Asia and Oceania sharply discriminates the countries with very early marriage (SMAM under 20 years in development groups III and IV) from those with moderate or late marriage age (SMAM of 21.8-25.1 in groups I and II).

Trends in age at first marriage

The use of retrospective data from WFS for an analysis of trends in age at first marriage is problematical because it depends upon recall of an event in the past, in some cases more than 20 years before the survey. One common error observed in Asia and Oceania is understatement of age at marriage by older women; this distortion is often not very large, however, by comparison with the amount of trend reflected in other sources, as well as in the WFS

Figure 14. **Singulate mean age at marriage, by region and level of development**

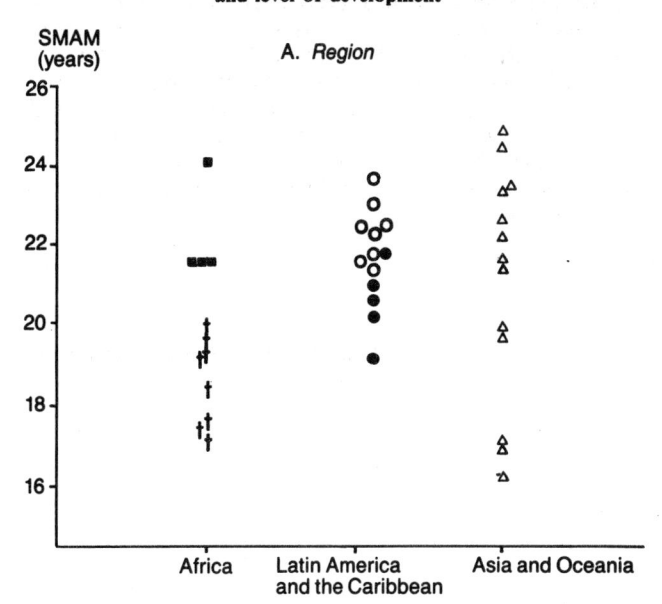

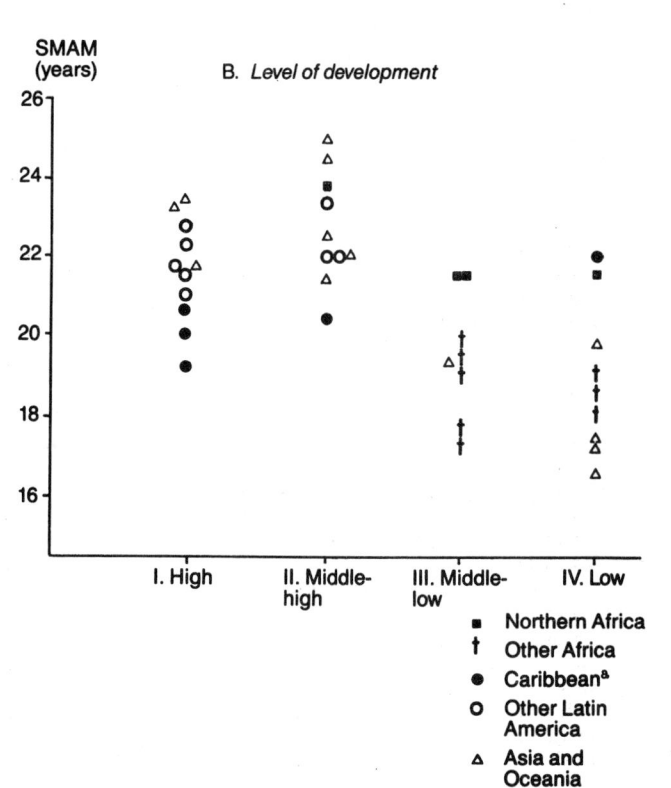

Source: Table 43.
NOTE: SMAM = Singulate mean age at marriage.
[a] Including Guyana.

marriage histories (Smith, Shahidullah and Alcantara, 1983). In contrast, in Africa and in Latin America and the Caribbean, the opposite error is found—older age groups may have overstated their age at first marriage, possibly due to omission of informal unions during the teen-age years (Goldman, Rutstein and Singh, 1985, and United Nations, 1983a). In addition, Coale (1983) suggests that, in the case of Egypt, where reporting errors appeared similar to the Asian error pattern, age misstatement alone without any distortion in the reporting of marriage duration could have produced a bias in the observed trend in the age at marriage.[5] To minimize the effect of these reporting errors on the observed trends, only the data based on the reports of women aged 20-39 are discussed below, though the upper age groups are also included in the tables and figures.

In the case of samples restricted to ever-married women (see Introduction to this volume), household data on proportions ever married were used. In certain cases, proportions married may have been understated in the household data, because of proxy reporting by the head of the household. For example, women who are currently separated, widowed or divorced, particularly if they are young, or if the union was short-lived or informal, may be reported as never married (Timaeus, 1984). A further source of error is the tendency to underestimate the age of unmarried women or overestimate the age of those who have married, which can affect the estimated proportions ever married. This is especially crucial at ages 15-24, which largely determines the mean age at first marriage since, in the majority of these countries, most women are married by age 25.

TABLE 44. PERCENTAGE MARRIED BY EXACT AGE 20, ACCORDING TO FIVE-YEAR CURRENT AGE GROUP, BY REGION, COUNTRY AND LEVEL OF DEVELOPMENT

	20-24	25-29	30-34	35-39	40-44	45-49	Assessment of quality of marriage history data[a]
Africa							
Benin	74	71	71	71	64	57	C
Cameroon	81	78	80	72	73	62	C
Côte d'Ivoire[b]	79	77	78	77	73	72	C
Egypt	54	58	69	76	76	77	B
Ghana	72	69	71	72	68	71	C
Kenya	65	70	76	76	74	68	B
Lesotho	70	67	69	66	68	70	A
Mauritania	72	80	82	83	83	78	C
Morocco	53	64	76	85	85	86	B
Senegal	77	79	90	90	88	88	C
Sudan	57	75	80	77	76	76	C
Tunisia	29	44	59	61	59	55	A
AVERAGE	65	69	75	76	73	72	
Latin America and the Caribbean							
Colombia	42	45	49	52	45	42	B
Costa Rica	40	35	41	44	42	37	B
Dominican Republic	61	70	67	70	69	64	C
Ecuador	46	46	52	52	54	50	C
Guyana	62	68	73	72	72	69	C
Haiti	48	52	52	51	56	41	C
Jamaica	77	70	74	63	57	48	C
Mexico	47	49	52	53	56	50	A
Panama	46	51	56	56	61	57	B
Paraguay	41	46	46	48	55	48	B
Peru	37	45	49	52	50	47	C
Trinidad and Tobago	56	61	60	65	71	68	B
Venezuela	45	51	53	58	59	60	B
AVERAGE	50	53	56	56	57	52	
Asia and Oceania							
Bangladesh	93	97	99	98	98	98	C
Fiji	48	56	66	67	66	67	A
Indonesia	72	81	84	86	87	85	C
Jordan	54	64	71	75	75	79	C
Malaysia	37	43	55	65	72	75	A
Nepal	86	85	86	82	83	81	C
Pakistan	72	77	83	87	89	92	C
Philippines	30	37	41	45	49	46	B
Republic of Korea	15	18	26	46	70	88	A
Sri Lanka	27	34	48	51	57	59	B
Syrian Arab Republic	50	56	64	59	56	60	B
Thailand	42	46	49	52	56	52	B
Yemen	84	80	82	80	76	74	C
AVERAGE	55	59	66	68	72	74	
Level of development							
I. High	47	50	56	59	62	62	—
II. Middle-high	42	49	54	56	56	56	—
III. Middle-low	68	70	75	77	75	74	—
IV. Low	73	77	81	80	79	76	—
ALL COUNTRIES	56	60	65	66	67	66	—

Source: Smith (1980), and Ebanks and Singh (1984).
[a] From table 24: A = good quality; B = acceptable quality; C = less reliable.
[b] Formerly called the Ivory Coast.

Chapter I presents an overview of findings with respect to the quality of the marriage history data (see table 24). It was determined through both internal consistency checks and external comparisons that some of the trends implied by the retrospective marriage histories are exaggerated. This conclusion, however, could be more confidently drawn in the case of certain Asian countries because of the comparability of the definition of marriage between previous censuses and WFS, whereas in Africa and in Latin America and the Caribbean, differences in the definition of unions between the census and the survey make comparison difficult. While the actual extent of the trends may be subject to some doubt for certain countries, other sources provide independent evidence that the direction of trends found in the WFS data is approximately correct (Smith, Shahidullah and Alcantara, 1983; Henry and Piotrow, 1979).

Figure 15. Percentage married by exact age 20, five-year current age groups, by region and level of development

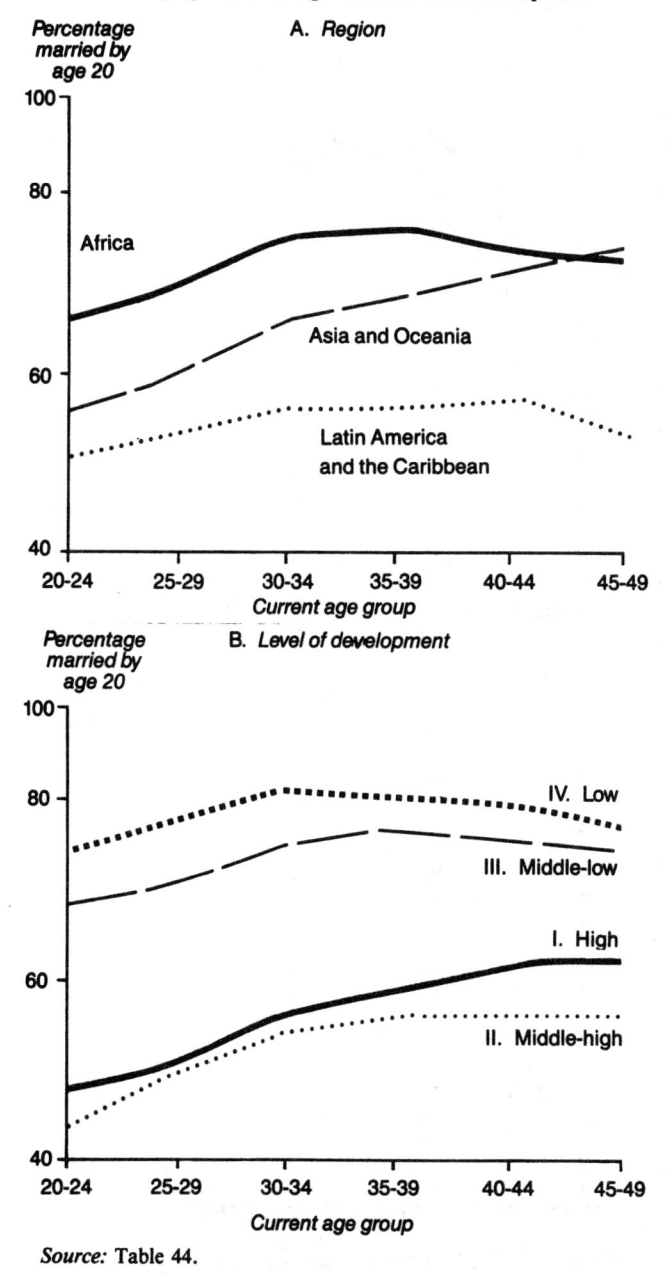

Source: Table 44.

Despite problems with the quality of retrospective data from some surveys, these data provide some idea of changes over time in the proportion ever married and in the age at first marriage. Five-year cohorts of women have been compared as a means for estimating change over time, under the assumption that the experience of older age groups largely characterizes earlier time periods, although the cohort and time measures are clearly not identical, given the spread in age at marriage for every age group of women.

Table 44 shows the proportion ever married by exact age 20, according to age groups over current age 20, for individual countries and by region and level of development. The proportions are derived using life-table analysis to obtain the cumulative proportions ever married by single years of age for each five-year age group (see Smith, 1980). Regional averages show declines in the proportion ever married from older to younger cohorts, in all three regions, but declines are relatively small in Latin America and the Caribbean (figure 15); and in most of the countries of sub-Saharan Africa, they are non-existent. Patterns by level of development differ somewhat. Development groups I and II show much the same pattern, with the lowest proportions married by age 20, in all age cohorts and with total declines of 12 and 14 percentage points, respectively, when comparing the 20-24 and 35-39 cohorts. Development groups III and IV show smaller declines in the proportion ever married.[6] As in the case of age at marriage, these regional averages conceal substantial inter-country variation.

A further measure of changes in the pattern of marriage over time, the Coale and McNeil model estimates of the mean age at marriage of each five-year age group of women is presented in table 45, for groups of countries (Coale, 1971; Coale and McNeil, 1972; Rodríguez and Trussell, 1980). The model is premised on the finding that the distribution of the age at marriage in a female cohort takes the same basic form across populations. Differences occur because of variations in the initial age at marriage, in the rate at which marriage occurs and in the proportion eventually marrying. This model uses the observed behaviour of each cohort as far as possible (e.g., ages at marriage up to age 25 for those aged 25 at the survey) to estimate the parameters of the model.[7] These parameters are then used to obtain hypothetical rates of marriage for the rest of the cohorts' reproductive years, for which no data are available. Predictions will be more accurate for age groups with more data; and because of this, the means for ages 20-24 should be used with caution. For some surveys, problems were noted in the fit of the model to the data (Trussell and Reinis, 1984); none the less, these results are useful as a description of the approximate time trends.

These fitted means show an average rise in the age at first marriage of nearly one year in Africa and in Latin America and the Caribbean, and a larger rise of about 1.5 years in Asia and Oceania, when comparing age group 20-24 with those aged 35-39. As seen from the results for SMAM, Latin America and the Caribbean continues to have the highest average age at first marriage. Development groups I and II are very similar, and both show a rise of about 1.5 years in the mean age from the oldest to the youngest cohort. Groups III and IV experienced a much smaller rise and also began with substantially lower mean ages.

TABLE 45. ESTIMATES OF MEAN AGE AT MARRIAGE, BASED ON THE COALE-MCNEIL MODEL, FOR FIVE-YEAR AGE GROUPS, BY REGION AND LEVEL OF DEVELOPMENT

	\multicolumn{6}{c	}{Mean age at marriage for age groups}	Difference between ages 35-39 and 20-24 (years)
	20-24	25-29	30-34	35-39	40-44	45-49	
Region							
Africa	18.9	18.7	18.0	18.0	18.2	18.5	0.9
Latin America and the Caribbean	20.8	20.6	20.2	20.0	20.0	20.5	0.8
Asia and Oceania	19.9	19.4	18.7	18.4	18.0	17.9	1.5
Level of development							
I. High	21.1	20.8	20.2	19.7	19.5	19.5	1.4
II. Middle-high	21.5	21.1	20.4	20.0	20.0	20.1	1.5
III. Middle-low	18.8	18.7	18.1	18.0	18.3	18.2	0.8
IV. Low	17.5	17.1	16.7	17.0	16.8	17.5	0.5
ALL COUNTRIES	19.9	19.5	18.9	18.9	18.8	18.9	1.0

Source: Trussell and Reinis (1984).

These various measures agree in showing a fairly strong relationship between the proportions who delay the first marriage and the level of socio-economic development. They also suggest that the more rapid increases in the age at marriage are occurring in the more developed of these countries. Lastly, although regional averages conceal substantial country variations, it is interesting to note that these data show larger and more persistent increases in the age at first marriage in Asia and Oceania, although Latin America and the Caribbean currently has the highest mean age at first marriage. The near universality of marriage over age 30 in all regions is also worth emphasizing (table 43).

Current marital status and disruption of marriages

After the first marriage, fertility may be affected by loss of exposure time due to the dissolution of unions—"voluntarily" by separation or divorce and "involuntarily" by death of the husband. In this section, the distribution of women of reproductive ages according to current marital status is presented and the effect of marriage dissolution on loss of potential reproductive time is discussed.

The percentage currently married shows slightly different age patterns by region than did the proportion single, when women under age 30 are examined. Whereas both Latin America and the Caribbean, and Asia and Oceania show similar proportions single at ages 20-29, the former region had a noticeably lower proportion currently married, because dissolution of unions is more common in this region. Africa shows the highest level of current marriage (see figure 16), as well as the highest proportions ever married. Across all countries, the proportion of women who were married, but are not currently married, increases steadily with age:

15-19	20-24	25-29	30-34	35-39	40-44	45-49
1	5	6	7	10	13	19

Figure 16. Percentage of women currently married, by age group, for regions and selected countries

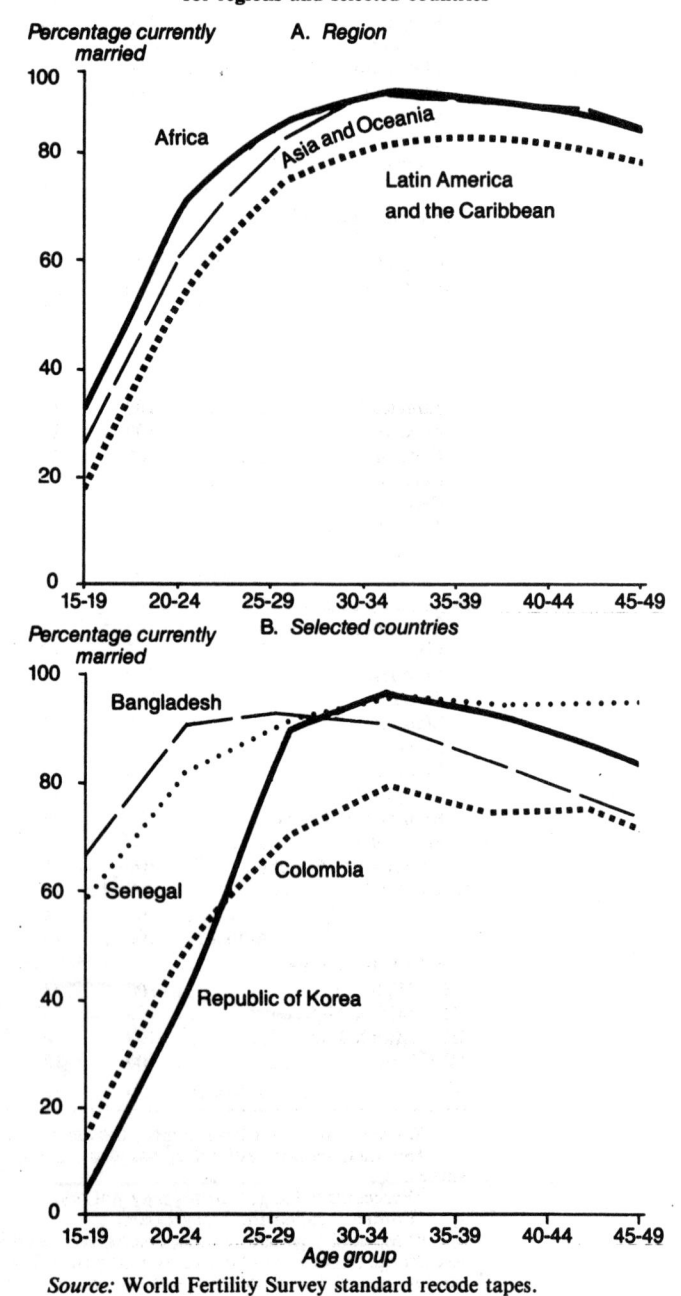

Source: World Fertility Survey standard recode tapes.

An important contributor to this rise is widowhood, which accounts for almost half of total marital dissolution over age 35. Figure 16 shows a few of the more extreme examples with respect to current marital status: two countries, Bangladesh and Senegal, with high proportions married at young ages; and Colombia and the Republic of Korea, with low proportions married at young ages. In Senegal, about 55 per cent of age groups 15-19 were currently married, and from age 25 onward, more than 90 per cent of women were currently married. The rapid decrease in the percentage currently married with age in Bangladesh is probably due to the combination of high mortality and low widow remarriage; this situation contrasts with Senegal, where mortality is high

TABLE 46. PERCENTAGE OF WOMEN'S REPRODUCTIVE YEARS EXPECTED TO BE SPENT IN VARIOUS MARITAL STATES,[a] BY REGION, COUNTRY AND LEVEL OF DEVELOPMENT

	Total[b]	Single	Married Total	First union	Later union	Divorced or separated	Widowed
Africa							
Benin	100	10	86	69	17	2	2
Cameroon	100	10	81	69	12	4	5
Côte d'Ivoire[c]	100	9	84	63	21	5	2
Egypt	100	19	72	65	7	3	6
Ghana	100	13	78	61	17	7	2
Kenya	100	14	77	71	7	4	4
Lesotho	100	15	72	70	2	4	8
Mauritania	100	15	68	50	19	13	4
Morocco	100	19	73	61	12	4	4
Senegal	100	9	87	62	25	3	1
Sudan	100	19	73	64	9	4	4
Tunisia	100	26	70	67	4	1	1
AVERAGE	100	15	77	65	12	4	4
Latin America and the Caribbean							
Colombia	100	28	61	53	8	8	3
Costa Rica	100	29	62	57	5	7	2
Dominican Republic	100	17	66	45	21	15	2
Ecuador	100	25	66	58	8	6	3
Guyana[d]	100	17	73	52	21	10	..
Haiti[d]	100	21	65	39	26	13	..
Jamaica[d]	100	13	71	34	37	15	..
Mexico	100	22	69	64	6	6	3
Panama	100	21	67	50	16	11	1
Paraguay	100	25	66	57	9	9	1
Peru	100	26	66	58	7	6	2
Trinidad and Tobago[d]	100	19	72	46	26	9	..
Venezuela	100	22	64	52	12	12	2
AVERAGE	100	22	67	51	16	9	2
Asia and Oceania							
Bangladesh	100	5	82	72	10	3	11
Fiji	100	20	74	64	10	3	3
Indonesia	100	16	72	48	24	6	6
Jordan	100	20	75	72	3	1	4
Malaysia	100	24	69	60	9	3	4
Nepal	100	8	84	84	0	1	7
Pakistan	100	14	80	75	4	2	4
Philippines	100	30	66	63	3	1	2
Republic of Korea	100	24	69	66	3	2	5
Sri Lanka	100	30	63	60	3	2	5
Syrian Arab Republic	100	22	75	72	3	1	3
Thailand	100	24	69	61	8	4	3
Yemen	100	8	86	71	15	3	3
AVERAGE	100	19	75	67	7	2	4
Level of development							
I. High	100	21	69	55	14	8	2
II. Middle-high	100	25	68	61	7	5	3
III. Middle-low	100	14	77	64	12	4	5
IV. Low	100	12	79	65	14	5	4
ALL COUNTRIES	100	18	73	60	12	5	3

Source: Calculated from Smith, Carrasco and McDonald (1984); and Smith and Balkaran (1984).
[a] Synthetic-cohort estimates, based on age-specific marital status distributions at the time of the survey.
[b] Percentages for categories may not add up to 100 because of rounding.
[c] Formerly called the Ivory Coast.
[d] "Married" includes visiting unions. In this table, the distinction between first and later unions refers to a change of partner rather than of union type. The "divorced or separated" column refers to all dissolved unions; reason for dissolution was not ascertained.

but remarriage must also be high, because the percentage of currently married remained consistently high, at about 95 per cent up to age 50. Colombia represents another extreme, in which no age group had more than 80 per cent currently in a union. In contrast to Colombia, the Republic of Korea shows one of the highest proportions married after age 30 due to a low incidence of divorce and widowhood.

A useful summary index of the proportion of the reproductive years spent in the different marital statuses may be derived by assuming that current five-year age groups represent a synthetic cohort. Their cross-sectional experience is used to estimate the lifetime pattern of cohorts, in much the same way as current fertility behaviour across age groups is used to estimate the total number of children women will bear (i.e., the total fertility rate). It must be borne in mind that these are simple estimates of time spent married, widowed, divorced or single; and no attempt is made to weight time lost by the relative level of fertility at particular ages. Table 46 shows these results for individual countries and for groups of countries. The percentage of reproductive years (15-49) spent in a given marital status is obtained by summing the relevant percentages for the seven 5-year age groups and dividing by seven.

Across all countries, about 73 per cent of the average woman's reproductive years are spent within marriage, either a first or later marriage; and of the remaining 27 per cent of her time, two thirds is lost due to timing of the first marriage and only one third to dissolution of marriages. Regions differ somewhat from this overall average. Latin America and the Caribbean has the lowest proportion of time spent within marriage (67 per cent), compared with 77 per cent in Africa and 75 per cent in Asia and Oceania. All of these regional averages conceal variations among countries as well. About 80 per cent of reproductive time or more is spent married in several sub-Saharan countries, while Northern African countries average 72 per cent. Similarly, in the Southern Asian countries (Bangladesh, Nepal and Pakistan) and in Yemen, 80-86 per cent of time is spent married, compared with 63-75 per cent in other countries of Asia and Oceania. As expected, Latin America and the Caribbean had a greater amount of time in second and later unions (16 per cent of all reproductive time), compared with 12 and 7 per cent, respectively, in Africa and in Asia and Oceania.

In Latin America and the Caribbean, the countries that stand out as having the highest level of time lost due to dissolution (8-15 per cent) are mainly those in the Caribbean subregion or with Caribbean elements in their populations (the Dominican Republic, Guyana, Haiti, Jamaica, Panama, Trinidad and Tobago, and Venezuela). These countries also have a high proportion of time spent in second or later unions. In most sub-Saharan African countries, little time is lost to dissolution, with the notable exception of Mauritania. In these countries, it would appear that a high proportion of time is spent in second unions and that although dissolution is high, remarriage is rapid.

There is some relationship between level of development and proportion of time spent married: development groups I and II averaged about 68-69 per cent of time spent within marriage, compared with 77-79 per cent in groups III and IV. Most of this difference is due to

TABLE 47. PERCENTAGE DISTRIBUTION OF EVER-MARRIED WOMEN BY STATUS OF FIRST MARRIAGE, BASED ON WOMEN AGED 40-49, BY REGION, COUNTRY AND LEVEL OF DEVELOPMENT

	Total	First marriage		
		Undissolved First union	Dissolved Remarried	Not remarried
Africa				
Benin	100	65.6	27.8	6.6
Cameroon	100	65.0	20.5	14.6
Côte d'Ivoire[a]	100	55.5	36.4	8.1
Egypt	100	72.5	13.2	14.3
Ghana	100	60.4	29.5	10.2
Kenya	100	76.9	11.2	11.9
Lesotho	100	72.4	3.0	24.6
Mauritania	100	44.1	43.2	12.8
Morocco	100	65.6	24.3	10.1
Senegal	100	57.5	40.4	2.2
Sudan	100	69.6	17.7	12.7
Tunisia	100	85.0	7.5	7.4
AVERAGE	100	65.8	22.9	11.3
Latin America and the Caribbean				
Colombia	100	65.3	17.8	16.9
Costa Rica	100	75.3	11.5	13.3
Dominican Republic	100	47.4	38.9	13.7
Ecuador	100	70.1	18.2	11.7
Guyana[b]	100	55.3	34.7	10.0
Haiti[b]	100	46.7	44.0	9.2
Jamaica[b]	100	37.1	53.9	9.0
Mexico	100	75.1	10.9	14.0
Panama	100	56.2	32.6	11.2
Paraguay	100	70.7	19.9	9.4
Peru	100	73.9	15.5	10.5
Trinidad and Tobago[b]	100	52.7	38.5	8.8
Venezuela	100	58.1	27.2	14.7
AVERAGE	100	60.3	28.0	11.7
Asia and Oceania				
Bangladesh	100	63.6	16.7	19.8
Fiji	100	79.6	12.3	8.0
Indonesia	100	45.5	42.2	12.3
Jordan	100	84.6	6.1	9.3
Malaysia	100	66.6	21.7	11.7
Nepal	100	79.9	0.0[c]	20.1
Pakistan	100	81.2	7.6	11.3
Philippines	100	85.5	7.8	6.7
Republic of Korea	100	76.0	9.2	14.8
Sri Lanka	100	78.5	6.5	15.0
Syrian Arab Republic	100	86.1	5.9	8.0
Thailand	100	73.1	17.5	9.3
Yemen	100	68.5	25.0	6.5
AVERAGE	100	74.5	13.7	11.8
Level of development				
I. High	100	63.4	24.6	12.0
II. Middle-high	100	75.5	14.4	10.1
III. Middle-low	100	64.2	22.5	13.3
IV. Low	100	64.1	24.7	11.2
ALL COUNTRIES	100	66.9	21.5	11.6

Source: World Fertility Survey standard recode tapes.
[a] Formerly called the Ivory Coast.
[b] Refers to dissolution of relationship with first partner.
[c] The Nepal survey asked only about the most recent marriages, assuming the number of remarriages to be negligible. Accepting this assumption as reasonable, the value of 0.0 is included in the regional average. Omitting Nepal yields a regional average of 14.9 per cent for "remarried" and 11.1 per cent for "not remarried".

postponement of the first marriage, however, not to dissolution of marriages.

The percentage of time spent in divorce/separation or widowhood represents the net effect of dissolution and remarriage. Even high rates of dissolution will have little effect on time spent married, if remarriage is frequent and occurs soon after the end of the previous union. Both for the purpose of better understanding the summary measures given in table 46 and for a better description of cultural or regional variation in the prevalence of dissolution and remarriage, table 47 and figure 17 present, for women at the end of their reproductive years (ages 40-49), the proportion of first marriages dissolved and the proportion of these women who remarried at some time.

Figure 17. Percentage ever remarried among women aged 40-49 whose first marriage had been dissolved, by percentage of all first marriages ever dissolved, selected countries

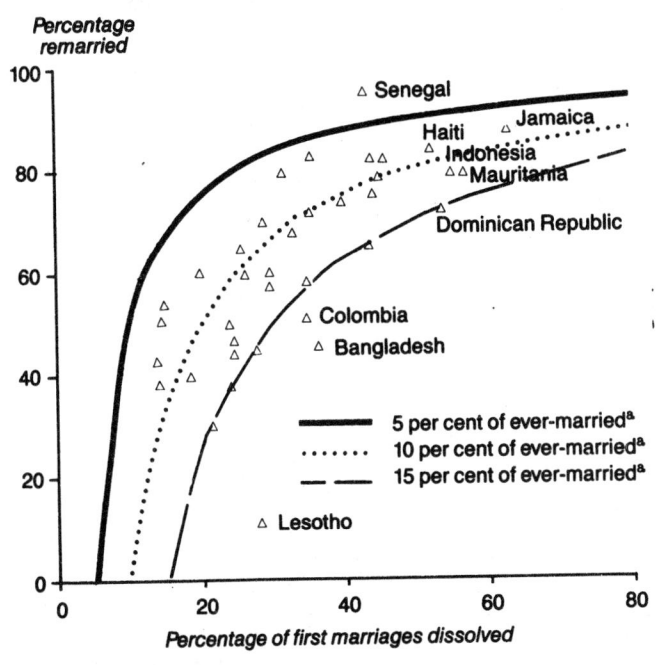

Source: Table 47.

[a] Curves show the set of points at which 5, 10 and 15 per cent of all ever-married women aged 40-49 had experienced marital dissolution and had not remarried.

Table 47 shows large regional contrasts in average level of dissolution of first marriage—25 per cent in Asia and Oceania, 34 per cent in Africa and 40 per cent in Latin America and the Caribbean. Most women whose first marriage had ended did remarry: two thirds in Africa and in Latin America and the Caribbean; and over one half in Asia and Oceania. A few of the more extreme cases are the Dominican Republic, Haiti, Indonesia, Jamaica and Mauritania, where over 50 per cent of first unions had been dissolved over the reproductive years. In all of these cases, however, over three fourths had remarried at some time during the reproductive years.

Figure 17 shows this relationship across countries: the proportion of broken marriages that end in remarriage is plotted against the proportion of first unions dissolved. Lines showing the combination of levels of disruption and of remarriage, which would imply that 5, 10 and 15 per cent of all ever-married women had not remarried following disruption of the first union, are superimposed on figure 17. This figure shows that a wide range of levels of disruption may result in the same amount of long-run non-exposure, depending upon the likelihood of remarriage. These results demonstrate the dangers of using the levels of dissolution alone to estimate effects on exposure to pregnancy. In addition, as a description of country variations in a very important aspect of family structure and marriage patterns, they are of interest in themselves.

In summary, synthetic-cohort or summary measures of marital patterns indicate that variations in the average amount of time spent within marriage are substantial and have the potential to influence fertility. Definite regional patterns emerge, with women in Latin America and the Caribbean losing the greatest proportion of potential reproductive time because of dissolution of marriages, mainly through separation and divorce, followed by Africa, where widowhood adds to separation and divorce; and lastly by Asia and Oceania, which has the lowest amount of time lost, with widowhood being a more important contributor than divorce or separation (United Nations, 1983). This synthetic-cohort measure reflects the levels of both dissolution and remarriage. However, analysis of lifetime levels of dissolution and remarriage suggests that regional differentials in both of these have a wider range than their net effects, because countries with higher levels of dissolution of marriages also have a greater likelihood of remarriage.

B. FERTILITY ACCORDING TO TIME SPENT MARRIED

The existence of variation among countries and groups of countries in the proportion of the reproductive years spent within marriage was demonstrated in the previous section. Since time spent outside marriage is one of the main constraints on fertility, a direct relationship may be expected across countries between the amount of time spent married and the overall level of fertility. In this section, age-specific and marital-specific fertility rates[8] are compared between regions to examine differences in the effect of proportions married. A further issue examined in this section is the effect on the current level of fertility of standardizing for the proportions currently married. In addition, differences among regions in the level of fertility within and outside unions are briefly discussed.

Age pattern of fertility

Figure 18 shows that the greater part of the difference between marital and overall fertility is at the young ages and mainly results from delay of the first marriage. While a woman reproducing at these average marital fertility rates during ages 15-49 would have 7.9 children (the average total marital fertility rate, TMFR), she would have 5.7 children (the average total fertility rate, TFR) if she experienced the average timing and prevalence of marriage, a reduction of nearly 30 per cent. Because of the smaller proportion married among women aged 15-24 in Latin America and the Caribbean and in Asia and Oceania, the gap between marital and overall fertility is larger in these two regions than in Africa. The overall effect of marriage among the three regions, estimated as $1-(TFR/TMFR)$, is, as expected, largest in Latin America and the Caribbean, where loss of marital exposure causes a fertility reduction of 34 per cent, and smallest in Africa, where the reduction in fertility is 22 per cent.

Figure 18. **Age-specific fertility rates for all women and marital age-specific fertility rates, averaged for all countries and for regions**

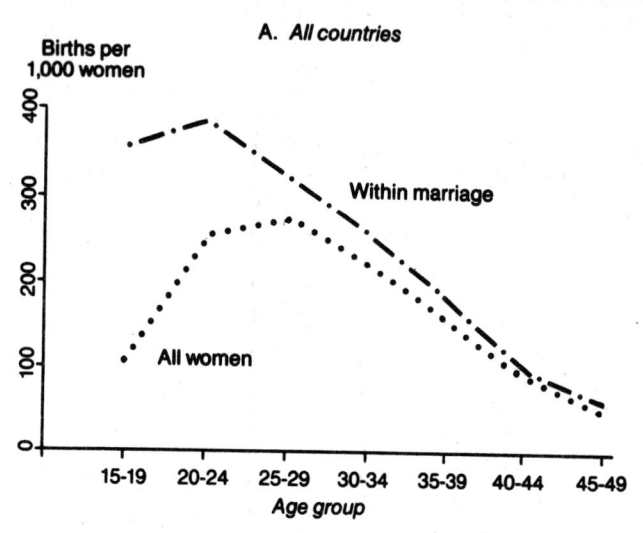

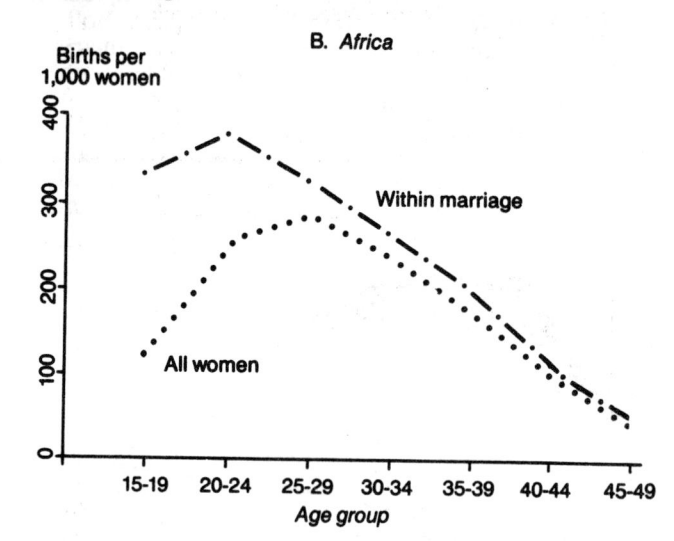

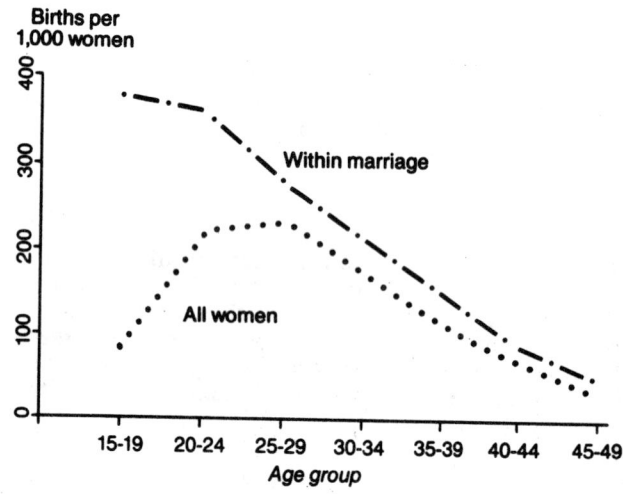

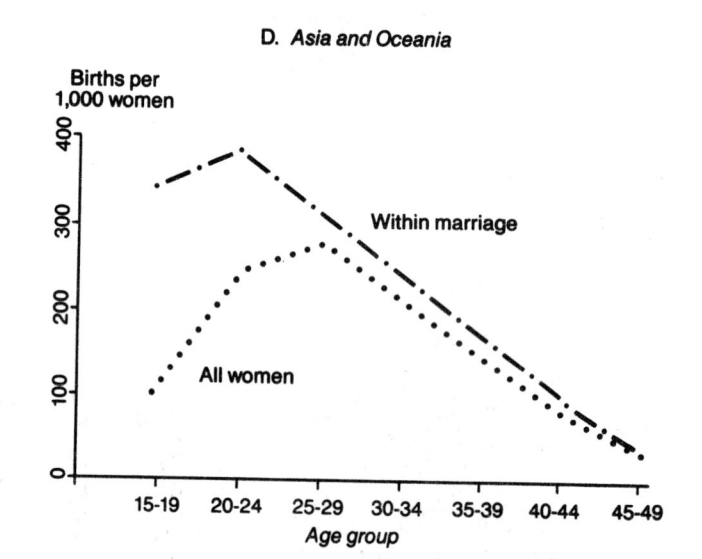

A. *All countries*

B. *Africa*

C. *Latin America and the Caribbean*

D. *Asia and Oceania*

— · — Marital age-specific fertility rate
· · · · · Age-specific fertility rate

Source: World Fertility Survey standard recode tapes.

Fertility outside of marriage

Given the wide definition of marriage adopted by the World Fertility Survey programme, which included any socially recognized sexual union as marriage, the proportion of births occurring outside of any union was not expected to be sizeable. In fact, even with this liberal definition, some countries, mainly in Africa and in Latin America and the Caribbean, have non-negligible levels of childbearing by unmarried women. Regional average rates are shown in figure 19. The age-specific fertility patterns given in figure 19, panel A, are the result of the levels of marital and non-marital fertility shown in panel B and the proportions of married women. The relatively high levels of non-marital fertility in Africa are largely found in sub-Saharan countries (Benin, Cameroon, Côte d'Ivoire,[9] Ghana, Kenya, Lesotho and Senegal), while rates in Egypt, Morocco, the Sudan and Tunisia are comparatively very low. A woman who spent all her reproductive years unmarried would have an average of nearly two children in Africa if she reproduced at the rates shown here. Most countries in Latin America

Figure 19. Average age-specific fertility rates and average rates within and outside marriage, by region

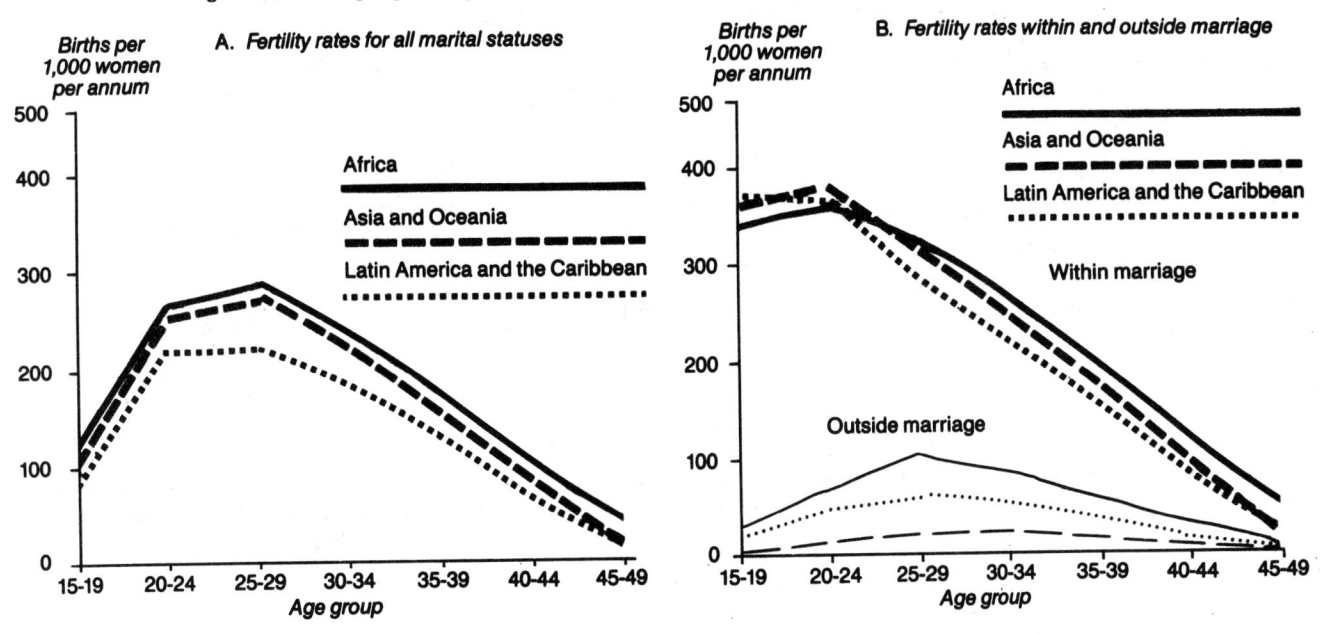

A. Fertility rates for all marital statuses

B. Fertility rates within and outside marriage

Source: World Fertility Survey standard recode tapes.

TABLE 48. PERCENTAGE DISTRIBUTION OF BIRTHS IN THE FIVE YEARS PRECEDING THE SURVEY, ACCORDING TO MARITAL STATUS OF THE MOTHER AT THE TIME OF BIRTH, BY REGION, LEVEL OF DEVELOPMENT AND STRENGTH OF FAMILY PLANNING PROGRAMME EFFORT

	Total	Married	Not married Total	Single	After union
Region					
Africa	100.0	95.2	4.8	2.4	2.4
Latin America and the Caribbean	100.0	93.9	6.5	2.6	3.8
Asia and Oceania	100.0	99.1	0.9	0.2	0.7
Level of development					
I. High	100.0	95.1	4.9	1.9	3.0
II. Middle-high	100.0	96.4	3.6	1.6	2.0
III. Middle-low	100.0	94.4	5.6	2.8	2.7
IV. Low	100.0	97.7	2.3	0.7	1.6
Strength of family planning programme effort					
1. Strong	100.0	95.0	5.0	2.4	2.6
2. Moderate	100.0	97.7	2.3	0.5	1.8
3. Weak	100.0	96.2	3.8	1.5	2.3
4. Very weak/none	100.0	95.4	4.6	2.1	2.5
ALL COUNTRIES	100.0	96.0	4.0	1.7	2.3

Source: World Fertility Survey standard recode tapes.

and the Caribbean have a moderate rate of childbearing among unmarried women, averaging about 1.2 children per woman over the reproductive years. In Asia and Oceania, fertility among unmarried women is at its lowest level, averaging under 0.5 child per woman.

The absolute contribution of childbearing by unmarried women to total fertility depends upon the amount of time spent unmarried. An estimate of this absolute contribution is made using the percentage of all births during the five years before the survey whose mothers were unmarried (never married or not currently married) at the time of the birth (table 48). This is an overestimate of births conceived outside unions, because births that occurred within nine months of the end of a previous marriage were conceived within marriage. A division of the "after union" category into less than and more than nine months after the end of marriage was carried out in a previous report (United Nations, 1983) for a subset of these surveys, and it suggests that in most of Asia and Oceania (except Fiji and Indonesia), nearly all these births were conceived within marriage. In Africa and in Latin America and the Caribbean, from 25 to 85 per cent of all after-union births were conceived more than nine months after the end of a previous marriage. The results shown in table 48 should be interpreted in the light of these findings. As expected, Africa and Latin America and the Caribbean have a much larger percentage of births occurring to unmarried women, 4.8 and 6.5 per cent, respectively, than Asia and Oceania (0.9 per cent), but even in the first two regions, this is not a particularly high proportion. In a few countries (Colombia, Costa Rica, Côte d'Ivoire, Jamaica, Kenya and Paraguay), 9-12 per cent of births occurred to unmarried mothers (not shown here); but these are the highest values, and as noted before, the proportion conceived outside of marriage is somewhat less than this. Development level and strength of family planning programme effort have little relationship to the level of non-marital fertility, as seen in table 48. This is clearly an aspect of the marriage/fertility pattern that is based on the social and cultural norms within particular societies.

Relationship between fertility and proportions currently married

Although other factors (mainly contraception and post-partum infecundability) also affect the level of fertility, it is nevertheless interesting to look at the direct relationship between a measure of current fertility and the proportion of time expected to be spent married by the average woman. The average total fertility rate for these 38 countries is 5.7 children; the range is from a high of 8.5 in Yemen to a low of 3.3 in Trinidad and Tobago. In figure 20, TFR is plotted against the percentage of time spent married. While there is some tendency for countries with a higher proportion of women's reproductive years spent married to have higher fertility, it is also striking to note the wide range of TFRs observed for countries with a similar percentage of reproductive years spent married. For instance, although women in Fiji, Jordan and the Syrian Arab Republic spend about the same amount of time in marriage, the rate in the latter two countries is 7.5-7.6, as compared with 4.2 in Fiji. Still, countries with over 80 per cent of time married have an average TFR of 6.7 children, while those with less than 66 per cent of time married have an average of 4.9. The

Figure 20. **Total fertility rates, by percentage of reproductive years married**

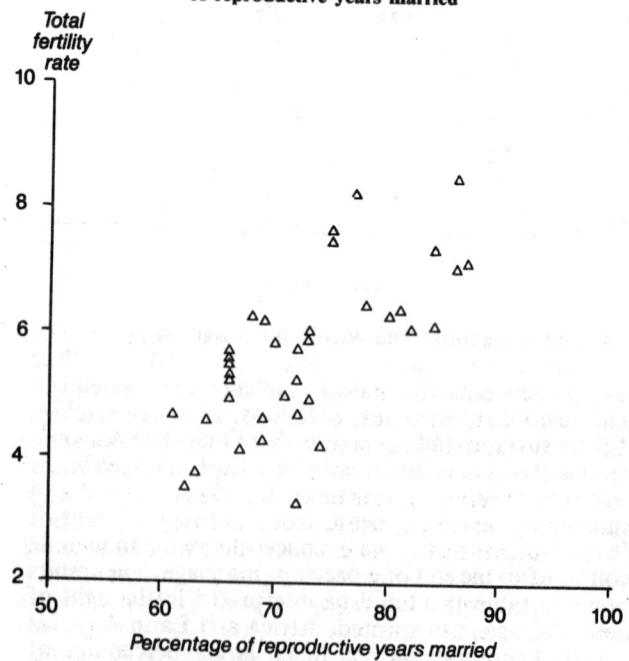

Sources: World Fertility Survey standard recode tapes; table 46, column (3); table 49, column (1).

TABLE 49. TOTAL FERTILITY RATES FOR THE FIVE YEARS PRECEDING THE SURVEY AND TOTAL FERTILITY RATES STANDARDIZED FOR PROPORTION CURRENTLY MARRIED IN EACH AGE GROUP, BY COUNTRY, REGION AND LEVEL OF DEVELOPMENT[a]

	Total fertility rate		Difference between total fertility rate and 38-country average (TFR = 5.65)	
	Observed	*Standardized*	*Observed*	*Standardized*

A. Individual countries

	Observed	Standardized	Observed	Standardized
Africa				
Benin	7.08	5.81	1.43	0.16
Cameroon	6.40	5.02	0.75	−0.63
Côte d'Ivoire[b]	7.36	5.79	1.71	0.14
Egypt	5.26	5.06	−0.39	−0.59
Ghana	6.46	5.57	0.81	−0.08
Kenya	8.25	6.81	2.60	1.16
Lesotho	5.76	5.08	0.11	−0.57
Mauritania	6.25	5.61	0.60	−0.04
Morocco	5.90	5.64	0.25	−0.01
Senegal	7.15	5.72	1.50	0.07
Sudan	6.03	5.54	0.38	−0.11
Tunisia	5.85	6.20	0.20	0.55
Latin America and the Caribbean				
Colombia	4.69	4.98	−0.96	−0.67
Costa Rica	3.53	3.83	−2.12	−1.82
Dominican Republic	5.71	5.44	0.06	−0.21
Ecuador	5.32	5.40	−0.33	−0.25
Guyana	4.95	4.41	−0.70	−1.24
Haiti	5.51	5.62	−0.14	−0.03
Jamaica	4.99	4.25	−0.66	−1.40
Mexico	6.20	6.10	0.55	0.45
Panama	4.11	4.21	−1.54	−1.44
Paraguay	4.97	5.12	−0.68	−0.53
Peru	5.57	6.02	−0.08	0.37
Trinidad and Tobago	3.30	3.07	−2.35	−2.58
Venezuela	4.60	4.81	−1.05	−0.84
Asia and Oceania				
Bangladesh	6.08	4.70	0.43	−0.95
Fiji	4.22	4.06	−1.43	−1.59
Indonesia	4.73	4.16	−0.92	−1.49
Jordan	7.64	7.15	1.99	1.50
Malaysia	4.65	5.01	−1.00	−0.64
Nepal	6.15	5.07	0.50	−0.58
Pakistan	6.28	5.45	0.63	−0.20
Philippines	5.24	5.90	−0.41	0.25
Republic of Korea	4.27	4.77	−1.38	−0.88
Sri Lanka	3.75	4.60	−1.90	−1.05
Syrian Arab Republic	7.48	7.16	1.83	1.51
Thailand	4.63	4.87	−1.02	−0.78
Yemen	8.51	7.05	2.86	1.40

B. Means for groups of countries

	Observed	Standardized	Observed	Standardized
Region				
Africa	6.48	5.65	0.83	0.00
Latin America and the Caribbean	4.88	4.87	−0.76	−0.77
Asia and Oceania	5.66	5.38	0.01	−0.27
Level of development				
I. High	4.48	4.45	−1.16	−1.19
II. Middle-high	5.52	5.70	−0.13	0.05
III. Middle-low	6.26	5.38	0.61	−0.27
IV. Low	6.56	5.62	0.92	−0.03
ALL COUNTRIES	5.65	5.29	0.00	−0.36

Source: World Fertility Survey standard recode tapes.
NOTE: *TFR* = total fertility rate.
[a] The standard distribution of proportions married was the unweighted average for all 38 countries. For each country, the total fertility rate was standardized using its own marital fertility rates and the standard proportions married. Group results are the unweighted averages of the countries within the group.
[b] Formerly called the Ivory Coast.

correlation (r) between the percentage of time married and the total fertility rate is 0.70.

Thus, the variation in TFR across countries observed in figure 20 is only partially due to differences in the proportions married. Differences between countries in the level of marital fertility interact with marital exposure to produce the observed pattern. In order to separate these factors more clearly, the effect of country variations in the proportion married is removed, in table 49, by applying a standard set of proportions married by age to each country's age-specific marital fertility rates. This standard is the average proportion married for each five-year age group, across all 38 countries. Both observed and standardized total fertility rates are shown in table 49, as well as the difference between the average observed TFR and these rates.

One important result of standardization is a reduction of the difference between groups (table 49, panel B). For example, whereas the total fertility rate in Africa exceeded that of Latin America and the Caribbean by 1.6 children, the standardized rates differ by only 0.8 child. A similar narrowing of differences is found among the development and family planning effort groups. The conclusion is that differences in proportions married are significant contributors to group differences in overall fertility. Within-region differences are also reduced by standardization for Africa and for Asia and Oceania, but remain about the same for Latin America and the Caribbean (table 49). Indeed, in Latin America and the Caribbean, standardization has comparatively little effect on individual countries, as was found for the regional average also. For all countries considered together, the variance in the standardized total fertility rates is about one half as large as that of the observed rates.

There is some tendency for countries with high rates of marital fertility to have high proportions married. As a result, there is a positive correlation between the percentage of reproductive years spent in marriage and the standardized TFRs; this correlation is, however, weak ($r = 0.31$) by comparison with that observed between the unstandardized rate and proportion of reproductive years married ($r = 0.70$).

The correlation across countries between the total fertility rate and the singulate mean age at marriage is, as might be expected, negative ($r = -0.54$) but somewhat weaker than that between TFR and the estimate of reproductive years spent within marriage—the latter measure takes account of time lost to permanent celibacy and marital disruption as well as that lost to delayed marriage. None the less, the association between recent fertility levels and average marriage age is substantial. It is therefore surprising to note that no similar cross-national association exists between average marriage age of older women and their cumulative fertility (figure 21). For ever-married women currently aged 40-49, the correlation between mean number of children ever born and mean marriage age is essentially zero ($r = -0.06$). Recent declines in marital fertility have occurred predominantly in conjunction with increased marriage age (as in parts of Asia) or in countries where the marriage age was already later than average (as in much of Latin America and the Caribbean), so that the pattern of cross-national associations has changed profoundly in a relatively short period.

An alternative, more indirect measure of loss of reproductive time after the first marriage may be obtained by classifying women by the status of their first marriage—still in the first marriage, dissolved but remarried, and dissolved but did not remarry—and then looking at the mean number of children born to women who have nearly completed their childbearing (those aged 40-49). On the assumption that age at marriage did not vary much across the three categories, it is expected that women who are still in their first marriage would have the largest amount of time spent within marriage, followed by those who had remarried after the dissolution of their first marriage, and lastly by those who had not remarried after the dissolution of their first marriage. Across all countries and groups,

Figure 21. **Age at marriage and family size**

A. *Ever-married women aged 40-49*

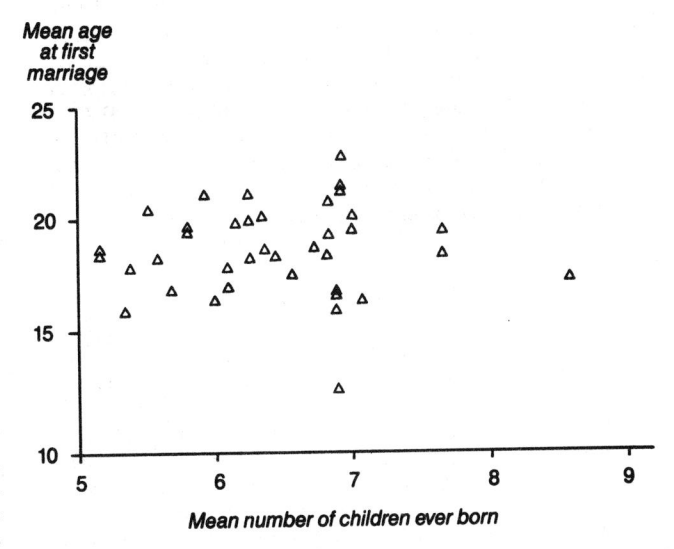

B. *Synthetic measures, all women aged 15-49*

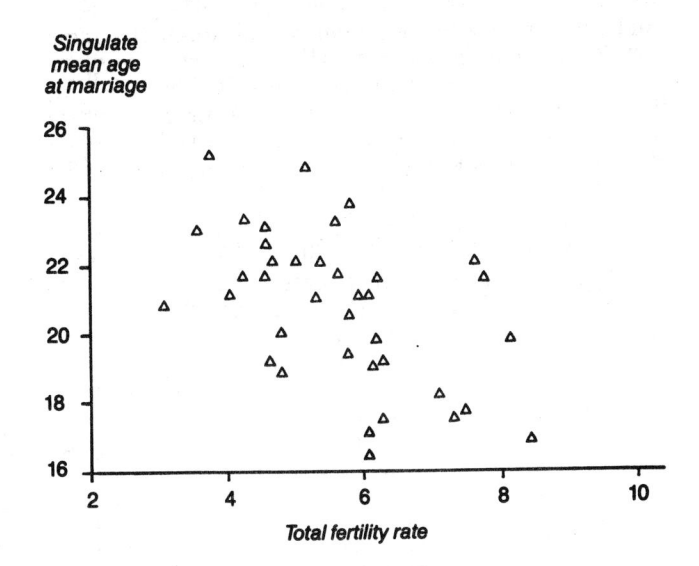

Source: World Fertility Survey standard recode tapes.

TABLE 50. MEAN NUMBER OF CHILDREN EVER BORN TO EVER-MARRIED WOMEN AGED 40-49, ACCORDING TO STATUS OF FIRST MARRIAGE, BY REGION, LEVEL OF DEVELOPMENT AND STRENGTH OF FAMILY PLANNING PROGRAMME EFFORT

	Total	Still in first marriage	First marriage dissolved		
			Total	Remarried	Not remarried
Region					
Africa	6.43	6.88	5.52	5.41	5.55
Latin America and the Caribbean	6.41	6.68	6.02	6.47	5.11
Asia and Oceania	6.61	6.99	5.53	5.71	5.29
Level of development					
I. High	6.16	6.37	5.68	5.93	5.11
II. Middle-high	6.88	7.18	6.07	6.44	5.54
III. Middle-low	6.31	6.81	5.41	5.25	5.44
IV. Low	6.48	7.04	5.51	5.71	5.04
Strength of family planning programme effort					
1. Strong	6.14	6.47	5.52	5.75	5.05
2. Moderate	6.31	6.72	5.43	5.64	5.12
3. Weak	6.81	7.21	5.97	6.28	5.46
4. Very weak/none	6.55	6.92	5.77	5.81	5.44
ALL COUNTRIES	6.48	6.85	5.70	5.88	5.29

Source: World Fertility Survey standard recode tapes.

dissolution has a noticeable effect; continuously married women aged 40-49 had 1.2 children more than those whose first union had ended (table 50). As expected, women who had not remarried after dissolution had the smallest completed family size—a difference of 1.5 children, across all countries, compared with about 1.0 child for those who had remarried. In almost all groups, these relationships hold, although remarriage makes little difference in Africa and in development group III. One reason may be that those who do not remarry consist largely of women who experienced dissolution later in life. In addition, in societies that place a high value on ability to bear children, such as in sub-Saharan Africa, infecundity may lead to marital dissolution and might also make remarriage less likely.

Latin America and the Caribbean also has some unusual results, showing the smallest difference between dissolved and continuous marriages, 0.7 child, but most of this is due to those who do not remarry. Women who remarry have almost the same family size as the continuously married. One plausible explanation is that use of contraception differs between women with intact unions and those with dissolved unions; married women are increasingly likely to stop childbearing when the desired number of children is attained; i.e., they plan their families. Remarried women lose some reproductive time, but they may want to have children with each new husband/partner and are unlikely to control fertility in the same way as continuously married women. Their loss of time is balanced against the greater motivation in a stable marriage to control fertility. Results from the Caribbean support this hypothesis (Lightbourne and Singh, 1982). This motivational difference can be expected to produce higher fertility for remarried women only if other women limit fertility. An earlier study found that in countries where contraceptive practice was widespread, remarried women did tend to have higher fertility rates than women in first marriages; in other countries, remarried women usually had lower-than-average marital fertility rates (United Nations, 1983).

Using a sample of 30 countries and separately analysing large ethnic subgroups within countries, McDonald (1984) evaluated the effect of dissolution on fertility, taking into account effects of marriage age and several other factors that were not controlled in table 50. Comparison of the number of children borne by continuously married women aged 40-49 with the number borne by all women confirmed that the inclusion of those whose first union was dissolved generally reduced the overall level of fertility slightly. The effect was as much as a 17 per cent reduction in Indonesia but more typically varied between 1 and 8 per cent. Small increases appeared in three cases. This reduction was effected mainly through the younger age at last birth of women with dissolved first unions. The fact that the fertility impact of dissolution was not larger was explained by the tendency for women whose marriages had dissolved to have had relatively early ages of marriage, as well as the small total amount of time lost in disruption in many of the countries. Thus, a variety of analytical approaches confirm that marital dissolution rarely has a large effect on the national level of fertility.

C. AGE AT MARRIAGE AND FERTILITY

Age at marriage is expected to be related to fertility in various ways. It can affect cumulative fertility directly, by limiting the number of years available for childbearing. However, populations with a later age at marriage are likely to have a higher average level of education, to be more urbanized; and, in general, to have a higher level of socio-economic development. These characteristics are associated with higher contraceptive use; thus, in the aggregate, populations with later ages at marriage may show quite low levels of fertility, not only because of their lost reproductive years but because of deliberate limitation of marital fertility. At the individual level, a related line of argument may also be put forward: women who marry late tend to have other characteristics associated with contraceptive use, such as above-average education. Late marriage in itself may allow women the opportunity to develop career or personal interests which compete with the childbearing role when they do get married. Thus, indirectly, delayed age at marriage in itself may enhance the motivation for family planning after marriage. Whatever the reasons, women who marry late are more likely

TABLE 51. CUMULATIVE PERCENTAGE OF WOMEN HAVING A FIRST BIRTH WITHIN SPECIFIC PERIODS SINCE FIRST MARRIAGE, ACCORDING TO AGE AT FIRST MARRIAGE, BY REGION AND LEVEL OF DEVELOPMENT

| | Women aged under 20 at first marriage ||||||| Women aged 20 or older at first marriage |||||||
| | Percentage with birth by month: ||||| Excluding pre-marital conceptions[a] || Percentage with birth by month: ||||| Excluding pre-marital conceptions[a] ||
	0 (1)	7 (2)	12 (3)	18 (4)	36 (5)	60 (6)	12 (7)	60 (8)	0 (9)	7 (10)	12 (11)	18 (12)	36 (13)	60 (14)	12 (15)	60 (16)
Region																
Africa	7	14	34	51	77	88	23	86	22	30	52	68	88	94	31	91
Latin America and the Caribbean	6	14	46	64	88	95	37	94	12	20	55	72	91	96	44	95
Asia and Oceania	2	4	26	44	72	86	23	85	5	10	40	61	85	94	33	93
Level of development																
I. High	5	11	42	62	86	94	35	93	10	18	53	71	91	96	43	95
II. Middle-high	4	11	42	62	87	94	35	93	8	15	54	73	92	97	46	96
III. Middle-low	8	16	35	51	76	87	23	85	24	32	53	69	88	95	31	93
IV. Low	3	6	19	35	64	81	14	80	13	17	35	52	80	91	22	89
ALL COUNTRIES	5	11	35	53	79	90	27	89	13	20	49	67	88	95	36	94

Source: World Fertility Survey standard recode tapes.

[a] Assumed to be those births which occurred less than eight months after marriage.

to use contraception (McDonald, 1984). Although the relationship is by no means straightforward, it is nevertheless interesting to look at differentials within countries in various measures of fertility, according to age at first marriage. These differentials have implications for those countries where direct manipulation of the age at marriage by government policy is possible and where Governments may more indirectly attempt to affect age at entry into the first marriage through the provision of alternative opportunities for women.

Age at first marriage and first birth interval

Women who marry at older ages usually have a shorter first birth interval than those who marry at younger ages. Contributory reasons are a higher level of non-permanent infecundity among adolescents, due to physical immaturity, and a greater likelihood that pre-marital conceptions lead to marriage among older women. The incidence of pre-marital births may also be greater for those who marry late, especially where informal unions are common. Although a long first birth interval might, in more economically advanced societies, be due to deliberate delay of the first birth, this is not a likely explanation for the longer first intervals of young wives in these developing countries, where brides often face strong cultural incentives to demonstrate their fecundity as quickly as possible. In fact, in the WFS countries, women who marry early are less likely than others to use contraception before the first birth.[10]

Table 51 shows the percentage of ever-married women who had their first birth by given durations up to 60 months since first marriage, for women aged under and over 20 years at the first marriage. The table excludes women married less than five years before the survey, in order to ensure 60 months of observation for those included in the table; marriages that occurred more than 14 years before the survey were excluded because of the presumed lower quality of reported dates. Especially during the early months of marriage, the figures are affected by the number of pre-marital conceptions and births; columns (7)-(8) and (15)-(16) control for much of this effect by removing women with a birth less than eight months after marriage.[11]

All regional and development groups show a more rapid pace of early childbearing for women who married at age 20 or over. A detailed analysis using more refined age-at-marriage groups by McDonald (1984) also supports this conclusion. Since Africa and Latin America and the Caribbean show a higher level of pre-marital conceptions (as measured by first births occurring less than eight months after the first marriage) than Asia and Oceania, the 12-month interval is more useful for making comparisons across regions. All three regions show a substantial difference in the proportion who have had their first birth within 12 months of marriage, according to age at the first marriage. The existence of greater absolute differences in Africa and in Asia and Oceania is probably due largely to a younger average age at marriage among the under-20 groups, compared with Latin America and the Caribbean, where the proportion marrying at very young ages, e.g., under 18, is very low. The age-at-marriage differential in the percentage with a birth within 12 months after marriage is smaller if women with a probable pre-marital conception are excluded (columns (7) and (15)) than if all women are considered (columns (3) and (11)).

The differential between younger and older age-at-marriage groups persists up to 60 months after the first marriage although it does narrow considerably, almost disappearing in Latin America and the Caribbean, five years after the first marriage.

Although the size of the age-at-marriage differential does not show a consistent pattern across development levels, there is a marked tendency for first births to occur more rapidly in the upper development groups, and in Latin America and the Caribbean, within each age-at-marriage category. For example, in the "20+" marriage category, the percentage with a birth at 12 months is 53-54 per cent in development groups I-III and 35 per cent in group IV; with pre-marital conceptions excluded (column (15)), the percentages decline from 43-46 in groups I and II to 22 per cent in group IV. For the "under 20" marriage category, such a pattern might be attributed to differences between development groups in the relative numbers of very early marriages, where adolescent infecundity delays the first birth. This is not likely to be an influence for women who marry after age 20, however. The results thus suggest higher fecundity for women in the relatively developed countries, and for women in Latin America and the Caribbean (see Hobcraft and McDonald, 1984; Goldman, Westoff and Paul, 1985). There is, in addition, a suggestion of above-average levels of primary sterility in the low development group (IV), since even at five years since marriage the percentage with a birth is relatively low, controlling for age at marriage. Additional information relating to primary sterility is presented in a later section of this chapter.

Although table 51 shows that the pace of early childbearing differs between the two age-at-marriage groups, this does not necessarily imply that cumulative fertility will differ greatly. The effect of a difference of a few years in the age at first marriage on cumulative fertility can be cancelled out by shorter birth intervals (for example, if women who marry later also have less traditional behaviour patterns, such as shorter duration of breast-feeding) and also by later termination of childbearing.

Age at first marriage and marital fertility rates

In effect, the shorter first birth interval for women who marry at older ages means that their fertility rates during the first few years of marriage are higher than those of women married at younger ages. Age-specific fertility rates within marriage for the two large age-at-marriage groups can be examined across ages 15-49 to see whether marital fertility differences persist even at older ages. These marital age-specific rates are based on the five-year period preceding the survey.

The WFS data indicate that there is a small but pervasive tendency for women who marry late to have higher marital fertility rates in some or all age groups (table 52 and figure 22). The total marital fertility rate provides a summary of the age-specific rates; it represents the number of children that the average woman would bear, during the age ranges indicated in table 52, if she experienced the observed marital fertility rates shown in the table.[12] For all countries, the total marital fertility rate for ages 20-49 averages 6.6 births per woman for those who married later and 6.1 for those who married under age 20. For groups of countries, the difference in TMFR (20-49) between the two marriage categories is in the range

TABLE 52. AGE-SPECIFIC MARITAL FERTILITY RATES,[a] ACCORDING TO AGE AT FIRST MARRIAGE, BY REGION, LEVEL OF DEVELOPMENT AND STRENGTH OF FAMILY PLANNING PROGRAMME EFFORT

	Age at first marriage and age group																
	Women aged under 20 at first marriage									Women aged 20 or older at first marriage							
	Age-specific rate							TMFR[b]		Age-specific rate							TMFR[b]
	15–19 (1)	20–24 (2)	25–29 (3)	30–34 (4)	35–39 (5)	40–44 (6)	45–49 (7)	15–49 (8)	20–49 (9)	15–19 (10)	20–24 (11)	25–29 (12)	30–34 (13)	35–39 (14)	40–44 (15)	45–49 (16)	20–49 (17)
A. Region																	
Africa	379	403	359	285	200	107	37	8.8	7.0	..	365	347	289	241	154	72	7.3
Latin America and the Caribbean	385	361	271	212	156	77	16	7.4	5.5	..	373	302	228	159	80	27	5.8
Asia and Oceania	357	379	295	245	174	86	24	7.8	6.0	..	374	351	272	193	109	30	6.6
B. Level of development																	
I. High	387	355	250	187	125	56	10	6.8	4.9	..	375	300	210	131	60	16	5.5
II. Middle-high	416	404	313	256	193	93	21	8.5	6.4	..	421	355	271	202	103	38	7.0
III. Middle-low	338	346	303	241	176	105	41	7.8	6.1	..	362	332	273	222	141	68	7.0
IV. Low	339	412	365	307	211	111	35	8.9	7.2	..	314	344	302	242	161	55	7.1
C. Strength of family planning programme effort																	
1. Strong	390	356	252	188	132	61	15	7.0	5.0	..	392	310	218	143	66	21	5.8
2. Moderate	357	367	278	213	151	65	15	7.2	5.4	..	375	313	230	169	75	32	6.0
3. Weak	345	368	310	247	183	96	23	7.9	6.1	..	353	337	270	202	126	44	6.7
4. Very weak/none	392	415	355	302	212	117	40	9.2	7.2	..	369	355	303	243	154	60	7.4
ALL COUNTRIES	374	381	307	246	176	90	26	8.0	6.1	..	371	332	263	197	113	42	6.6

Source: World Fertility Survey standard recode tapes.
[a] Rates are for the five years preceding the survey and are based on all births occurring within marriage and years lived within marriage during those five years.
[b] *TMFR* = total marital fertility rate calculated for ages indicated.

Figure 22. Age-specific marital fertility rates, by age at marriage and by region, level of development and strength of family planning programme effort

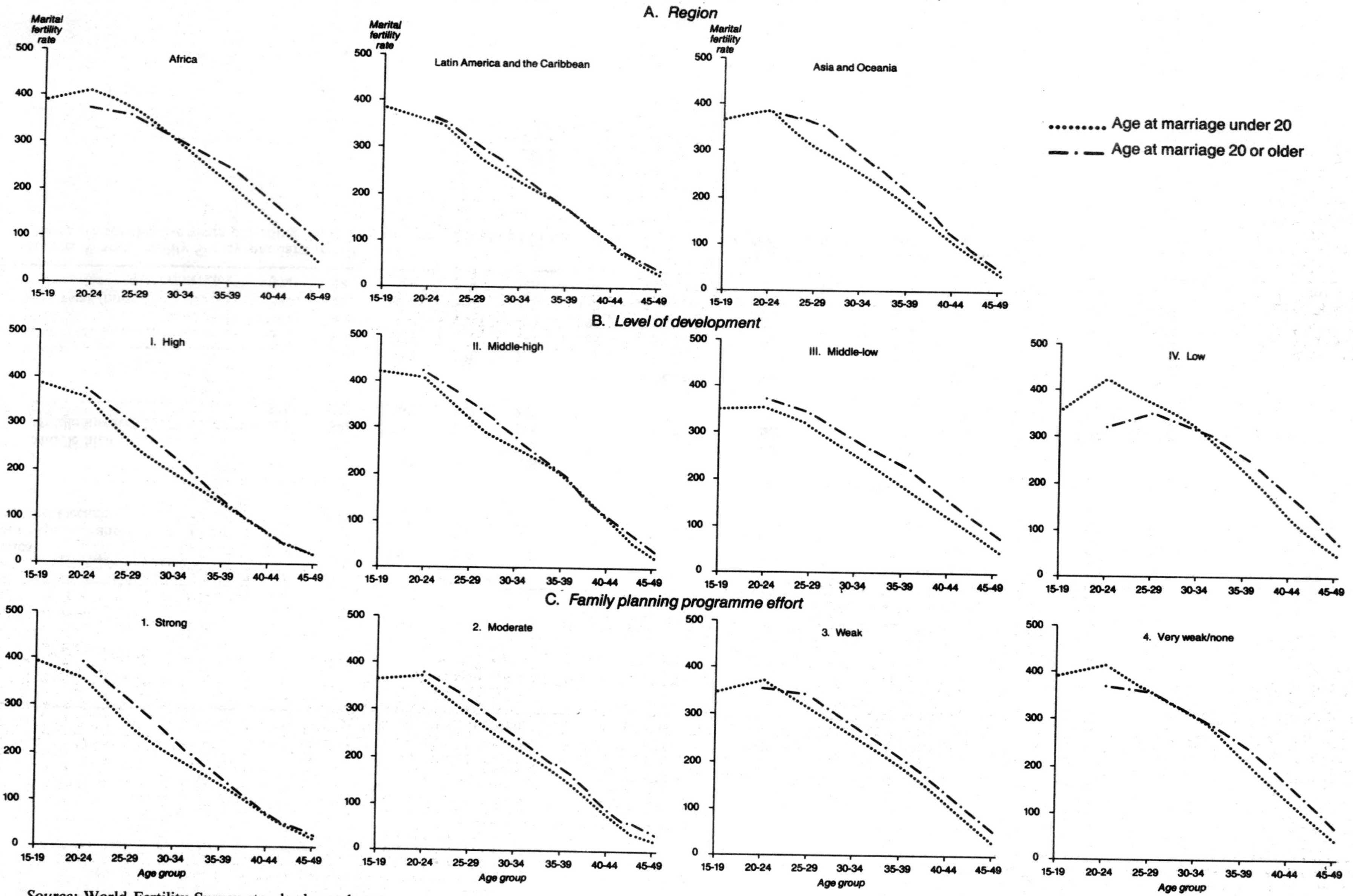

Source: World Fertility Survey standard recode tapes.

of 0.5-0.9 birth per woman in most cases, but is smaller in Africa and in Latin America and the Caribbean, and at the low development level and the very weak/none family planning programme effort. These differences in marital fertility rates are not large enough to compensate fully for the longer amount of time spent within marriage by women who marry early. At typical marital fertility rates of 0.35-0.40 birth per woman per year in age groups 15-25, from two and a half to three years of early marriage is sufficient to ensure at least one additional child, on average.

Figure 22 shows that the ages at which differences between marital fertility rates are the greatest are not the same for all groups of countries. In many cases, the absolute difference is greatest at relatively young ages, particularly ages 25-29: Asia and Oceania, and Latin America and the Caribbean; development groups I and II; and the strong and moderate family planning effort groups. A quite different pattern characterizes Africa, the very weak/none family planning group; and in particular, development group IV. In these countries, the fertility rates of women who married later fall below those of the other group at ages below 30 and above them for the higher age groups. Furthermore, the age profile of rates for women in development group IV who married later is highly unusual, in that the average marital fertility rate at ages 20-24 is slightly lower than at ages 25-29. This pattern, if genuine, might be attributable to irregular sexual exposure immediately after marriage; perhaps some women did not live with their husbands continuously from the reported marriage date but spent part of the early marriage years with their own parents.[13] Such a pattern of marital rates might also arise through reporting errors—certainly development group IV contains many countries where date reporting was problematical (see chapter I).[14] Whatever the reasons, the variations in age patterns shown in figure 22 suggest that the mechanisms responsible for the age-at-marriage effect may differ somewhat between regions and levels of development.

A variety of explanations can be advanced for these results. It is not possible at this point to determine which combination of influences provides the correct explanation, but a study by McDonald (1984), based on 30 of these countries, provides evidence on several points. One idea that at first seems plausible is that women who have been married longer by the time they reach a given age are more likely to control fertility. Women who marry early usually do have more children within each age group, and they are more likely to say they want no more children (McDonald, 1984). Despite their apparent motivation to control fertility, however, women who marry early are less likely to be using contraception at the time of the survey. More precisely, McDonald found appreciably higher contraceptive prevalence among women who married later (currently aged 35-44) in about half the populations in his study, including most of those with moderate-to-high overall contraceptive prevalence. There was very little difference by age at marriage in countries where the overall prevalence of contraception was low, plus a few of those with moderate prevalence levels. Thus, in the absence of contraceptive use, the difference in marital fertility rates according to age at marriage would probably be larger than observed, particularly in countries where contraceptive practice is common (Latin America and the Caribbean, development groups I and II, and the strong and moderate family planning efforts).

McDonald found that the higher age-specific fertility rates of women who married late could be attributed mainly to a later age at last birth (among women currently aged 40-49), rather than to shorter intervals between births. The association between age at marriage and age at last birth was pronounced in most countries but was absent or weak in much of Latin America and the Caribbean and a few countries of other regions. Although there may be particular country exceptions to any generalization, McDonald's results strongly suggest that factors that exert their influence on marital fertility rates primarily through their effect on birth intervals—duration of breast-feeding, for instance—cannot explain most of the fertility rate difference according to marriage age. (Consistent with this, McDonald found that reported duration of breast-feeding differed little by age at marriage.) A decrease in frequency of intercourse with marriage duration would also affect birth intervals and thus seems unlikely to account for the whole of the observed difference.[15] Although "terminal" abstinence for women who have become grandmothers has been reported in the anthropological literature for some societies and could in principle account for an earlier cessation of childbearing by women who marry young, there is no evidence that this practice is sufficiently widespread to produce the pervasive effects seen in these data; furthermore, the WFS data from questions about terminal abstinence (Benin, Cameroon, Côte d'Ivoire, Ghana and Kenya) suggest that the practice was very uncommon in these societies (Singh and Ferry, 1984; Cleland and Kalule-Sabiti, 1984).

Another factor that has received attention in this connection is sterility. Recent evidence from historical European data suggests that women who married early tended also to become sterile at relatively early ages (Trussell and Wilson, 1985). While the mechanism is not completely clear, infection and trauma associated with childbirth in unsanitary conditions is a likely possibility. In modern developing countries, childbirth clearly presents health risks—it is a major cause of death among women of reproductive ages. Although little direct evidence exists, there may be many non-lethal infections and other effects of childbirth that impair later fertility, particularly where modern medical care is not available. Women who marry young are exposed to such hazards from an earlier age.

Age at marriage and cumulative fertility

The long-run effect of differing ages at first marriage on fertility may be estimated by considering the average number of children ever born to women aged 40-49 years who have nearly completed childbearing (table 53). Here, four age-at-marriage groups are compared, as well as the simpler breakdown between the two larger marriage groups (under 20 and 20 or older). This older cohort of women was, in most countries, little affected by strong fertility and marriage changes, which are relatively recent. The cohort may therefore show weaker contrasts than those that now exist. However, this is an empirical question, because recent declines in overall marital fertility may not have affected age-at-marriage groups differentially.[16]

The average results for all countries show a substantial effect of age at marriage: across all countries there is a monotonic decline in completed family size, from 7.3 children for women married under age 17 to 4.1 children for those married at age 25 or older. This monotonic decline is found in all groups of countries but varies in size. In

TABLE 53. MEAN NUMBER OF CHILDREN EVER BORN TO EVER-MARRIED WOMEN AGED 40-49, ACCORDING TO AGE AT FIRST MARRIAGE, BY REGION, COUNTRY AND LEVEL OF DEVELOPMENT

	Total	Under 17	17-20	21-24	25+	Under 20	20+
Africa				(number of children)			
Benin	6.2	6.8	6.0	5.9	5.0	6.5	5.6
Cameroon	5.2	5.3	5.8	5.3	4.4	5.3	5.0
Côte d'Ivoire[a]	6.8	7.0	6.5	6.6	6.3	6.9	6.4
Egypt	6.6	7.4	6.3	5.0	3.0	7.2	4.6
Ghana	6.4	7.1	6.2	5.6	4.5	6.9	5.3
Kenya	7.7	8.2	7.5	7.5	6.2	8.0	7.0
Lesotho	5.2	5.5	5.4	4.8	3.4	5.5	4.5
Mauritania	6.0	6.3	6.3	4.3	3.9	6.4	4.4
Morocco	7.1	7.4	6.8	6.6	4.2	7.3	6.3
Senegal	6.9	7.2	6.9	5.1	(4.7)	7.2	5.2
Sudan	6.1	6.2	6.0	6.6	4.5	6.2	5.9
Tunisia	6.8	7.7	7.0	6.2	4.6	7.5	5.8
AVERAGE	6.4	6.8	6.4	5.8	4.6	6.7	5.5
Latin America and the Caribbean							
Colombia	6.9	8.5	7.7	6.4	4.2	8.2	5.7
Costa Rica	6.9	9.0	7.9	6.2	4.3	8.5	5.7
Dominican Republic	6.7	7.6	7.1	5.1	3.3	7.5	4.9
Ecuador	7.0	8.6	6.7	6.0	4.3	8.2	5.5
Guyana	6.5	7.3	6.5	4.9	3.0	7.2	4.7
Haiti	5.9	6.5	6.8	5.5	4.0	6.6	5.2
Jamaica	5.5	6.5	5.7	4.9	3.8	6.4	4.5
Mexico	7.0	8.2	7.5	6.0	3.9	8.1	5.4
Panama	5.8	7.3	5.5	4.7	3.3	6.8	4.3
Paraguay	6.3	8.1	6.8	4.9	3.6	7.7	4.6
Peru	6.8	8.3	7.1	6.1	4.0	7.9	5.6
Trinidad and Tobago	5.6	6.8	5.0	4.2	2.4	6.3	3.9
Venezuela	6.3	7.8	6.6	5.1	3.0	7.3	4.7
AVERAGE	6.4	7.7	6.7	5.4	3.7	7.4	5.0
Asia and Oceania							
Bangladesh	6.9	7.0	6.4	..	(7.5)	7.0	6.2
Fiji	6.3	7.2	5.9	5.5	3.6	6.9	5.1
Indonesia	5.3	5.4	5.2	4.5	2.9	5.4	4.2
Jordan	8.7	9.5	8.1	7.2	4.7	9.1	7.0
Malaysia	6.1	6.5	6.6	5.3	3.1	6.6	4.8
Nepal	5.7	6.0	5.3	5.0	4.0	5.9	4.7
Pakistan	6.9	7.1	6.8	5.5	4.2	7.1	5.4
Philippines	6.9	8.6	7.4	6.2	3.8	8.1	5.6
Republic of Korea	5.4	6.0	5.1	4.1	3.3	5.8	4.2
Sri Lanka	5.8	6.9	6.0	5.1	2.9	6.7	4.4
Syrian Arab Republic	7.7	8.7	8.1	7.1	4.4	8.6	6.3
Thailand	6.4	7.3	6.6	5.8	3.8	7.1	5.4
Yemen	6.9	7.1	6.5	7.0	(5.2)	7.1	6.3
AVERAGE	6.5	7.2	6.5	5.6	4.1	7.0	5.4
Level of development							
I. High	6.2	7.4	6.4	5.2	3.5	7.1	4.8
II. Middle-high	6.9	8.1	7.1	6.0	4.0	7.8	5.5
III. Middle-low	6.3	6.7	6.2	5.7	4.4	6.6	5.4
IV. Low	6.4	6.7	6.3	5.6	4.8	6.7	5.4
ALL COUNTRIES	6.5	7.3	6.5	5.6	4.1	7.1	5.3

Source: World Fertility Survey standard recode tapes.
NOTE: Means based on 10-24 observations are shown in parentheses. Means for categories with fewer than 10 observations are not shown and were excluded in calculation of group averages.
[a] Formerly called the Ivory Coast.

absolute terms, Africa and development groups III and IV have differences of from two to three children between the youngest and oldest age-at-marriage categories; by comparison, in Latin America and the Caribbean and in Asia and Oceania, development groups I and II have larger differences of 3.5-4.0 children. The relative difference across marriage groups (100 − (25+ marriage category/17 marriage category)) is also greater for the latter groups of countries—usually 50-55 per cent, compared with 30-40 per cent for Africa and development groups III and IV. These cumulative differentials in children ever borne are a reasonable estimate of age-at-marriage effects, incorporating the direct effects of loss of exposure due both to postponement of the first marriage and to periods spent between marriages, as well as the indirect effect of late marriers exercising greater fertility control within marriage.

Delay in the age at first marriage may also be related to an increased proportion permanently childless if it results in postponement until very late ages. The percentage

TABLE 54. PERCENTAGE OF EVER-MARRIED WOMEN AGED 40-49 WHO WERE CHILDLESS, ACCORDING TO AGE AT FIRST MARRIAGE, BY REGION AND LEVEL OF DEVELOPMENT

	Total	Under 17	17-20	21-24	25+	Under 20	20+
Region							
Africa	4.9	4.6	4.4	4.7	9.2	4.6	6.0
Latin America and the Caribbean	3.7	1.8	2.6	4.0	12.1	1.9	6.5
Asia and Oceania	3.3	2.7	3.0	2.7	8.9	2.7	4.8
Level of development							
I. High	4.0	2.3	3.3	4.4	12.6	2.6	6.8
II. Middle-high	3.0	1.7	2.1	2.3	9.8	1.7	4.6
III. Middle-low	5.5	5.4	4.7	5.2	10.9	5.1	6.9
IV. Low	3.7	3.2	3.5	3.7	6.9	3.4	5.1
ALL COUNTRIES	4.0	3.0	3.3	3.8	10.1	3.0	5.8

Source: World Fertility Survey standard recode tapes.

childless among ever-married women aged 40-49, by age at marriage, is shown for groups of countries in table 54. Among all countries, delays in the age at marriage up to age 25 have relatively little effect on the percentage remaining childless. However, those who marry at age 25 or older do have a substantially higher proportion childless—10 per cent across all countries, compared with 3.0-3.8 per cent among earlier marriers. This differential is substantial in all country groups, but is especially strong in Latin America and the Caribbean, and in development groups I and II. Results for the two large age-at-marriage categories show a much smaller effect, given the averaging of ages over 20. McDonald (1984) also found that only at very late ages at marriage did cumulative fertility decline and attributed this not only to reductions in exposure time but to an increased likelihood of infertility and subfecundity as age at marriage increased.

The much larger effect for women married at age 25 or older is probably due mainly to the onset of problems in conceiving, rather than to a decision to remain childless. This group is open-ended, and includes some who marry in their thirties, when proportions sterile are higher than for younger women. The variations in percentage childless for this age-at-marriage category (from 6.9 per cent for the least developed countries to 12.6 per cent for the high development group) is probably due mainly to differences in the distribution of those who marry after age 25, by age at marriage. Other factors may be operating though, since the development groups with above-average proportions childless for the highest marriage category also have slightly above-average proportions for women who married at age 21-24.

Age, duration of marriage, age at first marriage and fertility

The foregoing analyses have concentrated on age at marriage only, considering its direct relationship with fertility, and in some cases also introducing current age. The difference in age-specific marital fertility by age at marriage (table 52) might be equally well regarded as an effect of marriage duration or as an effect of age at entry into unions, since women who marry late necessarily have shorter marriage durations by the time they reach any particular age. Other investigations of the WFS data have focused more directly on the relation between marriage duration and fertility; and one (Hobcraft and Casterline, 1983) has assessed the separate effects of age, age at marriage and marital duration. While it is beyond the scope of this report to carry out a joint analysis of all three of these demographic factors and their effect on fertility, the relevant findings of the WFS Cross-National Summaries of surveys dealing with these relationships are summarized here.

When duration-specific fertility rates for age-at-marriage groups were examined (Goldman and Hobcraft, 1982; Singh, 1984a), it was found that fertility during the first five years of marriage was much the same for women who married after age 15. Women who marry at very young ages (usually at 15 or under, but occasionally this difference is evident up to age at marriage of 17) tend to have lower fertility during the first five years of marriage, because of subfecundity during these adolescent years. The effect of adolescent subfecundity persists for some time. Even by duration 15-19 years after the first marriage, as many as one third of the 40 countries showed a lower cumulative number of children for the youngest age-at-marriage quartile than for older age-at-marriage groups. Typically, the mean number of children was lower for the oldest than for intermediate age-at-marriage groups, producing a curvilinear relationship. As already shown, however, completed family size (approximated by the number of children borne to women aged 40-49, table 53) usually declines monotonically with increasing age at marriage. Thus, at least for marriages occurring after 17 or 18 years of age, the effects of adolescent subfecundity and of lower average age-specific fertility (table 52) are eventually outweighed by the influence of longer exposure time before the onset of menopause.

A more rigorous analysis of the joint effect of age, marriage age and duration was carried out for nine WFS countries by Hobcraft and Casterline (1983).[17] This report focuses on the effects of the set of demographic controls on the speed of reproduction, not on completed family size. However, one application in the report does present estimated differences in completed family size. Results for these nine countries, chosen to cover the range of fertility levels, show that age is a better differentiator of fertility rates than duration since first marriage; and the age pattern of rates also appeared to reflect the degree of voluntary fertility control more closely than did increasing duration of marriage. Duration did have a statistically significant and separate effect, however: among women of the same age, those who were married for a shorter time had somewhat higher fertility rates. This is consistent with the more descriptive analysis of fertility rates in the five years preceding the survey, shown in table 52, and with the findings based on reproductive histories of older women (McDonald, 1984).

The Hobcraft and Casterline analysis also shows that when age, duration and period are controlled, the age at entry into the first marriage has little or no effect on reproductive timing. In the context of their analysis, a separate age-at-marriage effect would exist if some age-at-marriage groups showed a pattern of age or duration effects that differed from those of other women. For example, if women who married at extremely young ages were much more likely to become sterile after the first birth, due to exceptional trauma associated with giving birth at a very young age, then the lowest age-at-marriage group might show a more rapid decrease with duration in their fertility rates than would be expected, based on the age and duration effects estimated from other age-at-marriage groups. Instead, Hobcraft and Casterline found that different age-at-marriage groups behaved similarly in these respects (that is, no statistically significant age-at-marriage effect).[18] These results do not mean that age at entry does not affect completed fertility. Indeed, the age at entry determines the age at which each duration segment is experienced and also defines the length of the exposure period: "Both sets of effects, especially the age effects, are non-linear, and hence the effect of a change in age at entry, which determines the pairings of age and duration categories, will not be the same through the whole range of typical ages at entry" (Hobcraft and Casterline, 1983, p. 23).

In the application of results from the model to obtain estimates of completed fertility for different ages at first marriage (i.e., an attempt to capture a more realistic picture, by combining age and duration effects), the authors find substantial predicted effects: comparing first marriage centred on ages 15, 20 and 25 showed completed family sizes of 6.9, 6.1 and 4.8, respectively, averaged for the nine countries. The effect of age at marriage centred on age 25 in relation to 20 is much larger than that for ages 20 and 15. The authors conclude that these results suggest that delays in the age at first marriage under age 18 are unlikely to have substantial effects on completed fertility, while delays after age 18 can have a marked effect.

In summary, this section examined the effect of variation in the age at marriage on several measures of fertility. The measures of fertility fall into two categories, the rate or tempo of fertility (the first birth interval, duration-specific fertility rates, age-specific marital fertility rates) and cumulative fertility (children ever born and the percentage permanently childless). The evidence presented here suggests that age at marriage has different effects on these two aspects of fertility. Women who marry at later ages tend to have somewhat higher rates of premarital births and conceptions, and shorter first birth intervals. However, their fertility rates (marital duration or age-specific) are about the same or only marginally higher than those of early marriers.

On the other hand, age at marriage has a stronger relationship with cumulative fertility, or the eventual completed family size. This effect is due to reduction of the time exposed to sexual relationships rather than to lower marital fertility. Using a similar current status measure of fertility to that employed here, Hobcraft and Casterline (1983) estimated that while an increase from an age at first marriage centred on 15 to one centred on 20 had only a small effect, an increase from 20 to 25 had a much more substantial impact on completed family size. Results in this report also show that women aged 40-49, who have almost completed childbearing, do show noticeable differences in children ever born by age at marriage. Strong evidence of adolescent subfecundity was also found, as women who married very early had longer first birth intervals and had slightly lower cumulative fertility at duration 15-19 years, compared with women who married later (Goldman and Hobcraft, 1982; Singh, 1984a). Women who marry early also tend to have slightly below-average age-specific marital fertility rates throughout life, mainly due to an earlier cessation of childbearing (McDonald, 1984). The reasons for this are not clear, but the effect does not appear to be due to voluntary restriction of family size. Among older women, a higher age at marriage, especially age 25 or older, was found to be associated with somewhat higher proportions childless by ages 40-49. While these results suggest that age at first marriage is related to completed family size, it is mainly delays above an average age at first marriage of 20 years that appear to have a substantial impact.

D. MARRIAGE AND CHILDBEARING AMONG ADOLESCENTS

Apart from interest in the relation between marriage and the level of fertility among all women, attention has recently been increasingly focused on marriage and childbearing among adolescents. Awareness of the special consequences for adolescents of early marriage and childbearing has grown: there is some evidence to suggest that childbearing during the younger teen-age years has negative effects on the health of both the mother and child. Equally important, marriage or motherhood during the teen-age years eliminates or greatly reduces educational and labour force options for women.

In chapter I, period age-specific fertility rates for age group 15-19 were presented by single years. In this section, women aged 20-24 at interview are examined separately for their experience during the teen-age years, including proportions who had married by ages 15, 16, 18 and 20 and who became mothers by ages 15, 18 and 20. The group currently aged 15-19 could not be directly analysed for these same exact ages, because of incomplete exposure over the teen-age years. Use of women aged 20-24 avoids this problem, while still providing recent experience that is similar to that of teenagers at the time of the survey. Ages 15, 16 and 18 were chosen because these are the most common legal minimum ages for marriage in the countries covered in this report, and because it is relevant for policy-makers to be aware of the extent of entry into unions (not always legal marriage) and of motherhood below minimum legal marriage ages.

Proportions who had married by exact ages 15, 16, 18 and 20 are shown in table 55. In Africa and in Asia and Oceania, substantially higher proportions married at young ages: 25 per cent by age 16, compared with 15 per cent for Latin America and the Caribbean. Differentials are even larger among levels of development (a range of 11-41 per cent), but the range is about the same across family planning programme effort groups as for regions, 13-28 per cent. These differentials are much wider among individual countries than among regions—for example, by age 16, in a few countries over 40 per cent of teen-aged girls were married (Mauritania, Nepal, Senegal and Yemen, and the extreme case, Bangladesh, where 80 per

TABLE 55. PERCENTAGE WHO HAD MARRIED OR HAD GIVEN BIRTH BY SPECIFIC AGES, BASED ON WOMEN AGED 20-24, BY COUNTRY, REGION, LEVEL OF DEVELOPMENT AND STRENGTH OF FAMILY PLANNING PROGRAMME EFFORT

	Minimum legal age at marriage for women	Married by age 15	16	18	20	Birth by age 15	18	20
A. *Individual countries*								
Africa								
Benin	None	9	17	42	74	3	21	52
Cameroon	15	21	36	61	81	6	38	65
Côte d'Ivoire[a]	16	18	33	60	80	7	44	71
Egypt	16	11	19	39	53	3	21	37
Ghana	None-21[b]	9	20	48	72	3	29	56
Kenya	9-18[b]	13	22	45	65	7	38	63
Lesotho	16	6	14	39	69	3	17	43
Mauritania	..	39	47	62	72	15	39	54
Morocco	15	11	19	36	53	3	19	36
Senegal	16	28	42	62	77	5	40	65
Sudan	None	26	33	47	57	11	31	44
Tunisia	17	1	2	13	30	0	3	16
Latin America and the Caribbean								
Colombia	12	7	12	26	42	3	17	37
Costa Rica	15	4	9	23	40	1	15	34
Dominican Republic	15	13	22	43	61	3	23	44
Ecuador	12	6	12	29	46	3	20	37
Guyana	14	8	19	42	62	2	19	39
Haiti	None	8	14	30	48	1	11	23
Jamaica	16	13	29	59	77	3	36	57
Mexico	14	8	15	32	51	3	20	41
Panama	12	8	13	26	46	2	19	36
Paraguay	12	4	9	25	41	1	13	31
Peru	14	5	9	23	37	2	14	30
Trinidad and Tobago	12-14[b]	9	18	37	56	1	14	29
Venezuela	12	7	12	28	45	2	18	34
Asia and Oceania								
Bangladesh	16	73	82	90	93	21	64	79
Fiji	16	3	6	24	49	1	10	29
Indonesia	16	25	35	59	71	6	30	51
Jordan	17	10	20	39	53	2	23	43
Malaysia	14	4	8	21	37	1	10	25
Nepal	16	36	47	70	84	2	23	46
Pakistan	16	25	38	57	69	4	30	48
Philippines	14[c]	3	6	17	31	0	9	22
Republic of Korea	16	0	0	4	15	0	1	6
Sri Lanka	12-16[b]	4	7	16	27	1	8	18
Syrian Arab Republic	..	12	18	35	50	3	19	37
Thailand	17	3	8	25	41	1	12	28
Yemen	16	35	48	71	84	7	33	56
B. *Mean values for groups of countries*								
Region								
Africa		16	25	46	65	6	28	50
Latin America and the Caribbean		8	15	32	50	4	21	38
Asia and Oceania		18	25	41	54	2	18	36
Level of development								
I. High		6	13	30	47	2	16	33
II. Middle-high		6	11	26	42	2	14	31
III. Middle-low		14	25	48	68	5	30	53
IV. Low		32	42	60	73	8	33	52
Level of family planning programme effort								
Strong		8	13	29	45	2	16	33
Moderate		7	13	30	48	1	14	29
Weak		20	28	46	62	5	26	45
Very weak/none		17	26	47	64	5	28	50
ALL COUNTRIES		14	22	40	57	4	22	41

Source: For percentages married or with a birth, World Fertility Survey standard recode tapes. For minimum legal age at marriage, except as shown separately, United Nations (1985, table 24). For Cameroon, Jamaica, Lesotho and Senegal, Paxman (1980, table 24). For Benin, Ghana, Guyana, Kenya, Thailand, and Trinidad and Tobago, Henry and Piotrow (1979). For Côte d'Ivoire, Haiti and the Sudan, Nortman (1982, table 3, pp. 27-37). For Morocco and Yemen, Chamie (1985, table 5.1, p. 118). For Bangladesh, Indonesia, Nepal and Pakistan, Shah (1985, table 5.1, p. 87). For the Republic of Korea and Sri Lanka, Sihombing and Finlay (1979, pp. 65, 119).

NOTE: Legal minimum age represents most recent available information. The legal minimum generally requires parental consent.

[a] Formerly called the Ivory Coast.

[b] Varies according to major administrative divisions, or religious or ethnic groups.

[c] Non-Muslim population. For Muslims, the minimum is the age of puberty, presumed to be 15 years (Henry and Piotrow, 1979).

cent were married). In contrast, however, in several countries fewer than 8 per cent were married by age 16 (Fiji, the Philippines, the Republic of Korea, Sri Lanka and Tunisia). By age 20, fewer than 40 per cent of women were married in Malaysia, Peru, the Philippines, the Republic of Korea and Sri Lanka.

The proportion of women aged 20-24 who had become mothers by ages 15, 18, and 20 is also shown in table 55. In general, the percentage who were mothers by given ages (15, 18, 20) is somewhat lower than the proportion who were married by these ages. In Africa, however, in development groups III and IV and the very weak/none family planning effort group, 45-52 per cent of age group 20-24 had at least one child by age 20. Although other groups of countries had lower proportions who had become mothers by this age, the percentages were also substantial, ranging from 29 to 38 per cent. Childbearing among girls under age 15 was extremely uncommon (less than 2 per cent) in Asia and Oceania and in the two upper development and family planning effort groups.

These results show that even by age 15, the proportion who had married was by no means negligible in some groups of countries (Africa, Asia and Oceania, development groups III and IV, and the lowest family planning effort group), although motherhood by this age is much less likely. These results imply that legal minimum ages are not always reflected in actual behaviour (Henry and Piotrow, 1979), because many of the countries in Africa and Asia and Oceania, where 25 per cent or more of women aged 20-24 reported themselves to have been married by 15, have legal minimum ages of marriage of 16.[19] Among these same groups of countries, 40-60 per cent of adolescent girls marry by age 18; and across all countries, the average is 40 per cent. The more serious implication, however, is that many of those who marry or become mothers before age 18 are likely to lose the opportunities to complete secondary school, to develop interests outside the home and to gain labour force skills.

E. SUMMARY AND CONCLUSIONS

The analysis in this chapter has focused on marriage as a means of measuring regular exposure to sexual intercourse and to the risk of pregnancy and childbearing. With this aim in mind, all socially sanctioned unions were uniformly considered to be "marriages", a qualification that is relevant to many countries in Africa and in Latin America and the Caribbean, where legal marriage is not the primary or the only form of union that exists. However, descriptions of marital status composition, age at first marriage, dissolution of marriages and remarriage, level of fertility outside marriage, and adolescent marriage and childbearing also have many applications for policy-makers, other than those strictly related to family size and population growth. It is clear that the formation of unions or the institution of marriage itself has important links with several aspects of social behaviour, of social control and of the maintenance of social groups, in addition to its role in procreation.

Following the pattern of this volume, marriage behaviour was described for groups of countries. Region (Africa, Latin America and the Caribbean, Asia and Oceania) is highly relevant for a study of marriage, given the importance of cultural variation for this topic. It is also rewarding to look at variations in marriage patterns by level of development, since age at marriage is one of the means through which modernization affects fertility. Because strength of family planning programme effort is not directly relevant to descriptions of marital behaviour, its role was examined only in the analysis of the marriage/fertility interrelationship.

Results for these 38 developing countries show large regional and inter-country differences in the amount of time spent single, either due to delaying the first marriage or to dissolution of marriages. The African region has the lowest proportion of time spent single at the young ages, 15-24, while Latin America and the Caribbean, and Asia and Oceania are more similar, with higher proportions delaying first marriage. The percentage of time spent single increases with level of development. For all groups of countries, however, the majority of women (90-99 per cent) marry by age 30-34 and marriage is nearly universal by age 40-44 (95-99 per cent). The differences at the young ages are directly reflected in the current average age at first marriage, which is highest in Latin America and the Caribbean and lowest in Africa; and highest for development groups I and II (column (1) of table 56). There is a fairly strong relationship between level of development and the likelihood of young women delaying their first marriage. Part of this is probably due to increased

TABLE 56. SUMMARY MEASURES OF MARRIAGE PATTERNS AND FERTILITY, BY REGION AND LEVEL OF DEVELOPMENT

	Singulate mean age at marriage (1)	Mean AGFM, women aged 40-49 ever married (2)	Percentage time lost to marital dissolution, ages 15-49 (3)	Percentage of recent births outside marriage (4)	Difference in CEB if AGFM is 20 versus 20+ (5)	Total fertility rate[a] (6)	Total marital fertility rate[a] (7)
Region							
Africa	19.8	18.1	8	5	1.2	6.48	7.94
Latin America and the Caribbean	21.5	20.1	11	7	2.5	4.88	6.98
Asia and Oceania	21.0	17.7	6	1	1.7	5.66	7.69
Level of development							
I. High	21.6	19.3	10	5	2.3	4.48	6.49
II. Middle-high	22.7	19.9	8	4	2.3	5.52	8.11
III. Middle-low	19.5	18.0	9	6	1.2	6.26	7.58
IV. Low	18.7	16.9	9	2	1.2	6.56	7.91
ALL COUNTRIES	20.8	18.7	8	4	1.8	5.65	7.52

Sources: Tables 43, 46, 48 and 53; and World Fertility Survey standard recode tapes.
NOTE: *AGFM* = age at first marriage; *CEB* = children ever born.
[a] Ages 15-19.

education, but changes in the role of women and greater labour force participation in the modern sector may also be contributing factors. In addition, the upward trend over time in age at first marriage is greater for the more developed groups of countries. Development groups I and II had increases of about 1.5 years in the mean age at first marriage, from the cohort of women currently aged 35-39 to those aged 20-24, compared with 0.8 and 0.5 year, approximately, for development groups III and IV. The proportion married by age 20 declined by 14-15 per cent between age groups 35-39 and 20-24 among more developed countries, compared with about 7 per cent among the less developed. Another way to estimate the trend over time is to compare the mean age of marriage for women currently aged 40-49 (column (2) of table 56) with the singulate mean age at marriage (column (1)). This comparison also shows a greater rise in the mean age among relatively developed countries. Nevertheless, it is apparent that all groups of countries have experienced substantial increases in age at marriage, or increases in time spent unmarried, during the recent two decades.

In contrast, some aspects of marriage are not strongly related to level of development. Instead, they are determined more by the norms and customs of particular societies and therefore are more strongly related to region. The prevalence of dissolution of the first marriage (column (3) of table 56), remarriage and the level of fertility outside marriage are three such aspects (table 50 and column (4) of table 56). Africa and Latin America and the Caribbean are the two regions with the highest levels of dissolution, proportions in informal unions and childbearing outside marriage. By comparison, Asia and Oceania has more continuous exposure within marriage, and most of the time lost to dissolution is to widowhood. In terms of reducing exposure time and affecting fertility, however, it is the joint prevalence of dissolution and of remarriage which must be taken into account, because together they determine the percentage of time spent outside marriage after the date of the first marriage. Since remarriage is very common in Africa and in Latin America and the Caribbean, the percentage of time lost does not differ as much as might be expected (column (3) of table 56).

The relationship between marriage and fertility was examined in some detail. These results argue that delays in age at marriage after age 20, for example, have relatively little effect on the rate of fertility in the early years of marriage. There is some tendency for women who marry late to have higher levels of pre-marital births and conceptions than other women and to have slightly higher or about the same fertility rates early in marriage. However, a delayed age at first marriage does reduce the completed family size (column (5)). The effect of reducing family size is even larger if a later age at marriage is considered, e.g., 25 years. The reduction in completed family size is mainly due to the reduction in time available for childbearing, since age-specific fertility rates are much the same among the two main age-at-marriage groups (under 20 years and 20 or older, table 52). In fact, women who marry later usually have the higher age-specific rates.

The effect of reductions in marital exposure (both because of delays in first marriage and dissolution of marriage) may be summarized as the difference between the total marital fertility rate and the total fertility rate. This difference is as large as 2-2.5 children in the most economically advanced of these countries (see table 56, columns (6) and (7)), and in Latin America and the Caribbean, and Asia and Oceania, compared with 1.3-1.7 children in the other groups of countries.

The relationship between national average marriage age and the level of fertility has become stronger over time. Among ever-married women aged 40-49 years, the national mean age at first marriage bears little relationship to family size. The correlation coefficient across countries is very weak, -0.06. However, the singulate mean age at marriage, which is based on current proportions ever married, and current fertility (TFR) have a stronger correlation, a coefficient of -0.54.

Despite the support found for a relationship between age at first marriage and completed family size, it is evident that a delayed age at marriage cannot be the main means of reducing fertility to a low level in countries where lower fertility is a desirable goal. Even countries with the highest ages at first marriage, a mean age of 23 years or older, have total fertility rates of 3.5-3.8 children (figure 21, panel B). It is clear that increasing the age at marriage within a practical range (e.g., with a maximum mean of 25) is not in itself a sufficient means of greatly reducing fertility. Nevertheless, delaying the first marriage has the potential to cause fertility decline to the extent that it allows women time to develop alternative roles to childbearing and motherhood, either in the workforce or in other areas. These competing roles or activities may result in greater fertility control within marriage in order to limit the amount of time devoted to motherhood.

One area where an increase in the legal minimum age for marriage might have a large effect is in reducing adolescent marriage and childbearing. It is still true that early marriage is very common: on average, in these 38 countries, 22 per cent of women aged 20-24 had entered a union by age 16 years, 40 per cent by age 18 and almost 60 per cent by age 20. Moreover, 30 per cent had their first child by age 18 and nearly 60 per cent by age 20. However, marriage behaviour is difficult to influence directly by public policy; one sign of this is the lack of any clear tendency for developing countries with relatively late legal minimum age at marriage to have low proportion in unions at ages below the minimum. Marriage age may respond to other policy actions, such as support for continued education for girls and measures to increase job opportunities for women.

The description of marital status and its relation to childbearing can also be useful to policy-makers in other ways. Family planning policy-makers may find it useful to have information on the age at which women begin to be exposed to the risk of pregnancy and on the level of fertility outside unions, in directing their services to the population in need. Departments of government concerned with social welfare may be interested in information on the level of break-up of marriages, of remarriage, and again, of childbearing outside marriage, because of their implications for divorce law, child support and related social problems. Descriptions of existing marriage patterns are also a necessary foundation for developing any policy measures to improve women's status.

NOTES

[1] At the other extreme, a very late average age at marriage (e.g., over 25) implies that a substantial proportion of women marry in their thirties, and this may result in a quite different type of problem: some

proportion of late marriers may not be able to have children when they decide to do so. This may not be a societal problem in terms of population growth, but it implies that costs for medical treatment of these women may rise. This issue is being increasingly recognized in the developed countries, where both postponement of the first birth within marriage and delay of marriage itself are contributing causes (Baldwin and Nord, 1984).

[2] Useful sources for those seeking more information on the World Fertility Survey (WFS) programme than contained in this publication are Smith (1980), McCarthy (1982), United Nations (1983), McDonald (1984); Smith, Shahidullah and Alcantara (1983); Smith and Balkaran (1984), and Ebanks and Singh (1984). For those seeking corroborations of WFS findings against independent sources, such references include Henry and Piotrow (1979); Smith, Shahidullah and Alcantara (1983); and United Nations (1983a).

[3] In this chapter, Guyana, a country in Tropical South America, is discussed with the countries of the Caribbean. Visiting unions are prevalent in Guyana as well as in much of the Caribbean.

[4] The singulate mean age at marriage, SMAM, is calculated as

$$SMAM = (S - 50\ U)/(1.0 - U)$$

where S is an estimate of the mean number of person-years spent single between birth and age 50, calculated here by summing the proportions single in each five-year age group 0-4, ..., 45-49 and multiplying by five; U is an estimate of the proportion never marrying (before age 50), and $50\ U$ is thus an estimate of the person-years contributed to S by persons who never marry. U is calculated here as the average of the proportions single at ages 45-49 and 50-54, or where marital status information was taken from the individual interviews, as the proportion single at ages 45-49. Since the age at marriage and proportions ever marrying often show substantial change over time, SMAM may not give an accurate view of the mean age at marriage of actual birth cohorts. Migration and age misstatement may also affect SMAM. It is, however, a convenient measure for use in broad comparisons; and large differences among countries in SMAM generally correspond to sizeable differences in age at marriage of actual cohorts. Trends in age at marriage and cohort measures of age at marriage, as calculated from the World Fertility Survey data, are discussed in Smith (1980).

[5] If women are better able to recall marriage duration than date of marriage (the datum requested in the interview), interviewers are likely to use current age and marriage duration to estimate the date of marriage and hence, age at marriage. This means, however, that distortions in the current age distribution, which in some World Fertility Survey countries are quite marked, would be translated into distorted reporting of age at marriage, with the amount and direction of error varying from one age group to the next.

[6] The pattern of overstatement by older women (aged 40-49), mentioned above, is especially marked in development group IV.

[7] The computer program NUPTIAL was developed by Rodríguez and Trussel to operationalize a reformulated version of the model, tailored to suit the data obtained in the WFS type of survey. This version uses the reported data to obtain the three parameters: the mean and standard deviation of the age at marriage among those who eventually marry; and the proportion who ever marry.

[8] All births occurring within marriage and exposure time within marriage are used to calculate marital fertility rates shown in this chapter. These marital fertility rates are slightly higher than those shown in chapter I, which were based on all births and time since marriage, including time spent after a marital dissolution.

[9] Formerly called the Ivory Coast.

[10] Use of contraception before the first birth is fairly common in Latin America and the Caribbean, but uncommon in most countries elsewhere or other regions (see chapter V). Among women who had been married less than five years, had no child and were not currently pregnant, the 38-country average percentage using contraception at interview was 10 per cent for women who married under age 20, 13 per cent for those who married at 20 or over. In Africa, the average proportions were 3 and 4 per cent, respectively; in Asia and Oceania, 5 and 7 per cent; and in Latin America and the Caribbean, 22 and 27 per cent (detail not shown). The percentage who had ever used contraception was higher—19 per cent for the under-20 marriage group and 25 per cent for the over-20 group, on average—but presumably this reflects any use that had occurred before the first recorded union began.

[11] The percentage shown in table 51 refers to the middle of the month shown, e.g., the percentage for month 0 refers to one-half month since marriage. These figures differ slightly from statistics shown in Hobcraft and McDonald (1984), where numbers refer to the complete number of elapsed months. The base population to which the percentages apply is also different.

[12] In fact, most women who marry under age 20 are not in sexual unions for the full period 15-49 years, nor are most of those who marry at ages over 20 in unions from exact age 20. These rates should be viewed as summaries of the age-specific rates rather than as estimates of completed family size for marriage cohorts of women.

[13] Countries showing marital fertility rates for the "20+" marriage group that are at least as high at ages 20-24 as 25-29 include six or nine countries in development group IV—Bangladesh, Haiti, Nepal, Pakistan, Senegal and the Sudan—plus Ghana (group III) and the Syrian Arab Republic (group II). It should be noted that the rates for the "20+" group are subject to substantial sampling variations in most of these countries, because most women marry before age 20.

[14] The pattern of fertility rates for "20+" marriage cohort in development group IV might be due to reporting error if current age of some women was overstated and if recorded age at marriage had been estimated by comparing women's recollection of marriage duration with their current age. In such a case many of those coded as marrying at ages 20 and above would really have been younger at marriage, and younger at interview, than stated. There is no direct evidence that this occurred, however.

[15] Tabulations for four World Fertility Survey countries that asked about coital frequency suggest that there may be some decline in frequency with marriage duration, independent of age. The patterns are irregular and difficult to interpret, however. (See Cleland and Kalule-Sabiti, 1984.)

[16] Indeed, at one extreme overall fertility declines may be due to the shifting of larger proportions of women into higher age-at-marriage categories, with fertility differences across marriage groups remaining the same.

[17] This report also incorporates other demographic controls (period and cohort effect), using a "rates model" (log-linear) approach.

[18] The authors point out, however, that their measure of age at entry may be problematical, in that 10-year age categories are used.

[19] In some cases, however, these women may have married prior to more recent marriage legislation, and the statistics given in table 55 are not in any case confined to legal unions.

References

Baldwin, Wendy H. and Christine Winquist Nord (1984). *Delayed Childbearing in the U.S.: Facts and Fiction*. Population Bulletin, vol. 39, No. 4. Washington, D.C.: Population Reference Bureau.

Chamie, Mary (1985). *Women of the World: Near East and North Africa*. Office of Women in Development report WID-3. Washington, D.C.: United States Department of Commerce, Bureau of the Census.

Cleland, J. G. and I. Kalule-Sabiti (1984). Sexual activity within marriage: the analytic utility of World Fertility Survey data. World Fertility Survey Technical Bulletin, TECH.2265. Voorburg, the Netherlands, International Statistical Institute (mimeographed).

Coale, Ansley J. (1971). Age patterns of marriage. *Population Studies* 25(2): 193-214.

_____ (1983). Assessment of fertility trends in Egypt, taking account of the Egyptian Fertility Survey. Unpublished manuscript.

_____ and Donald R. McNeil (1972). The distribution of age of the frequency of first marriage in a female cohort. *Journal of the American Statistical Association* 67(340):743-749.

Ebanks, G. W. and Susheela Singh (1984). Socio-economic differentials in age at marriage. Draft for World Fertility Survey Comparative Studies; Cross-National Summaries. Voorburg, The Netherlands, International Statistical Institute (unpublished).

Gilks, W. R. (1979). The examination of a model of marital fertility depending on both age and duration of marriage. Unpublished Master of Science thesis, University of Southampton, Department of Social Statistics.

Goldman, Noreen and John Hobcraft (1982). *Birth Histories*. World Fertility Survey Comparative Studies, No. 17; Cross-National Summaries. Voorburg, The Netherlands: International Statistical Institute.

_____, Shea Oscar Rutstein and Susheela Singh (1985). *Assessment of the Quality of Data in 41 WFS Surveys: A Comparative Approach*. World Fertility Survey Comparative Studies, No. 44. Voorburg, The Netherlands: International Statistical Institute.

_____, Charles F. Westoff and Lois E. Paul (1985). Estimation of fecundability from survey data. *Studies in Family Planning* 16(5): 252-259.

Hajnal, John (1953). Age at marriage and proportions marrying. *Population Studies* 7(2):111-136.

Henry, Alice and Phyllis T. Piotrow (1979). *Age at Marriage and Fertility*. Population Reports, vol. VII, No. 6; Special Topic, Series M, No. 4. Baltimore, Maryland: Population Information Program of The John Hopkins University.

Hobcraft, John and J. B. Casterline (1983). *Speed of Reproduction*. World Fertility Survey Comparative Studies, No. 25. Voorburg, The Netherlands: International Statistical Institute.

_____ and John McDonald (1984). *Birth Intervals*. World Fertility Survey Comparative Studies, No. 28; Cross-National Summaries. Voorburg, The Netherlands: International Statistical Institute.

Jemai, Hedi and Susheela Singh (1984). Question design for measurement of selected demographic events. Paper submitted to the World Fertility Symposium, London, 24-27 April 1984.

Lightbourne, R. E. and Susheela Singh (1982). Fertility, union status and partners in the WFS Guyana and Jamaica Surveys, 1975-76. *Population Studies* 36(2):201-225.

Little, Roderick J. A. (1982). *Sampling Errors of Fertility Rates from the WFS*. World Fertility Technical Bulletin, No. 10. Voorburg, The Netherlands: International Statistical Institute.

McCarthy, James (1982). *Differentials in Age at First Marriage*. World Fertility Survey Comparative Studies, No. 19; Cross-National Summaries. Voorburg, The Netherlands: International Statistical Institute.

McDonald, Peter (1984). *Nuptiality and Completed Fertility: A Study of Starting, Stopping and Spacing Behaviour*. World Fertility Survey Comparative Studies, No. 35. Voorburg, The Netherlands: International Statistical Institute.

Nortman, Dorothy L., with assistance of Joanne Fisher (1982). *Population and Family Planning Programs, A Compendium of Data Through 1981*. 11th ed. New York: The Population Council.

Page, Hilary J. (1977). Patterns underlying fertility schedules: a decomposition by both age and marriage duration. *Population Studies* 31(1): 85-106.

Paxman, J. M. (1980). *Law and Planned Parenthood*. A handbook compiled and edited for the International Planned Parenthood Federation Panel on Law and Planned Parenthood. London: International Planned Parenthood Association.

Rodríguez, Germán and James Trussell (1980). *Maximum Likelihood Estimation of Coale's Model Nuptiality Schedule from Survey Data*. World Fertility Survey Technical Bulletin, No. 7. Voorburg, The Netherlands: International Statistical Institute.

Shah, Nasra M. (1985). *Women of the World: Asia and the Pacific*. Office of Women in Development report WID-4. Washington, D.C.: United States Department of Commerce, Bureau of the Census.

Sihombing, J. E. and H. A. Finlay, eds. (1979). *Lawasia, Family Law Series*. Singapore: Singapore University Press for the Law Association for Asia and the Western Pacific.

Singh, Susheela (1984). *Comparability of Questionnaires: Forty-one WFS countries*. World Fertility Survey Comparative Studies, No. 32, Cross-National Summaries. Voorburg, The Netherlands: International Statistical Institute.

_____ (1984a). Birth histories: levels and trends in fertility in 41 WFS countries. Draft for World Fertility Survey Comparative Studies; Cross-National Summaries. Voorburg, The Netherlands, International Statistical Institute (unpublished).

_____ and Benoît Ferry. (1984). *Biological and Traditional Factors That Influence Fertility: Results from WFS Surveys*. World Fertility Survey Comparative Studies, No. 40; Cross-National Summaries. Voorburg, The Netherlands: International Statistical Institute.

Smith, David P. (1980). *Age at First Marriage*. World Fertility Survey Comparative Studies, No. 7; Cross-National Summaries. Voorburg, The Netherlands: International Statistical Institute.

_____ (1980a). *Life Table Analysis*. World Fertility Survey Technical Bulletin, No. 6. Voorburg, The Netherlands: International Statistical Institute.

_____ and S. Balkaran. (1984). Marriage dissolution and remarriage: additional tables. Draft for World Fertility Survey Comparative Studies. Voorburg, The Netherlands, International Statistical Institute (unpublished).

_____, Enrique Carrasco and Peter McDonald (1984). *Marriage Dissolution and Remarriage*. World Fertility Survey Comparative Studies, No. 34; Cross-National Summaries. Voorburg, The Netherlands: International Statistical Institute.

Smith, Peter C. (1984). The impact of age at marriage and proportions marrying on fertility. In Rodolfo A. Bulatao and Ronald D. Lee, eds., with Paula E. Hollerbach and John Bongaarts, *Determinants of Fertility in Developing Countries*, vol. 2, *Fertility Regulation and Institutional Influences*. Report of the National Research Council Committee on Population and Demography, Panel on Fertility Determinants. New York: Academic Press, 473-531.

_____, Mohammed Shahidullah and Adelamar N. Alcantara (1983). *Cohort Nuptiality in Asia and the Pacific: An Analysis of WFS Surveys*. World Fertility Survey Comparative Studies, No. 22. Voorburg, The Netherlands: International Statistical Institute.

Timaeus, Ian (1984). Estimation of fertility and mortality from WFS household surveys. Background paper submitted to the World Fertility Survey Symposium, London, 24-27 April 1984.

Trussell, J. and K. Reinis (1984). Age at first marriage and age at first birth. Draft for World Fertility Survey Comparative Studies; Cross-National Summaries. Voorburg, The Netherlands, International Statistical Institute (unpublished).

_____ and C. Wilson (1985). Sterility in a population with natural fertility. *Population Studies* 39(2):269-286.

United Nations (1983). Department of International Economic and Social Affairs. Population Division. *Marital Status and Fertility: A Comparative Analysis of World Fertility Survey Data for Twenty-one Countries*. Non-sales publication ST/ESA/SER.R/52. New York.

_____ (1983a). *Fertility Levels and Trends as Assessed from Twenty World Fertility Surveys*. Non-sales publication ST/ESA/SER.R/50. New York.

_____ (1985). Department of International Economic and Social Affairs. Statistical Office. *Demographic Yearbook, 1983*. New York. Sales No. E/F.84.XIII.1.

IV. BREAST-FEEDING AND RELATED ASPECTS OF POST-PARTUM REPRODUCTIVE BEHAVIOUR

Abstract

Data from 38 World Fertility Survey (WFS) countries show that the large majority of women breast-feed their babies, with prevalence ranging from more than 99 per cent of mothers in some countries of Western Africa and Southern Asia to 83 per cent in Malaysia. The duration of breast-feeding, however, varies widely both within and between regions and is strongly related to levels of development. On average, women in Africa and in Asia and Oceania nurse their babies for about 18 months, while in Latin America and the Caribbean, women nurse for about 9-10 months. The range in durations is particularly large in Asia, where some countries in Southern Asia had durations of over 30 months, while the average duration in Malaysia was only six months. Women in the least developed countries breast-fed, on average, two and a half times longer than those in the high development group.

No differentials in the incidence and duration of breast-feeding by sex of child were observed although duration was positively related to the age and parity of the mother. These differentials persist at all levels of development and regardless of family planning programme strength.

A strong negative relationship was found between contraceptive use and both the incidence and the duration of breast-feeding. The data show consistent patterns within countries: women who did not use any contraception breast-fed the longest, followed by those who used traditional methods, while women who used modern methods breast-fed for the shortest durations. Nevertheless, substantial proportions of breast-feeding women are exposed to the risk of another birth as only from one fifth to one quarter (fewer in Africa) of women who were currently breast-feeding were also using some form of contraception.

Special data on full breast-feeding, amenorrhoea and abstinence are available for 13 WFS countries. Full breast-feeding represents only a small part of total breast-feeding, the average duration among all 13 countries being between four and five months. The mean duration of amenorrhoea was over 10 months, ranging from 7 months in the Syrian Arab Republic to 13 months in Benin, Cameroon, Ghana and Haiti. Post-partum amenorrhoea in general extends for longer periods than full breast-feeding. The average duration of post-partum abstinence varies considerably. In most cases, the mean duration is low, from two to four months, but it is of potential importance in some African countries where it extends beyond the end of the amenorrhoeic period.

In recent years, the impact of breast-feeding on birth intervals has received increased attention in fertility research. It is known that lactation delays the return of ovulation following a birth, thereby contributing to longer birth intervals than would occur in the absence of lactation. There is increasing evidence that the incidence and duration of breast-feeding are declining in some developing countries. This decline is of concern as it could lead to shorter birth intervals and higher fertility, particularly among women who already have high fertility rates, in addition to resulting in adverse effects on infant and maternal health. A major part of the documentation of these trends has come from a number of small surveys or hospital studies and data from health care centres. Recently, however, because of increased interest in the subject, more nation-wide fertility surveys have included questions on breast-feeding. The World Fertility Survey (WFS), which also included questions on breast-feeding in the core questionnaire, provided an opportunity to study breast-feeding patterns from both global and regional perspectives. Although it is not possible to obtain trend information from World Fertility Survey data, comparisons can nevertheless be made of breast-feeding patterns in different regions and at different levels of socio-economic development.

Breast milk has long been considered the best form of nutrition for the new-born as it contains a complete range of nutrients and is also more easily digested by infants than milk substitutes. Breast milk also contains active agents that provide immunological protection against childhood illnesses. Diarrhoeal diseases, for instance, which are a major infant health problem, are less common among breast-fed infants, as are staphylococcal and viral infections.[1] Breast milk alone usually meets all the nutritional needs of infants for at least from four to six months after birth (McCann and others, 1981). The term used when the infant is fed only with breast milk is "full breast-feeding". The infant is subsequently "weaned", during which time breast-feeding continues while semi-solids and later solid food are introduced into the baby's diet.

Physiologically, the amount of milk a woman produces depends more upon the frequency, duration and intensity of infant suckling than upon maternal nutrition, age or parity. Although several studies have suggested that poor nutrition of the mother affects the volume and probably also the fat and vitamin content of breast milk, poorly nourished women, except at extremes of starvation or malnutrition, are able to breast-feed their children adequately (Jelliffe and Jelliffe, 1978; Hambraeus, 1979; Whitehead, Paul and Rowland, 1980).

Frequent suckling, including night feeding, activates the production of hormones which suppress ovulation and menstruation. The more frequently the infant suckles, the greater the amount of hormones released. Some studies have shown that feeding "on demand" releases higher levels of hormones than "schedule" feeding; and, in particular, night feeding releases higher levels of hormones (Simpson-Herbert and Huffman, 1981). As suckling diminishes, so does the amount of hormones released; and protection against pregnancy consequently is reduced.

The link between breast-feeding and the delay of the return of ovulation and menstruation is important for population growth. In countries where breast-feeding is universal but where there is little use of modern contraception, breast-feeding provides added protection against pregnancy. A decline in the incidence and duration of breast-feeding in these countries increases the risk of conception, thereby leading to shorter birth intervals and higher fertility levels. Studies of some population groups have shown that where women are exposed to modernizing influences, fertility may already be increasing, largely because of declines in breast-feeding without compensatory increases in use of contraception. Such increases are usually suggested by a shortening in the length of birth intervals, particularly among more "modern" groups.[2]

A trend towards shorter breast-feeding durations has been noted in a number of developing countries. Evidence from Malaysia (Butz and DaVanzo, 1981), Mexico (Mexico, 1981), the Republic of Korea (Coale, Cho and Goldman, 1979) and Thailand (Knodel and Debavalya, 1980) all point to declining breast-feeding durations. Among several reasons given for the decline in the intensity and duration of breast-feeding is the increasingly widespread availability of formulas for feeding infants. While the infant formula by itself has no harmful effects and indeed may be a useful supplement to breast milk after from four to six months, and frequently even earlier, the lack of facilities properly to sterilize bottles and nipples or to refrigerate mixed formulas or milk may result in gastrointestinal diseases for the child.[3]

Another probable reason for the decline in breast-feeding durations in developing countries is that because of urbanization and industrialization, more women now work in non-agricultural jobs which are frequently in a place away from home where it is difficult to breast-feed "on demand" even if breast-feeding on schedule is continued. Several studies have shown that urban women are less likely than rural women to initiate breast-feeding and when they do breast-feed, they are likely to do it for shorter durations than rural women (McCann and others, 1981).

In developed countries, recent trends in the incidence and duration of breast-feeding are in the opposite direction to that observed in the developing countries. Several studies, including those carried out in Australia, Sweden and the United States of America, have observed an increase in the incidence of breast-feeding though no changes have been reported in durations (which remain short). A survey conducted in 1980 in the United States reported a dramatic increase in the percentage of women breast-feeding: 51 per cent of white mothers fed their children exclusively by breast-feeding in 1980, as against only 19 per cent in 1979 (United States of America, 1984). The current movement towards breast-feeding reflects new attitudes among women in developed countries about the physiological and psychological advantages of breast-feeding over milk substitutes.[4]

Although breast-feeding has the known effect of delaying ovulation, it may prove an unreliable method of avoiding conception for the individual woman if it is used alone. During the period of full breast-feeding, the use of contraception may be unnecessary, especially if feeding is "on demand", but when breast-feeding is reduced or terminated, the period of lactational amenorrhoea ends soon after. Ovulation may occur before the onset of the first menstruation or it may occur after the first or subsequent menstrual cycles. The uncertainty surrounding the time of return of the first ovulatory cycle makes breast-feeding an unreliable method of contraception for the individual woman. Therefore, contraceptive protection may be required as early as six months after birth or even earlier if pregnancy is to be avoided.

In general, non-hormonal contraceptives, such as the intra-uterine device (IUD), voluntary sterilization and withdrawal, do not have any effect on lactation. However, certain types of contraceptives are known to influence the quantity and composition of breast milk. Combined estrogen-progestin pills are known to reduce the volume of milk in some cases, though the available evidence is not conclusive (World Health Organization, 1983). They may also have a detrimental effect on the composition of breast milk and may result in the excretion of exogenous steroids in the milk. In some countries, oral contraception is not available to lactating women, while in others, it is available with the restriction that oral contraception cannot be used during the first several months of lactation (with the number of months varying in different countries) (Nortman, 1982). In Costa Rica, it is recommended that physicians do not supply oral contraceptives to breast-feeding women, while in Thailand, a low-dosage preparation is prescribed immediately post-partum and a regular dosage for women one month post-partum. The World Health Organization (1981) recommends that programmes advocating hormonal methods only should, nevertheless, provide a variety of non-hormonal methods for breast-feeding women.

In some developing countries, especially those in sub-Saharan Africa and parts of Asia, sexual intercourse is not culturally sanctioned for breast-feeding mothers. In some countries, this taboo is rationalized as a means of avoiding pregnancy in order to protect the health of the mother and infant; and, in other countries, so that breast milk does not become "contaminated". In either case, the effect keeps birth intervals long. Sexual abstinence is known to have been practised among some groups for as long as from two to three years: for example, the Yoruba of Nigeria and the Javanese of Indonesia

(Kent, 1981). The duration and incidence of post-partum abstinence, however, is thought to be declining in most of these countries (Caldwell and Caldwell, 1981; Hull, 1980; McCann and others, 1981). While the reasons for this decline are not clear, its impact on fertility has already been felt in some countries. In this context, it is important to know the incidence and duration of abstinence in different populations so that appropriate recommendations for contraceptive protection can be made.

Fifteen countries participating in the World Fertility Survey programme collected data on full breast-feeding, abstinence and amenorrhoea, using the module for factors other than contraception affecting fertility (FOTCAF). This information is also analysed in this chapter. Unfortunately, an analysis of trends was not possible as information was collected only for the last and penultimate births.

Prior to the World Fertility Survey, most information on breast-feeding came from studies carried out at the village level or from observations from health centres and clinics; and although data were available on patterns and differentials of breast-feeding, these usually pertained to select subpopulations. Estimates of breast-feeding patterns and differentials are necessary at the national level so that Governments can formulate policies relating to breast-feeding for the country as a whole, as well as for subgroups if necessary. Policies relating to the availability of breast-milk substitutes, the provision of contraceptives to breast-feeding women and the education of women with respect to the positive effects of breast-feeding can also be better formulated if based on nation-wide information. In this chapter, the prevalence, duration and patterns of breast-feeding are examined for all WFS countries. In addition, for each country, breast-feeding differentials by age of mother, parity and sex of the breast-fed child are presented.

The WFS data also facilitate the study of some other aspects of the breast-feeding and fertility relationship. Data on post-partum amenorrhoea, full breast-feeding and post-partum abstinence are available, and the incidence and duration of these factors and their relationship to each other are also examined. Breast-feeding differentials by contraceptive use are also analysed. Information is summarized by region, level of development and strength of family planning programme effort.

A. DATA AND METHODOLOGY

Information on breast-feeding was collected in the core questionnaire by all countries. The questions on breast-feeding, however, were restricted to the last closed birth interval and the open birth interval, except in Fiji, where women were only asked about their last live birth. Respondents were asked whether the child was breast-fed; and if so, the number of months that the child was breast-fed. Details on the questions asked and the variations in questions between countries are well presented in a WFS publication on the comparability of questionnaires (Singh, 1984). In some countries (Cameroon, Ghana, Haiti, Kenya, Lesotho, the Philippines, Senegal, the Sudan, the Syrian Arab Republic, Tunisia and Yemen), pregnancies and not live births were used to define intervals. Questions on breast-feeding therefore related to the last and penultimate pregnancies. In these cases, no breast-feeding questions were asked if the outcome of the pregnancy was not a live birth.

Fifteen of the WFS countries included the FOTCAF module in their basic questionnaire: Benin; Cameroon; Côte d'Ivoire;[5] Egypt; Ghana; Haiti; Kenya; Lesotho; Mauritania; the Philippines; Senegal; the Sudan; the Syrian Arab Republic; Tunisia; Yemen. The FOTCAF module included questions on post-partum abstinence, post-partum amenorrhoea and age of child at weaning, that is, the duration of full breast-feeding, for both the open and last closed birth interval. While some countries modified some of the questions suggested by WFS, others collected additional information. The questions canvassed by countries that included the FOTCAF module and the responses that were coded are also presented in the WFS publication on comparability of questionnaires (Singh, 1984).

Although parameters of the breast-feeding distribution can be obtained from data on the last live birth and the penultimate live birth, it has been shown that the distributions derived from these intervals tend to be biased. An alternative method of describing the distribution, which utilizes data on current breast-feeding status, has fewer problems than those associated with either the open or closed birth interval. All three methods—open interval, last closed interval and current breast-feeding status— and their limitations are discussed in detail in two WFS publications (Page, Lesthaeghe and Shah, 1982; and Ferry and Smith, 1983). The advantages and disadvantages of the different methods are summarized here.

Women whose birth intervals are longer than average tend to be overrepresented in the open birth interval. At the individual level, the chance that the survey date cuts across a woman's longer birth interval is higher than having the survey date cut across one of her shorter intervals. Therefore, those intervals which are longer than average have a higher chance of being included in the survey as the open interval. Another source of bias towards longer open intervals arises from the peculiar coding of intervals of pregnant women used by WFS. In the WFS data sets, women who are currently pregnant at the time of interview are considered to have a closed birth interval for purposes of recording duration of breast-feeding. In other words, for currently pregnant women who had breast-fed their last child, the duration of breast-feeding of their last child is coded as if it were their penultimate child. Women with short birth intervals will therefore be underrepresented in the open birth interval because the probability of being pregnant at the time of the survey and therefore of being excluded from the open-interval data set is higher for women with short intervals. Besides giving biased estimates of the duration of breast-feeding, one researcher has noted that differentials in breast-feeding duration between the open and the closed interval within a given country have a low degree of consistency (Lesthaeghe, 1982).

Data for the last closed birth interval underrepresent women with longer than average birth intervals, using the reasoning outlined above. Both the open and closed birth intervals therefore give biased estimates of breast-feeding durations. A combination of the two intervals might arrive at a more accurate estimate, but it is not certain that the biases actually cancel each other. Another bias results from recall problems, which can be associated with both the open and the last closed birth interval when the births occurred further in the past. This is more likely to occur for older women. Recall problems can be associated with whether a woman breast-fed at all; and if she did, with the duration of breast-feeding. Most breast-feeding distributions show heaping on multiples of 6 or 12 months. While it is possible that a tendency to stop breast-feeding at these intervals may exist and that the peaks are genuine, it is more likely that it is a reporting problem. Proportions who were still breast-feeding at the time of the survey do not show heaping on multiples of 6 and 12, as one might expect if the heaping were genuine (Page, Lesthaeghe and Shah, 1982).

The third method of arriving at a mean duration of breast-feeding, and the one used almost exclusively in this chapter, is to consider data for all births for a given period immediately preceding the survey.[6] This estimate is derived from information on breast-feeding status at the time of the survey and is limited to births that had occurred within 48 months (or some specified period) prior to the survey. The proportion of children breast-fed at a given duration is obtained by dividing the number of currently breast-feeding children born that many months ago, by the number of births that occurred in that month. Therefore, its accuracy depends upon the correct reporting of children's birth dates. The proportion of children currently being breast-fed among births occurring d months ago is similar to the life-table value l_x and can be taken as an estimate of the same. This proportion estimated from the birth history, $P(d)$, also includes in the denominator births that were not breast-fed at all to begin with and therefore is an estimate of l'_x, which is the life-table l_x for all children, regardless of whether they were breast-fed.

The mean duration of breast-feeding in months ($\bar{y}$) can therefore be estimated as

$$\bar{Y} = 0.5E + \sum_{d=1}^{n} P(d)$$
$$= 0.5E + \sum_{x=1}^{n} l'_x$$

where E is the proportion ever breast-fed. As the interest is in the proportion of children being breast-fed at different ages among all children and not just breast-fed children, E, the proportion ever breast-fed, is included in the equation.

By ordering the proportions breast-feeding at progressively longer durations (up to 48 months in this example), a synthetic life table of breast-feeding is obtained. The median and quartiles can be obtained by summation of proportions. Unlike the life-table l_x values, the $P(d)$ values often do not decline monotonically because the number of births in each month has a high degree of variability, largely because of small sample sizes and also because of the reporting of birth dates. If the $P(d)$ values do not decline monotonically, it may not be possible to identify unique values for the median and quartiles. For presentation, the data are blocked into categories that are three months wide and centred on 3, 6, 9 etc. months by taking three-month averages. Even after the blocking of data it is sometimes not possible to obtain a unique median or quartile; in these cases, the average of the values was taken to be the median or quartile, as the case may be.

By considering the number of children born in a specified period, the reference is to a sample of children, not a sample of women. If, for example, there are breast-feeding differences associated with the age of the mother, the difference should be interpreted as the difference in the breast-feeding experiences of children born to mothers in different age groups. The difference between the two interpretations is slight (Singh and Ferry, 1984); and in the subsequent analysis, the latter interpretation is always meant, if not always explicitly stated.

Several assumptions are made about children who were currently breast-fed. For twin births, it is assumed that only one twin was currently breast-fed, although both might have been.[7] Another assumption is that only the oldest child was currently being breast-fed. In other words, for the purposes of the estimate, each woman could have only one child currently being breast-fed although she might in fact have been breast-feeding more than one.

The response on current breast-feeding status was obtained from the question on duration of breast-feeding in the open interval. A separate category for women who were still breast-feeding was created. It is possible that some women misinterpreted the question and gave a duration up to the date of interview instead of saying that they were still breast-feeding. Whether this occurred frequently cannot be determined from these data. Lastly, in WFS, currently pregnant women were coded as having a closed birth interval, the interval being closed by the yet unborn child. This does not follow the conventional definition of open and closed birth intervals in which currently pregnant women would have their last birth interval coded as being an open birth interval. In this study, birth intervals of currently pregnant women are recoded to reflect the more conventional definition.

The "current status" method of estimating mean breast-feeding durations does not have recall problems on the reporting of duration associated with means derived from retrospective reporting of duration in the open or closed birth interval. Heaping on multiples of 6 and 12 months is not apparent in this method, which depends upon the reporting of children's date of birth in the period under consideration. However, the displacement of birth rates towards the survey date and/or away from the survey date, as has been observed in some countries in the period from one to two years prior to the survey date, may result in a bias in estimated durations (United Nations, 1983).

The current status method is also used for measurement of the duration of full breast-feeding, amenorrhoea and abstinence for those countries that used the FOTCAF module. As in the case of breast-feeding duration estimates described above, the period under consideration was 48 months before the survey, except for Bangladesh, Indonesia, Nepal and Sri Lanka, where the period was 60 months. For the latter countries, a period of 60 months was chosen because an examination of the distribution of children currently breast-fed showed that a fair number of babies born more than four years prior to the date were still being breast-fed at the time of the survey.

All women in the sample who had had one or more surviving births and who had been between 15 and 49 years old at the time of birth were included in this study. Estimates of durations based only on surviving births as opposed to all births are expected to be slightly longer since breast-feeding can continue only if the child survives. Women whose last child was dead at the time of survey may have intended to breast-feed longer but due to the premature deaths of these children it was not possible. In populations with low infant mortality, the difference in estimates is small but it is somewhat larger in countries with high infant mortality. Usually

TABLE 57. MEAN, MEDIAN, FIRST AND THIRD QUARTILES OF BREAST-FEEDING DURATION FOR ALL BIRTHS
AND MEAN BREAST-FEEDING DURATION ONLY FOR BIRTHS THAT WERE BREAST-FED

Region and country	All births — Percentage ever breast-fed (1)	Mean (2)	Median (3)	First quartile (4)	Third quartile (5)	Mean duration of only births that were breast-fed (6)
Africa						
Benin	98.5	21.2	19.9	15.3	27.1	21.5
Cameroon	98.8	18.9	18.2	14.0	23.9	19.3
Côte d'Ivoire[a]	98.8	19.3	20.2	13.9	24.5	19.5
Egypt	96.9	18.8	17.8	11.7	23.8	19.4
Ghana	99.6	19.2	17.8	13.8	23.7	19.3
Kenya	99.0	17.9	16.6	12.7	22.4	18.1
Lesotho	98.1	20.9	21.0	18.4	26.1	21.3
Mauritania	99.3	17.0	17.7	15.0	20.7	17.1
Morocco	96.1	15.6	16.6	9.6	21.5	16.2
Senegal	99.4	19.9	19.7	17.5	23.3	20.0
Sudan	98.8	17.0	17.1	12.8	20.9	17.2
Tunisia	97.6	14.9	15.8	6.7	19.8	15.3
AVERAGE	98.4	18.4	—	—	—	18.7
Latin America and the Caribbean						
Colombia	94.5	9.7	7.4	3.1	14.5	10.3
Costa Rica	85.3	5.2	1.9	0.5	9.2	6.1
Dominican Republic	92.6	9.0	7.7	3.1	13.4	9.7
Ecuador	96.1	13.1	12.5	7.0	18.2	13.6
Guyana	93.6	7.0	4.0	1.6	9.9	7.5
Haiti	97.1	16.9	18.6	11.7	20.8	17.4
Jamaica	97.3	8.8	9.1	2.9	12.0	9.0
Mexico	88.0	9.6	7.9	1.6	16.0	10.9
Panama	89.1	7.6	3.8	1.2	13.5	8.5
Paraguay	95.3	11.6	12.1	6.9	16.5	12.2
Peru	94.7	14.2	13.8	6.2	20.9	14.9
Trinidad and Tobago	87.4	6.1	3.4	1.1	7.9	7.0
Venezuela	90.2	7.6	4.1	1.3	12.4	8.4
AVERAGE	92.4	9.7	—	—	—	10.4
Asia and Oceania						
Bangladesh	99.2	33.5	32.1	23.3	43.5	33.8
Fiji	87.6	9.7	9.2	2.1	14.2	11.1
Indonesia	98.2	26.3	26.0	17.0	34.3	26.8
Jordan	95.8	11.8	10.7	4.8	18.1	12.3
Malaysia	83.3	5.8	2.7	0.8	10.2	7.0
Nepal	99.2	30.5	26.8	21.0	37.9	30.7
Pakistan	97.7	21.9	20.8	16.5	26.9	22.4
Philippines	88.8	13.7	14.1	4.6	19.4	15.6
Republic of Korea	97.1	17.0	17.3	9.9	23.4	17.5
Sri Lanka	97.8	22.3	21.7	12.3	30.0	22.8
Syrian Arab Republic	91.6	11.7	10.2	5.5	17.8	12.8
Thailand	95.5	19.9	19.4	10.8	28.4	20.8
Yemen	96.0	12.9	9.4	5.2	21.7	13.4
AVERAGE	94.5	18.2	—	—	—	19.0

Source: World Fertility Survey standard recode tapes.
[a] Formerly called the Ivory Coast.

no more than one month is added to the mean (Singh and Ferry, 1984).

B. GENERAL CHARACTERISTICS

Incidence

The proportion of women who had ever breast-fed their children varies from country to country. In some countries, breast-feeding is very much a part of the cultural practices surrounding childbirth and almost all women breast-feed, though some may breast-feed for shorter durations than others. In other countries, breast-feeding is not so closely tied to traditional practices surrounding childbirth. In these countries, women tend to wean their children earlier or not to breast-feed at all if other alternatives are available. Time spent breast-feeding may compete with other uses of time, and work-dictated separation of the child from the mother soon after birth may make breast-feeding inconvenient. One would expect this to be the case mainly in those countries where more women are working away from home and where infant food supplements are readily available and affordable. However, there has not been sufficient evidence from other sources to determine if this is the case.

The WFS data show that there is considerable variation across countries in the proportion of women who had ever breast-fed their children. Figure 23 shows the proportion of women who did not breast-feed their last children for countries grouped by region. This proportion is estimated using data from both the open and closed interval. Women who had breast-fed in either one of the intervals

Figure 23. **Percentage of women who had never breast-fed, by country**

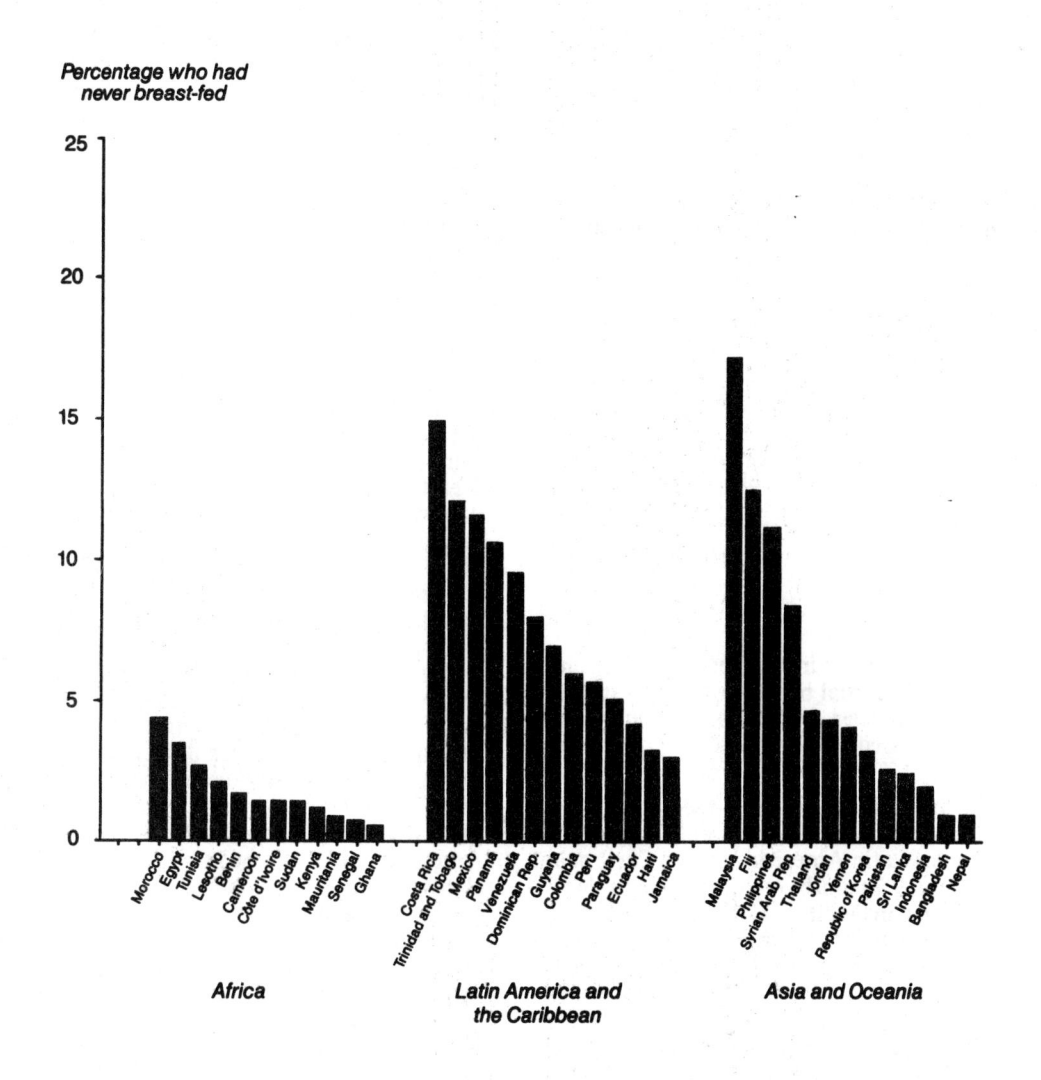

Source: Table 57.

were considered to have ever breast-fed. Women in countries of Africa are more likely to breast-feed than those in Latin America and the Caribbean or Asia and Oceania (table 57, column (1); and figure 23). On average, 98.4 per cent of women with at least one birth had ever breast-fed in African countries. In Latin America and the Caribbean, the corresponding percentage is 92.4; and in Asia and Oceania, 94.5. In Africa, there is not much variation in the proportion of women who had ever breast-fed. In the Northern African countries, Tunisia, Egypt and Morocco, 97.6, 96.9 and 96.1 per cent, respectively, of women had ever breast-fed, while in Ghana, Kenya, Mauritania and Senegal, the proportion was about 99 per cent. There is much more variation among countries in Latin America and the Caribbean and in Asia and Oceania. In Costa Rica, Mexico, Panama and Trinidad and Tobago, fewer than 90 per cent of women had ever breast-fed; and in Haiti and Jamaica, about 97 per cent. In Asia and Oceania, 98 per cent or more of women in the Southern Asian countries—Bangladesh, Nepal, Pakistan and Sri Lanka—and in Indonesia in South-eastern Asia, had ever breast-fed. In contrast, only about 83 per cent of the women in Malaysia had ever breast-fed.

Unfortunately, the WFS data do not permit the study of trends in the prevalence of breast-feeding, as information on breast-feeding was obtained only for the last two births in almost all countries. Mixed evidence of trends in the prevalence of breast-feeding comes from a few nation-wide surveys and a number of smaller studies (McCann and others, 1981). Although some of the data are not comparable across studies, the various studies suggest a decline in the proportion of women who breast-feed their children. In Thailand, there was little change in the proportion of women who breast-fed between 1969 and 1979, although the average duration of breast-feeding declined by almost five months (Knodel and Debavalya, 1980). In Malaysia and Mexico, on the other hand, some decline in the proportion of women who had ever breast-fed has been recorded. In Malaysia, from before 1960 to 1974, there was a drop both in the proportion of women who had ever breast-fed (from 89 to 74 per cent) and in the duration of breast-feeding (Butz and DaVanzo, 1981). In Mexico, the decline in proportion breast-feeding was from 80 to 78 per cent over a three-year period from 1973 to 1976 (Mexico, 1981).[8]

The incidence of breast-feeding, as grouped by level of development and strength of family planning programme effort, can be seen in table 58. It is clear that fewer women initiate breast-feeding in the more developed of these countries, but the differences are not large. This finding is consistent with the findings of declining levels of incidence described above. Countries with strong family planning programmes, however, have only slightly lower incidence levels than other countries.

TABLE 58. INCIDENCE OF BREAST-FEEDING, BY LEVEL OF DEVELOPMENT AND STRENGTH OF FAMILY PLANNING PROGRAMME EFFORT

Level of development	Percentage	Strength of programme effort	Percentage
I. High	90	1. Strong	91
II. Middle-high	95	2. Moderate	95
III. Middle-low	98	3. Weak	96
IV. Low	98	4. Very weak/none	97

Source: Table 57.

Duration

In this section, the total duration of breast-feeding, including both full and partial breast-feeding, is studied. As information on full breast-feeding is not available for all countries, it is discussed below with other post-partum variables.

The average mean duration of breast-feeding is similar in Africa and in Asia and Oceania, 18.4 and 18.2 months, respectively, while in Latin America and the Caribbean, it is about half as long, 9.7 months (column (2) of table 57). In other words, women in the first two regions stop breast-feeding, on average, when the child is about 1.5 years old, while in Latin America and the Caribbean, they stop when the child is about 10 months old. The range of mean breast-feeding durations is the smallest among countries in Africa and the largest among those in Asia and Oceania. Mean durations in Africa range from 15 months in Morocco and Tunisia to 21 months in Lesotho. In Asia and Oceania, women in Bangladesh and Nepal breast-feed for more than 30 months, on average, while women in Fiji and Malaysia breast-feed for less than 10 months. The Southern Asian countries of Bangladesh, Nepal, Pakistan and Sri Lanka, and Indonesia in South-eastern Asia, have longer average durations (about 20 months) than other Asian countries. In most Latin American and Caribbean countries, except for Ecuador, Haiti, Paraguay and Peru, women had breast-fed for less than 10 months, with a range of mean durations from 5 months in Costa Rica to about 17 months in Haiti.

The amount of variation in breast-feeding durations among women within any one country is measured by the difference between the first and third quartile (columns (4) and (5) of table 57). On average, countries in Africa had more concentrated distributions than those in the other two regions. Benin, Egypt, Mauritania and Tunisia had slightly larger spreads (more than 10 months) than other countries in Africa. Asian countries, particularly those in Southern Asia, had the largest spread in their distribution. Among Latin American and Caribbean countries, the spread was between 10 and 15 months for most countries, except Costa Rica, Guyana, Haiti, Jamaica, Paraguay, and Trinidad and Tobago. In sharp contrast, all Asian countries, except Malaysia, had a spread of over 10 months. In Malaysia, the spread was nine months. Nearly half the 13 countries in Asia and Oceania had spreads of over 15 months; Bangladesh and Sri Lanka had particularly large spreads of 20 months.

The pattern of breast-feeding among countries is presented in table 59 and in figure 24. Table 59 shows the proportion of women who were still breast-feeding after specified intervals from birth for each country and averaged over regions. The proportions who were currently breast-feeding, in three-month intervals from 0 to 48 months averaged by region, are graphed in figure 24. The pattern of breast-feeding among countries in Africa has a convex distribution, while that of Latin America and the Caribbean is concave, with Asia and Oceania somewhere between the two. For example, almost 80 per cent of the women in Africa were still breast-feeding children who were a year old, while only slightly over a third of Latin American and Caribbean women were breast-feeding children of that age (column (3) of table 59). Among women in Asia and Oceania, three fifths were still breast-feeding 12 months after the birth of the child. After 1.5 years, only about a fifth of the women in Latin America and the Caribbean were breast-feeding, compared with about half of those in Africa and in Asia and Oceania who were still breast-feeding. There is large variation among Asian countries in the proportions still breast-feeding at specified intervals. The Southern Asian countries, which include Bangladesh, Nepal, Pakistan and Sri Lanka, have a convex distribution, on average, more like African countries, compared with other Asian countries. The remaining nine countries in Asia and Oceania have a slightly concave distribution, more like Latin American and Caribbean countries. With development, changing patterns of contraceptive use and other factors, such as the availability of breast-milk substitutes, countries are expected to move from a convex to a concave pattern of breast-feeding.

Two aspects of breast-feeding durations may be distinguished: the breast-feeding duration of all children and the breast-feeding duration only of children who were breast-fed. Changes in breast-feeding durations for all children could be the result of changes in the proportion of children ever breast-fed and/or changes in the duration of breast-feeding of children who are breast-fed. Table 57 (columns (2) and (6)) shows that there is very little difference between the means of the two distributions. For example, although 14.7 per cent of women in Costa Rica had never breast-fed (column (1)), the mean breast-feeding duration for all children was 5.2 months (column (2)), whereas the mean among children who were breast-fed was 6.1 months (column (6)). The small differences observed are mainly due to the fact that in countries where the proportion of women who had breast-fed was high, the mean duration of breast-feeding was long and vice versa.

Mean durations of breast-feeding are clearly linked to level of development, as was the case for incidence, and, less strongly, to family planning programme effort. It is striking that women in the low development group of countries breast-feed, on average, more than two and a half times longer than those in the high development group. It is clear that, as suggested above, women move quickly to shorter breast-feeding periods as development proceeds, but only slowly to a pattern of no breast-feeding. The presence of family planning programmes

TABLE 59. PERCENTAGE OF WOMEN WHO WERE STILL BREAST-FEEDING AT VARIOUS DURATIONS FROM BIRTH

Region and country	3 (1)	6 (2)	12 (3)	18 (4)	24 (5)
Africa					
Benin	94	94	87	59	42
Cameroon	97	92	87	52	26
Côte d'Ivoire[a]	92	89	83	62	27
Egypt	91	88	74	49	24
Ghana	96	93	78	49	23
Kenya	97	93	80	41	19
Lesotho	96	93	85	79	31
Mauritania	94	92	74	47	14
Morocco	90	76	66	42	27
Senegal	99	98	94	73	22
Sudan	95	90	80	45	16
Tunisia	87	78	55	33	18
AVERAGE	94	90	79	53	24
Latin America and the Caribbean					
Colombia	75	56	40	16	2
Costa Rica	62	39	10	10	2
Dominican Republic	75	55	32	15	5
Ecuador	91	80	52	26	6
Guyana	58	35	22	7	6
Haiti	99	91	74	57	9
Jamaica	74	59	25	5	2
Mexico	63	55	42	21	4
Panama	53	42	34	12	3
Paraguay	80	70	51	16	5
Peru	84	76	61	39	13
Trinidad and Tobago	53	29	15	6	4
Venezuela	56	39	26	14	8
AVERAGE	71	56	37	19	5
Asia and Oceania					
Bangladesh	98	96	95	90	73
Fiji	70	53	31	16	6
Indonesia	96	93	87	72	54
Jordan	87	68	48	26	5
Malaysia	46	33	18	10	3
Nepal	99	99	96	84	65
Pakistan	99	94	91	70	36
Philippines	79	71	58	28	14
Republic of Korea	86	91	65	47	24
Sri Lanka	92	88	76	66	33
Syrian Arab Republic	88	72	45	24	6
Thailand	86	74	71	53	36
Yemen	82	72	39	34	9
AVERAGE	85	77	63	48	28
Average excluding Southern Asia[b]	80	70	51	34	17
Average for Southern Asia only[b]	97	94	89	78	52

Source: World Fertility Survey standard recode tapes.
[a] Formerly called the Ivory Coast.
[b] Including Bangladesh, Nepal, Pakistan and Sri Lanka.

TABLE 60. MEAN DURATION OF BREAST-FEEDING, BY LEVEL OF DEVELOPMENT AND STRENGTH OF FAMILY PLANNING PROGRAMME EFFORT

Level of development	Months	Strength of programme effort	Months
I. High	8.5	1. Strong	11.6
II. Middle-high	14.2	2. Moderate	15.4
III. Middle-low	19.7	3. Weak	17.5
IV. Low	21.1	4. Very weak/none	16.7

Source: Table 57.

with strong or moderate effort scores also appears to be associated with shorter mean durations, but the pattern is less clear-cut and may be due more to the positive relationship between development and programme effort than to the latter alone (see table 6 in the Introduction to this report).

Breast-feeding by sex of child

In some cultures, a strong preference for male children has been documented. It is possible that such an attitude may lead to preferential breast-feeding habits. In this section, the question of whether breast-feeding patterns vary by the sex of child is examined using data on breast-feeding behaviour in the open birth interval.[9]

Figure 24. **Proportion of women who were still breast-feeding after specified intervals from birth, by region**

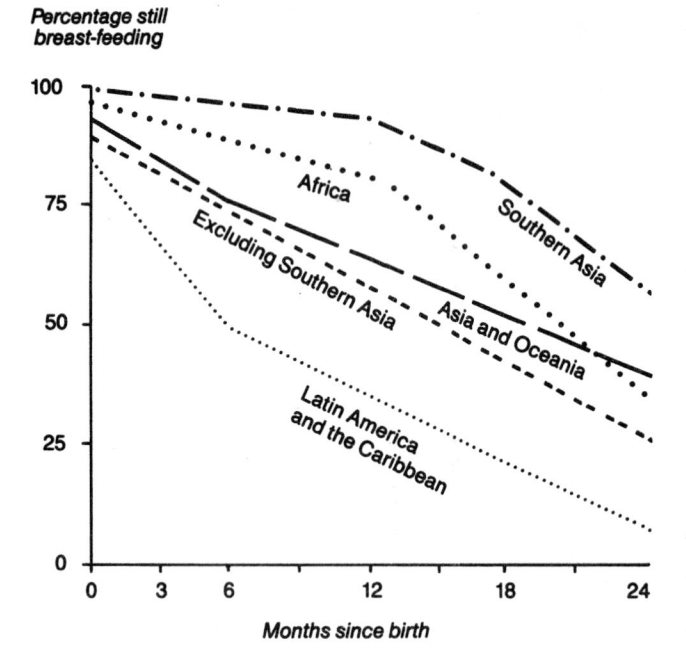

[Figure: Line graph showing percentage still breast-feeding on y-axis (0 to 100) vs months since birth on x-axis (0 to 24), with curves for Africa, Southern Asia, Excluding Southern Asia, Asia and Oceania, and Latin America and the Caribbean.]

Source: Table 59.

The proportions of male and female children (latest born) who were reported to have ever been breast-fed are shown in columns (1) and (2) of table 61. The most significant point to be noted is that differentials in initiating breast-feeding by sex of child are very slight or non-existent. In the majority of countries, less than half of one percentage point separates the sex-specific proportions never breast-feeding and only in five countries does the difference amount to as much as two percentage points. In fact, in only one country is this differential statistically significant.[10] Moreover, the small differences that are found do not show any systematic cross-national pattern by region or by level of development. Hence, it seems safe to conclude that in the WFS countries women do not generally make decisions about initiating breast-feeding based on the sex of their new-born children.

Mean durations of sex-specific breast-feeding are given in table 61, columns (3)-(4). In about half of the WFS countries, mean durations for male and female children are within 0.5 month and can be considered identical for all practical purposes (table 61, column (5)). In no WFS country does the mean breast-feeding duration for one sex exceed that of the other by more than two months, although in 13 countries, the difference is between one and two months. A simple statistical test[11] indicated that in all but six countries such variation could be attributed to random sampling. These countries are Jamaica and Jordan, where sons were breast-fed one month longer than daughters, and four Latin American countries (Costa Rica, Colombia, Panama and Paraguay), where the reverse was true. While in the case of Jordan it is tempting to attribute the difference to a cultural preference for sons, the opposite findings in the latter countries make such an explanation less appealing, especially since no significant differences were observed in several other countries with well-known son preferences. In any case, the similarities in sex-specific patterns are far greater than the slight differences in mean durations, which, in percentage terms, amount to less than 10 per cent except in some Latin American and Caribbean countries where the general level of breast-feeding is low to begin with.[12]

Regionally, comparisons of the means of sex-specific breast-feeding distributions reinforce earlier observations, namely, that women in Caribbean and Arab countries, as well as in Pakistan and the Republic of Korea, tend to breast-feed sons slightly longer, while in Hispanic Latin America, daughters are breast-fed somewhat longer on average. Sub-Saharan Africa and the remainder of Asia and Oceania show no consistent pattern. Breast-feeding differentials by sex of child are not related to other country characteristics, such as level of development, level of contraceptive use, strength of family planning programme effort or average duration of breast-feeding (results not shown). A fuller exploration of sex-specific breast-feeding differentials would be difficult since further subdivisions of the samples lead to small numbers of cases and correspondingly greater chance fluctuations in the results.

In conclusion, an investigation of breast-feeding patterns by sex of child reveals a greater similarity than diversity both in incidence and duration. While differences, on the order of from one to two months, are noted in some countries, no predominant pattern prevails when mean durations are compared—sons being favoured in several WFS countries and daughters in an equal number of other countries.

Breast-feeding by age of mother

Previous studies have generally shown longer breast-feeding durations among older women.[13] A multivariate analysis for eight WFS countries using reported durations, however, found that the positive association of length of breast-feeding and either age or parity of mother was largely attenuated once modernization variables, such as education and residence, were controlled (Jain and Bongaarts, 1981). This suggests that there exists a widespread trend to shorter breast-feeding durations that is related to modernization or general socio-economic development and only coincidentally to age (since age itself is related to such variables as education and rural or urban residence). Among the reasons to expect this outcome are an increased availability of substitutes for mother's milk, a growing importance of new ideas and attitudes which compete with traditional lactational practices and a higher level of income to be able to afford the milk substitutes. An alternative explanation, however, is that increased breast-feeding durations by age of mother may be related not so much to time trends as to physiological characteristics and/or common child-rearing practices. In extended-family households, for instance, younger women, who tend to have an inferior status, may sometimes find prolonged breast-feeding incompatible with their onerous work-load. Physiological evidence on this point is mixed and anthropological studies are lacking (McCann and others, 1981).

TABLE 61. PREVALENCE AND AVERAGE DURATION OF BREAST-FEEDING
BY SEX OF CHILDREN, USING CURRENT STATUS DATA

Region and country	Percentage ever breast-feeding Male (1)	Percentage ever breast-feeding Female (2)	Mean duration of breast-feeding Male (3)	Mean duration of breast-feeding Female (4)	Difference in mean duration between males and females (male − female) (months) (5)
Africa					
Benin	99	99	21.1	21.1	0.0
Cameroon	99	99	18.7	19.5	−0.8
Côte d'Ivoire[a]	99	99	19.1	19.6	−0.5
Egypt	96	96	19.4	18.2	1.2
Ghana	100	100	18.8	19.5	−0.7
Kenya	100	99	17.9	17.7	0.2
Lesotho	98	98	20.4	21.4	−1.0
Mauritania	99	100	17.7	16.4	1.3
Morocco	94	94	15.8	15.3	0.5
Senegal	100	100	19.6	20.2	−0.6
Sudan	99	99	16.7	17.1	−0.4
Tunisia	96	96	15.2	14.6	0.6
Latin America and the Caribbean					
Colombia	92	92	9.2	10.4	−1.2
Costa Rica	77	79	4.2	6.1	−1.9
Dominican Republic	90	89	8.6	9.3	−0.7
Ecuador	94	94	12.9	13.2	−0.3
Guyana	89	90	7.2	6.6	0.6
Haiti	96	97	16.4	17.4	−1.0
Jamaica	95	93	9.3	8.3	1.0
Mexico	81	82	9.4	9.8	−0.4
Panama	81	82	6.9	8.3	−1.4
Paraguay	93	94	10.8	12.3	−1.5
Peru	91	91	14.4	14.1	0.3
Trinidad and Tobago	81	81	6.2	5.9	0.3
Venezuela	86	84	7.8	7.4	0.4
Asia and Oceania					
Bangladesh	100	100	33.2	33.7	−0.5
Fiji	88	88	9.8	9.6	0.2
Indonesia	98	98	25.4	27.2	−1.8
Jordan	94	93	12.3	11.3	1.0
Malaysia	76	78	5.7	5.8	−0.1
Nepal	100	100	30.7	30.3	0.4
Pakistan	99	99	22.4	21.3	1.1
Philippines	86	86	13.6	14.1	−0.5
Republic of Korea	95	96	17.7	16.4	1.3
Sri Lanka	98	97	22.5	22.1	0.4
Syrian Arab Republic	83	83	11.8	11.6	0.2
Thailand	92	92	19.9	19.9	0.0
Yemen	96	95	13.2	12.6	0.6

Source: World Fertility Survey standard recode tapes.
[a] Formerly called the Ivory Coast.

The present section, in examining differences in incidence and mean breast-feeding duration by mother's age, addresses these questions. As before, current status data are used. Mother's age is taken as of the time of the birth. Dividing the samples into three age groups produces rather small numbers of births for each month since birth. Throughout the analysis, however, the minimum sample size used in computations was 25 births.

The size of differentials in incidence of breast-feeding (table 62, columns (1)-(3)) shows no systematic pattern by age of mother; and, in most cases, proportions of children ever breast-fed vary by only a few percentage points from one age group to another. In four countries, there are virtually no differences by age group; in four others, mothers aged 15-24 initiate lactation less often than those aged 25-34 and these less often than women aged 35-49; in three other countries, however, just the opposite is found: the oldest women are the least likely group to begin breast-feeding and the youngest the most likely. In the remaining countries, no clear-cut pattern emerges. Furthermore, there are about equal numbers of countries where age group 15-24 displays the lowest and the highest prevalence, and the same is true for age group 35-49. It seems safe to conclude, therefore, that incidence of breast-feeding is not related to age of mother.

Means of breast-feeding duration by mother's age are given in table 62, columns (4)-(6). Certain countries, particularly Benin, Cameroon, Ghana, Lesotho, Mauritania and the Sudan,[14] show little variation (about one month or less) in mean breast-feeding duration by mother's age, while others, particularly Indonesia, Nepal, Tunisia, Thailand and Venezuela (six months or more), have comparatively large differences. The Venezuelan differentials are notable in that the average length of breast-feeding among women aged 35-44 is more than twice that of women aged 15-24. Most of the differential in mean duration is found between age groups 25-34 and 35-49 (average differential, 2.5 months), while, as noted

TABLE 62. INCIDENCE AND MEAN DURATION OF BREAST-FEEDING BY AGE OF MOTHER, USING CURRENT STATUS DATA

Region and country	Proportion ever breast-feeding[a] in age group: 15-24 (1)	25-34 (2)	35-49 (3)	Mean duration of breast-feeding for age group: 15-24 (4)	25-34 (5)	35-49 (6)	Difference of means[b] (7)
Africa							
Benin	99	99	99	21.1	21.0	21.9	0.8
Cameroon	99	99	99	18.7	19.2	19.9	1.2
Côte d'Ivoire[c]	99	99	100	17.9	20.4	22.5	4.6
Egypt	96	95	97	17.9	18.8	22.0	4.1
Ghana	99	100	100	19.0	19.0	20.1	1.1
Kenya	99	99	99	16.7	18.0	20.4	3.7
Lesotho	99	98	98	20.7	20.9	21.1	0.4
Mauritania	100	100	99	16.9	17.4	17.0	0.1
Morocco	93	94	95	14.3	15.9	17.7	3.4
Senegal	100	100	100	19.9	19.6	21.6	1.7
Sudan	100	99	99	16.8	17.0	18.0	1.2
Tunisia	96	96	97	12.7	14.2	20.1	7.4
Latin America and the Caribbean							
Colombia	90	93	94	9.1	9.4	13.1	4.0
Costa Rica	75	81	76	4.1	5.7	6.7	2.6
Dominican Republic	91	88	92	8.0	9.4	11.6	3.6
Ecuador	95	94	94	12.3	13.2	15.3	3.0
Guyana	90	90	87	6.4	7.6	8.7	2.3
Haiti	96	97	98	15.4	17.5	17.8	2.4
Jamaica	95	93	96	8.5	8.4	10.7	2.2
Mexico	83	81	80	9.1	9.5	11.4	2.3
Panama	79	82	85	6.2	8.3	10.1	3.9
Paraguay	94	94	92	10.6	12.4	12.4	1.8
Peru	93	91	90	12.5	14.4	18.0	5.5
Trinidad and Tobago	80	82	80	5.7	5.7	8.1	2.4
Venezuela	86	84	87	6.6	7.4	14.2	7.6
Asia and Oceania							
Bangladesh	100	100	99	31.9	35.2	36.4	4.5
Fiji	88	88	86	8.6	10.0	12.8	4.2
Indonesia	99	98	98	24.5	26.3	32.3	7.8
Jordan	94	92	95	10.2	12.1	15.2	5.0
Malaysia	79	76	76	5.4	5.4	7.5	2.1
Nepal	98	97	98	28.4	30.8	36.0	7.6
Pakistan	99	98	99	20.1	22.3	24.7	4.6
Philippines	88	86	85	12.7	13.8	16.2	3.5
Republic of Korea	97	95	95	16.1	16.8	20.2	4.1
Sri Lanka	98	98	97	20.7	22.1	26.6	5.9
Syrian Arab Republic	88	82	79	10.7	11.6	14.6	3.9
Thailand	92	91	93	17.6	20.3	24.7	7.1
Yemen	96	96	95	12.0	13.6	15.3	3.3

Source: World Fertility Survey standard recode tapes.
[a] Proportion of women who breast-fed in the open interval, by current age group.
[b] Mean duration (35-49) minus mean duration (15-24).
[c] Formerly called the Ivory Coast.

above, the difference between age groups 15-24 and 25-34 is often less important (average differential, 1.2 months). In 12 countries,[15] in fact, this latter differential is either close to zero or the mean for younger women is actually slightly above the middle group. Mean breast-feeding duration is positively related to age of mother at all development and family planning programme effort groups (table 63). The size of the differential, however, increases very slightly with level of development and programme effort although the middle-high development group (II) and the moderate programme effort group (2) have the highest differential—7.3 and 5.1 months, respectively. An individual-level analysis of data from eight WFS countries found that the effect of age or parity of mother was largely attenuated once such factors as education and residence were controlled for (Jain and Bongaarts, 1981). The results given above indicate, however, that at the aggregate level the effects of age persist at all levels of development, although breast-feeding durations increase with increasing levels within all age groups.

In general, there is an increase in breast-feeding duration with age, although for most countries the size of the differential is small. Differentials persist even after controlling for level of development and programme effort. The increase is larger between the oldest two age groups than between those aged 15-24 and 25-34 years. One possible reason for the small differential in mean breast-feeding duration by age is that in countries where average breast-feeding durations are long, the length of the birth interval plays a part in determining duration as many women stop breast-feeding only when they become pregnant again. This would account, in part, for the shorter mean durations of breast-feeding among younger women (Ferry and Smith, 1983).

TABLE 63. MEAN DURATION OF BREAST-FEEDING OF CHILDREN BY AGE OF MOTHER: AVERAGES BY LEVEL OF DEVELOPMENT AND STRENGTH OF FAMILY PLANNING PROGRAMME EFFORT

	Age of mother		
	15-24 (1)	25-34 (2)	35-49 (3)
Level of development			
I. High	7.8	8.6	11.2
II. Middle-high	12.8	14.3	20.1
III. Middle-low	18.7	19.8	22.0
IV. Low	20.3	21.6	23.2
Strength of family planning programme effort			
1. Strong	10.6	11.6	14.4
2. Moderate	13.8	15.0	18.9
3. Weak	16.1	17.8	20.2
4. Very weak/none	15.8	16.8	18.3

Source: Table 62.

Breast-feeding by birth order of child

Most studies of breast-feeding differentials have treated age of mother and her parity as almost interchangeable variables. In countries where fertility is not consciously controlled, these two demographic variables are highly correlated, but in more modern countries where contraceptive use is widespread and marriage age is more variable, such a correlation may be far weaker. In a regression analysis of 28 WFS countries using current status information, Smith and Ferry (1984) found that either age or parity is significantly related to the duration of breast-feeding. When both age and parity are included in the regression, unstable regression coefficients result for some countries, as age and parity are highly correlated.

TABLE 64. INCIDENCE AND AVERAGE DURATION OF BREAST-FEEDING BY BIRTH ORDER, USING CURRENT STATUS DATA

Region and country	Proportion ever breast-feeding[a] for birth order:				Difference of proportions[b] (5)	Mean duration of breast-feeding[a] for birth order:				Difference of means[c] (10)
	1-2 (1)	3-4 (2)	5-6 (3)	7+ (4)		1-2 (6)	3-4 (7)	5-6 (8)	7+ (9)	
Africa										
Benin	99	99	99	99	0	20.6	21.4	22.0	21.3	0.7
Cameroon	99	99	100	99	1	18.7	19.1	19.3	19.3	0.6
Côte d'Ivoire[d]	99	99	99	100	1	16.9	19.9	21.4	22.0	5.1
Egypt	94	96	97	98	4	16.3	18.8	20.4	22.6	6.3
Ghana	99	100	100	100	1	18.7	18.8	19.9	20.1	1.4
Kenya	99	100	100	99	1	16.4	17.4	18.0	19.8	3.4
Lesotho	98	98	98	97	1	21.1	20.5	21.2	21.2	0.1
Mauritania	100	99	100	99	1	17.4	16.5	17.4	16.4	−1.0
Morocco	91	94	95	95	4	13.6	15.0	17.6	17.8	4.2
Senegal	100	99	100	100	1	19.5	19.4	20.6	20.4	0.9
Sudan	99	99	100	99	1	15.4	17.2	17.5	17.9	2.5
Tunisia	94	96	98	97	4	11.7	14.0	15.9	20.9	9.2
Latin America and the Caribbean										
Colombia	89	92	95	94	6	8.7	9.4	10.1	12.2	3.5
Costa Rica	72	81	82	81	10	3.6	5.6	7.5	8.5	4.9
Dominican Republic	86	90	92	93	7	7.1	9.8	10.8	11.5	4.4
Ecuador	92	94	96	96	4	11.4	13.2	14.4	16.0	4.6
Guyana	87	91	91	90	4	6.2	6.4	8.1	9.3	3.1
Haiti	95	98	98	98	3	15.2	17.6	18.0	19.8	4.6
Jamaica	93	95	95	96	3	7.3	9.7	10.5	10.0	2.7
Mexico	78	83	85	82	7	7.4	10.0	11.1	11.7	4.3
Panama	73	82	87	90	17	4.1	8.1	10.3	12.4	8.3
Paraguay	91	94	97	95	6	9.2	12.2	14.5	14.1	4.9
Peru	91	90	92	92	2	10.8	13.9	16.7	18.1	7.3
Trinidad and Tobago	78	81	84	86	8	5.0	6.0	7.1	8.8	3.8
Venezuela	82	86	86	88	6	5.4	7.7	9.6	12.3	6.9
Asia and Oceania										
Bangladesh	100	100	99	100	1	31.1	33.5	35.3	35.3	4.2
Fiji	85	87	90	90	5	7.9	9.5	11.7	13.5	5.6
Indonesia	98	98	98	98	0	24.3	25.6	27.8	30.6	6.3
Jordan	91	95	94	94	4	8.4	11.5	13.3	14.2	5.8
Malaysia	70	77	81	81	11	4.4	6.0	6.5	7.9	3.5
Nepal	94	97	97	95	3	29.3	30.5	31.1	34.0	4.7
Pakistan	99	99	99	99	0	19.6	21.6	22.7	24.1	4.5
Philippines	84	86	88	87	4	11.7	13.6	16.1	15.8	4.1
Republic of Korea	94	95	96	96	2	15.2	17.7	19.0	22.2	7.0
Sri Lanka	97	98	98	97	1	19.4	21.9	25.1	28.0	8.6
Syrian Arab Republic	85	85	83	80	5	10.3	11.3	12.6	13.6	3.3
Thailand	88	92	95	94	7	16.9	21.0	22.5	24.6	7.7
Yemen	94	97	97	95	3	11.7	12.6	14.1	14.4	2.7

Source: World Fertility Survey standard recode tapes.
[a] Proportion who breast-fed in the open interval.
[b] Maximum difference between parity groups.
[c] Mean duration (7+) minus mean duration (1-2).
[d] Formerly called the Ivory Coast.

Compared with mother's age, differentials in incidence of breast-feeding by child's parity show a distinct pattern, namely, that the proportion of children ever breast-fed rises with birth order (table 64, columns (1)-(4)). In almost four fifths of the WFS countries, children who are first or second born are the least likely to have been breast-fed, while children of parity 5 or higher are the most likely. Countries where this is not the case are generally those with uniformly high proportions breast-feeding (i.e., close to 100 per cent). The one exceptional case is the Syrian Arab Republic, where 85 per cent of low-parity children had ever been breast-fed, compared with 80 per cent of high-parity children. The size of parity-specific incidence differentials is generally higher than that of the corresponding age-specific differentials. Costa Rica, Malaysia and Panama, with differences of 10, 11 and 7 percentage points, respectively, between parity groups 1-2 and 7+ are notable in this regard.

First and second birth-order children were weaned at earlier ages than higher-parity children; and, in fact, this group stands out from the higher-parity groups. This finding contrasts with the analysis by age of mother where children with older mothers (aged 35-49) formed a distinctive, slower-weaning subgroup. As with incidence figures, the largest differentials in mean duration of lactation are found between the lower parity groups (see table 65).

TABLE 65. AVERAGE DIFFERENCE IN MEAN DURATION OF BREAST-FEEDING BY BIRTH ORDER

Parity groups compared	Mean duration of breast-feeding	Average difference in mean duration of breast-feeding (months)
Parity (3-4) − parity (1-2)	15.4 − 13.6	1.8
Parity (5-6) − parity (3-4)	16.8 − 15.4	1.4
Parity (7+) − parity (5-6)	18.0 − 16.8	1.2
Parity (7+) − parity (1-2)	18.0 − 13.6	4.2[a]

Source: Table 64.

[a] Difference of means tests, comparing parity group 1-2 with parity group 7+, were statistically significant for all World Fertility Survey countries (level of significance = 0.01) except Cameroon, Ghana, Lesotho and Senegal.

The child's birth order appears to have a stronger positive relationship with duration of breast-feeding than does age, and this differential persists at all levels of development and programme strength (table 66). One interpretation of these findings is that breast-feeding duration increases as parity progresses for a woman. In other words, the currently low-parity women will breast-feed for longer periods as they move to higher parities. Another interpretation that assumes that an individual woman breast-feeds all her children for the same duration is that breast-feeding norms have come to differ across parity groups through the influence of factors that reflect modernizing influences. Low-parity women therefore reflect the more modernized group and high-parity women the more traditional group that breast-feeds for longer durations. Both these interpretations are confounded by differences between parity groups in fecundability or exposure to conception. Younger women and women at low parities are more likely to stop breast-feeding at earlier durations than older women or women at higher parities because of a pregnancy interruption. Without trend data on breast-feeding duration, these alternative interpretations cannot be fully assessed.

TABLE 66. MEAN DURATION OF BREAST-FEEDING OF CHILDREN BY BIRTH ORDER OF CHILD: AVERAGES BY LEVEL OF DEVELOPMENT AND STRENGTH OF FAMILY PLANNING PROGRAMME EFFORT

	Birth order of child			
	1-2 (1)	3-4 (2)	5-6 (3)	7+ (4)
Level of development				
I. High	6.8	8.8	10.1	11.8
II. Middle-high	11.6	14.2	16.2	17.6
III. Middle-low	19.2	20.0	21.1	22.3
IV. Low	20.3	21.8	22.8	23.7
Strength of family planning programme effort				
1. Strong	9.7	11.7	13.3	14.8
2. Moderate	12.8	15.2	17.0	19.4
3. Weak	15.5	17.3	18.6	20.0
4. Very weak/none	15.2	16.5	17.8	18.0

Source: Table 65.

C. BREAST-FEEDING AND FAMILY LIMITATION

The reasons for prolonged breast-feeding observed in traditional societies may have little to do with keeping fertility low through long birth intervals, although the net result of prolonged breast-feeding is long birth intervals. The health of the infant and mother and a lack of substitutes of equal nutritional value for breast milk may be some of the underlying reasons for prolonged lactation and the customs and traditions surrounding it. None the less, in the absence of modern contraception, women may breast-feed for longer durations if they wish to avoid another pregnancy altogether or to space the next birth. These customs and traditions vary from country to country; and for any one country, there may be a breakdown in these traditions with the onset of modernization. In this section, the relationship between breast-feeding and contraceptive use is explored, with particular emphasis on the use of contraception by currently breast-feeding women.

Contraceptive use in last closed interval

Among the many questions on contraceptive use and knowledge, WFS asked women if they had used contraception in the open and closed birth intervals and if they were currently using contraception. In five countries— Colombia, Costa Rica, Egypt, Paraguay and Venezuela —the duration of use was also recorded. Unfortunately, it is not possible to determine from all of this information

TABLE 67. INCIDENCE AND MEAN DURATION OF BREAST-FEEDING AMONG WOMEN WHO HAD USED OR HAD NOT USED CONTRACEPTION DURING LAST CLOSED BIRTH INTERVAL

	Incidence (percentage)				Mean duration (months)			
	Had not used	Had used			Had not used	Had used		
Region and country	(1)	Traditional[a] (2)	Modern[b] (3)	Total (4)	(5)	Traditional (6)	Modern (7)	Total (8)
Africa								
Benin	95	97	c	97	20.4	24.0	c	23.7
Cameroon	97	95	c	94	27.7	20.3	c	20.7
Côte d'Ivoire[d]	95	98	91	98	27.6	18.9	c	18.8
Egypt	93	94	91	91	17.2	12.4	14.0	13.9
Ghana	98	98	98	98	19.4	17.7	14.9	16.7
Kenya	97	97	99	98	19.2	18.1	14.7	16.5
Lesotho	94	97	c	95	24.2	21.9	17.8	20.6
Morocco	92	c	90	89	14.5	c	13.4	12.0
Senegal	98	98	c	98	29.6	20.5	c	20.1
Sudan	97	c	98	97	22.4	c	15.1	15.1
Tunisia	96	94	91	92	22.8	16.8	19.4	18.7
Latin America and the Caribbean								
Colombia	91	88	88	88	9.6	7.6	6.4	6.9
Costa Rica	79	81	78	79	6.1	5.6	4.7	5.0
Dominican Republic	89	87	83	85	10.4	8.9	5.5	6.8
Ecuador	93	91	89	90	10.2	9.5	7.3	8.1
Guyana	89	92	88	88	10.1	8.6	6.6	7.0
Jamaica	95	95	93	93	8.6	7.0	6.8	6.8
Panama	86	82	77	79	9.6	8.2	4.8	5.9
Paraguay	92	91	90	90	11.7	10.4	8.4	9.3
Peru	91	88	87	88	12.4	10.3	6.7	9.2
Venezuela	85	87	84	85	8.0	5.8	6.5	6.0
Asia and Oceania								
Bangladesh	97	96	99	97	24.4	27.8	22.9	25.6
Indonesia	97	96	96	96	19.4	18.0	19.0	18.7
Jordan	94	90	88	89	12.8	9.6	9.4	9.5
Malaysia	81	69	70	69	6.6	4.5	3.7	4.1
Nepal	96	c	99	99	24.1	c	20.9	22.4
Pakistan	94	c	91	92	16.1	18.0	13.4	14.3
Philippines	88	85	83	84	24.0	22.0	22.0	22.0
Republic of Korea	94	96	95	95	19.4	17.8	18.9	18.7
Sri Lanka	95	96	95	96	16.3	17.2	14.2	16.3
Syrian Arab Republic	86	83	83	83	13.9	10.3	10.7	10.4
Yemen	92	c	c	c	20.5	c	c	c

Source: World Fertility Survey standard recode tapes.
[a] Including rhythm, withdrawal, abstinence, douche and country-specific folk methods.
[b] Including contraceptive sterilization, oral pills, injectables, intra-uterine devices, condoms, and female barrier and chemical methods (diaphragm, cervical cap, spermicidal foams, creams and jellies).
[c] Fewer than 25 cases.
[d] Formerly called the Ivory Coast.

how long after birth those women who were breast-feeding had begun using contraception or for how long women had continued breast-feeding while using contraception. These are important considerations for planners in family planning programmes in terms of the timing and type of contraception to recommend to breast-feeding women.

Data on breast-feeding and contraceptive use in the last closed birth interval will be used to study some of the relationships between breast-feeding and contraceptive use. Although other studies have cautioned against the use of the closed birth interval because of selection biases, it is assumed here that the biases would be the same among subgroups of the population, that is, users and non-users of contraception, and also that such biases should produce similar effects in all countries, thus not greatly influencing cross-national analysis. Five countries (Haiti, Mauritania, Mexico, Thailand, and Trinidad and Tobago) completely omitted the question on use of contraception in the last closed birth interval, while Fiji did not collect information on breast-feeding in the closed interval. These six countries are therefore excluded from the present analysis. In addition, some other countries were omitted from different parts of the analysis when the number of cases in certain subgroups became too low.[16] Women who used contraception in the last closed interval are more likely to be "spacers" than "limiters", unless the last birth resulted from a contraceptive failure. It is not certain what impact this has on the analysis, but readers should bear in mind that the contraceptive users here refer mainly to "spacers", not "limiters".

Data on the incidence of breast-feeding show that the proportion ever breast-fed is generally higher among women who did not use contraception in the last closed birth interval than among those who did in the majority of countries (table 67, columns (1)-(4)). This is true of countries in Latin America and the Caribbean and in Asia and Oceania, but not so of the African countries. Among the African countries, only women in Cameroon, Egypt, Morocco and Tunisia have lower incidence among those who used contraception than among those who did not. Differences, however, are not large; only Panama, Jordan and Malaysia have differences of more than five percentage points in the proportions ever breast-fed during the last closed birth interval. In Malaysia, the difference is as much as 12 points. Differences in incidence by the type of contraception used (modern versus traditional) are also not large, although in almost all countries proportionately more women who used a traditional method had breast-fed than women who used a modern method. In general, incidence is highest among women who had not used any contraception during the last closed birth interval, followed by women who had used traditional methods and lastly by those who had used modern methods, except in much of Africa, as noted above.

Table 67 (columns (5)-(8)) shows differences in breast-feeding duration among those who had used contraception in the last closed birth interval and those who had not. In almost all countries, women who had not used any contraception in the last closed birth interval breast-fed for longer durations than did women who had used contraception. Differences are largest among the African countries, an average difference of about five months. Large differences were recorded in Cameroon, Senegal and the Sudan—7.0, 9.5 and 7.3 months, respectively; while in Egypt, Ghana, Kenya, Lesotho and Tunisia, differences were on the order of from two to four months. Differences in breast-feeding duration are much smaller among women in Latin America and the Caribbean, the average being 2.5 months. In Asia and Oceania, the average difference is only 1.7 months, and in Bangladesh, women who did not use any contraception had stopped breast-feeding about one month before those who did use contraception. In several countries, the number of women who used contraception was so low that there were not enough cases to study the breakdown between those who had used a modern method and those who had used a traditional one. For those countries with a sufficient number of cases, women who had used modern methods of contraception breast-fed for shorter durations than those who used traditional methods, though differences are not large. In general, the information from the last closed birth interval points to longer breast-feeding durations among women who did not use any contraception, followed by those who used traditional methods, while women who used modern methods breast-fed for the shortest duration. The negative association between duration of breast-feeding and contraceptive use suggests that possible decreases in birth interval length due to declining breast-feeding will be partially or more than offset by contraceptive use.

Contraceptive use among current breast-feeders

It is difficult to establish when breast-feeding women began to use contraception because specific timing questions were not posed. However, questions were asked on current use of family planning and also on current breast-feeding status at the time of the survey. From these two pieces of information, it is possible to estimate the proportion of users of contraception among breast-feeders. These results are presented in table 68, where column (1) shows the percentage of women who were breast-feeding at the time of the survey among women with at least one live birth, and column (2) shows the percentage of women who were breast-feeding and using contraception. In Africa and in Asia and Oceania about one third of women with at least one live birth were breast-feeding at the time of the survey, while in Latin America and the Caribbean, the average was lower—17.6 per cent. The regional averages mask the large variation, especially among countries of Latin America and the Caribbean and of Asia and Oceania. In Bangladesh and Nepal, more than 50 per cent were breast-feeding at the time of the survey. In Africa and in Latin America and the Caribbean, under 5 per cent, on average, of women were breast-feeding and using contraception, while in Asia and Oceania, the corresponding figure was 5.3 per cent. Only in Indonesia and Sri Lanka were more than 10 per cent of women breast-feeding and using contraception. A comparison of the percentages given in columns (1) and (2) shows that there was a large pool of women who were breast-feeding but not using contraception, although some of them were post-partum infecund and some abstaining.

Focusing on the type of contraception used by breast-feeders, columns (4), (5) and (6) show, respectively, the percentages of all currently breast-feeding women who were using some form of contraception, using a modern method and using the pill. About one quarter of Latin American and Caribbean women and a fifth of women in Asia and Oceania who were currently breast-feeding were using contraception. In Africa, the corresponding percentage was less than 10 per cent. The proportions of breast-feeding women who were using modern methods of contraception showed a similar pattern across regions but at a lower level. Variation among countries within the regions is considerable. In Latin America and the Caribbean, for example, 41.6 per cent of breast-feeding women in Trinidad and Tobago were using modern methods, while in Haiti and Peru only 3.3 and 2.6 per cent, respectively, were using modern methods. More than 20 per cent of breast-feeding women in Fiji, Indonesia, Sri Lanka and Thailand in Asia and Oceania; and in Costa Rica, Jamaica, and Trinidad and Tobago in Latin America and the Caribbean were using modern methods of contraception. In Africa, only Egypt, Morocco and Tunisia in Northern Africa had more than 10 per cent of breast-feeding women using modern methods. The proportion of pill users among those breast-feeding is about 5 per cent in Latin America and the Caribbean and in Asia and Oceania, and 3 per cent in Africa. Indonesia stands out among all countries in that 20 per cent of breast-feeding women were currently using the pill. Relatively high percentages were also recorded in Egypt, Morocco, and Trinidad and Tobago.

In summary, the data from table 68 show that a high percentage of women were currently breast-feeding at the time of the survey. Although from one fifth to one quarter (less in Africa) of these women were using some form of contraception, a substantial proportion of breast-feeders were exposed to the risk of another birth. Some of these women would be post-partum infecund and some would be abstaining; nevertheless, a substantial proportion of them would still be exposed to the risk of another birth soon after the last. Although the percentage of pill users among breast-feeders was generally low (except for Indonesia and a few other countries), it is still not inconsequential.

The results of table 68 are summarized according to level of development and strength of family planning programme effort in table 69. Here, an inverse relationship can be observed between current breast-feeding status and socio-economic development and family planning programme strength. On the other hand, a positive relationship can be seen between the proportion of women who were using contraception among breast-feeders related to the two contextual measures (column (3)).

TABLE 68. PERCENTAGE OF WOMEN CURRENTLY USING CONTRACEPTION AMONG THOSE STILL BREAST-FEEDING AT THE TIME OF THE SURVEY

Region and country	Percentage of women with at least one live birth — Still breast-feeding (1)	Breast-feeding and using contraception (2)	Number of breast-feeders (3)	Percentage using contraception among breast-feeders — Total (4)	Modern (5)	Pill (6)
Africa						
Benin	47.3	13.4[a]	1 557	28.3[a]	0.4	0.1
Cameroon	36.3	0.5	2 264	1.5	0.2	0.1
Côte d'Ivoire[b]	41.0	0.8	1 922	1.9	0.1	0.1
Egypt	34.3	5.5	2 683	16.0	14.9	12.2
Ghana	37.7	2.3	1 735	6.1	2.8	0.8
Kenya	43.2	2.1	2 697	4.9	2.0	1.5
Lesotho	41.1	2.6	1 287	6.2	1.8	0.8
Mauritania	35.6	0.3	1 106	0.8	0.2	0.1
Morocco	30.5	4.1	1 105	13.3	11.4	10.0
Senegal	42.7	3.3	1 334	7.6	0.5	0.1
Sudan	38.0	1.6	1 051	4.3	3.2	2.8
Tunisia	31.7	5.8	1 196	18.4	14.0	4.9
AVERAGE	38.2	2.6[c]	—	7.4[c]	4.3	2.8
Latin America and the Caribbean						
Colombia	17.1	3.8	553	22.4	12.8	5.4
Costa Rica	6.5	2.8	198	43.4	30.3	8.6
Dominican Republic	17.3	2.6	347	15.3	10.4	2.0
Ecuador	25.3	4.3	1 088	17.0	11.7	5.6
Guyana	11.3	2.3	358	20.4	17.0	5.0
Haiti	33.8	6.1	674	18.0	3.3	1.9
Jamaica	14.0	4.3	345	30.7	28.1	7.2
Mexico	19.8	3.0	1 166	15.1	9.8	4.1
Panama	11.6	3.0	356	25.8	12.6	5.6
Paraguay	21.2	4.1	599	19.2	9.8	5.3
Peru	27.0	5.1	1 450	19.1	2.6	1.0
Trinidad and Tobago	8.7	4.0	246	45.9	41.6	14.1
Venezuela	15.3	3.7	381	24.4	16.5	4.5
AVERAGE	17.6	3.8	—	24.4	15.9	5.4
Asia and Oceania						
Bangladesh	51.1	4.8	2 851	9.3	5.1	3.9
Fiji	15.9	6.6	695	41.4	33.7	6.0
Indonesia	37.4	12.3	2 968	33.0	28.3	20.0
Jordan	29.8	4.2	994	14.1	7.5	5.7
Malaysia	10.1	1.5	591	14.7	8.8	7.4
Nepal	54.3	1.3	2 652	2.4	2.4	0.4
Pakistan	40.5	2.0	1 724	5.0	3.6	1.6
Philippines	26.7	8.4	2 356	31.6	10.4	1.9
Republic of Korea	24.0	4.9	1 218	20.4	16.7	5.3
Sri Lanka	33.0	11.4	2 055	34.6	21.0	1.6
Syrian Arab Republic	34.0	3.9	1 379	11.4	8.0	7.0
Thailand	31.2	7.9	1 095	25.3	21.5	8.3
Yemen	34.6	0.1	752	0.3	0.3	0.3
AVERAGE	32.5	5.3	—	18.7	12.9	5.3

Source: World Fertility Survey standard recode tapes.
[a] A large proportion of women who were practising post-partum abstinence were classified as contraceptive users in Benin. For more details, see chapter V.
[b] Formerly called the Ivory Coast.
[c] Excluding Benin.

Thus, countries with a high level of development and strong programme effort have lower proportions of breast-feeders but these women are more adequately protected by modern methods of contraception.

D. OTHER ASPECTS OF REPRODUCTIVE BEHAVIOUR ASSOCIATED WITH THE BREAST-FEEDING PERIOD

In addressing the question of the effect of breast-feeding on fertility, several more pieces of information are required than those available from the standard WFS questionnaire. The basic questions asked were "Did you feed at the breast?"; and, if yes, "For how many months did you breast-feed?". Although many of the biological interconnections remain only imperfectly understood, it is known that the return of post-partum ovulation (and of other physiological conditions necessary for reproduction) is linked hormonally to frequency and, possibly, duration of suckling (World Health Organization, 1983). Furthermore, intensity of suckling also seems to determine, at least partially, when menstruation returns following parturition and, importantly, whether ovulation precedes or follows first menstruation (Potter and others, 1971). In all cases, greater frequency, and possibly longer duration, of suckling leads to lower fertility by lengthening inter-birth intervals. Another very germane point is the extent of post-partum sexual abstinence, due

TABLE 69. PERCENTAGE OF WOMEN USING CONTRACEPTION AMONG THOSE STILL BREAST-FEEDING AT THE TIME OF THE SURVEY: AVERAGES BY LEVEL OF DEVELOPMENT AND STRENGTH OF FAMILY PLANNING PROGRAMME EFFORT

	Percentage of women with at least one live birth		Percentage using contraception among breast-feeders		
	Still breast-feeding (1)	Breast-feeding and using contraception (2)	Total (3)	Modern (4)	Pill (5)
Level of development					
I. High	14.0	3.6	27.7	20.7	6.6
II. Middle-high	27.7	5.8	20.6	11.7	4.3
III. Middle-low	37.7	3.8	10.4	7.7	5.7
IV. Low	42.0	3.7	8.4	2.1	1.2
Strength of family planning programme effort					
1. Strong	18.1	5.3	29.3	20.2	7.5
2. Moderate	26.0	6.2	25.9	20.6	7.2
3. Weak	32.5	3.4	13.0	8.3	3.8
4. Very weak/none	35.9	3.2	9.3	2.9	1.9

Source: Table 68.

to cultural mores, which may be associated with breast-feeding.

For the majority of WFS countries, such additional data are simply not available. In several surveys, however, all or parts of the FOTCAF module were added to the core questionnaire. While detailed questions concerning suckling patterns were not asked, valuable information was collected on the extent of full breast-feeding,[17] post-partum amenorrhoea and post-partum sexual abstinence. This section, which relies exclusively upon those countries where FOTCAF data are available, examines relationships between these additional factors in order to gain a better understanding of the role of breast-feeding in controlling fertility.[18] In each of the succeeding three subsections, it should be kept in mind that current status data is first examined, followed by analysis of data for the last closed birth interval.

Full breast-feeding

For all WFS countries where the pertinent data were collected (see table 70 and figure 25), full breast-feeding represents only a small part of the total period of breast-feeding. The simple average is between four and five months of feeding mother's milk without supplements, although there is considerable range in the mean duration of full breast-feeding among the 15 countries. In Egypt and Haiti, full breast-feeding lasts, on average, up to 1.3 months and 0.6 month, respectively, while in Mauritania, the Sudan, the Syrian Arab Republic, Tunisia and Yemen, the mean duration exceeds six months. These implausibly long mean durations of full breast-feeding among the Arab countries probably reflect the differences in the interpretation of the question on full breast-feeding. In the Arabic translation, "any other food" was taken to be a meal rather than the intended meaning, use of food as a partial supplement, even in small quantities and for occasional rather than regular feeding (Singh and Ferry, 1984). On average, about one quarter of the total breast-feeding period is encompassed by "full breast-feeding", except for the Arab countries (Mauritania, the Syrian Arab Republic and Yemen), where it amounts to about half of this period. Although no other direct data are available, it is probable that in countries where full breast-feeding is a small fraction of the entire period (see table 70, column (4), suckling intensity is maintained at close to the level of full breast-feeding for some time after partial weaning and probably is only gradually reduced as more supplementary food is added to the babies' diets. Indirect evidence of this is provided in the following section on amenorrhoea.

Further aspects of full breast-feeding are explored in table 71, which is based on reported durations in the last closed birth interval. As has been pointed out, data from the last closed birth interval are liable to errors and biases so that caution must be exercised in interpreting results. Since mean differences between the durations of breast-feeding and full breast-feeding from data on the last closed birth interval and current status data (columns (1) and (2) of table 71) agree quite well in pattern, if not in level, it seems safe to assume that the differentials apparent in table 71 are real, even if their values may not be accurate. In the Syrian Arab Republic, Tunisia and Yemen, a high percentage of women ceased breast-feeding shortly after they had stopped full breast-feeding (table 71, columns (3) and (7)). This is probably due to the translation of the question, as mentioned above. In some African countries, especially in Cameroon, Lesotho and Senegal, a long period of continued breast-feeding after partial weaning has occurred. In the three countries just mentioned, this period lasted 10 or more months for more than 75 per cent of the women sampled (column (6)).

Table 71 (columns (8)-(13)) also shows that longer periods of full breast-feeding were reported, in almost all countries and age groups, by non-contracepting women. The difference, compared with women who did report contraceptive use, was generally on the order of from one to two months, except in Kenya and Lesotho, where smaller, less significant differentials were found.

Post-partum amenorrhoea

Post-partum amenorrhoea is closely associated with post-partum sterility. If breast-feeding up to the time of first post-partum menses has been intensive, most evidence appears to indicate that ovulation, and probably other physiological conditions necessary for successful conception, are normally delayed until after the first two or three menstrual cycles (Short, 1982). In countries where this datum is available, the mean duration of amenorrhoea was over 10 months, on average, with a range

TABLE 70. DURATION OF FULL BREAST-FEEDING, POST-PARTUM AMENORRHOEA AND POST-PARTUM SEXUAL ABSTINENCE, USING CURRENT STATUS DATA

| Region and country | Full breast-feeding ||| | Amenorrhoea |||| Sexual abstinence ||||
| | Duration || Percentage of mean total breast-feeding period (4) | Duration || Third quartile (7) | Percentage of mean total breast-feeding period (8) | Duration ||| Percentage of mean total breast-feeding period (12) | Percentage of mean amenorrhoea period (13) |
	Mean (1)	Median (2)	Third quartile (3)		Mean (5)	Median (6)			Mean (9)	Median (10)	Third quartile (11)		
Africa													
Benin	2.9	2.2	3.9	13.7	13.1	12.3	17.5	61.8	17.8	17.0	25.6	84.0	135.9
Cameroon	5.3	4.1	5.8	28.7	13.0	12.8	18.1	68.1	16.0	16.2	20.7	83.8	123.1
Côte d'Ivoire[a]	6.0	4.6	7.6	31.1	12.2	11.9	17.2	63.2	15.9	14.6	23.6	82.4	130.3
Egypt	1.3	1.5	2.2	6.9	..	..	..	..	..	..	..	..	..
Ghana	5.1	3.6	5.7	26.6	13.3	12.4	17.4	69.3	11.4	6.1	15.4	59.4	85.7
Kenya	2.5	1.9	2.9	14.0	11.8	11.4	16.2	65.9	4.2	2.2	4.3	23.5	35.6
Lesotho	2.6	2.4	4.4	12.4	10.4	9.2	18.1	49.8	17.1	18.7	23.5	81.8	164.4
Mauritania	9.0	6.8	15.8	52.9	9.5	6.8	17.1	55.9	..	..	..	..	..
Senegal	5.6	4.6	6.8	28.1	..	..	..	..	..	..	..	..	..
Sudan	6.2	4.8	7.6	36.5	11.8	13.1	17.2	69.4	2.9	1.8	2.6	17.1	24.6
Tunisia	7.0	5.7	9.5	47.0	7.8	3.8	12.0	52.3	2.2	1.7	2.6	14.8	28.2
Latin America and the Caribbean													
Haiti	0.6	1.5	2.2	3.8	13.3	12.2	19.3	83.1	8.6	4.6	8.6	53.8	64.7
Asia and Oceania													
Philippines	3.7	2.8	5.1	28.9	8.9	7.2	13.9	64.0	3.8	2.2	4.0	27.3	42.7
Syrian Arab Republic	6.1	4.6	8.2	52.1	7.1	4.9	8.8	60.7	1.5	1.6	2.4	12.8	21.1
Yemen	6.4	3.0	8.8	49.6	9.0	6.2	15.2	69.8	3.8	1.9	2.8	29.4	42.2

Source: World Fertility Survey standard recode tapes.

[a] Formerly called the Ivory Coast.

Figure 25. **Proportions who were breast-feeding, full breast-feeding, amenorrhoeic and abstaining, using current status data**

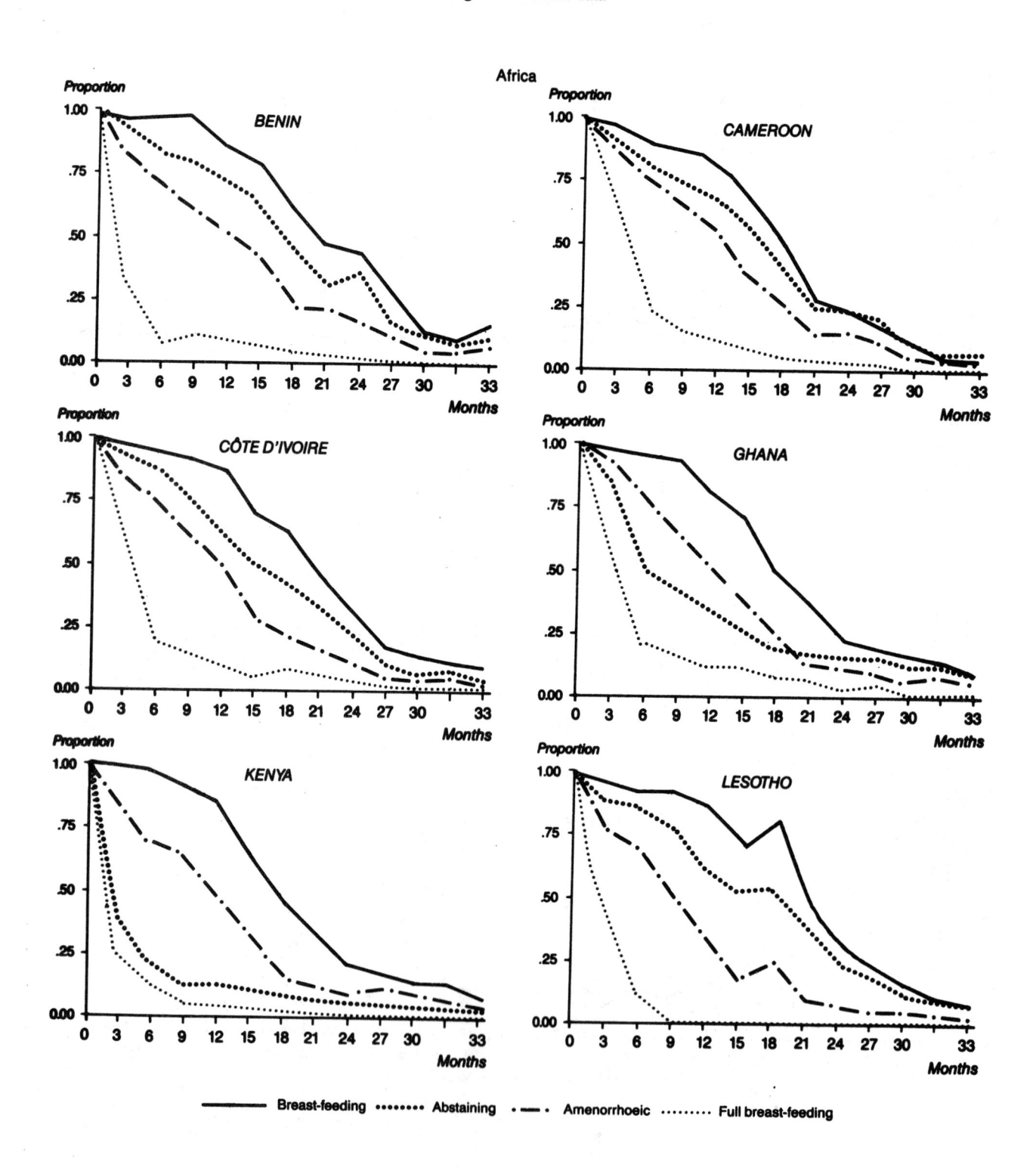

Africa

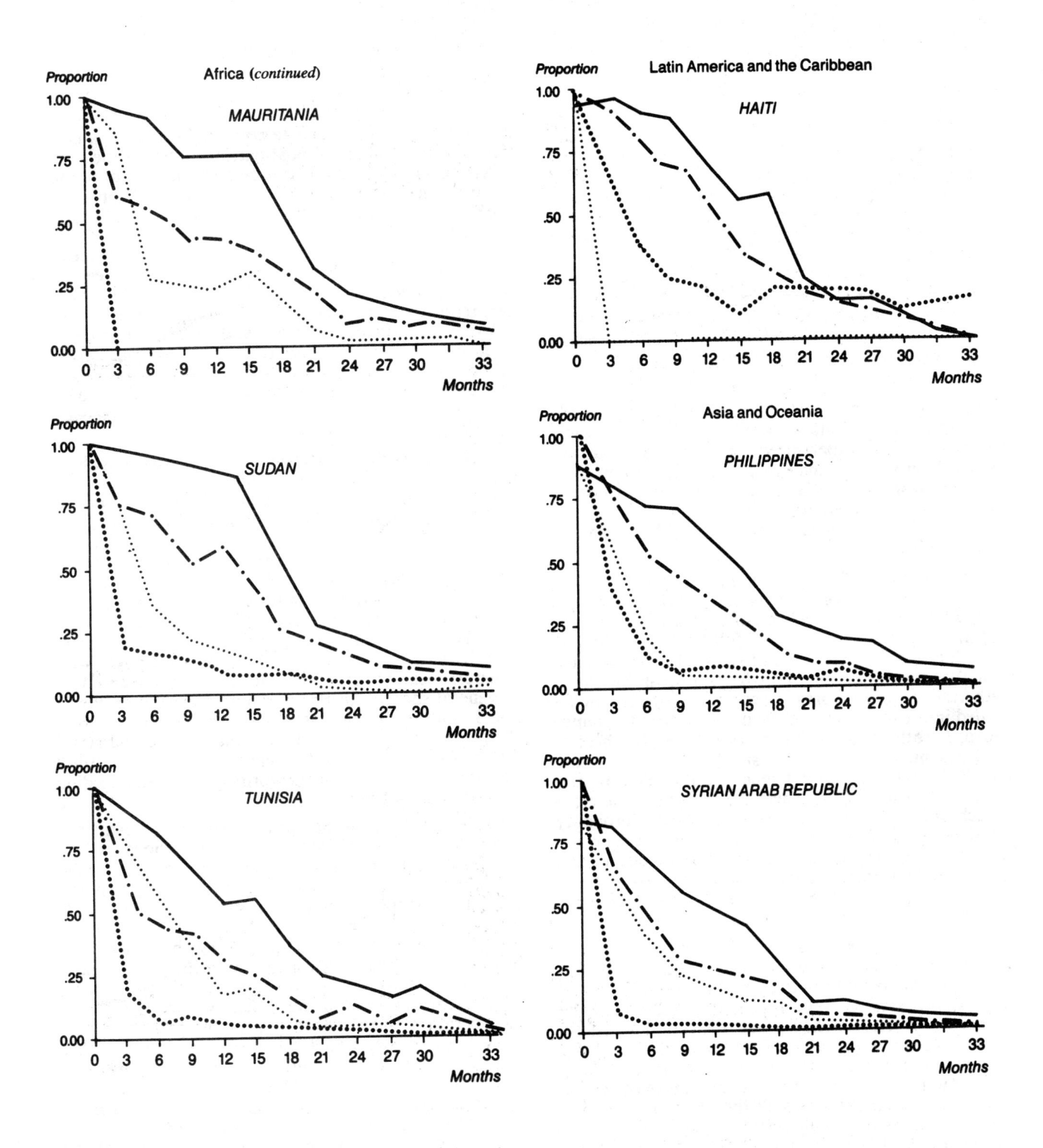

Figure 25 (*continued*)

Figure 25 (*continued*)

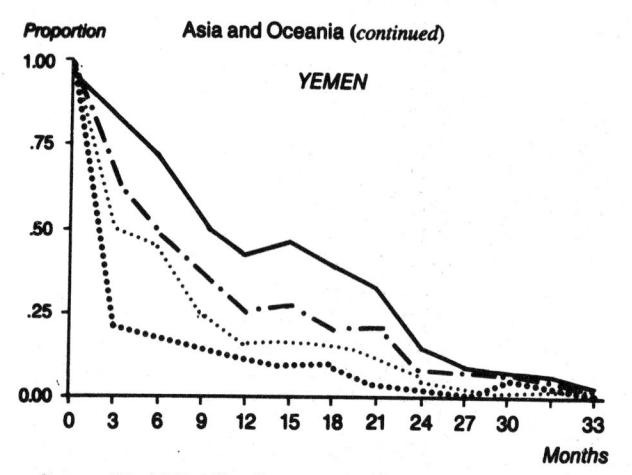

Asia and Oceania (*continued*)

YEMEN

Source: World Fertility Survey standard recode tapes.

of about 7-13 months (table 70). On average, for the countries for which data are available, half of the sampled women had experienced their first post-partum menses about nine months after a birth (range of median, 4-12 months) and three quarters of women about 14 months (range of 9-19 months) after a birth. In most cases, the duration of amenorrhoea appears to lengthen with age of the mother (not shown).

As can be seen in figure 25 and in columns (5) and (8) of table 70, the amenorrhoeic period generally occupies a substantially larger proportion of the time spent breast-feeding than does the period of full breast-feeding. At all durations from birth, the proportion amenorrhoeic is less than the proportion breast-feeding for all countries. With respect to full breast-feeding, countries can be divided into two groups: (*a*) Benin, Cameroon, Ghana, Kenya, Lesotho and the Philippines, where full breast-feeding is much shorter than post-partum amenorrhoea; and (*b*) the Syrian Arab Republic, Tunisia, Yemen and, to an extent, the Sudan, where the two curves lie close to each other. In the first pattern, weaning is probably a slow and gradual process; and suckling frequency is not likely to be immediately reduced after the end of the "full" breast-feeding period. The second pattern, as mentioned above, is probably due to the problem of the Arabic translation of the question.

Table 72 compares breast-feeding durations with post-partum amenorrhoea durations, using data from the last closed birth interval. The same qualifications mentioned above apply here as well. Interestingly, although the amenorrhoeic period is shorter than the period of general breast-feeding on average, as described above, more than one third of all women averaged for the countries included in fact reported that amenorrhoea lasted as long as or longer than the breast-feeding (full and partial) of their penultimate child. In some cases, this may be explained by relatively short durations of breast-feeding (since post-partum amenorrhoea will last a month or two even in the absence of lactation), but in other cases, such as the Sudan, where over 50 per cent of women reported durations for amenorrhoea equal to or longer than those for breast-feeding, these results mean that a strong link exists, among sizeable numbers of women, between the end of amenorrhoea and the cessation of breast-feeding. This group would presumably include those who decided to terminate breast-feeding at the first post-partum menses.

Post-partum sexual abstinence

Post-partum abstinence is of importance for the length of temporary post-partum sterility, when its duration exceeds either of the other factors discussed above, particularly the length of post-partum amenorrhoea. In table 70 and figure 25, it can be seen that the duration of abstinence is relatively short in Kenya, the Philippines, the Sudan, the Syrian Arab Republic, Tunisia and Yemen; moderate in Ghana and Haiti; and long in Benin, Cameroon, Côte d'Ivoire and Lesotho. The range of mean durations is larger than for either full breast-feeding or amenorrhoea. In the Syrian Arab Republic, for example, reported abstinence lasts, on average, for less than 1.5 months, whereas in Benin and Lesotho, it exceeds 17 months.[19] Another interesting feature evident in several of the curves in figure 25 is that even where post-partum abstinence is not widely practised, a small proportion of women avoid sexual relations for extended periods during breast-feeding.

Comparing full breast-feeding with post-partum abstinence, in Benin, Cameroon, Côte d'Ivoire, Ghana and Lesotho, the latter practice extends well beyond the period of full breast-feeding. In Kenya and the Philippines, the two curves are almost identical, implying perhaps that the taboo has been abridged to coincide with that part of lactation when the new-born is totally dependent upon breast milk. In the remaining countries, mainly Arab countries, abstinence was considerably shorter than the period of full breast-feeding; and, in fact, was not practised by a large proportion of couples. Compared with amenorrhoea, however, the duration of abstinence was in general shorter. In Benin, Cameroon, Côte d'Ivoire and Lesotho, however, sexual abstinence outlasts even the period of amenorrhoea; and this fact must be noted in any attempt to weigh the separate effects on fertility of its proximate determinants (principally, breast-feeding versus contraceptive use).

Differences in durations of post-partum abstinence compared with breast-feeding and amenorrhoea are also evident in table 73, which again uses data referring to the last closed birth interval. Abstinence throughout the lactational period is a practice found among significant proportions of WFS respondents in certain countries, especially in Benin, Cameroon and Lesotho, where over half of the sampled women followed this practice, and to a lesser extent in Ghana and Yemen. In these countries, post-partum abstinence must therefore be taken into consideration when accounting for the relative importance of proximate fertility determinants. In most other countries, however, this cultural norm, if it ever existed, has obviously lost sway: in Haiti, Kenya, the Sudan, the Syrian Arab Republic and Tunisia, two thirds or more of respondents reported that they had resumed conjugal relations seven or more months before the end of the general breast-feeding period (column (4)).

With regard to the relationship between post-partum amenorrhoea and abstinence, two similar cross-national patterns are evident in the last closed birth interval (table 73, columns (7) and (8)). In Western Africa and Lesotho, a large proportion of women abstained from sexual intercourse until after menstruation returned, the extreme cases being Lesotho and Benin, where 81 and

TABLE 71. DIFFERENCE IN DURATIONS OF GENERAL AND FULL BREAST-FEEDING AND MEAN DURATION OF FULL BREAST-FEEDING, BY AGE OF MOTHER AND USE OF CONTRACEPTION: DATA FOR LAST CLOSED BIRTH INTERVAL

	General minus full breast-feeding duration		Percentage: general minus full breast-feeding (percentage distribution)				Percentage of cases with general less than full breast-feeding (7)	Mean duration of full breast-feeding during last closed birth interval, by age group					
								15-24		25-34		35-49	
Region and country	Last closed birth interval (months) (1)	Current status data (2)	No difference (3)	Months				Yes[a] (8)	No[b] (9)	Yes[a] (10)	No[b] (11)	Yes[a] (12)	No[b] (13)
				1-3 (4)	4-9 (5)	10+ (6)							
Africa													
Benin	15.4	18.3	10	2	16	70	3	5.4	7.0	5.9	7.3	5.3	7.3
Cameroon	13.9	13.8	4	3	17	75	1	4.8	5.8	4.2	5.9	4.3	6.1
Côte d'Ivoire[c]	10.0	13.3	6	9	36	48	1	5.9	5.9	6.0	6.6	6.2	7.0
Ghana	10.1	14.0	5	6	44	44	2	4.1	5.0	4.4	5.4	5.0	5.8
Kenya	10.0	14.9	3	9	39	47	1	3.8	3.4	2.6	3.4	3.3	3.6
Lesotho	16.1	18.2	3	4	18	75	0	3.4	4.0	3.8	4.0	3.7	4.2
Mauritania	11.0	14.3	14	4	19	61	2	d	d	d	d	d	d
Senegal	13.6	10.6	5	2	15	78	0	5.7	6.4	5.8	6.2	5.4	6.6
Sudan	9.8	8.0	7	8	33	50	2	4.6	6.5	4.8	6.9	5.0	6.9
Tunisia	9.4	13.0	15	9	24	38	14	6.0	7.8	7.0	9.1	7.7	10.2
Asia and Oceania													
Philippines	8.5	9.1	8	15	42	35	0	4.0	4.9	4.1	4.8	4.2	5.2
Syrian Arab Republic	6.5	5.7	25	16	29	30	0	5.0	7.3	5.9	8.0	6.4	9.3
Yemen	6.6	6.5	38	13	16	33	0	3.0	6.0	6.5	6.9	3.7	8.7

Source: World Fertility Survey standard recode tapes.
[a] Had used contraceptive method during last closed birth interval.
[b] No use of contraception during last closed birth interval.
[c] Formerly called the Ivory Coast.
[d] No information on contraceptive use during last closed interval.

TABLE 72. DIFFERENCE IN DURATIONS OF GENERAL BREAST-FEEDING AND POST-PARTUM AMENORRHOEA: DATA FOR LAST CLOSED BIRTH INTERVAL

	Mean difference in duration: general breast-feeding minus amenorrhoea		Percentage of women		
Region and country	Last closed birth interval (1)	Current status data (2)	General breast-feeding less than amenorrhoea (3)	General breast-feeding equal to amenorrhoea (4)	General breast-feeding longer than amenorrhoea by seven months or more (5)
Africa					
Benin	7.5	8.1	11	18	46
Cameroon	7.8	6.1	9	17	52
Côte d'Ivoire[a]	7.0	7.1	11	10	48
Ghana	3.7	5.9	22	17	29
Kenya	4.1	6.1	15	18	30
Lesotho	10.7	10.5	7	14	60
Mauritania	8.4	7.5	7	24	55
Sudan	4.1	5.2	13	38	28
Tunisia	6.8	7.1	7	32	39
Latin America and the Caribbean					
Haiti	2.7	3.6	36	22	21
Asia and Oceania					
Philippines	4.5	5.0	19	17	33
Syrian Arab Republic	7.7	4.6	8	14	50
Yemen	5.3	3.9	16	25	38

Source: World Fertility Survey standard recode tapes.
[a] Formerly called the Ivory Coast.

80 per cent, respectively, did so. In sharp contrast, other African countries, particularly Kenya and the Sudan, do not follow this pattern, although even in these two countries more than one quarter of the women interviewed reported abstaining until the first post-partum menses.

In general, data on the post-partum factors show that full breast-feeding represents only a small part of the total breast-feeding period, while post-partum amenorrhoea, on average, extends longer than full breast-feeding. The period of amenorrhoea, however, is still somewhat less

TABLE 73. DIFFERENCE IN DURATIONS OF GENERAL BREAST-FEEDING, POST-PARTUM AMENORRHOEA AND POST-PARTUM ABSTINENCE: DATA FOR LAST CLOSED BIRTH INTERVAL

Region and country	Mean difference in duration: general breast-feeding minus abstinence — Last closed birth interval (1)	Current status data (2)	Percentage of women — General breast-feeding less than abstinence (3)	General breast-feeding longer than abstinence by seven months or more (4)	Mean difference in duration: amenorrhoea minus abstinence — Last closed birth interval (5)	Current status data (6)	Percentage of women — Amenorrhoea less than or equal to abstinence (7)	Amenorrhoea longer than abstinence by four months or more (8)
Africa								
Benin	3.9	3.4	49	30	−3.4	−4.7	80	14
Cameroon	3.8	3.1	57	30	−3.3	−3.0	76	14
Côte d'Ivoire[a]	4.0	3.4	39	30	−2.6	−3.7	76	12
Ghana	5.5	7.8	23	41	1.6	1.9	46	38
Kenya	9.3	13.7	10	66	4.8	7.6	27	50
Lesotho	4.1	3.8	55	26	−5.5	−6.7	81	10
Mauritania	..	..	—	—	..	..	—	—
Sudan	12.6	14.1	4	84	7.8	8.9	26	63
Tunisia	14.8	12.7	5	77	6.7	5.6	44	43
Latin America and the Caribbean								
Haiti	8.4	8.3	12	64	4.7	4.7	39	47
Asia and Oceania								
Philippines	10.2	10.1	9	73	4.5	5.1	32	48
Syrian Arab Republic	13.3	10.2	1	80	3.9	5.6	38	30
Yemen	9.5	9.1	24	60	3.7	5.2	41	37

Source: World Fertility Survey standard recode tapes.

[a] Formerly called the Ivory Coast.

than the total breast-feeding period, although for a large fraction of women (from one third to one half), amenorrhoea lasts as long as or longer than the breast-feeding period itself. It is possible that some women cease breast-feeding when menses return. The third post-partum factor studied, abstinence, varies considerably in duration between the countries studied. In most cases, mean duration is low, but it is of considerable importance in some African countries, where it extends beyond the end of the amenorrhoeic period. None the less, substantial proportions of women in all countries abstain for the entire amenorrhoeic period.

E. CONCLUSION

In this chapter, patterns and differentials in the incidence and duration of breast-feeding were examined for 38 countries. For a subsample of countries, 15 that canvassed the FOTCAF model, the incidence and patterns of other aspects of post-partum reproductive behaviour were studied. These included full breast-feeding, post-partum amenorrhoea and post-partum abstinence.

Although the incidence of breast-feeding is high in almost all countries, there is still a considerable amount of variation between countries. More than 99 per cent of babies in Bangladesh, Ghana, Mauritania, Nepal and Senegal were breast-fed, while under 85 per cent of those in Malaysia were breast-fed. Women from African countries are more likely to breast-feed than those in Latin America and the Caribbean or Asia and Oceania. Although fewer women initiate breast-feeding in the more developed of these countries, the differences between the more developed and less developed are not large.

The average mean duration of breast-feeding is similar in Africa and in Asia and Oceania (18.4 and 18.1 months, respectively), while in Latin America and the Caribbean, the average mean duration is about half as long, 9.6 months. These regional averages mask the substantial variation within regions, especially in Asia and Oceania, and to a lesser extent in Latin America and the Caribbean. Women in Southern Asian countries and Indonesia generally breast-feed for substantially longer periods than their other Asian counterparts or even women in other regions.

Mean durations of breast-feeding are strongly linked to level of development and less strongly to family planning programme effort. Women in the low development group (IV) breast-fed, on average, more than two and a half times longer than those in the high development group (I).

Differentials in the incidence and duration of breast-feeding by sex of child and by age and parity of mother were studied. No differentials in the incidence and duration of breast-feeding by sex of child were observed. The duration of breast-feeding was positively related to the age and parity of the mother, although the relationship was stronger with parity. These differentials persist at all levels of development and programme strength, although the size of the differentials is greatest in development groups I and II, and in countries with strong programmes.

The current status of breast-feeding was used in the estimation of mean breast-feeding durations; and therefore, it was not possible to arrive at conclusions about trends in breast-feeding durations. The interpretation of the positive relationship of breast-feeding durations with age and with parity of the mother cannot be conclusively related to trends in breast-feeding duration, although it is likely that the relationship in part reflects such trends.

A strong negative relationship was obtained between duration of breast-feeding and contraceptive use during the last closed birth interval. The relationship between incidence of breast-feeding and contraceptive use was also negative although not so strong. Women who did not use any contraception breast-fed the longest, followed by those who used traditional methods of contraception, while women who used modern methods breast-fed for the shortest durations. The negative association between contraceptive use and breast-feeding durations implies that part of the increase in fertility caused by declining breast-feeding durations will be offset by increased contraceptive use.

From about one fifth to one quarter (less in Africa) of the women who were currently breast-feeding were also using some form of contraception. This means that a substantial proportion of breast-feeding women were exposed to the risk of another birth soon after the last birth. Tabulations by duration of use since birth and the status of abstinence and amenorrhoea, which were not undertaken in this analysis, could further identify the proportion of women at greater risk. Pill users, among contraceptive users, were studied separately, given the possible effects of some types of pills on the volume of breast milk. The results show that although the percentage of pill users among breast-feeders was generally low, it is still not inconsequential in some countries.

Durations of full breast-feeding, amenorrhoea and abstinence were computed for a subsample of countries. Post-partum amenorrhoea, in general, extends for longer periods than full breast-feeding, which represents only a small part of the total breast-feeding period. For a large fraction of women, amenorrhoea lasts as long as or longer than the breast-feeding period although, on average, it is shorter than the breast-feeding period. Abstinence varies considerably in duration between countries. In most cases, the mean duration of abstinence is low but in some African countries it extends beyond the end of the amenorrhoeic period.

The evidence presented in this chapter enhances the knowledge of breast-feeding patterns and their variations across countries and at different levels of development, as well as about the interrelationships in the patterns of full breast-feeding, amenorrhoea and abstinence for some of the countries. Information is still lacking, however, on how lactation operates to suppress ovulation on the relationship between post-partum amenorrhoea and anovulation and on the effects of breast-feeding in suppressing conception after the resumption of menstruation. In this regard, more knowledge is also needed on the optimal timing and type of modern contraception that can be used during lactation. This type of knowledge would help women modify their behaviour in relation to their desires with regard to conception.

Although it was not possible to elicit information about trends in breast-feeding duration and in the incidence of breast-feeding, the strong negative correlation of breast-feeding duration with levels of development points to shorter breast-feeding durations and lower incidence of breast-feeding as products of increased development. For Governments wishing to induce fertility decline, an understanding of this relationship should be important to the design of educational programmes as well as maternal and child health and family planning programmes.

NOTES

[1] For an excellent coverage of literature on the immunological protection provided by breast milk, see McCann and others (1981).

[2] Such increases in fertility, thought to be only temporary, have been observed in the Republic of Korea (see Coale, Cho and Goldman, 1979). A discussion of this topic also appears in Nag (1979).

[3] During the Thirty-fourth World Health Assembly meetings in 1981, the World Health Organization approved an international code for the marketing of breast-milk substitutes which would inform the purchaser that human milk is the best food for infants under six months old (World Health Organization, 1981).

[4] It is believed that the physical contact involved in nursing promotes an emotional bond between mother and infant.

[5] Formerly called the Ivory Coast.

[6] Details of this method are given in Page, Lesthaeghe and Shah (1982), pp. 25-28.

[7] In case of multiple births, breast-feeding questions referred to only the first-born (Page, Lesthaeghe and Shah, 1982, p. 12).

[8] The estimation of the proportion ever breast-fed in these studies is different from that used in this chapter. Therefore, the proportions are not comparable with those given in table 57.

[9] Sex of child was reported by almost all women interviewed. Only 37 last-born children, out of more than 130,000 included in the analyses, did not have their gender coded. Such a small proportion would not have any noticeable effect on the analysis.

[10] In Jamaica, for example, the proportions of women who never breast-fed their most recent living child are 5 per cent for sons and 7 per cent for daughters. The chi-squared statistic in this sample is 2.67, not statistically significant (degrees of freedom = 1; level of significance = 0.01). The sole exception is Malaysia, where chi-squared, 7.12, attains statistical significance. This result, however, may be influenced by the sample size together with the large proportion of children who are never breast-fed in Malaysia.

[11] The difference of means test using the t-statistic (level of significance = 0.01).

[12] Differences in median durations give results similar to mean durations but are not presented because medians are less satisfactory than means as measures of central tendency, since breast-feeding distributions, while quite similar in shape in their entirety, may diverge considerably at any particular duration. The corresponding medians, therefore, must be expected to be more variable than mean values.

[13] See, for example, Ferry and Smith (1983) and Lesthaeghe (1982).

[14] These six African countries, plus Haiti, Paraguay and Senegal, were the only cases where simple difference of means tests between the averages for the youngest and oldest groups of mothers were not statistically significant (level of significance = 0.01).

[15] Benin, Cameroon, Colombia, Ghana, Jamaica, Lesotho, Malaysia, Mauritania, Mexico, Senegal, the Sudan, Trinidad and Tobago.

[16] The minimum sample size used was 25.

[17] The relevant question was "How many months old was the child when you began giving him/her additional food along with breast-feeding?". Although no other question was asked, it may be assumed that, for the majority of mothers who were full breast-feeding, babies were allowed to feed "on demand", including night-time sessions, and that the frequency of suckling was probably relatively high. In most cases, therefore, this period may be considered one of complete temporary sterility.

[18] For the most part, this section uses the same current status methodology as in other parts of this chapter, merely substituting the concepts, "full breast-feeding" etc. for "breast-feeding". In the final part of the section, however, durations in the last closed birth/pregnancy interval are used.

[19] The figure for Lesotho may be exceptionally high due to a large proportion of temporarily absent husbands working away from home.

REFERENCES

Butz, William P. and Julie DaVanzo (1981). Determinants of breast-feeding and weaning patterns in Malaysia. Paper presented at the Annual Meeting of the Population Association of America, Washington, D.C., 26-28 March 1981.

Caldwell, J. C. and P. Caldwell (1981). Causes and sequence in the reduction of postnatal abstinence in Ibadan City, Nigeria. In Hilary J. Page and Ron Lesthaeghe, eds., *Child-Spacing in Tropical Africa: Traditions and Change*. London and New York: Academic Press, 181-199.

Coale, Ansley J., Lee-Jay Cho and Noreen Goldman (1979). Nuptiality and fertility in the Republic of Korea. In Lado T. Ruzicka, ed., *Nuptiality and Fertility*. Proceedings of a seminar organized by the International Union for the Scientific Study of Population, Bruges, 8-11 January 1979. Liège: Ordina Editions, 43-60.

Ferry, Benôit and David P. Smith (1983). *Breastfeeding differentials*. World Fertility Survey Comparative Studies, No. 23: Cross-National Summaries. Voorburg, The Netherlands: International Statistical Institute.

Hambraeus, L. (1979). Maternal diet and human milk composition. In H. Aebi and R. Whitehead, eds., *Maternal Nutrition during Pregnancy and Lactation*. Vienna: Hans Hüber, 223-244.

Hull, Valerie J. (1980). Intermediate variables in the explanation of differential fertility: results of a village study in rural Java. *Human Ecology* 8(3):213-243.

Jain, Anrudh K. and John Bongaarts (1981). Breastfeeding: patterns, correlates and fertility effects. *Studies in Family Planning* 12(3):79-99.

Jelliffe, Derrick B. and E. F. Patrice Jelliffe (1978). The volume and composition of human milk in poorly nourished communities: a review. *American Journal of Clinical Nutrition* 31(3):492-515.

Kent, Mary Mederias (1981). *Breast-feeding in the Developing World: Current Patterns and Implications for Future Trends*. Reports on the World Fertility Survey, No. 2. Washington, D.C.: Population Reference Bureau.

Knodel, John and Nibhon Debavalya (1980). Breastfeeding in Thailand: trends and differentials, 1969-79. *Studies in Family Planning* 11(12):355-377.

Lesthaeghe, Ron (1982). Lactation and lactation-related variables, contraception and fertility: an overview of data problems and world trends. Paper submitted to the WHO/NRC Joint Workshop and Programme Policy Meeting on Breast-feeding and Fertility Regulation, Geneva, February 1982.

McCann, Margaret F. and others (1981). *Breast-feeding, Fertility, and Family Planning*. Population Reports, Series J, No. 24. Baltimore, Maryland: Population Information Program of The Johns Hopkins University.

Mexico (1981). Department of Welfare and Health. Breastfeeding: recent tendencies in the Mexico experience. Unpublished report by the Mother-child Health and Planning Divisions.

Millman, Sara (1981). Breastfeeding in Taiwan: trends and differentials, 1966-1980. Paper submitted to the Annual Meeting of the Population Association of America, Washington, D.C., 26-28 March 1981. The data in this paper refer to Taiwan, Province of China.

_____ (1985). Breastfeeding and contraception: why the inverse association? *Studies in Family Planning* 16(2):61-75.

Nag, Moni (1979). *How Modernization Can Increase Fertility*. Center for Policy Studies Working Paper, No. 49. New York: The Population Council.

Nortman, Dorothy L., with assistance of Joanne Fisher (1982). *Population and Family Planning Programs, A Compendium of Data Through 1981*. 11th ed. New York: The Population Council.

Page, H. J., R. J. Lesthaeghe, and I. H. Shah (1982). *Illustrative analysis: Breastfeeding in Pakistan*. World Fertility Survey Scientific Reports, No. 37. Voorburg, The Netherlands: International Statistical Institute.

Pebley, Anne R., Howard I. Goldberg and Jane Menken (1985). Contraceptive use during lactation in developing countries. *Studies in Family Planning* 16(1):40-49.

Perez, A. and others (1971). Timing and sequence of resuming ovulation and menstruation after childbirth. *Population Studies* 25(3):491-503.

Short, R. (1982). The biological basis for the contraceptive effects of breastfeeding. Paper submitted to the WHO/NRC Joint Workshop and Programme Policy Meeting on Breast-feeding and Fertility Regulation, Geneva, February 1982.

Simpson-Herbert, Mayling and Sandra L. Huffman (1981). The contraceptive effect of breastfeeding. *Studies in Family Planning* 12(4):125-133. Special issue entitled "Breastfeeding: program, policy and research issues"; Edward C. Baer and Beverly Winikoff, eds.

Singh, Susheela (1984). *Comparability of Questionnaires: 41 WFS countries*. World Fertility Survey Comparative Studies, No. 32; Cross-National Summaries. Voorburg, The Netherlands: International Statistical Institute.

_____ and Benôit Ferry (1984). *Biological and Traditional Factors That Influence Fertility: Results from WFS Surveys*, World Fertility Survey Comparative Studies, No. 40; Cross-National Summaries. Voorburg, The Netherlands: International Statistical Institute.

Smith, David and Benôit Ferry (1984). *Correlates of Breastfeeding*. World Fertility Survey Comparative Studies, No. 41. Voorburg, The Netherlands: International Statistical Institute.

United Nations (1983). Department of International Economic and Social Affairs. Population Division. *Fertility Levels and Trends as Assessed from Twenty World Fertility Surveys*. Non-sales publication ST/ESA/SER.R/50. New York.

United States of America (1984). Department of Health and Human Services. Public Health Services; Centers for Disease Control. Racial and educational factors associated with breastfeeding—United States, 1969 and 1980. *Morbidity and Mortality Weekly Report* 33(11):153-154.

Whitehead, R. A., A. A. Paul, and L. A. Rowland (1980). Lactation in Cambridge and in the Gambia. In B. A. Wharton, ed., *Proceedings of the Pediatric Conference of the Royal College of Physicians*. London: Pitman Medicals.

World Health Organization (1981). *International Code on Marketing of Breast-milk Substitutes*. Geneva.

_____ (1981a). *Contemporary Patterns of Breast-feeding*. Report on the WHO Collaborative Study on Breast-feeding. Geneva.

_____ (1983). Breast-feeding and fertility regulation: current knowledge and programme policy implications. Summary report of the WHO/NRC Joint Workshop and Programme Policy Meeting on Breast-feeding and Fertility Regulation, Geneva, February 1982. *Bulletin of the World Health Organization* 61(3):371-382.

V. CONTRACEPTIVE PRACTICE

ABSTRACT

This chapter describes levels of knowledge and practice of contraception and differentials in contraceptive use according to age, family size and desire for more children. Timing and method of first contraceptive use and the relation between levels of ever-use and current use are also discussed.

The World Fertility Survey data for the period from the mid-1970s to the early 1980s show that appreciable proportions of women in developing countries were attempting to control their fertility. The main exceptions are sub-Saharan Africa and four Asian countries (Bangladesh, Nepal, Pakistan and Yemen), where contraceptive prevalence (current use) was no more than 10 per cent of women of reproductive ages. Even awareness of modern contraceptive methods was limited in most of the low-prevalence countries. In the other countries of Asia and Oceania, contraceptive prevalence levels were 20-41 per cent of married women. Values in Latin America and the Caribbean were 30-64 per cent, except in Haiti, 19 per cent. Modern methods accounted for 18 of the overall average of 25 per cent of married women currently using contraception. Method distributions differ greatly among countries, but the pill was the most important single method, followed by female sterilization, intra-uterine devices, rhythm, the condom and withdrawal. The level of contraceptive use is strongly related to both level of development and strength of family planning programme effort, each has some separate effect on use levels.

Contraceptive prevalence was usually highest among women aged 25-40 years, and the level usually rose sharply up to a family size of two children but often varied little between women with moderate-sized families and those with large families. Although women who wanted no more children were more likely to use contraception, many used it to space wanted births; such use accounted for roughly 30, 40 and 65 per cent of all contraceptive practice in Asia and Oceania, Latin America and the Caribbean, and Africa, respectively. The pill was much more frequently the first contraceptive tried and was consistently used more by young than older women. The decreasing share of use due to the pill approximately balances the increasing resort to sterilization among older contraceptive users. Obviously excluding the permanent method of sterilization, the choice of methods tended to be similar between women who did and those who did not want more children.

The proportion of current users among those who had ever tried contraception tended to be high in the same groups of countries that had high levels of ever-use: relatively economically advanced countries and those with strong family planning programmes. Proportions of continuing users were especially low in sub-Saharan Africa, even for women who said they wanted no more children.

Information about contraception is of direct interest to policy-makers in most countries, as well as to demographers who study the dynamics of fertility. The gathering of data about contraception has grown along with the family planning movement in developing countries. Cross-sectional surveys of women of reproductive ages can yield information about contraceptive practice, the population's contact with family planning programmes, attitudes towards and knowledge about birth control and problems experienced with particular methods. These data provide an important supplement, useful for evaluation and monitoring, to records maintained by organized family planning programmes.

The World Fertility Survey (WFS) programme differed from most of the earlier Knowledge, Attitude and Practice (KAP) type of survey in several important respects.

One difference is that, compared with KAP surveys and also with their more recent relative, the Contraceptive Prevalence Survey, WFS devoted a smaller fraction of the interview to obtaining information directly about contraception. This practice was in keeping with the multiple purposes the WFS programme was intended to serve. The WFS questionnaires devoted little attention to measuring attitudes towards contraception, focusing instead mainly on contraceptive practice. Lessons learned from earlier surveys were taken into account in the design of the WFS questions, particularly in the decision to include in the core questionnaire a lengthy series of probe questions about particular methods. In order to accommodate the interests of countries with active family planning programmes, additional questions about contraception were included in the family planning module. The fertility regulation module, adopted by a majority of countries outside of sub-Saharan Africa, also contained some questions about past contraceptive use.

This chapter summarizes information about knowledge of contraception and past and current use of contraception. Differentials in contraceptive practice according to age, family size and desire for more children are examined here, while differential contraceptive practice according to socio-economic characteristics is examined in part two of this volume. Practice of induced abortion is not discussed, primarily because of data limitations.[1]

Section A describes the information about family planning that was gathered in WFS and mentions some problems relating to the definition, measurement and analysis of contraceptive use. Next, section B gives an overview of levels of contraceptive knowledge and use and their association with geographical region, level of socio-economic development and strength of family planning programme effort. Section C describes differences in the level of ever-use and current use of contraception according to marital status, age, family size and the respondent's stated desire for more children. Section D examines the specific contraceptive methods known and used in each country, and variations in type of method according to age, family size and desire for more children. Section E considers country differences in the extent of contraceptive discontinuation.

A. THE DATA

All WFS countries collected information about knowledge, ever-use and current use of specific contraceptive methods. The basic series of questions in the core questionnaire (World Fertility Survey, 1975) began with a general query about familiarity with and use of family planning. The interviewer then read a brief description of particular methods, omitting those the respondent had already mentioned, and asked whether the respondent had ever heard of and had ever used each of these methods. Next, there were additional open-ended questions about knowledge and use of any other methods. The core questionnaire included probe questions about 10 specific methods, or groups of methods: oral pill; intra-uterine devices (IUD); condom; female chemical and barrier methods (including diaphragm, cervical cap; and spermicidal foams, creams and jellies); rhythm or periodic abstinence; withdrawal or coitus interruptus; abstinence; douche; female sterilization; and male sterilization.

For female sterilization, there was an additional question to separate operations done solely for health reasons from those done at least partially for contraceptive reasons. In a few Latin American and Caribbean countries, a significant number of women reported a sterilization for health reasons.[2] In this chapter, statistics relating to sterilization refer only to operations performed for contraceptive reasons.

It may be noted that the catalogue of methods given above excludes breast-feeding, which has been listed as a contraceptive method in some other surveys. WFS treated breast-feeding as a separate topic, and it is discussed separately in this study (chapter IV). The possible overlap between another traditional birth-spacing method, post-partum abstinence, and contraceptive abstinence as measured in WFS, is discussed later.

The questions about contraceptive knowledge and ever-use were usually asked of all women interviewed, but some countries with all-women samples restricted these questions to women who had ever been in a union. The question about current use was asked of non-pregnant women who were currently in a union, except in countries that employed the module for factors other than contraception affecting fertility (FOTCAF). In most of the latter countries, the question about current contraceptive practice was skipped if the respondent had not resumed sexual relations since her last pregnancy.

Method-specific probe questions help to ensure that the respondents and the survey designers shall refer to the same range of practices when they speak of contraception. A study of responses in three WFS countries (Colombia, Sri Lanka and Thailand) found that the probe questions greatly increased the number of women reporting knowledge of each specific method (Vaessen, 1981). Furthermore, many of the women who later reported use of particular methods had not mentioned even knowing of the method when the initial open-ended question was asked. Apparent knowledge and use of the pill and IUD were affected relatively little by the probe questions, but familiarity with and practice of non-supply methods, such as rhythm, withdrawal and abstinence, was often many times higher after than before the probe questions were asked. The level of practice of sterilization would also be seriously affected by the omission of probes.

Most countries followed the recommended questions very closely. Twenty-three asked the probe questions dealing with knowledge and use of contraception for all 10 of the specific methods mentioned above. Twenty-two of the countries considered here added probe questions about knowledge and use of injectable contraceptives.[3] A few countries added probe questions about country-specific folk methods (see Singh, 1984).

The greatest departures from the standard questions occurred in Mauritania and Pakistan, both of which omitted all method-specific probe questions. Another 13 countries did not ask about one or more of the methods or did not include one or more methods in the final coding. The methods most often omitted were abstinence (seven countries), male sterilization (five countries) and female sterilization (four countries). Withdrawal, douche, rhythm and female barrier and chemical methods were also omitted by one or more countries.[4] Spontaneous mentions of methods for which probes were omitted may have been recorded under "other methods". However, the methods for which probes were most often omitted are among those which are least likely to be mentioned spontaneously.

Traditional birth-spacing mechanisms (mainly breast-feeding and lengthy post-partum abstinence) are rarely reported spontaneously by survey respondents as methods of contraception. However, surveys that include breast-feeding or abstinence in the list of contraceptive methods sometimes record appreciable numbers of users of these methods, though it is usually unclear whether contraceptive motives were the main reason for observance of these practices (see Laing, 1984).

In WFS, breast-feeding was not included as a contraceptive, but abstinence was.[5] Where lengthy post-partum abstinence is observed, there is a clear potential for overlap in reporting of contraceptive abstinence and post-partum abstinence. In most of the countries that asked about post-partum abstinence (which includes most of those with a tradition of extended abstinence), overlap between current practice of post-partum abstinence and contraception was avoided, by coding women who were abstaining post-partum as non-users of contraception.[6] However, post-partum abstinence may have been reported as past contraceptive use, since abstinence was listed in the standard sequence of probed contraceptive methods. In fact, the tendency to report post-partum abstinence as contraception appears to have varied between countries: in both Benin and Côte d'Ivoire,[7] most women observe extended periods of abstinence, averaging 15 to 16 months, but the percentage who reported ever-use of contraceptive abstinence was 68 in Côte d'Ivoire and 27 in Benin.

In a few countries, women who said they were abstaining post-partum were also asked whether they were currently using contraception. Responses for these countries (Benin, Fiji, Haiti, the Philippines) were examined for overlap between post-partum abstinence and current contraceptive use. The amount of overlap was judged to be serious enough to have a material effect on the analysis in Benin.[8] In this country, 20 per cent of currently married women were coded as current users of contraception, a markedly higher level than in the other sub-Saharan countries. However, this impression of higher contraceptive prevalence was an artifact of measurement: over half the "current users" in Benin had not resumed sexual relations since the last birth; and most of the contraceptive use they reported was abstinence itself. Had the same questioning and coding procedures been followed in Benin as in most of the other sub-Saharan countries, these women would have been treated as non-users of

TABLE 74. PERCENTAGES OF CURRENTLY MARRIED WOMEN AGED 15-49 WHO KNEW ANY CONTRACEPTIVE METHOD, KNEW A FAMILY PLANNING OUTLET, HAD EVER USED A METHOD AND WERE CURRENTLY USING MODERN AND TRADITIONAL METHODS, BY COUNTRY

Region and country	Age range (1)	Knew a method (2)	Knew a family planning outlet (3)	Had ever used contraception (4)	Currently using Any method (5)	Currently using A modern clinic or supply method (6)	Traditional and non-supply methods (7)
Africa							
Benin	15-49	40(21)	1[a]	36(14)	9(5)[b]	0[b]	9(4)[b]
Cameroon	15-49	34	..	11	2	1	2
Côte d'Ivoire[c]	15-49	85(26)	..	71(9)	3	0	2
Egypt	15-49	90	75	42	24	23	1
Ghana	15-49	69(62)	43	40(25)	10(6)	6	4(0)
Kenya	15-49	93	42	32(25)	7	4	2
Lesotho	15-49	65	27	23	5	2	3
Mauritania	15-49	8	..	2	1	0	1
Morocco	15-49	84	82	31	20	17	3
Senegal	15-49	60(39)	..	11(3)	4(1)	1	3(0)
Sudan	15-49	51	23	13	5	4	1
Tunisia	15-49	95	..	47	31	25	7
Latin America and the Caribbean							
Colombia	15-49	96	66	62	43	30	12
Costa Rica	20-49	100	89	84	64	53	11
Dominican Republic	15-49	98	..	50	32	26	6
Ecuador	15-49	90	..	54	34	26	8
Guyana	15-49	96	..	56	31	28	3
Haiti	15-49	85	..	37	19(15)	5	14(10)
Jamaica	15-49	98	..	66	38	36	2
Mexico	15-49	90	49	47	30	23	7
Panama	20-49	99	72	75	54	46	8
Paraguay	15-49	96	91	57	36	24	13
Peru	15-49	82	..	50	31	11	20
Trinidad and Tobago	15-49	99	92	80	52	46	6
Venezuela	15-44	98	95	70	49	38	12
Asia and Oceania							
Bangladesh	15-49	84	..	16	8	5	3
Fiji	15-49	100	..	69	41	35	6
Indonesia	15-49	80	53	39	26	23	3
Jordan	15-49	97	..	47	25	18	7
Malaysia	15-49	93	77	51	33	24	9
Nepal	15-49	23	6	4	2	2	0
Pakistan	15-49	76	33[d]	10	5	4	1
Philippines	15-49	94	77	58	36	16	20
Republic of Korea	15-49	98	86	59	35	27	8
Sri Lanka	15-49	92	..	45(42)	32(28)	19	13(9)
Syrian Arab Republic	15-49	78	..	34	20	15	5
Thailand	15-49	97	..	48	33	30	3
Yemen	15-49	24	..	3	1	1	0

Source: World Fertility Survey standard recode tapes.

NOTE: Percentage who knew or were using a method other than abstinence is shown in parentheses for countries where 3 per cent or more of married women knew about or used only abstinence.

[a] Percentage who knew a source for pills.

[b] Women who had not resumed sexual relations since the last pregnancy were counted as non-users.

[c] Formerly called the Ivory Coast.

[d] Assumes that all women who had ever used contraception knew of an outlet.

contraception. In the tables of this chapter, the level of current contraceptive use for Benin excludes women who were abstaining post-partum, in order to improve comparability of the figures for the sub-Saharan countries.

Another problem related to measurement of contraceptive abstinence surfaced during data analysis. Even though post-partum abstinence was excluded from current contraceptive use in most sub-Saharan countries, women who had resumed sexual relations at some time since the last birth could still report abstinence as the current contraceptive method. But in Côte d'Ivoire, Ghana and Kenya, a large majority of the women coded as abstaining for contraceptive reasons said, in response to another question, that they were having sexual relations "these days" (or "currently") (Cleland and Kalule-Sabiti, 1984). While it is not completely clear which variable is more at fault, the lack of consistency is disturbing.

Most of this chapter is based on responses to the basic questions on contraceptive knowledge and use, but some tables draw upon questions asked in a subset of countries. Many of the countries that had organized family planning programmes included questions about the respondent's knowledge of family planning outlets and her use of programme facilities. Some of the information pertaining to knowledge of outlets is included here. (For a comprehensive discussion, see Jones, 1984.) Countries that employed the family planning module usually included questions about the first use of contraception; some of this information is discussed in section E.

B. AN OVERVIEW OF LEVELS OF CONTRACEPTIVE KNOWLEDGE AND USE

Knowledge of any method

The type of knowledge indicated in column (1) of table 74 is simple recognition of at least one contraceptive method, after the interviewer described the methods. Given the liberality of this definition, it is not surprising that knowledge of contraception appears widespread in many developing countries—over 90 per cent of married women recognized a method, in 21 of 38 countries. More noteworthy, however, is that substantial proportions of women did not have even this minimal sort of knowledge in most of the African countries and in a few countries in other regions. In Mauritania, only 8 per cent of the women could name a contraceptive method; the descriptive probe questions about specific methods were not used there. But under one fourth of women in Nepal and Yemen knew of a method, despite inclusion of probe questions.

Knowledge of specific methods is discussed in more detail later, but it is worth noting at this point the role of abstinence in sub-Saharan Africa. Lengthy periods of post-partum abstinence are prescribed by tradition in many countries of this region; and, as chapter IV discusses, the practice is still widely observed in several. Although many women who follow this tradition did not report this practice when asked about contraception, abstinence was reported much more often in a few of the sub-Saharan countries than was any other method. The percentage who knew of a method other than abstinence is shown in parentheses in table 74, where this figure is at least three percentage points lower than the percentage when abstinence is included. In Benin, Côte d'Ivoire and Senegal, between 19 and 59 per cent of married women knew of "contraceptive abstinence" but no other method. Since a few of the sub-Saharan questionnaires did not include abstinence in the list of contraceptive methods, the percentage who reported knowledge of a method other than abstinence provides a better basis for comparison between the countries of this region, and it gives a better indication of the spread of information about non-traditional means of fertility control.

Knowledge of a family planning outlet

Nineteen of the surveys asked women whether they knew of a place to obtain family planning information or supplies. Answers to this question suggest that a lack of access to services (or possibly lack of information about the services that are available) is an important constraint to greater use of modern contraceptive methods in many of the WFS countries. One third or fewer of the women knew of an outlet in Lesotho, Pakistan and the Sudan, and between one third and one half in Ghana, Kenya and Mexico. Only in Paraguay, Trinidad and Tobago, and Venezuela did at least 90 per cent know of an outlet.[9]

Current use of contraception

On average, the level of current use of contraception, like the level of contraceptive knowledge, was lowest in Africa and highest in Latin America and the Caribbean (table 74, column (4)). There is, however, much variation within each major region. In three countries of Northern Africa —Egypt, Morocco and Tunisia—contraceptive prevalence (the level of current use among married women of reproductive ages) was moderate at 20-30 per cent, but all of the sub-Saharan countries had very low prevalence levels, 10 per cent or less. Four countries in Asia (Bangladesh, Nepal, Pakistan and Yemen) also had very low prevalence levels, while in the other Asian countries, from 20 to 36 per cent of married women were using contraception. The level was about 40 in Fiji, the one country in Oceania. Within Latin America and the Caribbean, over 30 per cent were currently using contraception, except in Haiti, 19 per cent.

If the 38 countries are grouped according to the level of current contraceptive use, the distribution is distinctly bimodal, with concentrations in the range from 30 to 39 per cent and under 10 per cent:

Percentage using contraception	*Number of countries*
0-9	12
10-19	2
20-29	5
30-39	13
40-49	3
50-59	2
60+	1

At the upper end, the values for Costa Rica, Panama, and Trinidad and Tobago overlap the range observed in developed countries, which is approximately 50-80 per cent currently using contraception (United Nations, 1984a).

Ever-use of contraception

For the simple descriptive purpose of distinguishing low, medium and high levels of contraceptive use, either the proportion who had ever tried contraception or the proportion who were currently using can be employed. The two measures are highly associated (the coefficient of correlation is 0.9), and the ranking of countries according to one measure is nearly the same as according to the other (see Sathar and Chidambaram, 1984), though there are a few exceptions, such as Côte d'Ivoire.

The level of ever-use of contraception is considerably raised by the inclusion of abstinence, probably mainly post-partum abstinence, in Côte d'Ivoire (the most extreme example) and several other sub-Saharan countries. Between 2 and 25 per cent of women in the sub-Saharan countries had used a contraceptive method other than abstinence. The higher values appear in Ghana, Kenya and Lesotho, all countries with officially sponsored family planning programmes. In the francophone African countries, whose past policies towards contraception had been heavily influenced by the restrictive position of French law in the colonial period, levels of ever-use of methods other than abstinence were under 15 per cent; the level of ever-use was also quite low in the Sudan and in those Asian countries with very low levels of current use.

At the other extreme, in most of the Latin American and Caribbean countries, and in several of those in Asia, a majority of women had tried contraception at some time. The highest values of all, 80 per cent or more, are observed in Costa Rica and in Trinidad and Tobago.

Current use of modern and traditional methods

Contraceptive prevalence is shown for two groups of methods in columns (5) and (6) of table 74. Modern clinic and supply methods include contraceptive sterilization, oral pills, injectables, intra-uterine devices, condoms and female barrier and chemical methods (diaphragm, cervical cap, spermicidal foams, creams and jellies). These methods can be highly effective in preventing pregnancy, though in practice the effectiveness of some of them is heavily dependent upon the motivation of users and their understanding of the correct method of use. These are the methods most often promoted by family planning programmes, and their use requires either regular supplies or access to modern medical services. The other group of methods, shown in column (6), includes rhythm (periodic abstinence, natural family planning), withdrawal, abstinence, douche and country-specific folk methods. These methods are relatively ineffective at preventing pregnancy (except for abstinence) and do not require supplies or medical services, although some family planning programmes do promote and provide instruction in newer variants of the rhythm method. For the sake of brevity, these two groups of methods are referred to as "modern" and "traditional" methods.

In most of the WFS countries, modern methods are more widely practised than traditional ones. At the same time, use of traditional methods contributes importantly to the overall prevalence of contraceptive use in many of the countries: in Peru and the Philippines, 20 per cent of married women were currently using traditional methods; and in six other countries (one in Asia and five in Latin America and the Caribbean), over 10 per cent were using one of these methods. In most of the sub-Saharan countries, traditional methods accounted for over half of the slight contraceptive use. They also contributed over half of total use in three of the countries with moderate levels of contraceptive prevalence—Haiti, Peru and the Philippines. Still, these are exceptional cases. On average (unweighted), 18 per cent of women in the 38 countries were currently using a modern method and 6 per cent were using a traditional method.

Relationship of contraceptive knowledge and use to level of development and strength of family planning programme effort

The average level of contraceptive knowledge, ever-use and current use is strongly related to both the level of socio-economic development and the strength of family planning programme effort (table 75). In the nine least developed countries (according to the index given in the Introduction to this volume), an average of 50 per cent of married women had heard of any method, 15 per cent had used a method and 6 per cent were currently using.

TABLE 75. AVERAGE PERCENTAGES OF WOMEN WHO KNEW ANY CONTRACEPTIVE METHOD, HAD EVER USED A METHOD AND WERE CURRENTLY USING MODERN AND TRADITIONAL METHODS, BY REGION, LEVEL OF DEVELOPMENT AND STRENGTH OF FAMILY PLANNING PROGRAMME EFFORT

	Knew a method	Had ever used contraception	Currently using any method	Currently using a modern method	Currently using a traditional method
A. Region						
Africa	65	30	10	7	3
Latin America and the Caribbean	94	60	40	30	9
Asia and Oceania	80	37	23	17	6
B. Level of development						
I. High	97	65	43	35	8
II. Middle-high	92	49	31	21	10
III. Middle-low	75	36	12	9	3
IV. Low	50	15	6	3	3
C. Strength of family planning programme effort						
1. Strong	95	62	41	32	9
2. Moderate	95	52	34	28	6
3. Weak	82	36	21	15	5
4. Very weak/none	61	31	12	6	5
TOTAL	80	43	25	18	6

Source: Table 74.

TABLE 76. PERCENTAGE WHO KNEW OF CONTRACEPTION AND PERCENTAGE WHO HAD EVER USED A METHOD, SINGLE AND CURRENTLY MARRIED WOMEN

	Percentage who knew						Percentage who had used						Number of women			
	Any method			A modern method			Any method			A modern method						
	Single	Married		Single	Married		Single	Married		Single	Married		Single	Married		
Region and country	Age 15-49	Age 15-49	Age 15-19	Age 15-49	Age 15-49	Age 15-19	Age 15-49	Age 15-49	Age 15-19	Age 15-49	Age 15-49	Age 15-19	Age 15-49	Age 15-49	Age 15-19	
Africa																
Benin	19	40	23	15	13	6	15	36	18	7	2	1	441	3 450	264	
Cameroon	48[a]	34	33	42[a]	28	27	13[a]	11	7	4[a]	2	2	773	6 326	768	
Côte d'Ivoire[b]	64	85	73	37	17	21	33	71	49	6	3	2	774	4 590	714	
Ghana	64	69	61	57	59	55	30	40	27	16	18	12	1 182	4 436	368	
Kenya	82	93	90	73	88	84	19	32	22	6	12	4	1 773	5 702	491	
Morocco	81	84	77	81	83	76	. .	31	15	. .	28	14	1 642	3 604	282	
Senegal	52	60	47	40	20	17	3	11	9	1	1	1	501	3 291	507	
MEAN	59	66	58	49	44	41	19[c]	33	21	7[c]	9	5	. .	. .	. .	
Latin America and the Caribbean																
Colombia	86	96	92	86	95	91	3	62	45	2	50	35	2 076	2 827	181	
Dominican Republic	97	98	97	97	98	97	0	50	31	0	39	18	858	1 808	170	
Haiti	66	85	88	64	82	86	0	37	40	0	12	9	1 077	1 903	114	
Mexico	87	90	81	87	89	80	4	47	26	2	37	19	1 055	5 640	436	
Paraguay	82	96	92	81	95	92	4	57	34	3	44	23	1 625	2 610	167	
Venezuela	94	98[d]	99	92	98[d]	98	2	70[d]	46	1	59[d]	35	1 645	2 280[d]	207	
MEAN	55	94	92	84	93	91	2	54	37	1	40	23	. .	. .	. .	

Source: World Fertility Survey standard recode tapes.
[a] Excluding women who had not reached menarche.
[b] Formerly called the Ivory Coast.
[c] Excluding Morocco.
[d] Ages 15-44.

At the other extreme, in the 11 most developed countries, nearly all women had heard of at least one method, 65 per cent had used a method and 43 per cent were currently using. The contrast between countries with a strong family planning programme and those with a very weak programme, or no programme, is nearly as large. Greater use of modern methods is responsible for most of the difference between more and less economically advanced countries, and between those with strong and weak programmes. However, use of traditional methods also tends to be higher in the countries with relatively high development levels or strong programmes.

Since strong family planning programmes are found mainly in the more economically advanced developing countries, the effects of these two variables are confounded in simple tabulations such as table 75. More elaborate cross-tabulations and multiple regression analysis have been employed by other researchers in an attempt to separate the independent influence of family planning programmes from effects of level of development. While most of these studies have employed fertility, rather than contraceptive practice, as the dependent variable, the effects of programme effort on fertility are presumed to reflect primarily the effects of family planning effort on contraceptive use. Results of these studies need not be reviewed here in detail, as they are discussed in the Introduction. Generally speaking, these studies have found that the level of development and the strength of programme effort each has an independent effect on fertility, though the size of the effect varies between studies.

TABLE 77. PERCENTAGE OF CURRENTLY MARRIED WOMEN WHO WERE CURRENTLY USING CONTRACEPTION, BY AGE GROUP

Region and country	Total	15-19	20-24	25-29	30-34	35-39	40-44	45-49
Africa								
Benin[a]	9	3	7	8	10	10	12	18
Cameroon	2	2	3	3	2	2	2	1
Côte d'Ivoire[b]	3	2	3	3	5	2	2	2
Egypt	24	4	13	24	33	34	33	20
Ghana	10	5	8	12	13	10	9	5
Kenya	7	2	6	6	10	7	10	6
Lesotho	5	2	3	8	8	9	3	2
Mauritania	1	0	0	1	2	1	1	2
Morocco	20	10	17	21	25	23	22	14
Senegal	4	5	3	6	4	4	2	0
Sudan	5	4	4	7	5	4	4	1
Tunisia	31	8	17	29	39	41	38	26
MEAN	10	4	7	11	13	12	12	8
Latin America and the Caribbean								
Colombia	43	27	41	46	56	47	40	22
Costa Rica	64	..	63	68	69	71	64	43
Dominican Republic	32	13	27	41	41	40	28	18
Ecuador	34	14	29	37	43	42	35	20
Guyana	31	18	25	34	43	40	32	23
Haiti	19	17	15	18	23	15	27	18
Jamaica	38	31	39	43	50	43	32	21
Mexico	30	14	27	39	38	38	25	12
Panama	54	..	44	59	57	58	56	49
Paraguay	36	19	36	44	41	41	38	20
Peru	31	17	29	37	41	35	29	16
Trinidad and Tobago	52	42	53	59	61	55	45	28
Venezuela	49	29	45	53	56	55	49	..
MEAN	40	22[c]	36	44	47	45	38	24[d]
Asia and Oceania								
Bangladesh	8	4	8	8	12	12	9	5
Fiji	41	21	32	41	50	51	45	28
Indonesia	26	13	27	33	34	30	23	12
Jordan	25	9	17	26	32	33	33	19
Malaysia	33	15	29	39	39	38	34	16
Nepal	2	0	1	2	5	5	3	2
Pakistan	5	0	2	5	7	10	7	7
Philippines	36	16	29	39	43	46	36	18
Republic of Korea	35	13	13	28	45	54	38	13
Sri Lanka	32	14	20	30	43	41	35	20
Syrian Arab Republic	20	9	15	19	24	31	24	15
Thailand	33	18	31	41	42	41	29	13
Yemen	1	0	1	2	1	2	1	1
MEAN	23	10	17	24	29	30	24	13
TOTAL MEAN	25	12[c]	21	27	30	29	25	15[d]

Source: World Fertility Survey standard recode tapes.
[a] Women who had not resumed sexual relations since the last pregnancy were counted as non-users.
[b] Formerly called the Ivory Coast.
[c] Excluding Costa Rica and Panama.
[d] Excluding Venezuela.

One recent analysis does examine the level of contraceptive prevalence directly (Lapham and Mauldin, 1984). The analysis is based on prevalence as measured at dates between 1977 and 1983, for 74 developing countries and areas. The study found results compatible with those for fertility rates; that is, both programme effort and socio-economic conditions had separate and substantial effects on contraceptive practice.

A similar linear regression analysis performed for this study (based on the 38 surveys) confirmed the Lapham and Mauldin results, using the family planning and development index described in the Introduction to this report. Each had a statistically significant relationship (at the 1 per cent confidence level) with contraceptive prevalence, when the other index was controlled.[10]

Figure 26. **Percentage of currently married women currently using contraception and percentage who had ever used, by age: averages by region**

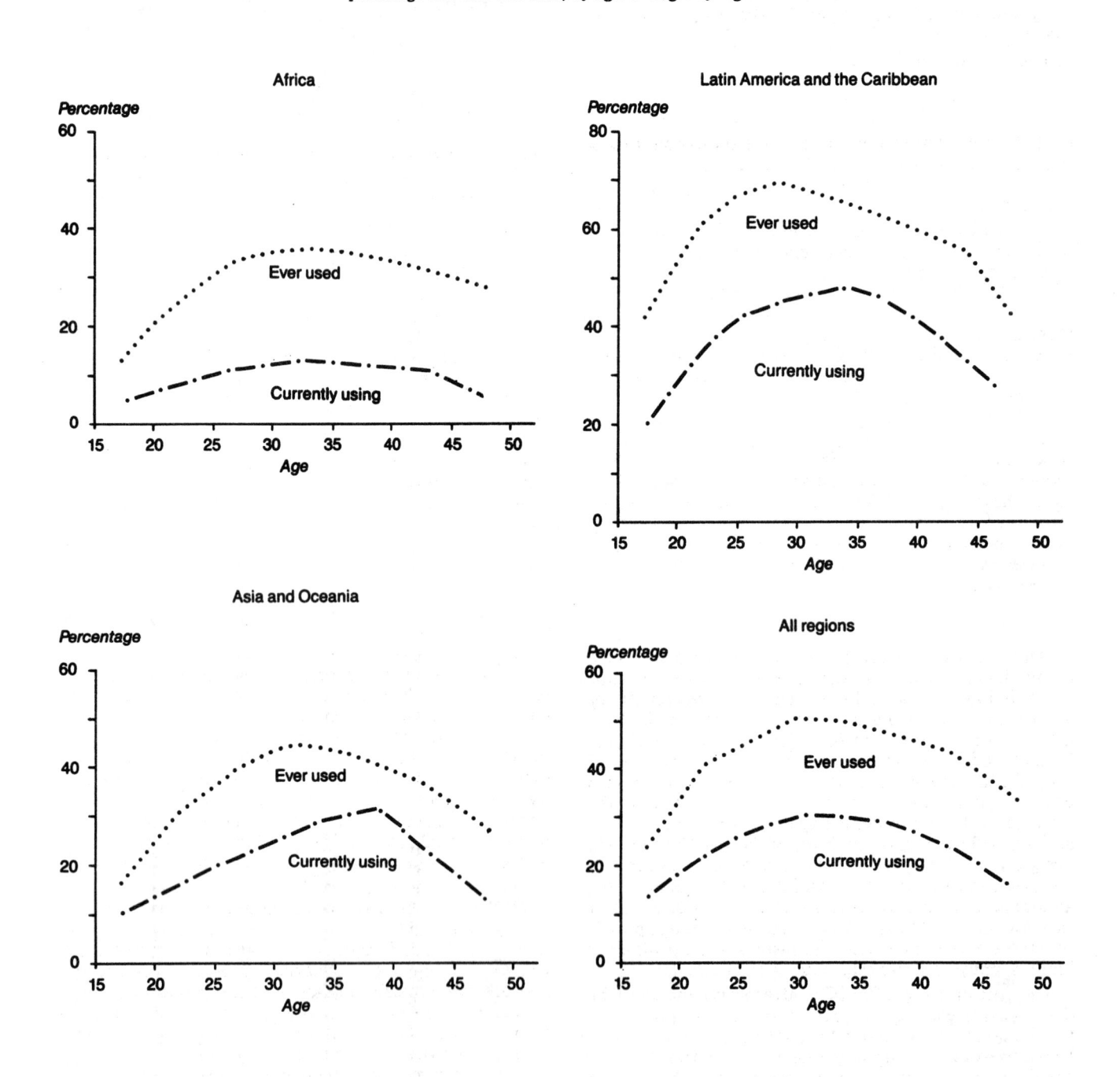

Sources: Table 77 and World Fertility Survey standard recode tapes.

C. DIFFERENTIALS IN USE OF ANY METHOD

Knowledge and use for single women

Many of the countries with all-woman samples in Africa and in Latin America and the Caribbean asked single women the standard question about contraceptive knowledge and ever-use (but not about current use). In table 76, the percentage of single women who reported knowledge and ever-use is compared with similar statistics for married women. Since single women are concentrated in the lower age groups, comparative statistics are given for young married women (ages 15-19) as well as for all married women.

There are major differences in results for Latin America and the Caribbean and for Africa. In the former region, although single women were less likely than married women to know about contraception, at least 80 per cent of single women knew of a modern method, except in Haiti. Few single women had used contraception, however—the highest level of use (for Mexico and Paraguay) was only 4 per cent.

In five of the six African countries with information available, more than 10 per cent of single women had used contraception (30-33 per cent in Ghana and Côte d'Ivoire). Although married women reported higher levels of use of any method (except in Cameroon), single women were more likely than young married women to have used a modern method and were usually more likely to report knowledge of a modern method as well. Moreover, even though the diffusion of knowledge about and use of modern contraceptives is much less complete in sub-Saharan Africa than in Latin America and the Caribbean, the percentage of single women who had used a modern method tends to be higher in the African countries. These regional differences in contraceptive use patterns provide further confirmation that the questions about marriage failed to separate sexually active from other women in many of the African countries (see chapter III).

Contraceptive use by age

Both ever-use and current use of contraception show a curvilinear relationship with age: the level of use was typically lowest at ages 15-19, reached a maximum for women in their thirties and then declined, particularly after age 45 (table 77 and figure 26). By ages 45-49, the level of current use among married women is frequently only slightly higher than at ages 15-19, and in several countries it is lower. The level of current use at the extremes of the reproductive ages is often less than half and is usually less than two thirds of the level for the peak age groups. All populations exhibit this curvilinear pattern, though there are minor variations; for instance, the ages of peak use are sometimes during the twenties rather than the thirties. The height of the peak in the age profile of contraceptive use varies; for instance, the profile for Haiti is unusually irregular and is relatively flat.

The typical age profile of contraceptive use must be due in part to changes in the need for contraception over the life cycle. The demand for contraception is likely to be relatively low among very young women who still have small families, while women aged over 40 may be at reduced risk of pregnancy because of infrequent sexual intercourse, and many women aged 45-49 have reached menopause. Indeed, the level of current use typically declines more steeply after age 40 than does the level of ever-use, suggesting a response to reduced levels of perceived risk of pregnancy.[11] When women who reported themselves to be infecund are excluded from the tabulation, the tendency for current use to decline at higher ages is reduced but not entirely eliminated (not shown).

The age pattern of both current contraceptive use and ever-use is probably influenced by recent trends in availability and social acceptability of contraception, as well as by life-cycle considerations. The oldest women in these samples typically passed through their most fecund years at a time when modern contraception was not widely available. Although some women do begin to use contraception during the later reproductive years, by age 40 or 45 many women who did not use contraception earlier have already gone for several years without a pregnancy and for this reason are probably not very likely to adopt contraception late in life. Older cohorts may also be less receptive to the idea of birth control, and they have a much lower average level of education than do younger women; as discussed in part two of this report, education shows a strong positive relationship to contraceptive use.

Contraceptive use by family size

In many developing countries, especially those in Africa and in Asia and Oceania, childless women are very unlikely to use contraception, even if contraceptive prevalence for women with children is fairly high (table 78). However, in six of the Latin American and Caribbean countries, as well as in Fiji and Ghana, between one fourth and one half of childless married women reported that they had used contraception at some time; and in Trinidad and Tobago, two thirds reported ever-use (Sathar and Chidambaram, 1984; Thompson and Chidambaram, 1984). In all of the countries with the Caribbean marriage pattern (Guyana, Haiti, Jamaica, and Trinidad and Tobago), the level of current use for childless women was nearly as high as for those with one child. In these countries, many of the childless women are in visiting unions, the least stable type of union; and they may wish to delay childbearing until they enter a legal or common-law union.

Since the proportion of women desiring no more children rises steadily with the number of children (see chapter II), it might be supposed that proportions practising contraception would also increase regularly with current family size. In fact, although there is almost always an increase in contraceptive use up to two or three children, there is usually no marked increase after that. In a majority of countries, the level of use for women with seven or more living children was lower than for women with moderate-sized families. The pattern usually persists if women who thought themselves infecund are excluded from the tabulation (not shown).

The contrast between the pattern of contraceptive use by family size and the pattern of desire for no more children is illustrated in figure 27 for several countries. For women with one or two children, the level of contraceptive use was typically higher than the proportion who wanted no more children, whereas the reverse is true at higher parities. This points, on the one hand, to substantial levels of use to delay births that are wanted eventually and, on the other hand, to incomplete protection against the risk of unwanted pregnancy—issues that are examined below.

Regional average patterns of current contraceptive use and ever-use by parity are depicted in figure 28. In all

TABLE 78. PERCENTAGE OF CURRENTLY MARRIED WOMEN WHO WERE CURRENTLY USING CONTRACEPTION, BY NUMBER OF LIVING CHILDREN

Region and country	Total	None	One	Two	Three	Four	Five	Six	Seven or more
Africa									
Benin	9	2	6	9	11	13	9	11	18
Cameroon	2	1	3	3	3	3	1	3	2
Côte d'Ivoire[a]	3	2	3	4	3	3	3	3	3
Egypt	24	1	16	27	28	32	32	32	29
Ghana	10	5	9	11	11	11	9	11	9
Kenya	7	1	3	6	7	7	9	9	9
Lesotho	5	1	2	6	8	8	8	7	8
Mauritania	1	1	0	0	1	1	0	2	2
Morocco	20	4	13	17	20	20	28	27	28
Senegal	4	0	6	4	4	3	3	3	5
Sudan	5	2	5	4	6	4	5	5	5
Tunisia	31	2	19	27	34	40	40	40	39
MEAN	10	2	7	10	11	12	12	13	13
Latin America and the Caribbean									
Colombia	43	13	39	50	49	51	49	42	39
Costa Rica	64	20	63	73	72	68	72	66	61
Dominican Republic	32	9	21	35	44	41	45	34	32
Ecuador	34	8	27	42	42	36	40	33	29
Guyana	31	17	20	31	34	34	41	41	40
Haiti	19	9	14	22	25	25	18	17	30
Jamaica	38	25	29	44	38	44	52	46	42
Mexico	30	6	27	39	37	37	31	31	28
Panama	54	19	46	59	60	61	60	60	50
Paraguay	36	14	37	50	49	43	36	25	27
Peru	31	7	27	39	38	35	31	29	27
Trinidad and Tobago	52	41	43	61	57	61	52	58	48
Venezuela	49	18	42	58	58	63	49	50	46
MEAN	40	16	34	46	46	46	44	41	38
Asia and Oceania									
Bangladesh	8	2	5	7	9	9	11	13	13
Fiji	41	6	27	38	43	53	56	58	53
Indonesia	26	2	20	31	35	32	33	33	37
Jordan	25	4	17	27	26	25	30	32	29
Malaysia	33	6	28	35	38	40	36	36	36
Nepal	2	0	1	2	3	4	7	6	7
Pakistan	5	0	2	3	5	6	8	10	12
Philippines	36	3	26	39	45	43	40	40	32
Republic of Korea	35	8	12	39	46	46	42	33	24
Sri Lanka	32	3	21	33	39	43	40	40	33
Syrian Arab Republic	20	3	14	21	24	25	27	21	21
Thailand	33	6	31	38	42	43	37	31	26
Yemen	1	0	0	2	0	2	2	2	4
MEAN	23	3	16	24	27	29	28	28	25
TOTAL MEAN	25	7	19	27	29	29	29	27	26

Source: World Fertility Survey standard recode tapes.
NOTE: Based on ages 15-49, except Costa Rica and Panama, ages 20-49; and Venezuela, ages 15-44.
[a] Formerly called the Ivory Coast.

regions, the shape of the curve for ever-use is similar to that for current use, at a higher level. In Latin America and the Caribbean, the level of use is usually at or near its maximum for women with two children, while in Asia and Oceania, it is more common for the peak or plateau level to occur at three or four children. In some countries, mainly those with low or moderate levels of use, the proportion using contraception does increase steadily through the larger family sizes, but only by a small amount. It is this pattern that dominates the average for Africa. Instances of lower levels of use for large rather than for moderate family sizes are more common where the general level of use is fairly high; this pattern dominates the average for Latin America and the Caribbean.

Lower levels of contraceptive use at the higher parities are likely to be due, at least in part, to the influence of contraceptive use on family size. To the extent that contraception is effective, users tend to remain at low or moderate parities, while women who do not adopt contraception—whether out of a desire for a large family or because of ignorance about, aversion to or lack of access to family planning services—progress to higher parities. As contraception practice becomes widespread and average family size falls, the women who are found at the higher parities are an increasingly atypical group, selected for their failure to control fertility.

Contraceptive use by desire for more children

On average, under one half of the exposed women (currently married, non-pregnant and fecund) who wanted

Figure 27. Percentage who wanted no more children and percentage who were using contraception, according to current family size, selected countries

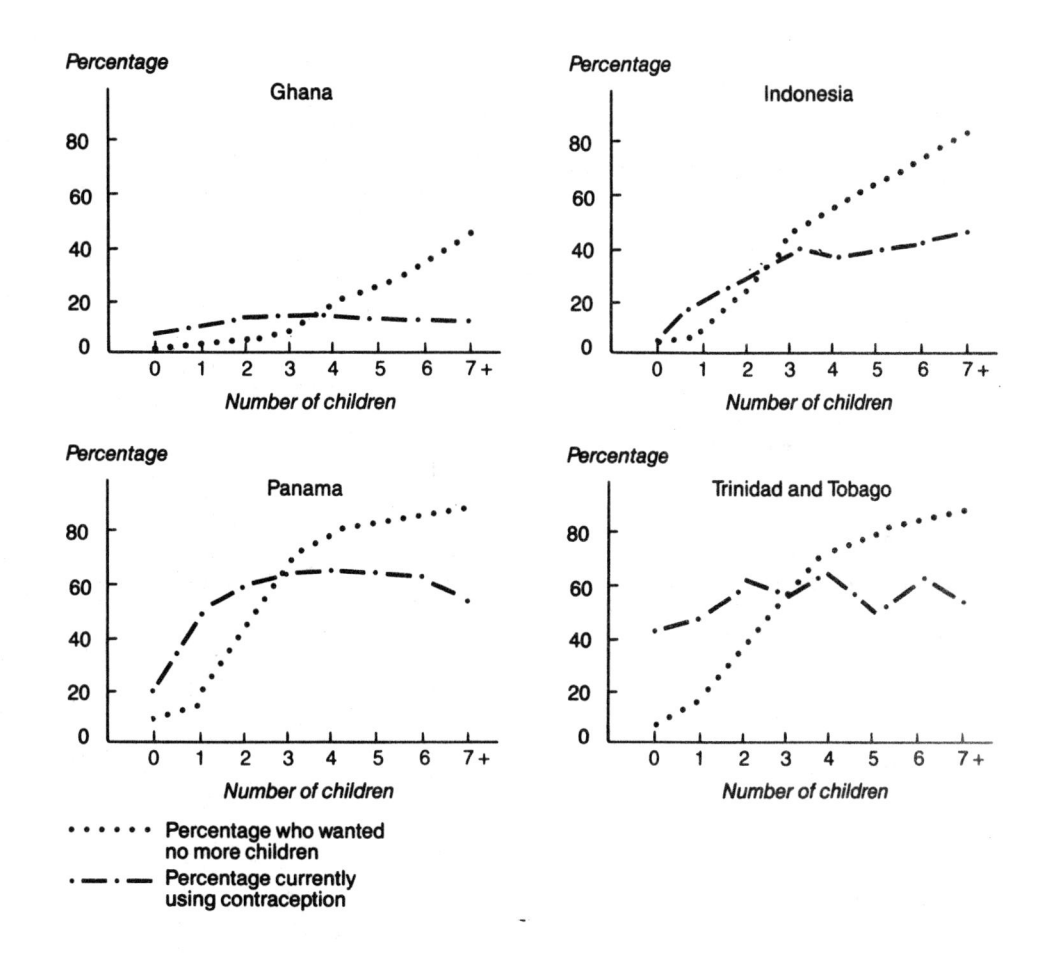

[Four panel charts: Ghana, Indonesia, Panama, Trinidad and Tobago, plotting Percentage vs Number of children (0 to 7+)]

······ Percentage who wanted no more children
—·—· Percentage currently using contraception

Source: World Fertility Survey standard recode tapes.

NOTE: Based on currently married fecund women. For the percentage who wanted no more children, the number of living children includes the current pregnancy, if any.

no more children were currently using contraception.[12] The average is only 23 per cent in Africa, 43 per cent in Asia and Oceania, and 57 per cent in Latin America and the Caribbean. The proportion exceeds 75 per cent only in Costa Rica and is above 65 per cent in only four other countries (table 79, column (5)). By contrast, in 11 developed countries, on average, 87 per cent of exposed women who wanted no more children were found to be using contraception (Berent, 1982, table 4).[13]

These statistics demonstrate a large gap in most developing countries between stated fertility preferences and adoption of means to limit family size. The existence of such gaps has been widely interpreted as indicating a substantial need for improved information about contraceptives and improved delivery of family planning services. The percentage using contraception, among exposed women who wanted no more children, does tend to be low in those countries where low proportions of women knew about modern contraceptives, and the percentage is strongly related both to the strength of national family planning effort and to the level of socio-economic development:

Strength of programme effort	*Percentage using*
1. Strong	62
2. Moderate	57
3. Weak	36
4. Very weak/none	24
Level of development	
I. High	61
II. Middle-high	55
III. Middle-low	29
IV. Low	14

Of course, exposed women who wanted no more children did not in all cases make up a large proportion of all married women of reproductive ages. The percentage

Figure 28. **Percentage of currently married women currently using contraception and percentage who had ever used, by number of living children: averages by region**

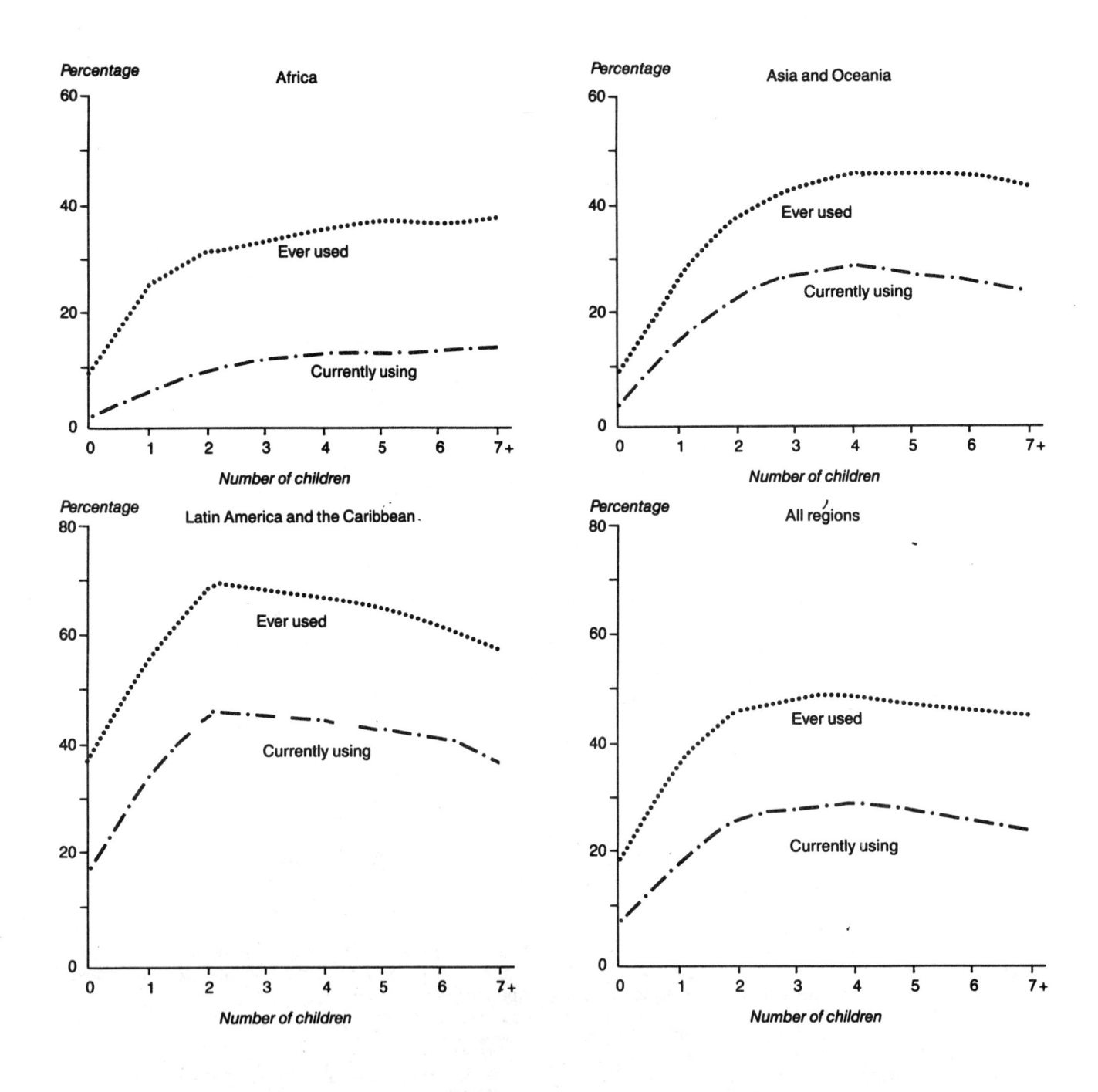

Source: Table 78 and World Fertility Survey standard recode tapes.

of currently married women who were exposed to risk of pregnancy, wanted no more children and were not using contraception ranges from 3 per cent (in Côte d'Ivoire) to 26 per cent (Pakistan) and averages 15 per cent (table 79, column (7)). This percentage tends to be low in sub-Saharan Africa, mainly because relatively few women there wanted no more children; of the countries where fewer than 10 per cent of married women had "unmet need" for purposes of birth limitation, only Costa Rica has a low value because the level of contraceptive practice was high, rather than because the percentage who wanted no more children was low. This measure of "need" is also rather weakly related to strength of family planning effort and level of development: values

TABLE 79. EVER-USE AND CURRENT USE OF CONTRACEPTION BY EXPOSED WOMEN, BY DESIRE FOR MORE CHILDREN

Region and country	Percentage of exposed[a] who wanted no more children[b] (1)	Percentage who had ever used contraception among exposed women:[a] Who wanted more children (2)[b]	Percentage who had ever used contraception among exposed women:[a] Who wanted no more children (3)[b]	Percentage currently using contraception among exposed women:[a] Who wanted more children (4)	Percentage currently using contraception among exposed women:[a] Who wanted no more children (5)	Of those who were using contraception, the percentage who wanted more children (6)	Percentage of currently married with unmet need for contraception to prevent future birth[c] (7)	Index of contraceptive use for birth-spacing[d] (8)
Africa								
Benin	8	40	36	12[e]	15[e]	90[e]	5[e]	83[e]
Cameroon[f]	8	10	15	3	4	89	6	75
Côte d'Ivoire[g]	4	71	79	4	11	89	3	34
Egypt	54	20	68	12	49	18	21	31
Ghana	12	39	61	11	23	79	7	50
Kenya	16	29	46	7	21	63	9	36
Lesotho	14	20	51	5	21	60	8	28
Mauritania	11	1	6	1	3	67	9	26
Morocco	42	21	60	15	50	29	14	33
Senegal[h]	6	11	19	5	11	87	4	50
Sudan	15	11	26	5	16	62	9	29
Tunisia	48	39	70	30	58	36	15	58
MEAN	20	26	45	9	23	64	9	44
Latin America and the Caribbean								
Colombia	61	61	69	45	56	34	22	85
Costa Rica	52	86	92	71	84	43	7	87
Dominican Republic	52	41	69	25	57	29	17	48
Ecuador	55	50	67	32	52	33	21	65
Guyana	54	53	63	28	45	35	25	65
Haiti	42	31	51	17	36	39	20	49
Jamaica	48	63	76	36	55	42	18	67
Mexico	56	46	60	34	48	36	21	75
Panama	63	68	84	50	74	29	14	72
Paraguay	32	60	67	45	52	64	12	91
Peru	61	47	59	33	46	32	25	75
Trinidad and Tobago	46	80	85	56	66	49	13	86
Venezuela	55	67	79	51	68	39	14	80
MEAN	52	58	71	40	57	39	18	73
Asia and Oceania								
Bangladesh[h]	30	11	30	6	20	41	19	33
Fiji	50	63	87	35	69	33	12	58
Indonesia	40	35	63	26	53	42	13	56
Jordan	42	37	73	22	59	34	12	40
Malaysia	46	45	68	34	53	43	17	69
Nepal	30	1	13	1	9	13	21	9
Pakistan	43	4	25	2	15	12	26	13
Philippines	54	50	77	33	60	31	16	58
Republic of Korea	74	33	79	16	56	9	25	30
Sri Lanka	62	31	65	22	54	20	22	47
Syrian Arab Republic	38	22	63	16	52	33	12	34
Thailand	61	41	67	29	56	25	20	58
Yemen	19	2	8	1	5	41	12	19
MEAN	45	29	55	18	43	29	17	40
TOTAL MEAN	40	38	57	23	42	43	15	53

Source: World Fertility Survey standard recode tapes.

[a] Exposed = currently married, non-pregnant women who reported that they were able to have children, plus those sterilized for contraceptive reasons.

[b] Women who were uncertain whether they wanted more children were counted with those who wanted more.

[c] Percentage of currently married women who were exposed, wanted no more children and were not using contraception.

[d] Ratio (× 100) of percentage who were using contraception among women who wanted more children to percentage who were using among women who wanted no more. Restricted to exposed women with at least one birth.

[e] Women who had not resumed sexual relations since the last pregnancy were counted as non-users.

[f] Women were counted as wanting no more children if either the desired family size was less than or equal to the current number of living children, or the respondent stated that she wanted no more. (Most women were asked only one of these questions.)

[g] Formerly called the Ivory Coast.

[h] Women were counted as wanting no more children if the desired family size was less than or equal to the number of living children.

tend to be low in the less developed countries and in those with very weak family planning programmes, or no programme.[14]

There is reason to think, however, that this measure might give a poor indication of the number of women in need of improved family services and, what is particularly important in the present comparative context, that it distorts the pattern across countries in the relative level of unmet need. The most serious problem is that the measure takes no account of the need for contraception to space births. Since most of these surveys did not inquire about desired timing of the next birth (for several exceptions, see Lightbourne, 1985), it is difficult to give an estimate of the number of women in need of contraception for birth-spacing. Omission of this part of total "need" is likely to be an especially serious problem in the countries where most women wanted more children, notably sub-Saharan Africa. The problem of measuring unmet need has engendered considerable debate, and estimates for the same country often vary widely. The matter is of great practical importance, but a thorough discussion of the issue is beyond the scope of this chapter (see Westoff and Pebley, 1981; Nortman, 1982; Nortman and Lewis, 1984; Boulier, 1985).

The earlier discussion of differential contraceptive practice according to age and family size suggested that many women had adopted contraception before having all the children they eventually wanted to have. Table 79 shows that this is indeed the case. On average, for all 38 countries, 38 per cent of exposed women who wanted more children had tried contraception and 23 per cent were currently using. The highest levels of current use were over 50 per cent (in Costa Rica, Panama, Trinidad and Tobago, and Venezuela). In all the countries of Latin America and the Caribbean, except Haiti, at least one fourth of exposed women who wanted more children were current users, and 25 per cent or more were also currently using in the four countries of South-eastern Asia, in Fiji and in Tunisia.

Furthermore, women who wanted more children usually accounted for a large proportion of all current contraceptive use. The proportion was, not surprisingly, highest where most women wanted to have more children (table 79, columns (1) and (6)). In all the sub-Saharan African countries, women who wanted more children made up at least 60 per cent of total current contraceptive users, and from 85 to 90 per cent in Benin, Cameroon, Côte d'Ivoire and Senegal. In the sub-Saharan countries, only from 4 to 16 per cent of exposed women said they wanted no more children. In other regions, a larger proportion of women already had at least as many children as they wanted; still, women who wanted more children in most cases accounted for at least 30 per cent of all current contraceptive use. Only in Egypt, Nepal, Pakistan and the Republic of Korea was the share of use for birth-spacing below 20 per cent.

Although desire to increase birth-spacing is frequently the reason for adopting contraception, without exception the level of current use was higher for women who wanted no more children than for those who wanted more. This is due in part to lower levels of ever-use among those who wanted more children (table 79) and in part to a lower level of contraceptive continuation, defined as the proportion of ever-users who were contracepting at the time of the survey (Lightbourne and Singh, 1982, table 14). The lower level of ever-use may indicate that some women perceived no need for wider birth-spacing than that provided by traditional mechanisms, such as breast-feeding and post-partum abstinence, while the lower percentage of continuing users is to be expected since, by the time of the interview, some women had undoubtedly already experienced a sufficiently long delay and had interrupted use in order to become pregnant.

The amount of contraceptive practice for birth-spacing must be determined, to a large extent, by the same factors that influence the level of use among those who wished to stop bearing children, for the two use levels tend to vary together. The correlation (r) between the percentage who were using contraception for women who wanted more children and the percentage for women who wanted no more (columns (4) and (5) of table 79) is 0.9. The common determinants of contraceptive use for birth-spacing and limiting are presumably the extent of availability and the quality of family planning services, and knowledge about and attitudes towards the practice of birth control. At the same time, it can be seen that the gap in current use levels between women who did and those who did not want more children tended to be largest not where the average level of use for birth limitation was highest, in Latin America and the Caribbean, but in Asia and Oceania and in Northern Africa, where most countries had a moderate level of use among women who wanted no more children.

One factor that might influence contraception for birth-spacing more than for family limitation is the practice of extended breast-feeding; the perceived need for contraception to space births is likely to be greatest where birth intervals would otherwise be short. In order to test this idea, the proportionate difference between current use levels for spacing and limiting (rather than the absolute difference) is employed here as an indicator of the relative amount of contraceptive use for birth-spacing.[15] The "index of contraceptive use for birth-spacing" (table 79, column (8)) is 100 times the ratio of the current use level for exposed women with one or more births who wanted more children, to the level for those who wanted no more.[16]

The index of contraceptive use for birth-spacing does, as hypothesized, tend to be highest where a substantial fraction of women either do not breast-feed or else breast-feed for a few months only (figure 29). The correlation between the index and the percentage who breast-fed for at least six months is moderate in strength, -0.66. The index of socio-economic development shows the same strength of relationship to the index of use for spacing ($r = 0.65$), and the development score is also highly correlated with the percentage who breast-fed for at least six months ($r = 0.87$). It is plausible to interpret these relationships as indicating that level of development operates to decrease the proportion of women who breast-feed for lengthy periods and that the decline in breast-feeding in turn increases the need women feel to prolong birth intervals through contraceptive use. However, the high degree of statistical association between these variables makes it difficult to determine the separate roles.[17]

All these variables are also strongly associated with region (figure 29). Most countries in Latin America and the Caribbean have high values of the index of contraceptive use for birth-spacing and relatively low proportions of women who breast-fed for more than six months, while most countries in Africa and in Asia and Oceania have lower index values and high proportions who practised extended breast-feeding. Only for Asia and Oceania is there an appreciable relationship within the region between the index and breast-feeding values.

Multivariate analysis

Since age, family size and desire for more children are strongly associated, it is natural to ask whether each of these variables has an independent effect on contraceptive use. For example, the tendency of contraceptive prevalence to rise between ages 15 and 35 might be entirely a response to increased family size. If so, the two age groups should exhibit the same level of contraceptive use after statistical control for family size. Multiple classification analysis can be employed to gain a better under-

Figure 29. **Index of contraceptive use for birth-spacing, by percentage of women who had breast-fed for at least six months**

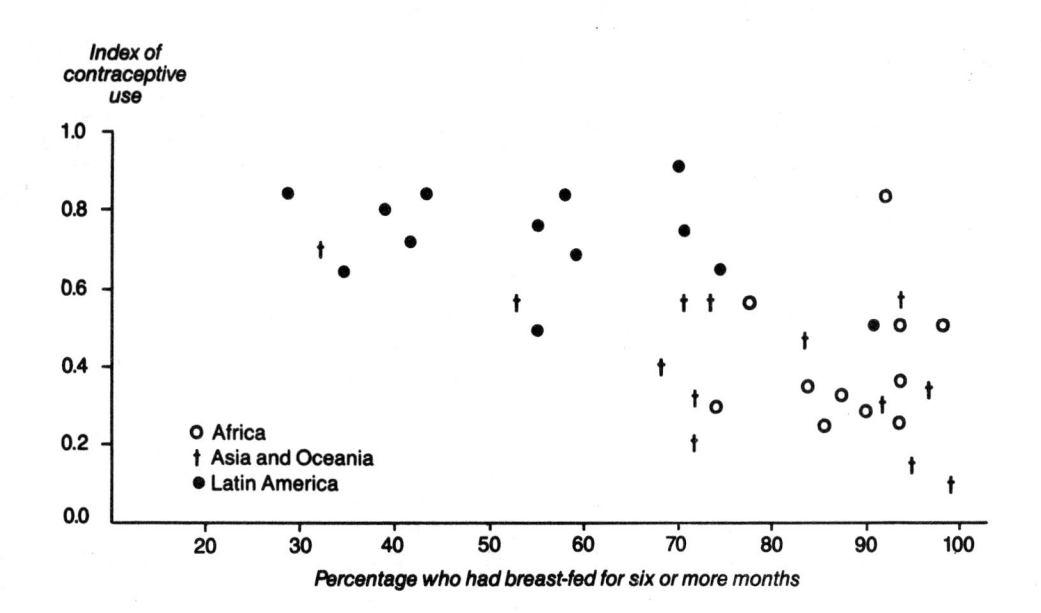

Sources: Table 79 and World Fertility Survey standard recode tapes.

Figure 30. **Average pattern of current contraceptive use, by age and family size, adjusted for other variables**

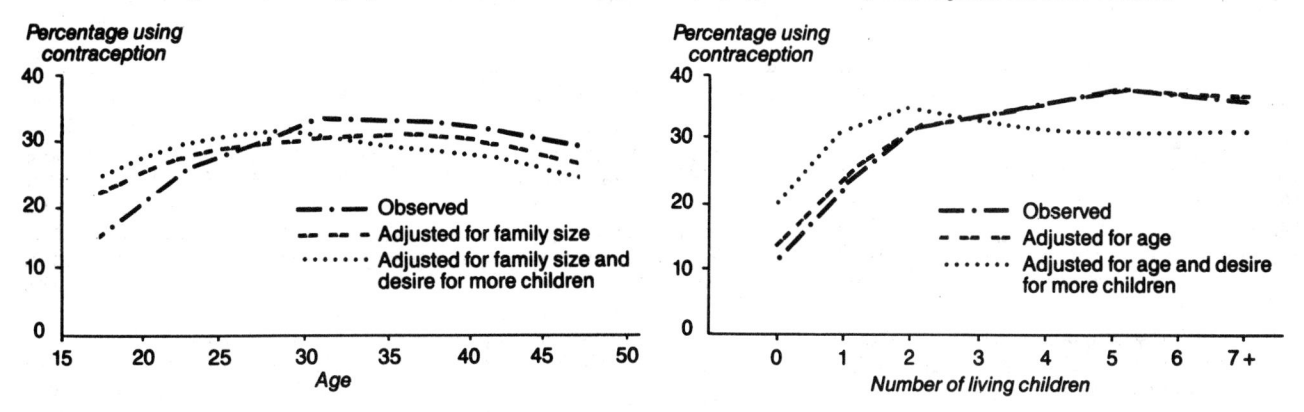

Source: World Fertility Survey standard recode tapes.
NOTES: Based on exposed women aged 15-49 years.
Adjustment for the factors indicated was carried out in each country using multiple classification analysis. Results shown are averaged over the 38 countries.

standing of these interrelationships. For exposed women in each country, current use of contraception was regressed on age, current family size and desire for more children.[18] Selected results, averaged for all countries, are shown in figure 30; and the main findings are summarized below, stressing consistency across countries in the types of patterns seen, rather than the statistical significance of the results.

The difference in level of current contraceptive use between women who wanted more children (or were undecided) and those who wanted no more was virtually the same after statistical controls for age and family size as before (not shown). Thus, although desire for more children is certainly influenced by age and family size, as discussed in chapter II, the attitudinal variable has a systematic effect on contraceptive use which is largely independent of age or family size.

TABLE 80. PERCENTAGE OF CURRENTLY MARRIED WOMEN AGED 15-49 WHO KNEW SPECIFIC CONTRACEPTIVE METHODS

Region and country	Any method	Any modern	Any traditional	Sterilization Female	Sterilization Male	Pill	Injectable	Intra-uterine device	Condom	Female barrier methods	Rhythm	Withdrawal	Abstinence	Douche	Other
Africa															
Benin	40.3	13.1	38.8	..	..	8.1	..	8.8	6.3	4.5	11.0	12.1	31.8	7.9	0.1
Cameroon	34.1	27.6	25.8	..	..	19.7	..	18.1	12.8	4.1	19.3	13.5	..	5.1	5.0
Côte d'Ivoire[a]	84.6	17.5	83.8	..	..	13.7	..	6.8	9.1	4.5	11.7	8.2	81.4	7.0	9.3
Egypt	90.5	90.4	26.8	43.2	6.1	90.2	15.8	70.8	26.7	14.0	14.3	9.9	9.7	8.0	7.5
Ghana	68.6	59.4	53.3	30.5	4.1	47.5	22.6	35.0	29.1	24.4	20.8	18.7	48.6	8.0	..
Kenya	93.5	88.0	85.1	58.6	15.5	78.4	60.8	54.6	41.9	21.8	54.2	26.5	49.0	12.8	73.0
Lesotho	64.9	59.4	46.7	34.8	10.2	45.5	31.7	21.2	27.0	10.1	11.5	41.8	..	8.4	1.4
Mauritania	8.2	6.4	3.1	0.6	0.9	5.6	..	0.6	0.3	0.8	0.3	1.0	0.1	0.2	1.6
Morocco	83.7	82.9	46.5	51.3	..	81.6	3.8	54.9	31.6	8.0	26.4	26.8	9.8	10.2	20.6
Senegal	60.0	20.3	57.3	..	..	17.0	4.3	9.0	7.8	1.9	10.3	..	51.5	..	25.4
Sudan	50.8	49.8	14.4	23.8	2.7	47.9	25.0	13.9	6.0	3.0	9.5	5.1	6.4	4.0	1.8
Tunisia	95.2	95.0	50.1	90.5	33.9	89.8	60.8	83.9	46.3	36.7	30.0	29.4	..	15.8	16.8
MEAN	64.5	50.8	44.3	41.7	10.5	45.4	28.1	31.5	20.4	11.2	18.3	17.6	32.0	7.9	14.8
Latin America and the Caribbean															
Colombia	95.9	95.0	74.6	72.7	39.7	90.5	71.1	82.8	60.2	56.7	57.6	47.6	27.6	40.5	8.9
Costa Rica[b]	99.7	99.7	91.3	93.9	67.8	98.0	88.4	91.8	91.4	71.3	81.7	67.5	31.2	59.7	7.1
Dominican Republic	97.6	97.6	74.6	94.6	31.0	90.7	68.6	78.6	71.4	60.5	42.9	56.5	..	46.6	12.1
Ecuador	90.3	89.5	71.6	76.0	24.5	82.7	72.5	73.2	46.3	54.8	55.6	43.4	20.6	43.1	8.1
Guyana	95.6	95.3	70.6	79.3	22.5	79.2	39.6	80.1	73.0	44.7	46.5	48.2	31.4	35.9	11.0
Haiti	84.8	81.6	74.0	37.8	14.3	74.5	..	51.2	51.2	29.8	55.1	48.6	41.2	31.0	55.7
Jamaica	98.1	98.1	77.4	88.1	40.5	94.6	86.3	84.3	89.4	67.6	39.7	58.9	37.7	43.1	2.4
Mexico	89.5	89.2	62.6	68.2	38.7	82.6	68.5	75.3	41.8	46.7	48.2	47.1	..	37.3	4.3
Panama[b]	98.8	98.6	85.8	93.9	64.5	95.5	26.0	88.8	75.5	56.4	65.6	60.4	34.8	61.8	4.2
Paraguay	95.8	94.8	76.9	47.3	14.3	90.5	72.9	78.2	58.4	29.9	49.2	47.1	..	53.5	27.5
Peru	82.2	77.8	68.9	59.8	19.1	63.5	61.4	42.7	39.6	31.1	55.1	40.3	23.8	47.4	10.9
Trinidad and Tobago	98.8	98.6	85.6	90.0	55.1	93.6	79.7	85.7	94.0	76.4	59.2	71.1	33.2	54.1	8.6
Venezuela[c]	98.4	97.8	92.3	87.5	32.2	94.0	9.1	88.5	78.5	55.4	60.6	60.9	..	69.8	83.9
MEAN	94.3	93.4	77.4	76.1	35.7	86.9	62.0	77.0	67.0	52.4	55.2	53.7	31.3	48.0	18.8
Asia and Oceania															
Bangladesh	83.8	81.0	42.5	54.6	53.1	66.3	..	41.7	32.1	10.5	22.5	16.4	29.6	12.3	5.1
Fiji	99.8	99.8	87.3	95.9	39.9	98.5	49.5	97.0	83.6	41.0	57.0	55.8	56.6	..	51.4
Indonesia	79.7	78.1	35.5	12.1	8.5	73.9	18.3	52.6	43.6	4.6	12.6	7.8	13.2	3.6	29.6
Jordan	97.3	97.2	81.6	79.0	19.0	96.1	..	76.5	50.9	21.4	50.8	54.8	32.8	20.0	55.7
Malaysia	93.0	91.3	62.5	74.5	35.4	88.8	49.5	41.5	53.6	27.5	39.8	31.1	31.0	..	19.5
Nepal	23.4	22.5	5.6	13.5	16.6	12.8	13.4	6.6	5.2	..	0.3	0.3	4.9	..	1.0
Pakistan	75.8	75.3	3.8	7.0	1.9	63.9	..	48.8	14.5	6.6	66.3	65.8	2.3	21.2	1.2
Philippines	94.3	94.0	79.3	74.9	70.0	90.4	5.1	86.6	87.8	40.2	59.8	37.8	36.5	27.7	4.1
Republic of Korea	97.7	97.5	68.9	66.5	84.5	94.7	44.0	91.8	76.9	0.5	45.1	20.9	25.8	9.1	2.3
Sri Lanka	91.8	91.0	56.9	83.6	38.8	80.6	14.8	62.9	52.2	11.3	41.7	33.3	31.8	22.4	3.0
Syrian Arab Republic	77.9	77.1	50.8	28.3	8.3	75.5	71.6	40.5	28.1	43.5	31.9	22.9	18.0	17.0	3.6
Thailand	96.6	96.3	56.0	87.5	71.1	92.2	15.4	86.4	49.1	22.7	0.9	1.1	36.4	0.3	3.4
Yemen	24.3	24.1	2.8	4.8	2.9	22.7	..	3.3	2.2	0.1	35.7	29.0	0.8	14.8	0.8
MEAN	79.7	78.9	48.7	52.5	34.6	73.6	31.3	56.6	44.6	19.2	36.9	34.4	24.6	25.6	13.9
TOTAL MEAN	79.9	75.0	57.1	59.0	29.9	69.2	43.1	55.7	44.6	28.2	36.9	34.4	28.7	25.6	15.9

Source: World Fertility Survey standard recode tapes.
[a] Formerly called the Ivory Coast.
[b] Ages 20-49.
[c] Ages 15-44.

TABLE 81. PERCENTAGE OF CURRENTLY MARRIED WOMEN AND CURRENT CONTRACEPTIVE USERS AGED 15-49 WHO WERE CURRENTLY USING EACH METHOD

A. *Based on currently married*

Region and country	Total	Modern	Sterilization Female	Sterilization Male	Pill	Injectable	Intra-uterine device	Condom	Female barrier methods	Rhythm	Withdrawal	Abstinence	Douche	Other
Africa														
Benin[a]	9.2	0.5	0.0	0.0	0.2	0.0	0.1	0.1	0.1	1.3	2.5	4.7	0.2	0.0
Cameroon	2.4	0.6	0.0	0.0	0.2	0.0	0.1	0.2	0.0	1.1	0.4	0.0	0.0	0.3
Côte d'Ivoire[b]	2.9	0.5	0.0	0.0	0.4	0.0	0.1	0.0	0.0	0.3	0.1	1.8	0.1	0.1
Egypt	24.2	22.8	0.7	0.1	16.5	0.1	4.0	1.1	0.2	0.5	0.4	0.1	0.1	0.3
Ghana	9.5	5.5	0.5	0.0	2.4	0.1	0.3	0.6	1.6	0.7	0.2	3.1	0.0	0.0
Kenya	6.8	4.3	0.8	0.0	2.0	0.6	0.7	0.1	0.0	1.1	0.1	1.1	0.0	0.0
Lesotho	5.2	2.5	0.8	0.0	1.2	0.2	0.1	0.1	0.1	0.1	2.5	0.0	0.0	0.0
Mauritania	0.8	0.3	0.2	0.0	0.0	0.0	0.0	0.0	0.0	0.1	0.4	0.0	0.0	0.0
Morocco	19.7	16.6	0.8	0.0	13.9	0.0	1.6	0.3	0.0	1.1	1.0	0.0	0.1	0.8
Senegal	3.8	0.6	0.0	0.0	0.3	0.0	0.1	0.1	0.0	0.4	0.0	2.5	0.0	0.3
Sudan	4.6	3.9	0.3	0.0	3.1	0.2	0.1	0.1	0.1	0.4	0.1	0.1	0.0	0.0
Tunisia	31.4	24.8	7.5	0.0	6.5	0.2	8.7	1.3	0.7	3.8	2.0	0.0	0.1	0.7
MEAN	10.0	6.9	1.0	0.0	3.9	0.1	1.3	0.3	0.2	0.9	0.8	1.1	0.1	0.2
Latin America and the Caribbean														
Colombia	42.5	30.4	4.0	0.2	13.3	0.4	8.5	1.7	2.3	5.1	4.7	0.9	0.5	0.8
Costa Rica[c]	64.4	53.5	12.3	1.0	22.5	2.0	5.2	8.8	1.7	5.1	4.6	0.5	0.3	0.4
Dominican Republic	31.8	26.0	11.9	0.1	7.8	0.2	2.8	1.5	1.6	1.2	3.7	0.0	0.5	0.3
Ecuador	33.6	25.8	7.8	0.2	9.5	0.8	4.8	1.0	1.6	4.8	2.3	0.4	0.3	0.1
Guyana	31.4	28.2	8.5	0.1	9.0	0.3	5.6	2.9	1.9	1.0	1.1	0.6	0.0	0.4
Haiti	18.9	5.3	0.2	0.1	3.5	0.0	0.4	1.0	0.1	4.8	4.7	3.4	0.5	0.1
Jamaica	38.3	36.1	8.1	0.0	11.8	6.2	2.0	6.6	1.5	0.3	1.4	0.4	0.0	0.0
Mexico	30.3	23.2	2.7	0.2	10.8	1.7	5.7	0.8	1.4	3.1	3.6	0.0	0.2	0.2
Panama[c]	54.1	46.1	21.2	0.4	17.2	0.7	3.7	1.2	1.8	2.6	3.0	1.4	0.7	0.4
Paraguay	36.4	23.5	2.1	0.1	11.9	1.7	5.4	1.5	0.8	4.2	2.4	0.0	1.9	4.4
Peru	31.4	11.2	2.8	0.0	4.2	1.0	1.3	1.0	0.8	10.9	3.3	2.1	3.3	0.6
Trinidad and Tobago	51.5	45.7	4.3	0.2	17.9	1.0	2.2	15.0	5.0	2.3	2.8	0.3	0.3	0.0
Venezuela[d]	49.3	37.7	7.6	0.1	15.3	0.2	8.5	4.8	1.0	4.0	4.7	0.0	2.3	0.5
MEAN	40.0	30.2	7.2	0.2	11.9	1.2	4.3	3.7	1.7	3.8	3.3	0.8	0.8	0.6
Asia and Oceania														
Bangladesh	8.0	4.9	0.3	0.5	2.9	0.0	0.4	0.8	0.0	1.1	0.5	1.2	0.1	0.2
Fiji	40.8	35.1	15.8	0.1	8.2	0.3	4.7	6.0	0.0	2.3	2.8	0.3	0.0	0.4
Indonesia	26.4	22.9	0.3	0.0	14.9	0.3	5.6	1.8	0.1	0.8	0.3	1.0	0.1	1.2
Jordan	25.2	17.8	1.8	0.1	11.9	0.4	2.0	1.4	0.1	2.1	3.3	0.4	0.0	1.6
Malaysia	33.2	23.9	3.4	0.4	16.2	0.2	0.7	2.7	0.1	3.5	1.9	1.7	0.0	2.2
Nepal	2.5	2.4	0.1	1.7	0.4	0.0	0.1	0.2	0.0	0.0	0.0	0.0	0.0	0.0
Pakistan	5.3	3.8	0.9	0.1	1.0	0.2	0.6	1.0	0.2	0.1	0.1	1.2	0.0	0.1
Philippines	36.0	16.0	4.6	0.7	4.5	0.0	2.3	3.5	0.1	8.5	9.4	1.8	0.2	0.0
Republic of Korea	34.9	27.0	1.7	3.3	8.4	0.2	8.0	5.1	0.3	4.6	2.6	0.4	0.3	0.0
Sri Lanka	31.7	18.8	9.2	0.7	1.5	0.3	4.7	2.3	0.0	7.9	1.5	3.5	0.0	0.0
Syrian Arab Republic	19.8	15.1	0.3	0.1	11.8	0.3	0.6	0.6	1.3	2.8	1.6	0.0	0.2	0.1
Thailand	33.1	30.4	6.3	2.1	13.7	1.9	5.9	0.4	0.1	0.9	0.9	0.7	0.0	0.3
Yemen	1.1	1.1	0.1	0.1	0.6	0.0	0.1	0.1	0.0	0.0	0.0	0.0	0.0	0.0
MEAN	23.0	16.9	3.5	0.8	7.4	0.3	2.7	2.0	0.2	2.7	1.9	0.9	0.1	0.5
TOTAL MEAN	24.5	18.3	3.9	0.3	7.8	0.6	2.8	2.1	0.7	2.5	2.0	0.9	0.3	0.4

145

TABLE 81 (continued)

B. Based on current contraceptive users

Region and country	Total	Modern	Sterilization Female	Sterilization Male	Pill	Injectable	Intrauterine device	Condom	Female barrier methods	Rhythm	Withdrawal	Abstinence	Douche	Other
Africa														
Benin[a]	100	5	0	0	2	0	1	1	1	14	27	51	2	0
Cameroon	100	24	0	0	10	0	6	8	0	47	16	0	1	12
Côte d'Ivoire[b]	100	17	0	0	14	0	2	0	0	12	3	62	5	2
Egypt	100	94	3	0	68	0	17	5	1	2	2	1	1	1
Ghana	100	58	5	0	25	1	3	7	17	7	2	32	0	0
Kenya	100	63	12	1	30	8	10	2	0	16	2	16	0	1
Lesotho	100	48	15	0	23	4	3	2	1	2	47	0	0	0
Mauritania	100[e]	33	22	0	4	0	0	0	7	11	56	0	1	4
Morocco	100	84	4	0	71	1	8	1	0	6	5	0	0	0
Senegal	100	15	1	0	8	1	4	0	0	10	0	67	1	8
Sudan	100	85	6	0	67	3	2	3	2	10	2	2	0	0
Tunisia	100	79	24	0	21	1	28	4	2	12	6	0	0	2
MEAN	100	51	8	0	29	2	7	3	3	12	14	19	1	3
Latin America and the Caribbean														
Colombia	100	72	9	0	31	1	20	4	5	12	11	2	1	2
Costa Rica[c]	100	83	19	2	35	3	8	14	3	8	7	1	0	1
Dominican Republic	100	82	38	0	25	1	9	5	5	4	12	0	2	1
Ecuador	100	77	23	1	28	3	14	3	5	14	7	1	1	0
Guyana	100	90	27	0	29	1	18	9	6	3	4	2	0	1
Haiti	100	28	1	0	18	0	2	6	1	26	25	18	3	1
Jamaica	100	94	21	1	31	16	5	17	4	1	4	1	0	0
Mexico	100	77	9	0	36	6	19	3	5	10	12	0	1	1
Panama[c]	100	85	39	1	32	1	7	2	3	5	6	3	1	1
Paraguay	100	65	6	0	33	5	15	4	2	12	7	0	1	1
Peru	100	36	9	0	13	3	4	4	3	35	10	7	5	12
Trinidad and Tobago	100	89	8	0	35	2	4	29	10	5	5	1	1	0
Venezuela[d]	100	76	15	0	31	0	17	10	2	8	10	0	5	1
MEAN	100	73	17	0	29	3	11	8	4	11	9	3	2	2
Asia and Oceania														
Bangladesh	100	62	4	6	37	0	5	9	1	14	6	15	1	2
Fiji	100	86	39	0	20	1	12	15	0	6	7	1	0	1
Indonesia	100	87	1	0	56	0	21	7	0	3	1	4	0	5
Jordan	100	71	7	0	47	2	8	6	1	8	13	2	0	6
Malaysia	100	72	10	1	49	1	2	8	0	10	6	5	0	6
Nepal	100	98	4	67	16	0	2	9	0	0	0	2	0	7
Pakistan	100	72	18	1	18	0	12	19	3	2	2	22	1	0
Philippines	100	45	13	2	13	0	6	10	0	24	26	5	0	2
Republic of Korea	100	77	5	9	24	1	23	15	1	13	7	1	1	0
Sri Lanka	100	59	29	2	5	1	15	7	0	25	5	11	0	0
Syrian Arab Republic	100	76	2	0	59	2	3	3	7	14	8	0	1	0
Thailand	100	92	19	6	41	6	18	1	0	3	3	2	0	1
Yemen	100[e]	96	12	10	57	3	7	7	0	0	4	0	0	0
MEAN	100	76	12	8	34	1	10	9	1	9	7	5	0	2
TOTAL MEAN	100	67	13	3	31	2	10	7	3	11	10	9	1	2

Source: World Fertility Survey standard recode tapes.

[a] Women who had not resumed sexual relations since the last pregnancy were counted as non-users.
[b] Formerly called the Ivory Coast.
[c] Ages 20-49.
[d] Ages 15-44.
[e] Based on fewer than 50 contraceptive users.

146

As might be expected, part of the association of age with contraceptive use was found to be attributable to effects of family size and desire for more children (figure 30). On average, before control for other variables, the percentage who were using contraception is more than 20 points lower for exposed women aged 15-19 than for those aged 30-34; over half of this differential can be explained by the differences between the age groups in family size and attainment of desired family size. There appears, however, to be some additional tendency for young women to use contraception less than those in their thirties; and control for the other variables has little effect on the amount of decline in use levels at the highest ages.[19]

Family size also has some independent association with contraceptive use. Statistical control for age alone has almost no effect on the pattern of use according to family size, but the pattern is significantly altered when desire for more children is brought into the analysis. The only large difference in use levels remaining after control for the motivational variable is that between women with no children and those with one or more. The contrast in contraceptive practice between childless women and the rest may be due to differences in desire to delay wanted births, a factor not controlled in this analysis: childless women in most developing countries are likely to want the first child as soon as possible after marriage, but they are less likely to want subsequent children as quickly as is biologically possible.

It was noted earlier that, particularly in countries with high levels of contraceptive use, women with large families were frequently somewhat less likely to be using contraception than those with moderate numbers of children. Statistical control for desire for more children increases the number of countries showing this pattern. After control for age and desire for more children, the peak level of use occurs, on average, at a family size of two children.

D. KNOWLEDGE AND USE OF SPECIFIC CONTRACEPTIVE METHODS

Knowledge and use among currently married women

Individuals' choices among contraceptive methods can be influenced by many factors. The relative availability of the various modern methods is certainly a major consideration in most developing countries, although its influence is not easy to separate from other forces, such as the pronouncements of religious or political leaders about the morality of use of particular methods and individuals' perceptions of method-effectiveness, and of the medical or other drawbacks associated with each method. It is clear, however, that simple awareness of various methods is a pre-condition for use. The percentage of married women who knew of each method is shown in table 80. Table 81 shows levels of current use of particular methods.

There is a great deal of variety in the specific contraceptive methods that women knew about and that they had adopted. The pill is the most widely known single method in 28 of the countries; in 24 at least three quarters of married women had heard of it. Frequently, the percentage who reported knowledge of any method is not much higher than the percentage who knew of this one method. Female sterilization and IUDs are the methods next most widely known, after the pill. In 16 countries, at least three fourths of women had heard of IUDs; and in 14, female sterilization was that widely recognized. Over three fourths of women knew of the condom in 8 countries, injectables in 3, and rhythm and male sterilization in 1 country each. The striking predominance of modern methods in this list of widely known methods undoubtedly reflects the publicity efforts of organized family planning programmes.

Questions about knowledge of methods may not be a good guide to the ability of women actually to obtain contraceptives. Questions about knowledge of outlets for particular methods (included in only a few surveys)[20] show that, in some instances, a majority of those who reported hearing of a method did not know of a supply source. For instance, in Benin, only 12 per cent of those who had heard of the pill knew where it could be obtained. The proportions in the Sudan were 28-30 per cent of those who knew of female sterilization, injectables, IUDs or condoms, and slightly under half for the pill. In Morocco under half, and in Egypt about 60 per cent, of those who knew of IUDs knew of a source. In these African countries, the proportions who knew of a source for the pill tended to be substantially higher than for any other method, and the pill was frequently the only method for which a source was known. By contrast, in Paraguay, the Philippines and Venezuela, at least 80 per cent of those who had heard of female sterilization, the pill, IUDs or condoms also knew where to obtain these methods.

The percentage of women who reported knowledge of any of the traditional and non-supply methods was, in most countries, lower than the percentage who knew of a modern method. While it might seem that the ability of abstinence and withdrawal to prevent conception would be obvious everywhere, on average, fewer than half of the women reported knowledge of these methods. It should be noted that the survey questions asked whether women had heard of these methods actually being used to prevent or space births, not whether women believed that such practices, if adopted, would be effective. The use of traditional abstinence in sub-Saharan Africa was discussed earlier. Extended post-partum abstinence is not always reported as contraception, but the percentage who reported knowledge of "contraceptive abstinence" tended to be relatively high in the sub-Saharan countries.

The percentage who knew of rhythm, withdrawal or douching tended to be highest in countries where most women also knew about a modern clinic or supply method. The percentage who reported knowledge of "other methods" was low in most countries but was in the range of 50-85 per cent in some of the countries where the survey included probe questions describing particular folk methods. In some cases, these folk methods include medicinal or mechanical means of inducing abortion.

The method most widely known, the pill, was also the most widely used (table 81, panel 8). It accounted for approximately one third of all current contraceptive use, averaged over all countries. In 26 countries more women had tried the pill than had used any of the other methods (United Nations, 1986), and in 21 the pill was also the method most widely used at the time of the survey. On average, for all 38 countries, about one fifth of all currently married women had tried the pill (United Nations, 1986), and 8 per cent were currently using it.

An average of from 9 to 11 per cent of married women had tried the condom, rhythm and withdrawal (United

Nations, 1986), but only 2-2.5 per cent were using each of those methods at the time of the interview. IUDs and female sterilization were, next to the pill, the methods most commonly used at the time of the survey; from 3 to 4 per cent of women were using each of these methods, on average.

The average figures for all countries combined do not give an adequate summary of the information about specific methods, because very few countries have method distributions that closely resemble the average. For any particular contraceptive method, it is possible to find at least one country where the level of use is essentially nil, but at the same time, even the methods that are little used in most countries find a substantial number of users in a few. Figure 31 is a box-and-whisker plot displaying the median level of current use of each method and summarizing the amount of variation around the median. The upper and lower "whiskers" extend to the highest and lowest levels of use of each method among currently married women. (The lowest value observed is always zero per cent.) The length of the "box" extends from the twenty-fifth to the seventy-fifth percentile, and the line across the box marks the median value for all 38 countries. For example, figure 31 shows that the percentage of married women who had been contraceptively sterilized ranges from zero to about 21 per cent (in Panama). The level was under 0.3 per cent of married women for one fourth of the countries and over 7.5 per cent for another one fourth. The median percentage sterilized was a little under 2 per cent.

It can be seen that although the pill was used by the greatest number of women, on average, it is also the method with the greatest range in levels of use, from barely above zero per cent of married women in Benin and Mauritania to 22.5 per cent in Costa Rica. The interquartile range (the length of the "box") is also greater for the pill than for any other method.

For many methods, there are one or two countries with prevalence levels far above those observed in other countries. For example, although in three fourths of the countries the prevalence of condom use was below 2.5 per cent of couples, in Trinidad and Tobago, it was 15 per cent; and in Costa Rica, 7.5 per cent.

In most countries, no one method accounts for more than half of all contraceptive use. In six countries, however, the pill was the choice of more than half of current contraceptive users (table 81, panel B). Abstinence accounted for over half of use in two countries, and withdrawal and male sterilization in one country each. But the countries with method distributions highly skewed in favour of one method tended to have low or, at most, moderate levels of contraceptive prevalence, so that the percentage of all married couples who were using the preferred method is often not especially high by comparison with prevalence levels for that method in other countries. For instance, although withdrawal accounted for over half of all reported use in Mauritania, only 0.4 per cent of married women said they were using withdrawal, as opposed to over 9 per cent in the Philippines, where

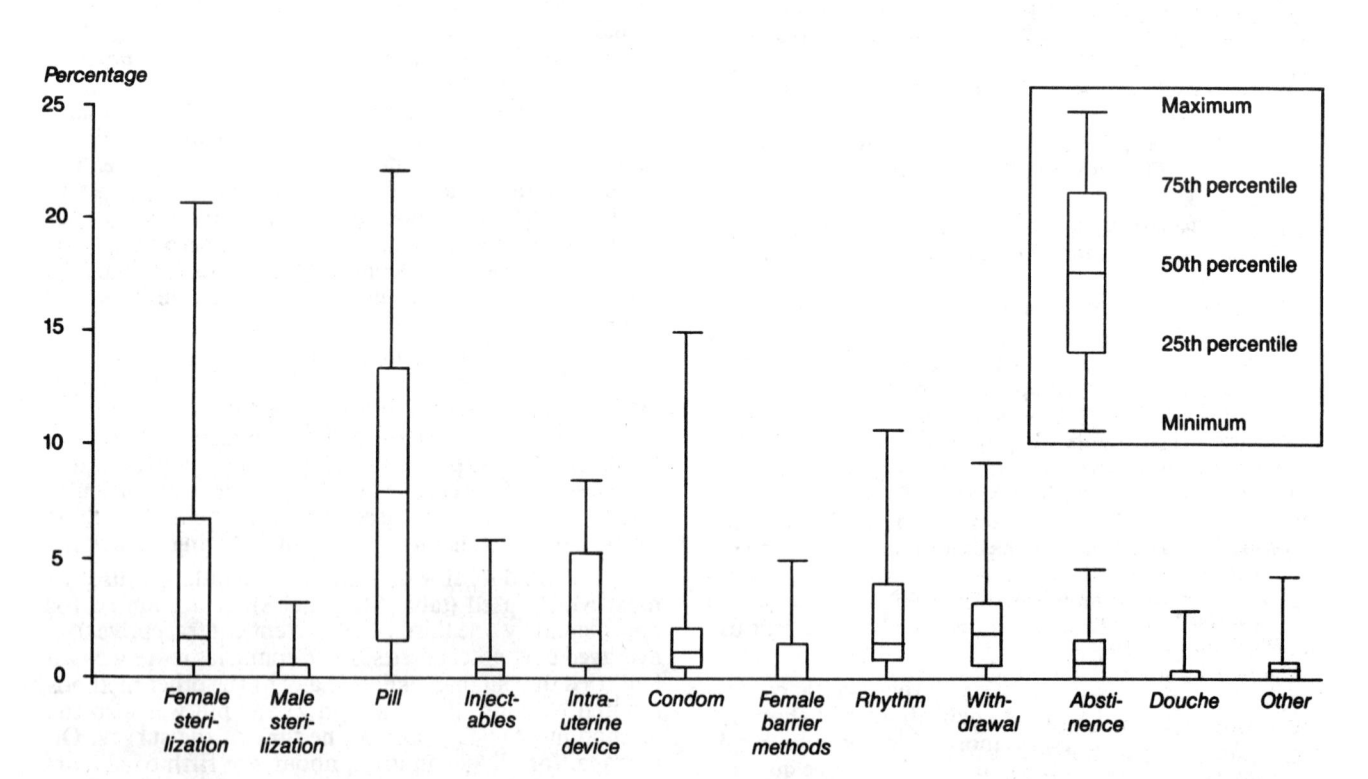

Figure 31. **Percentage of currently married women aged 15-49 currently using specific contraceptive methods: extreme values for 38 countries and 25th, 50th and 75th percentiles**

Source: Table 81.

148

withdrawal was responsible for only about one fourth of total contraceptive use. Similarly, the percentage of married women who were using the pill was higher in Costa Rica, where the pill accounted for about one third of all use, than in any of the six countries where the pill constituted over half of current contraceptive practice.

One way to summarize the amount of difference between method distributions is to consider what percentage of contraceptive users in one country would have to switch to another method in order for the method distribution to equal that of another particular country. The value of this measure, known as the index of dissimilarity, can range from zero, in the case where the two percentage distributions shown in table 81, panel B, are exactly equal, to 100, in the case where all the contraceptive users in the first country employed methods that no one in the second country used.[21] With 38 countries, a large number of such pair comparisons can be made, and only a few representative values are mentioned here. The mean value of the index of dissimilarity between method distributions, computed for all distinct pairs of countries, is 49. Thus, on average, about half of the contraceptive users in one country would have to switch to another method in order to make the method distribution equal to that of another arbitrarily chosen country.

To the extent that method choice depends upon cultural values and that geographical groupings correspond to cultural differences, one might expect contraceptive method distributions to be more similar within regions than between them. However, method distributions may be determined less by deep-seated preferences of couples than by laws regulating availability of particular methods and administrative decisions of family planning providers to stress particular methods. These legal and administrative decisions may also be made on the basis of the experience of neighbouring countries, though certainly this is not always the case.

As the following summary figures show, there are some regional subgroups in which the average values of the index of dissimilarity are relatively low, indicating a degree of similarity in method choice within the region:

	Average values of the index of dissimilarity comparing pairs of contraceptive method distributions
Within Africa	60
Within Northern Africa (Egypt, Morocco, Sudan, Tunisia)	33
Within rest of Africa	63
Within Latin America and the Caribbean	34
Within Asia and Oceania	42
Within Southern Asia (Bangladesh, Nepal, Pakistan, Sri Lanka)	56
Within Western Asia (Jordan, Syrian Arab Republic, Yemen)	27
Within rest of Asia	42
Comparisons of Africa, and Latin America and the Caribbean	53
Comparisons of Africa, and Asia and Oceania	56
Comparisons of Latin America and the Caribbean, and Asia and Oceania	42
All pair comparisons of countries	49

Latin America and the Caribbean, Western Asia and Northern Africa have average within-region index values in the range 27-34. In some other cases, method distributions within regions are no more similar than the average values of 42-53 found when countries of different regions are compared. Over all, the degree of within-region heterogeneity in method choice is as striking as the modest degree of clustering that can be observed in a few specific regional groups.

Current use of specific methods by age

Some of the factors governing choice of a particular contraceptive method are subject to change over the life cycle. Sterilization, which is for all practical purposes an irreversible procedure, is adopted only by couples who want no more children. Sterilization should thus be quite an uncommon choice for young women. Among the reversible methods as well, some types of contraception may be regarded as more suited than others for use by young women or by those interested in delaying rather than preventing births. The health risks of one method —the pill—have been found to increase with age; and in many countries, health workers now advise older women to try other methods. Whether this is desirable in developing countries depends not solely upon the objective health risks of long-term pill use (which may in any case differ between developed and developing countries) but upon the availability and acceptability of other effective methods and upon the health risks associated with accidental pregnancy, should women switch to less effective methods (see Schearer, 1983). Although there can be no general judgement about the advisability of pill use by older women in the current circumstances of the countries included in this report, the medical findings do suggest that the age pattern of pill use, and the factors influencing this age pattern, should be given special attention.

Variations with age in the use of various specific contraceptive methods are shown in figure 32. Both the average pattern based on currently married women and the average based on current users are illustrated.

Figure 33 illustrates the range of difference in percentages of younger and older users who were employing specific methods and the amount of consistency among countries in the direction of the age difference. More specifically, figure 33 is based on tabulations of the method distribution (as in table 81, panel B) done separately for contraceptive users aged under and over 30 years; the figure shows the difference between the two age groups in the percentage using each of seven methods. Larger dots denote values for countries where the method accounted for at least 20 per cent of total contraceptive practice, and smaller dots denote countries where the method made up 5-19 per cent. (Countries where the method accounted for under 5 per cent of use are not shown.) It can be seen, for example, that in every country where sterilization accounted for at least 5 per cent of contraceptive use ($N = 27$ countries), this method was relatively more important for older women, by amounts ranging from 7 to 43 percentage points. As might be expected, the absolute size of the age differential tends to be greater in countries where sterilization accounted for a large percentage of all contraception (large dots). One thing not evident from the figure is that, even among the younger women, sterilization was sometimes a major method. In the Dominican Republic, Sri Lanka and Thailand, sterilization accounted for over 20 per cent of contraceptive use among women under age 30 (United Nations, 1986).

Figure 32. Current use of specific contraceptive methods, by age group and number of living children: average distributions for 38 countries

A. Based on currently married women

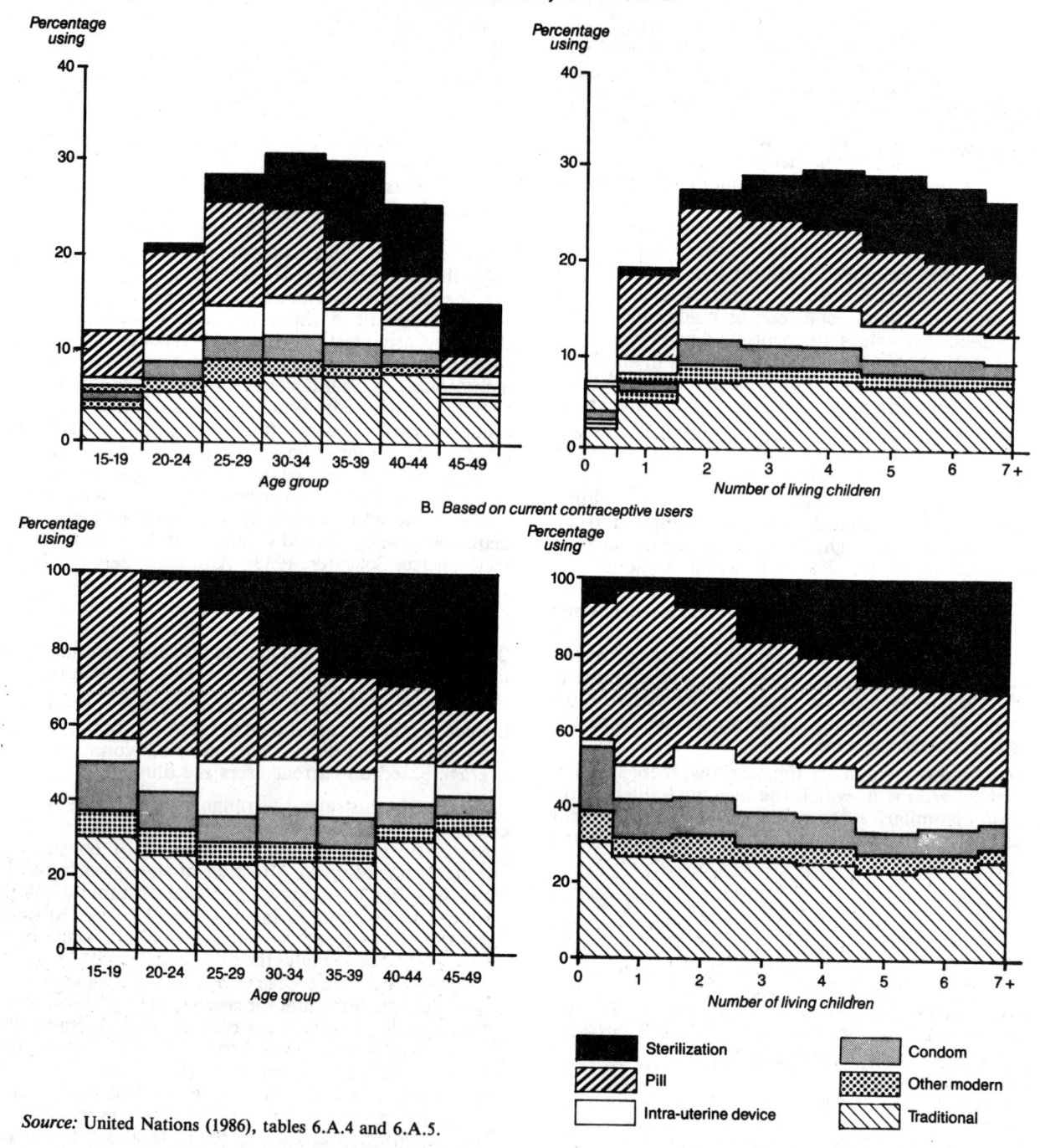

B. Based on current contraceptive users

Legend:
- Sterilization
- Pill
- Intra-uterine device
- Condom
- Other modern
- Traditional

Source: United Nations (1986), tables 6.A.4 and 6.A.5.

Since sterilization, once adopted, cannot be abandoned, the percentage sterilized necessarily increases as a birth cohort of women ages. However, in a cross-section composed of women of differing birth cohorts, the oldest women need not necessarily show the highest prevalence of sterilization. Figure 32 shows that the percentage of married women sterilized was indeed higher, on average, for women aged 35-44 than for the oldest age group, 45-49. This finding is an indirect reflection of the recency and rapidity with which sterilization services, and sterilization adoption, have spread in developing countries.

This method will plainly continue to grow in overall prevalence among women of reproductive ages, as the older women (with somewhat lower prevalence rates) leave those ages and are replaced by cohorts who, even by ages 35-39, already have reached higher cumulative rates of sterilization. In addition, the average age at acceptance of sterilization appears to be declining in developing countries, further suggesting that sterilization

Figure 33. **Age differences in percentage of current contraceptive users employing specific methods,[a] individual countries**

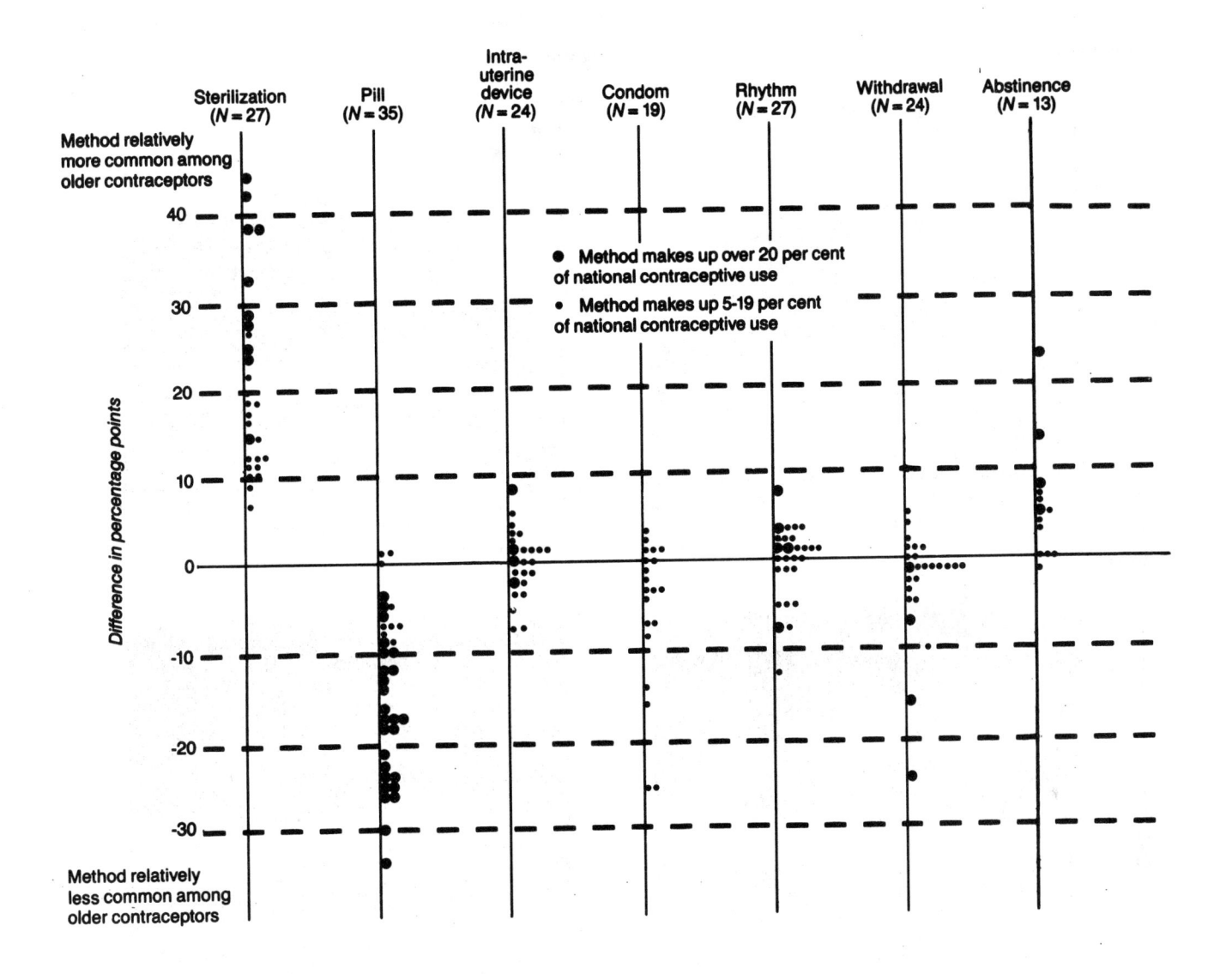

Source: World Fertility Survey standard recode tapes.
NOTE: Percentage difference shown only for countries where the specific methods accounted for at least 5 per cent of total contraceptive use. Number of countries shown in parentheses. Mauritania and Yemen excluded.

[a] For each method, M, the percentage point difference is 100 times: (number of users of M aged 30+ divided by total contraceptors aged 30+) minus (number of users of M aged under 30 divided by total contraceptors aged under 30).

prevalence will continue to grow (Ross, Hong and Huber, 1985).

With few exceptions, the pill accounted for a substantially larger fraction of total contraceptive use among women under 30 than among users over age 30 (figure 33). On average, the decreases with age in proportion of users who were employing the pill nearly offset the increases in use of sterilization (figure 32, panel B). Other methods typically show less marked shifts with age, but in a majority of countries the condom and withdrawal accounted for a larger proportion of contraceptive use among young women; and in the few countries where abstinence accounted for a substantial fraction of total use, this method tended to be more common for older women (figure 33). The IUD and rhythm methods did not consistently account for a larger fraction of use in one age group than in the other.

Although the pill almost always accounts for a lower proportion of total contraceptive practice for older than for younger women, the amount of change with age varies considerably. A crucial factor appears to be whether older women adopt sterilization. Two fairly extreme examples are shown in figure 34, Egypt and Panama. Panama had the highest prevalence of sterilization of all the WFS countries, but the pill also was an important method; it was used by 17 per cent of currently married women. In Panama, and in other countries where both sterilization and the pill are important methods, the percentage of older women using the pill tended to be quite low.

Figure 34. **Percentage of currently married women using sterilization, the pill and other methods, by age: Egypt and Panama**

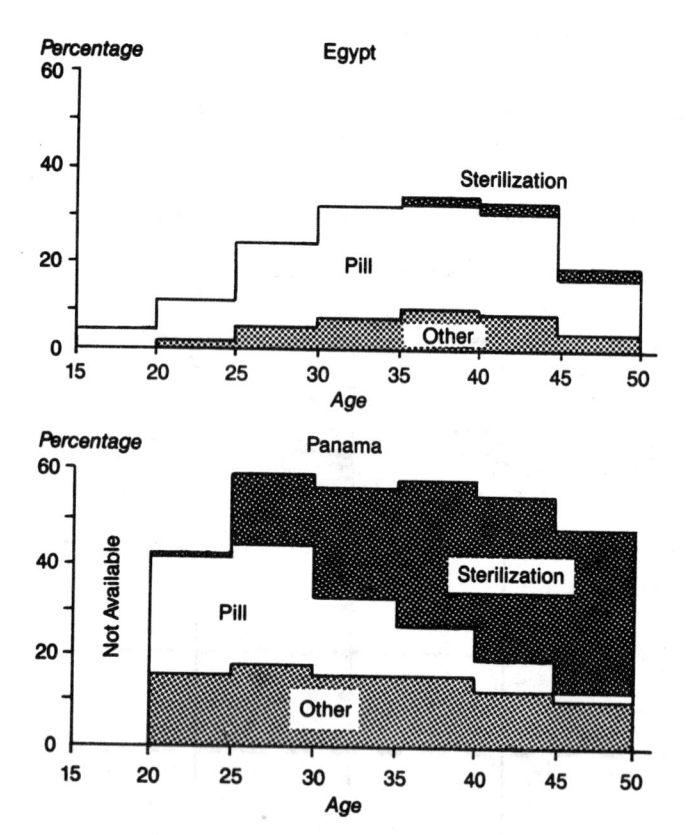

Source: United Nations (1986), table 6.A.4.

Although prevalence of reversible methods other than the pill also declined somewhat at higher ages, in Panama (and in several other countries with high levels of sterilization), the main trade-off was plainly between sterilization and the pill. In Egypt, the overall prevalence of the pill was slightly lower than in Panama, but this method accounted for a much higher proportion of contraceptive use than in Panama, and sterilization was especially uncommon. In Egypt and in other countries where the pill was a major method but sterilization was not, the pill accounted for a large percentage of total use even among older women. In fact, although several of the Latin American and Caribbean countries had a higher overall prevalence of pill use, in Egypt, the percentage of married women using the pill was higher at ages 30 and over than in any other WFS country (United Nations, 1986).

It is difficult to say on the basis of the WFS data alone whether persistence of relatively high levels of pill use into the older age groups in such countries as Egypt, Indonesia, Morocco and the Syrian Arab Republic is due primarily to the lack of general availability of other modern methods and particularly of sterilization. IUD use has been promoted by family planning programmes in some of these countries, but it is probably not as readily available as the pill. (Only 24 per cent of women knew of a source for IUDs in Morocco and 41 per cent in Egypt, while a source for the pill was known by 56 and 73 per cent, respectively.) Older women in these countries showed little tendency to turn to use of traditional and non-supply methods in place of the pill; indeed, levels of awareness of most such methods appears low (table 80).

The age differential in use of sterilization and the pill cannot be attributed solely to the fact that age is correlated with family size and desire for more children. Figure 35 summarizes the results of multiple classification analysis of the percentage of current contraceptive practice due to the pill, sterilization and other methods.[22] On average, and in most individual countries, the statistical adjustment for family size and desire for more children has almost no effect on the age differential in relative use of the pill and explains only part of the increased reliance of older contraceptive users upon sterilization. On average, older contraceptive users are somewhat more likely to choose methods other than the pill and sterilization than are younger users with similar family size and similar proportions desiring more children.

The most notable feature of these results is the persistence, after control for the other variables, of the strong negative relationship between pill use and age.[23] It is less surprising that a residual relationship between age and use of sterilization persists after the other variables are statistically controlled; among those women who had reached their desired family size (the only women for whom sterilization is an option), those who were relatively old at interview were likely, on average, to have reached the desired size longer ago and thus to have had more time to consider and adopt the permanent method of sterilization.

Current use of specific methods by family size

The distribution of contraceptive users by method chosen varies with family size in a manner generally similar to the changes according to age, as is shown in figure 32. On average, sterilization becomes more common at higher family sizes, until an approximate plateau is reached for families of five or more. The pill and condom account for a lower proportion of use for women with large than for those with small families. These features of the average pattern also appear in most individual countries (United Nations, 1986), and countries with relatively large contrasts in method distributions according to age usually also show large contrasts according to family size.

One notable feature of the method distributions by family size is the difference between women with no children and one child. Whereas the importance of the pill in relation to other methods decreases with family size among those who have children, contraceptive users with no children are, on average, somewhat less likely to choose the pill than those with one child. In most developed countries, by contrast, the pill accounts for an especially large proportion of use by childless women (Economic Commission for Europe, forthcoming). Childless

152

Figure 35. **Average percentage of current contraceptive users employing the pill, sterilization and other methods, by age and family size, adjusted for other variables**

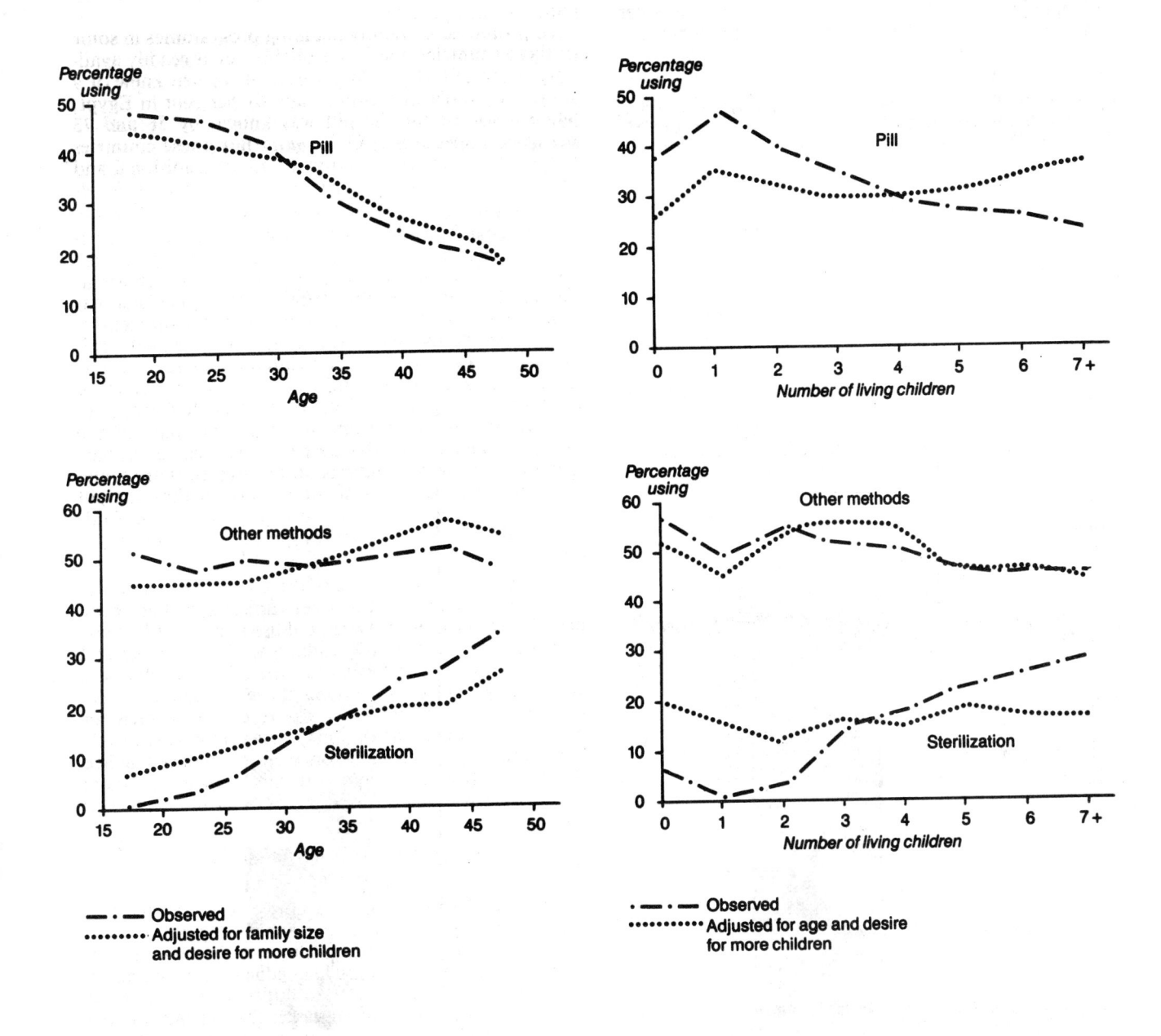

Source: World Fertility Survey standard recode tapes.
NOTES: Adjusted for the factors indicated using multiple classification analysis.

Results shown are averaged over the 25 countries where contraceptive prevalence was over 15 per cent of currently married women.

women are also extremely unlikely to be using an IUD. This may result partially from the reluctance of some medical authorities to recommend this method for women without children, because above average levels of pelvic inflammatory disease have been reported for zero-parity IUD users (Schearer, 1983).[24]

Among contraceptive users, choice of the pill, sterilization or some other method does not, in general, depend heavily upon family size *per se*, apart from the effects of family size that operate through desire for more children and the associated effects of age. Once the latter two variables are controlled statistically,[25] the average percentage of contraceptive users employing the pill, sterilization and other methods is nearly constant for women with differing numbers of children, as is shown in figure 35.[26] This contrasts with the results for age differentials in method choice, which could not be adequately explained by reference to family size and desire for more children.

Current use of specific methods by desire for more children

Couples who want no more children have a wider choice of methods than those who want more—the former can choose sterilization, which is for all practical purposes an irreversible procedure. Over all, sterilization of the husband or wife accounted for about one fourth of the total contraceptive practice in WFS countries, among couples where the wife wanted no more children. This corresponds to 11 per cent of exposed women who wanted no more children, on average, but proportions as high as 40-41 per cent were recorded in Fiji and Panama (United Nations, 1986).

Other contraceptive methods can be used either to space or to limit family size, but it is possible that some methods might be favoured for relatively short periods of use, suited for birth-spacing but not for limiting family size. No direct information is available from WFS about women's preferences in this regard, but distributions of

Figure 36. **Average percentage of exposed women and current contraceptive users employing specific methods, by desire for more children**

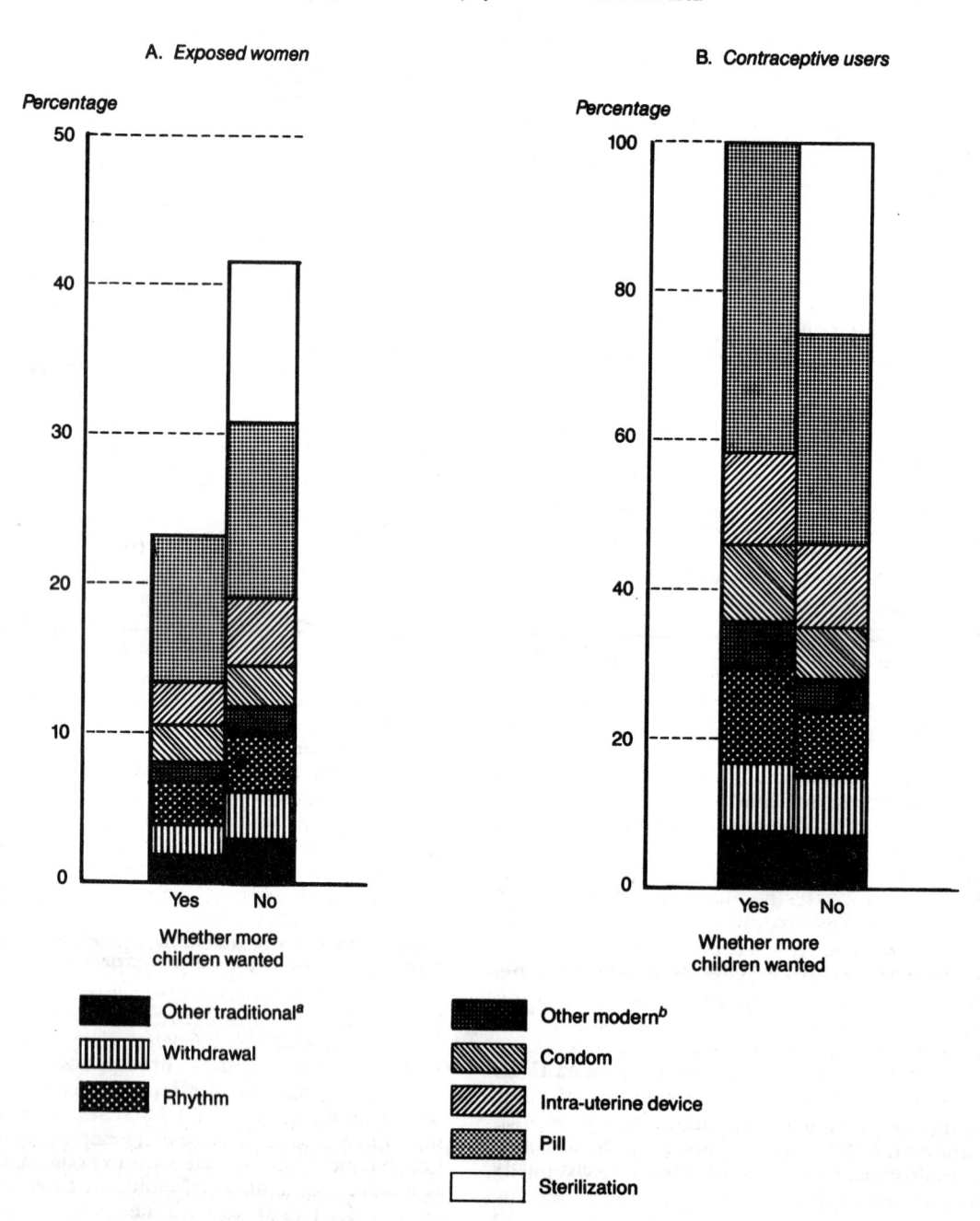

A. *Exposed women*

B. *Contraceptive users*

Legend:
- Other traditional[a]
- Withdrawal
- Rhythm
- Other modern[b]
- Condom
- Intra-uterine device
- Pill
- Sterilization

Source: United Nations (1986), table 6.A.6.
[a] Including abstinence, douche and folk methods.
[b] Including injectables and female barrier methods.

methods in current use can be examined according to desire for more children, to see if a particular method was in fact more heavily used for one purpose than for another. All-country averages, illustrated in figure 36, reveal that the pill was by far the most widely used reversible method for both groups of women. Among women who wanted more children it accounted for 42 per cent of contraceptive use, on average, and 28 per cent among women who wanted no more children (slightly higher than the percentage of use attributable to sterilization). Furthermore, examination of country-specific statistics (United Nations, 1986) shows that whenever a particular method was common among women who wanted more children, it was almost always common also among women who wanted no more children. If only those women who were using reversible contraceptive methods are considered, the percentage distribution according to method used is usually very similar between women who did and those who did not want more children. Thus, the purpose for which contraception is used—birth-spacing or birth limitation—does not appear to be an important factor in determining which reversible method to use.

E. CONTRACEPTIVE DISCONTINUATION AND METHOD-SWITCHING

When organized family planning programmes first began to conduct follow-up studies of their clients, it was recognized, at first with dismay, that a large proportion of couples who accepted a method abandoned it within a year or two, despite a continuing desire to avoid pregnancy. Although accidental pregnancy was often the reason for giving up certain methods, most women who discontinued use did so for other reasons: in the case of the pill or IUD, the experience of side-effects or the fear of eventual serious physical harm from long-term use, or expulsion of an IUD; in the case of other methods, inconvenience, interference with intercourse or fears of method failure. Further investigation led to the observation that many women who stopped using one method turned to another. These studies have made it clear, however, that the contraceptive methods currently available did not meet the needs of many couples and have led to calls for increased research to develop better contraceptives and to recognition of a need for availability of a wide range of methods, if couples are to have effective control over their fertility (United Nations, 1984, recommendations 25 and 69; *Family Planning in the 1980's*, 1981). Analysis of rates of contraceptive discontinuation and reasons for discontinuation and method-switching remain important for assessing the need for family planning services and for evaluation of the types of services currently offered.

The WFS results contain varying amounts of information about contraceptive discontinuation and method-switching. The information is not comparable to that obtained from follow-up studies, which have thus far provided most of the data on these topics; to some extent the two types of data source complement each other.

All the surveys in the WFS programme obtained information about which methods were ever used and all yielded a crude indicator of continuation—the proportion who were currently using a method, of those who had ever used (referred to below as the "continuation ratio"). The analytical utility of this measure is limited by a lack of information about the duration of use; apparent differences in levels of discontinuation might be due to differences in the average time since adoption of contraception, rather than to more fundamental differences in the propensity of contraceptors to abandon contraceptive practice.

The crude measures, however, are at least adequate to show that discontinuation is frequent with all reversible methods. The percentage of ever-users of specific methods who were currently using the method (averaged for all 38 countries) is: pill, 38; injectables, 27; IUD, 44; condom, 23; female barrier methods and spermicides, 17; rhythm, 24; withdrawal, 18; abstinence, 13; douche, 9.[27]

On average, fewer than half of the women who had tried any particular reversible method were currently using that method, and under one fourth for methods other than the pill, IUDs and injectables. Yet, on average (and for most individual countries), at least 50 per cent of ever-users of each particular method were currently using some type of contraceptive (not shown).

First use of contraception and subsequent fertility

In some of the surveys, respondents were asked about the number of children at first contraceptive use and the method first used. Although this information is available for only nine countries,[28] it adds importantly to understanding of the evolution of contraceptive practice over time. By consulting dates in the birth history, the approximate date of first use can be inferred from knowledge of the number of children at first use.[29] This additional information is employed below, in part to give a description of demographic characteristics of contraceptive users at first use and at the interview, and in part to decide whether the continuation ratio for all methods combined is sensitive to the amount of time elapsed since first use. Because the answer to this question is important for attempts to interpret country differences in the continuation ratio, the discussion turns next to examination of the additional information for nine countries and later returns to measures available for all 38 countries.

Table 82 describes the average demographic characteristics of contraceptive users at first use and at the interview. It should be noted that six of the nine countries for which this information is available are located in the Latin America and the Caribbean region, and only one country (Nepal) had a very low level of current contraceptive practice. Contraceptive users in the Latin American countries studied had, on average, from two to three living children when they first used contraception. In Egypt, Nepal and Sri Lanka, the average family size was from three to three and a half children. Average age at first use was also somewhat lower in the Latin American countries (23-25 years) than in the other countries shown (26-28 years). First use occurred, on average, from about 5.5 years (Nepal) to 8.6 years (Panama) prior to the survey.

For a majority of women, the adoption of contraception does not mean a total cessation of childbearing. In all of the countries except Nepal, the average number of living children was from 1.0 to 1.2 children greater at the interview than when contraception had first been used.[30] Family size had increased from 50 to 60 per cent of the contraceptive users (except in Nepal, 29 per cent). The proportion with an unwanted birth since first use of contraception varied from 5 to 8 per cent (in Paraguay) and

TABLE 82. AVERAGE DEMOGRAPHIC CHARACTERISTICS OF WOMEN AT FIRST USE OF CONTRACEPTION AND AT INTERVIEW, FOR WOMEN WHO HAD EVER USED CONTRACEPTION, NINE COUNTRIES

	Mean age at First use (1)	Mean age at Survey (2)	Mean years since first use (3)	Mean number of living children at First use (4)	Mean number of living children at Survey (5)	Percentage with more living children than at first use Total (6)	More children and last birth unwanted Measure A[a] (7)	More children and last birth unwanted Measure B[b] (8)
Africa and Asia								
Egypt	25.7	34.0	8.3	3.0	4.0	59	37	33
Nepal	27.8	33.3	5.5	3.6	4.1	29	..	9
Sri Lanka	26.4	34.5	8.1	3.0	4.0	49	22	14
Latin America								
Colombia[c]	24.3	31.7	7.4	2.6	3.7	56	27	18
Costa Rica	24.5	33.0	8.5	2.6	3.8	59	18	11
Mexico[c]	24.8	31.6	6.8	2.9	4.0	55	..	17
Panama	24.3	32.9	8.6	2.6	3.7	57	21	14
Paraguay[c]	24.2	32.2	8.0	2.1	3.3	57	8	5
Venezuela[c]	23.0	30.1	7.1	2.2	3.4	59	21	12

Source: World Fertility Survey standard recode tapes.

[a] Unwanted according to a direct question about whether the woman had wanted ever to have more children at the time the last child was conceived.

[b] Birth after first contraceptive use and current number of living children greater than total number desired.

[c] Including single women who used contraception.

from 33 to 37 per cent (in Egypt), depending upon the measure used (columns (7) and (8)).

An earlier study using WFS data for five Latin American and Caribbean countries (Colombia, Costa Rica, Dominican Republic, Panama and Peru) estimated the risk of bearing either an unwanted child or a child born sooner than desired taking into account the amount of time spent at risk (Goldman and others, 1983).[31] In these five countries, between 21 and 45 per cent of women who used contraception in the birth interval studied had an unwanted or mistimed pregnancy within three years of the preceding birth. (By comparison, approximately 80 per cent of women who did not use contraception became pregnant within three years.) Women who used the pill, IUD or injectables had a much lower risk of pregnancy than those who used other reversible methods, and differences between countries in pregnancy rates of contraceptors could be adequately explained by differences in the types of methods employed.[32] Thus, although contraceptive practice greatly reduces the rate at which pregnancies occur, the risk of an unwanted or mistimed pregnancy is still fairly high for women who adopt contraception.

Table 83 shows the percentage distribution of women who had ever used contraception according to the first method chosen (panel A) and, for comparison, the average distribution for the nine countries according to the current contraceptive method (panel B). Sterilization was a relatively uncommon choice as the first method, except in Nepal. On average, male and female sterilization accounted for 8 per cent of first contraceptive use but 23 per cent of current use. IUDs also grew in relative importance, from 8 per cent of first use to 13 per cent of current use. Increased reliance upon these methods was compensated by a substantial decline in use of the pill (from 43 per cent of first use to 32 per cent of current use) and declines of from 1 to 3 per cent in the relative importance of most other methods. The pattern of change from first to current method corresponds roughly to the pattern of differential use according to age (figure 32), except that the cross-sectional data do not show a consistent tendency for IUD use to increase in relative importance with advancing age.

Table 83 also shows, in panel C, that for most methods other than the pill a majority of women who had tried the method had turned to it only after having become dissatisfied with their first choice. On average, under 40 per cent of ever-users of female sterilization, injectables, condoms, female barrier methods (diaphragm, cervical cap, spermicides), withdrawal, abstinence and douching had adopted these as the first method.

By contrast, about three fourths of women who had ever used the pill had tried this method first. In part, this reflects the fact that the pill was in most countries the first choice of such a large number of women that relatively few women could choose this as the second or later method. However, even in Sri Lanka, where the pill was a relatively uncommon first choice, about 80 per cent of women who had ever used the pill had chosen it as their first method. The unique popularity of the pill as the first method may be responsible for much of the association between current pill use and age mentioned earlier. All reversible methods are subject to substantial levels of discontinuation, and a method such as the pill that is usually adopted first and while women are relatively young (see Nortman, 1982, table 18) is likely to become less prevalent as women age.

Continuation of contraception by time since first use

Two aspects of continuation of contraceptive use are examined here: whether the first method was currently used at the interview; and whether any method was currently used.[33] The discussion is restricted to women who had chosen a reversible method (that is, a method other than sterilization) at first use of contraception.

On average, for the nine countries, only about one third of women who had chosen a reversible method first were currently using the same method at the interview (table 84). The proportion using any method was between 58 and 76 per cent, except in Nepal, where only 28 per cent of the women were currently using contraception.

TABLE 83. SELECTED INDICATORS OF FIRST USE AND CURRENT USE OF SPECIFIC CONTRACEPTIVE METHODS, NINE COUNTRIES

Region and country	Total	Sterilization Female	Sterilization Male	Pill	Injectable	Intra-uterine device	Condom	Female barrier methods	Rhythm	Withdrawal	Abstinence	Douche	Other
A. Percentage distribution of currently married ever-users according to first method
Africa and Asia
Egypt	100	1	0	82	0	9	3	1	1	1	0	0	2
Nepal	100	2	39	35	0	3	9	0	0	0	5	0	5
Sri Lanka	100	12	1	15	1	12	5	0	35	6	12	0	0
Latin America
Colombia	100	1	0	39	2	13	4	5	16	13	2	2	3
Costa Rica	100	5	0	40	3	5	18	3	12	11	1	1	1
Mexico	100	1	0	42	6	6	6	5	13	18	0	3	1
Panama	100	12	0	44	1	4	6	5	9	10	3	4	2
Paraguay	100	0	0	44	7	7	4	1	10	6	0	7	13
Venezuela	100	3	0	42	0	10	11	3	11	13	0	7	1
Average for nine countries	100	4	4	43	2	8	7	3	12	9	3	3	3
B. Percentage distribution of current contraceptive users according to current method
Average for nine countries	100	15	8	32	2	13	6	2	9	7	2	2	2
C. Of all ever-users of each method, percentage who chose that method first
Average for nine countries[a]	..	30	56[b]	76	34	43	39	32	47	37	25	26	..

Source: World Fertility Survey standard recode tapes.
[a] Average for each method based on percentages for countries with at least 20 ever-users of the method.
[b] Average based on figures for three countries only.

TABLE 84. PERCENTAGE WHO WERE CURRENTLY USING THE FIRST METHOD AND PERCENTAGE USING ANY METHOD, BY TIME SINCE FIRST USE, NINE COUNTRIES

Region and country	Total[a] Observed	Total[a] Standardized[b]	Years since first use 0	1	2-4	5-9	10+
A. First method
Africa and Asia
Egypt	41	42	70	55	39	39	36
Nepal	20	18	----- 28 -----		29	------ 10 ------	
Sri Lanka	41	41	69	50	46	36	33
Latin America
Colombia	37	36	60	50	40	33	26
Costa Rica	32	34	61	45	36	31	24
Mexico	34	32	55	48	36	29	20
Panama	29	31	62	46	40	26	15
Paraguay	36	36	55	51	41	32	26
Venezuela	35	34	62	39	37	30	27
B. Any method
Africa and Asia
Egypt	58	58	78	64	49	55	62
Nepal	28	26	----- 36 -----		40	------ 14 ------	
Sri Lanka	65	65	74	63	66	67	62
Latin America
Colombia	68	68	71	68	63	71	67
Costa Rica	76	76	81	78	71	77	77
Mexico	64	64	69	63	62	69	60
Panama	69	68	72	64	68	68	70
Paraguay	63	63	65	66	64	64	61
Venezuela	69	70	71	59	63	73	76

Source: World Fertility Survey standard recode tapes.
NOTE: Based on currently married women who had chosen a reversible method as the first contraceptive.
[a] Excluding women for whom timing of first use was not ascertained.
[b] Standardized on the average distribution of time since first use for the nine countries.

The percentage currently using the first method decreases steadily with the number of years since first use, with the greatest drop occurring shortly after adoption. Figure 37 shows average values and the range of values for the eight countries other than Nepal. The much lower percentages for Nepal are shown separately. Among women who had adopted a reversible method less than a year before the survey, the proportion using the method had already dropped to between 55 and 70 per cent in countries other than Nepal. The percentage continues to decline with increasing duration, at first relatively rapidly, then slowly. An average of one fourth of women who had adopted a reversible method 10 or more years before the survey were using that method at the interview. (Note that they may have tried other methods in the meantime.)

Figure 37. **Percentage currently using the first method and percentage using any method, by years since first use of contraception**

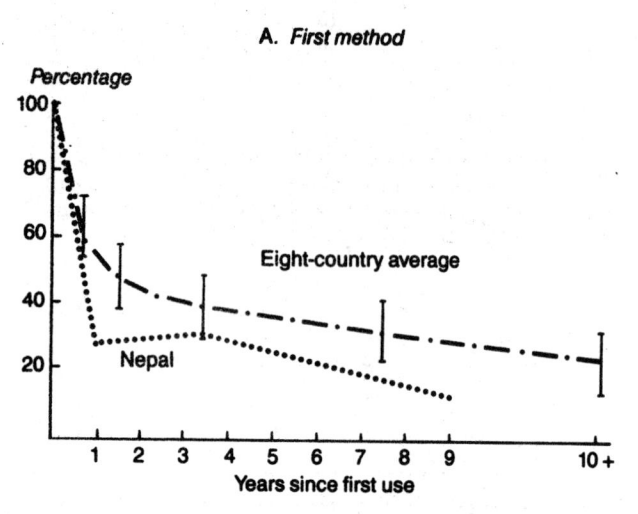

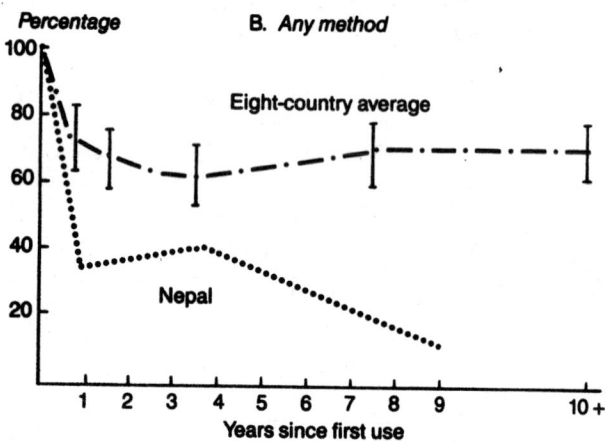

A. *First method*

B. *Any method*

Source: Table 84.
NOTES: Based on currently married women who had chosen a reversible method as the first contraceptive.
Vertical bars show range of values for the eight countries other than Nepal.

In contrast to the pattern for the first method, the percentage who were using any contraceptive method usually had changed very little with duration since first use, after the first year or so. An appreciable number of women had stopped using contraception shortly after initial use; the average proportion using a method among women who had adopted contraception less than one year before the survey was 73 per cent in countries other than Nepal. The percentage was from 66 to 88 at longer durations, slightly lower at from two to four years. In Egypt, the dip from two to four years is pronounced (table 84). Only in Nepal is there an indication of a decline at the longer durations.[34] The lack of variation in the all-method continuation ratio according to duration probably conceals numerous changes of status, from use to non-use and back, by individual women. Thus, although at any time since first use about one third of ever-users, on average, were observed not to be currently practising contraception, the number who had given up contraceptive practice permanently may be considerably lower than this.

Even though the first-method continuation ratio, and the all-method ratio for Nepal, decline somewhat with increasing duration, these ratios are affected very little by standardization for country differences in the distribution of time since first use (table 84). It is assumed in the next section that this applies to other countries as well. Although there are many other possible sources of variation in the overall continuation ratio, the large differences observed are almost certainly not simply an artifact of differing average amounts of time since adoption of contraception.

Up to this point no attention has been given to the quality of measurement of the continuation ratio. There is some reason to suspect that women who had tried contraception only briefly might tend to report that they had never used, particularly if a traditional, non-supply method was the only method employed.[35] This would bias the continuation ratio upward. For the purposes of this discussion and the consideration below of continuation ratios for all 38 countries, bias in the ratio would not necessarily invalidate the conclusions drawn, unless the bias were of a nature to distort the direction of differences in continuation ratios between countries or to undermine the conclusion that pronounced differences in the overall ratio are not due to differences between countries in the average duration since first use. Unfortunately, little independent evidence exists on these points. What little there is at least provides no reason to suspect the patterns across countries of being grossly distorted and provides a modest amount of support for the finding that the all-method continuation ratio is insensitive to average duration since first contraceptive use.[36]

Contraceptive continuation ratios and method change: 38 countries

On average, only 53 per cent of ever-users of contraception were currently practising: 36 per cent in Africa; 59 per cent in Asia and Oceania; and 64 per cent in Latin America and the Caribbean.[37] The continuation ratio increases markedly with level of development and strength of family planning programme effort (table 85).

Contraception may be discontinued for reasons that have nothing to do with inadequacies of methods or family planning services: a couple may want another child; or the need for contraception may have ceased. The level of discontinuation among exposed women who want no more children may therefore be a more useful indicator than the overall continuation ratio. Women who want no more children are indeed more likely than others to be continuing users (Lightbourne and Singh, 1982, p. 41).

TABLE 85. SELECTED INDICATORS OF CONTRACEPTIVE CONTINUATION AND USE OF MULTIPLE METHODS

Region and country	Percentage currently using a method, among women who had ever used contraception — Currently married women (1)	Percentage currently using a method, among women who had ever used contraception — Exposed women[a] who wanted no more children (2)	Of currently married women who had ever used contraception, percentage who had tried two or more methods (3)
A. Values for individual countries			
Africa			
Benin	26	43	21
Cameroon	23	30[b]	33
Côte d'Ivoire[c]	4	14	11
Egypt	58	71	33
Ghana	24	37	44
Kenya	21	45	41
Lesotho	23	41	27
Mauritania	48	53	16
Morocco	63	83	30
Senegal	34	57[b]	12
Sudan	36	63	32
Tunisia	68	82	45
Latin America and the Caribbean			
Colombia	68	81	60
Costa Rica	77	92	66
Dominican Republic	64	82	59
Ecuador	63	78	58
Guyana	56	71	52
Haiti	51	70	55
Jamaica	54	73	61
Mexico	65	80	57
Panama	73	88	55
Paraguay	64	78	51
Peru	63	79	60
Trinidad and Tobago	65	77	71
Venezuela	71	85	54
Asia and Oceania			
Bangladesh	51	65[b]	44
Fiji	59	80	53
Indonesia	69	85	29
Jordan	53	81	60
Malaysia	66	77	39
Nepal	57	72	17
Pakistan	51	61	28
Philippines	62	79	62
Republic of Korea	59	71	59
Sri Lanka	70	83	43
Syrian Arab Republic	59	82	56
Thailand	69	84	39
Yemen	36	65	17
B. Region			
Africa	36	52	29
Asia and Oceania	59	76	42
Latin America and the Caribbean	64	79	58
C. Level of development			
I. High	65	79	57
II. Middle-high	63	81	53
III. Middle-low	35	51	31
IV. Low	43	61	27
D. Strength of family planning programme effort			
1. Strong	66	81	53
2. Moderate	66	80	48
3. Weak	55	71	44
4. Very weak/none	38	56	34
TOTAL	53	69	43

Source: World Fertility Survey standard recode tapes.
[a] Currently married, non-pregnant women who believed themselves to be fecund, plus those who had been contraceptively sterilized.
[b] See table 79 for explanation of measurement of desire for no more children.
[c] Formerly called the Ivory Coast.

On average, the continuation ratio for exposed women who wanted no more children was approximately 70 per cent (table 85, column (2)). Although considerably higher than the ratio for all currently married ever-users, it nevertheless indicates a substantial amount of discontinuation. Continuation ratios for women who wanted no more children varied with region, level of development and strength of family planning programme effort in approximately the same way as the ratios for all ever-users.

Reasons for non-use of contraception were not gathered in the interviews. Conditions that may lead many couples to give up contraceptive use include unreliable or poorly accessible supply and follow-up services, and a lack of choice among methods; low levels of social support for fertility control or weak motivation on the part of users; local beliefs that may exaggerate the dangers associated with use of particular methods; and cultural attitudes that may make common side-effects of some methods, such as alteration of menstrual flow, unacceptable. Many of these same conditions seem likely to produce low levels of family planning acceptance, suggesting that low levels of couple continuation may be associated with low levels of ever-use.

Figure 38 examines the idea that the level of ever-use of contraception and the continuation ratio are related. The figure gives some support to this idea, but it is apparent that there is also a regional dimension to the relationship: all the sub-Saharan African countries had low continuation ratios (ranging from 14 to 57 per cent for exposed women who wanted no more children). The low

Figure 38. Contraceptive continuation ratio, by percentage of women who had ever used contraception, for exposed women who wanted no more children

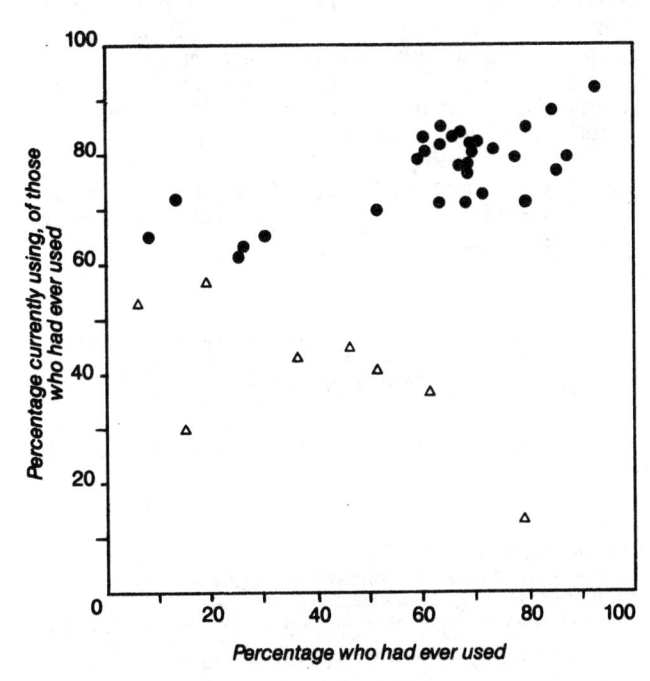

△ Africa, excluding Northern Africa
● Northern Africa, Latin America and the Caribbean, Asia and Oceania

Sources: Tables 79 and 85.

continuation ratios in this subregion may be partially an artifact of the way contraceptive abstinence was treated in WFS (described at the beginning of this chapter). However, those sub-Saharan countries which excluded abstinence as a contraceptive method (Cameroon, Lesotho) also exhibited low continuation rates. The reasons for these unusually low proportions of continuing contraceptive users deserve further investigation, but other sources of data will be required. Outside this subregion there is a positive relationship between the level of ever-use and the continuation ratio. For women who wanted no more children, countries where the level of ever-use was 30 per cent or less had continuation ratios of from 61 to 72 per cent; those where the level of ever-use was above 70 per cent had ratios between 71 and 92 per cent.

Since, as discussed earlier, most ever-users of any particular reversible method had given it up (ranging from an average of 56 per cent for IUDs to 91 per cent for douche), adoption of other methods is evidently crucial for maintenance of high levels of contraceptive continuation. On average, for all 38 countries, 43 per cent of ever-users reported trying two or more contraceptive methods (table 85, column (3)). In all the Latin American and Caribbean countries and in several of those in Asia and Oceania, over half had tried more than one method. As with the other measures shown in table 85, there is a marked relation between the percentage who had tried two or more methods and region, level of development and strength of family planning programme effort. There is also a direct relationship between the continuation ratio and the percentage of ever-users who had tried two or more methods. (The correlation (r) between column (3) and either column (1) or column (2) of table 85 is 0.6.) Furthermore, within countries there is a fairly consistent tendency for current contraceptive users to have tried more contraceptive methods than past users (not shown); on average, 36 per cent of past users and 50 per cent of current users had tried two or more methods. While hardly conclusive, all these relationships provide indirect support for the idea that availability of a range of methods is important for continued contraceptive use. (It is undoubtedly important also for attracting a large number of first-time users.) More direct investigation of the factors conducive to high or low rates of continuation will require other data.

F. SUMMARY AND CONCLUSIONS

The WFS data show that from the mid-1970s to the early 1980s appreciable proportions of women in most developing countries were attempting to control their fertility. The main exceptions are sub-Saharan Africa and four countries of Southern and Western Asia (Bangladesh, Nepal, Pakistan and Yemen), where the level of contraceptive prevalence was no higher than 10 per cent of currently married women of reproductive ages. Even awareness of modern, relatively effective contraception was limited in most of the low-prevalence countries, and the percentage who knew of a place to obtain family planning services, where this was measured, ranged from 1 to 43 per cent (in Benin and Ghana, respectively).

The countries in Asia and Oceania, other than the four already mentioned, had contraceptive prevalence levels between 20 and 41 per cent of married women. The values in Latin America and the Caribbean were between 30 and 64 per cent, except in Haiti (19 per cent). Several of the countries in this region had values within the lower part of the range seen in developed countries, which is roughly from 50 to 80 per cent using contraception (United Nations, 1984a).

The level of contraceptive practice was found to be strongly related to the strength of the country's family planning programme and to the level of development. Both these factors had an independent influence on use levels, as has also been reported in studies that were not confined to WFS data.

Various evidence suggests that these contraceptive prevalence levels are far from the maximum consistent with current fertility desires. Indeed, it is already clear that contraceptive practice continued to grow rapidly after WFS in many of the countries studied (United Nations, 1984a). The present report, however is confined to patterns evident from WFS itself.

One type of evidence of unmet need is the limited awareness of family planning services, already mentioned for countries with low levels of contraceptive practice. Twenty of the surveys asked about awareness of a family planning outlet; in all but three, under 90 per cent of married women knew of an outlet and the average percentage was about 60. Much higher proportions had heard of contraception (on average, 75 per cent knew of at least one modern method), but even this minimal awareness was lacking for a majority of women in several of the African countries and in Nepal and Yemen.

Other indicators of unmet need concern exposure to the risk of unwanted fertility, as well as the direct reports of unwanted births reviewed in chapter II. Over half (58 per cent) of women who wanted no more children and were exposed to the risk of pregnancy were not using contraception at the time of the survey—77 per cent in Africa, 57 per cent in Asia and Oceania and 43 per cent in Latin America and the Caribbean (calculated from table 79). Women who were exposed, wanted no more children and were not using contraception amounted to 17-18 per cent of all women of reproductive ages, on average, outside sub-Saharan Africa (but only 4-9 per cent in the sub-Saharan countries). The potential for further increase in contraception is likely to be underestimated by considering only those women who wanted no more children, because when contraceptive use expands among the latter group, it tends to increase also for women who wanted more children. Women who were using contraception to delay wanted births made up about 40 per cent of all current users, on average. Over the short term, the potential for large increases in contraceptive use in sub-Saharan Africa depends mainly upon the interest of couples in longer spacing between births.

This chapter also discussed patterns of contraceptive use according to age, family size and desire for more children. In all countries, the level of contraceptive use was higher for women aged from 25 to 40 than for those near the beginning or end of the reproductive years. This pattern is largely, though probably not entirely, the result of changing need for contraceptive protection over the life cycle. Intergenerational shifts in attitudes towards, and knowledge about, birth control may also be reflected in these data.

Patterns of contraceptive practice according to family size differ in some respects from country to country. Childless married women were usually much less likely than all others to have ever tried or to be currently using contraception, but that was not so in those Caribbean countries where many women were in visiting unions. In some countries, especially where overall contraceptive prevalence was low, the level of use increased steadily with the number of children. More often, it peaked at two, three or four children, with the peak tending to occur at lower family sizes in Latin America and the Caribbean than in Asia and Oceania. The peak tended to be more pronounced in countries with high overall prevalence levels, and it probably reflects the effects of past contraceptive use on both current contraceptive practice and on family size—women who had used contraception in the past tended to have moderate-sized families at the time of survey, while those who had not had progressed to higher parities.

The relation between contraceptive use and desire for more children was mentioned earlier, in the context of unmet need for family planning services. However, the use of contraception for birth-spacing deserves further comment. Of exposed women who wanted more children, an average of 23 per cent were currently using contraception, as compared with 42 per cent for women who wanted no more. In Latin America and the Caribbean, the level of use for birth-spacing tended to be especially high, both absolutely and in relation to the level of use for women who wanted no more children. A relatively high propensity to use contraception to space births was found in countries where the average length of breastfeeding was short and where the level of socio-economic development was high.

Limited data indicate that although most single women in Latin America and the Caribbean knew about contraception, only a small percentage had used it. In sub-Saharan Africa, although knowledge of contraception was much more limited, the percentage of single women who had used a modern method was higher than in Latin America and the Caribbean, and was close to the level observed among married women in the sub-Saharan countries. This is a further sign that the questions about marriage failed to capture many informal unions in Africa (see chapter III).

This chapter also discussed the specific contraceptive methods known and used. In most countries, one or more modern methods were recognized by more respondents than knew about any of the older methods, such as withdrawal. Modern methods tended to dominate contraceptive practice as well, though not in all countries. On average, 18 per cent of married women of reproductive ages were currently using methods requiring supplies or clinic services and 6 per cent were using other methods. Choice of specific methods differed greatly from country to country, but the pill was the most widely used over all, accounting for nearly one third of current contraceptive use. Female sterilization was the next most common method in WFS countries.[38] Other methods that protected over 1 per cent of married respondents, on average, are IUDs, rhythm, condoms and withdrawal, in order of importance.

There are a few broad similarities among countries in the way the mix of contraceptive methods changes with age and family size. Use of the two main methods, pill and sterilization, is strongly associated with these characteristics. On average, the increased reliance upon sterilization at higher ages and family sizes is approximately compensated by decreased reliance upon the pill. Pill use decreased with age even where sterilization was rarely employed, though the decrease tended to be larger where sterilization was an important method. These age differences in method choice remained after statistical control for family size and desire for more children. Family-size differentials in method choice, by contrast, showed no consistent pattern across countries once age and desire for more children were controlled.

One reason that the pill consistently accounts for a larger proportion of contraceptive practice among relatively young women may be simply that it is a very popular choice as the first method. All reversible methods are subject to substantial levels of discontinuation—indeed, follow-up studies indicate that for no reversible method is the average period of use more than from one to three years (Ross, 1983). The available WFS data indicate that about three quarters of the women who had ever tried the pill chose it as the first method, a much higher proportion than for other methods.

In the nine countries with information available, the first use of contraception had occurred, on average, from five to nine years before the survey. Since then, between 30 and 60 per cent of the contraceptive users had had at least one more child, and from 5 to 37 per cent at least one unwanted birth. The WFS data about first contraceptive use provide the opportunity to examine contraceptive practice many years after initial use, in contrast to contraceptive follow-up surveys, which offer much more detailed information but usually only for a few years after adoption of a method. The percentage of women currently using the first contraceptive method was found to decrease steadily with length of time since first use. However, an appreciable proportion of women—on average, about one quarter—were using the first method 10 or more years since first use of contraception. The proportion who were currently using any method was much higher and usually had changed very little with increased duration, after the first one or two years since initial use.

The factors contributing to high levels of contraceptive continuation must remain subject to speculation, although some suggestive relationships were noted in the chapter. Country values of the continuation ratio—the proportion of ever-users who were currently using—ranged from 4 per cent in Côte d'Ivoire to 77 per cent in Costa Rica (from 14 to 92 per cent for exposed women who wanted no more children). It was concluded that national differences in the continuation ratio, as measured in cross-sectional surveys of women of reproductive ages, are generally not due to differences in the average time since contraception was adopted. Although the values of the ratio in some of the African countries were probably artificially low for technical reasons relating to measurement of abstinence, the sub-Saharan countries appeared to have genuinely lower continuation ratios than those observed elsewhere; this finding deserves further study. For other countries, continuation ratios tended to be highest where the level of ever-use was high (including the more highly developed countries and those with strong family planning programmes) and where many contraceptive users had tried more than one method. It has long been thought that availability of a wide range of methods raises both contraceptive acceptance levels and couple continuation rates; these data are certainly consistent with this view.

NOTES

[1] Many of the surveys asked no questions about induced abortion (see Singh, 1984). In addition, interview surveys have been found to produce serious underestimates of the extent of practice of induced abortion, even in countries where the procedure is legal on broad social grounds and is known, from health record systems, to be widely practised (Tietze, 1983). Some statistics relating to abortion, as reported in the World Fertility Survey, can be found in Casterline and others (1984, table 19).

[2] Costa Rica (4.4 per cent of women currently in a union), Panama (3.6 per cent), Dominican Republic (2.2 per cent) (United Nations, 1984a, table A.II-1).

[3] Table 76 shows which countries asked about injectables.

[4] Countries that omitted questions about one or more methods are indicated in table 80. The questionnaire for Lesotho, reproduced in the main country report (Lesotho, 1981), indicates that although the question about contraceptive abstinence was asked, that method is not shown in the detailed tables of the report or on the standard recode tape used for this study.

[5] The possible counting of post-partum abstinence as contraception was eliminated in some sub-Saharan countries where lengthy abstinence is practised: Cameroon and Lesotho did not count abstinence as a contraceptive method.

[6] Two of the sub-Saharan countries, Mauritania and Senegal, did not inquire about post-partum abstinence; and any women currently abstaining would necessarily have been asked about current contraceptive use. Unlike Benin, which is discussed in the next paragraph, both countries recorded a low prevalence of contraceptive abstinence. One reason is that the typical period of post-partum abstinence is shorter in these countries than in Benin (see Schoenmaeckers and others, 1981), so that fewer women would report post-partum abstinence as a current contraceptive method. In Mauritania, reporting of abstinence was further discouraged by omission of probe questions about specific methods—abstinence is rarely mentioned spontaneously as a contraceptive method.

[7] Formerly called the Ivory Coast.

[8] In Benin, 10.5 per cent of currently married women were reported to be practising post-partum abstinence and currently using contraception. In Fiji, Haiti and the Philippines, the percentages were 1.8, 2.5 and 0.8, respectively. Of the overlap between contraception and post-partum abstinence, about 90 per cent in Benin, and about half in Haiti and the Philippines, was apparently due to post-partum abstinence being reported as contraception. In Fiji, the overlap was chiefly due to contraceptive sterilization, which is often performed post-partum. Some women who were coded as still abstaining post-partum were also coded as current practitioners of coitus-dependent methods, such as rhythm, withdrawal or condom, an inconsistency; such cases amounted to 1.4 per cent of the currently married in Benin and 1.1 per cent in Haiti.

[9] In several of the Latin American and Caribbean countries, the level of knowledge of an outlet may have been understated, because the questions about family planning outlets were asked before the questions about knowledge of specific methods. The latter series helped define the meaning of "family planning" and "contraception". Countries that posed the questions about knowledge of outlets first were Colombia, Costa Rica, Mexico, Panama, Trinidad and Tobago, and Venezuela. Effects of question order and wording are discussed more fully in Jones (1984).

[10] The estimated regression coefficients were as follows:

$$C = -2.62 + 0.16FP + 0.12DV$$

where C is the estimated percentage of currently married women currently using contraception; and FP and DV are, respectively, the family planning and development score values shown in the Introduction to this report. Standardized regression coefficients were 0.27 for the family planning score and 0.71 for the development score. R^2 for the regression was 0.82 ($N = 38$), and both predictors were significant at the 0.01 level. This cannot be viewed as an independent test of the relationships reported by Lapham and Mauldin (1984), since the family planning effort score employed here is based on that developed by those researchers, and Lapham and Mauldin employed World Fertility Survey data for some of the contraceptive prevalence measures in their analysis.

[11] The level of ever-use is shown, for each country, by age, in Sathar and Chidambaram (1984) and in Thompson and Chidambaram (1984).

[12] The population examined is restricted to exposed women because of this group's relevance to the estimation of unmet need for family planning services. (In addition, women who believed themselves to be infecund were not asked about desire for more children.) Reliance upon self-reported fecundity produces an overestimate of the actual percentage fecund (Vaessen, 1984), and this can have a large effect on estimates of unmet need. A range of estimates produced by varying assumptions about fecundity and other parameters is shown, for 18 of the countries examined here, in Westoff and Pebley (1981, 1984).

[13] Sterilized women were excluded from those considered "exposed" in the study of developed countries, but the effect of this was probably small, on average, because contraceptive sterilization was uncommon in most of the countries.

[14] The average percentage of married women who were exposed, wanted no more children and were not using any method of contraception for the four categories of development level, from low to high, is 14, 10, 17, and 17 per cent. For the four categories of family planning programme effort, from very weak or none to strong, the percentages are 10, 18, 18 and 17 per cent.

[15] Since, for reasons mentioned earlier, the level of use among women who want no more children usually exceeds that among women who want more, the ratio of the two proportions normally varies between zero and one. Assuming that many of the forces that limit the societal level of contraceptive practice, such as poor availability of family planning services, affect similar proportions of women who do and of those who do not want more children, the influence of common factors will tend to cancel when the ratio is formed, producing a measure that is relatively free of the confounding effects of factors that influence use for both spacing and limiting purposes.

[16] Since the focus here is directed towards breast-feeding as a determinant of the relative amount of contraceptive use for birth-spacing, attention is restricted to women who have had a chance to breast-feed, that is, women who have given birth.

[17] When the development score and the breast-feeding measure are included in a multiple regression predicting the value of the spacing index, neither predictor is statistically significant at the 0.05 level, even though, considered separately, both are highly significant.

[18] The analysis was conducted separately for each country, and the adjusted and unadjusted percentages using contraception were then averaged to produce figure 30. The categories of age, family size and desire for more children were the same as those shown in preceding tables of this chapter.

[19] The average difference in prevalence between exposed women aged 30-34 and those aged 40-49 is nine points before control for other variables and 10 points after.

[20] Information about knowledge of supply outlets for specific methods was available for eight of the countries: Benin; Egypt; Ghana; Morocco; Paraguay; the Philippines; the Sudan; Venezuela. The number of methods for which the question was asked varied from one (the pill, in Benin) to six in Ghana, with questions about the pill, intra-uterine device and female sterilization (in that order) being the most frequently asked. Detailed statistics for five countries are shown in Jones (1984).

[21] The index of dissimilarity (ID) for a pair of percentage distributions is calculated as:

$$ID = 1/2 \sum_{i=1}^{n} |P_{ai} - P_{bi}|$$

where n = the number of categories (in this case, the number of contraceptive methods);

$|P_{ai} - P_{bi}|$ = absolute value of the difference between distributions a and b, in the percentage in category i.

[22] Figure 35 is based on the countries where over 20 per cent of currently married women were currently using contraception, in order to eliminate countries with a very small number of users in particular age or family-size groups, for which random variations would be especially large. A multiple classification analysis was conducted for each country separately, and unadjusted and adjusted percentages were then averaged.

[23] This is not a universal pattern, but it is a very common one. Countries in which other methods (particularly condoms), as well as the pill, are markedly less common for users over 30 include Fiji, the Republic of Korea and Sri Lanka (United Nations, 1986, tables 6.A.4 and 6.A.5).

[24] It may be mentioned that in many countries a small number of childless women are coded as contraceptively sterilized (United Nations, 1986). Costa Rica and Panama recorded the highest levels—2 per cent of married women with no living children. While this may be correct, there may have been occasional cases of confusion between non-contraceptive and contraceptive sterilization, despite the surveys' attempts to separate the two. Costa Rica and Panama also recorded higher levels of sterilization for health reasons than did other countries (United Nations, 1984a).

[25] Using multiple classification analysis, as described above.

[26] The near constancy of the adjusted percentages is not observed in all countries (though it does appear in many); however, the differences in method choice by family size that remain after control for the other variables are inconsistent in direction from one country to the next and tend to cancel when the results are averaged.

[27] Based on currently married ever-users. Calculated from table 81 and United Nations (1986, table 6.A.3).

[28] The relevant questions were asked in several additional countries, but the information was not available on the data tapes used for this report.

[29] Since the surveys did not ascertain the date of first use, only the number of children at the time, the average duration since use is known only approximately. In tables 82 and 84, it was assumed that the answer to the question about children at first use referred to living children and that use began immediately after that number was attained (or at marriage if use began before the first birth). In fact, many women probably did not begin using immediately; average duration is therefore overestimated by several months, and average age at first use is underestimated. In order to derive the durations, additional assumptions were made about timing of child deaths and about date of use if use began before a pre-marital birth. Of course, women's ages and the birth dates of children employed in these calculations are themselves subject to misstatement, and women's recollection of family size at first use is likely to be imperfect.

[30] In Nepal, the average was only 0.5 child greater, a fact that may be partially explained by the unusually large proportion of users in Nepal who adopted sterilization as the first method (table 83), as well as by the shorter average time elapsed since first use.

[31] The failure rates reported by Goldman and others (1983) are conceptually similar to "extended-use failure rates" often calculated from follow-up survey data. Several assumptions were required in order to calculate such rates from the World Fertility Survey data. Information about ever-use of contraception in the open birth interval and in the last closed birth interval was available from the fertility regulation module for the countries included in the study. For most women, these two intervals represent at least the three years before the survey. The pregnancy rates discussed by Goldman and others include births conceived after contraception was abandoned (for any reason other than a desire to get pregnant) as well as births conceived while contraception was employed.

[32] In addition, at short durations since the preceding birth, part of the difference in pregnancy rates was apparently due to country differences in breast-feeding duration.

[33] The continuation ratios presented here differ conceptually from the various types of continuation rates usually presented in reports of follow-up survey data. The ratios given here show current use of the first method, or of any method, without regard to whether a pregnancy had occurred since use began. In addition, whereas follow-up surveys typically examine use over time for a cohort of acceptors, the tabulations presented here pertain only to current contraceptive practice of women who had accepted contraception at various times before the interview.

[34] It should be noted that the figures for Nepal are based on substantially fewer cases than were available for the other countries.

[35] Several studies show that past use of contraception, especially past use of non-supply methods, is less reliably reported than is current use (Laing, 1984). The data are consistent with the idea that brief or sporadic use tends to be underreported to a much greater extent than long-established or consistent use, though direct evidence of this is rarely available.

[36] Few other studies have presented continuation ratios that are conceptually comparable to those shown here. Most prospective or follow-up studies have shown continuation up to the point of an interruption in use of the first method or of any method, or up to the point of occurrence of a pregnancy. One study in Mexico was based on retrospective data from a survey which included more detailed questions about periods of use and non-use than did the World Fertility Survey. This study found that nearly the same proportion (about 72 per cent) of women were using contraception at any time between two and five years after acceptance. This is somewhat higher than the continuation ratio for Mexico shown in table 84 for the period from two to four years since first use; part of the difference is due to exclusion from table 84 of women whose first method was sterilization (Keller and others, 1981). A follow-up study in the Philippines found that continuation rates conceptually similar to those presented here (that is, calculated without regard for intervening pregnancies) declined slowly with duration, after the first year or so (Laing, 1978). Although this study indicated somewhat less constancy with increased duration than that shown in figure 37, this study's results also give grounds for thinking that large differences in overall continuation rates are unlikely to be due to differences in the average duration since first use, for average durations of two or more years. Neither of these studies was able to follow acceptors beyond four or five years since adoption of contraception.

[37] Note that these continuation ratios show current use of contraception among all currently married ever-users, unlike those in table 84, which were based on women who chose a reversible method first.

[38] On a world-wide basis, it is the most common method. See United Nations (1984); Liskin and others (1985).

References

Berent, Jerzy (1982). *Family planning in Europe and USA in the 1970s*. World Fertility Survey Comparative Studies, No. 20; ECE Analyses of WFS Surveys in Europe and USA. Voorburg, The Netherlands: International Statistical Institute.

Boulier, Bryan L. (1985). Family planning programs and contraceptive availability: their effects on contraceptive use and fertility. In Nancy Birdsall, ed., *The Effects of Family Planning Programs on Fertility in the Developing World*. World Bank Staff Working Papers, No. 677; Population and Development Series, No. 2. Washington, D.C.: The World Bank.

Casterline, John B. and others (1984). *The Proximate Determinants of Fertility*. World Fertility Survey Comparative Studies, No. 39. Voorburg, The Netherlands: International Statistical Institute.

Cleland, J. G. and I. Kalule-Sabiti (1984). Sexual activity within marriage: the analytic utility of World Fertility Survey data. World Fertility Survey Technical Bulletin, TECH. 2265. Voorburg, The Netherlands, International Statistical Institute (mimeographed).

Economic Commission for Europe (forthcoming). *Fertility and Family Planning in the ECE Region: A Comparative Analysis of WFS Surveys*.

Family Planning in the 1980's: Challenges and Opportunities (1981). Proceedings of the International Conference on Family Planning in the 1980's, Jakarta, Indonesia, 26-30 April 1980. New York: United Nations Fund for Population Activities, International Planned Parenthood Federation and Population Council.

Goldman, Noreen and others (1983). Contraceptive failure rates in Latin America. *International Family Planning Perspectives* 9(2):50-57.

Jones, Elise F. (1984). *The Availability of Contraceptive Services*. World Fertility Survey Comparative Studies, No. 37. Voorburg, The Netherlands: International Statistical Institute.

Keller, Alan and others (1981). Limitations of life table analysis: empirical evidence from Mexico. *Studies in Family Planning*, 12(10): 341-345.

Laing, John E. (1978). Estimating the effects of contraceptive use on fertility: techniques and findings from the 1974 Philippine National Acceptor Survey. *Studies in Family Planning* 9(6):150-162.

_____ (1984). Measurement of contraceptive protection for fertility analysis. Paper submitted to the Seminar on Integrating Proximate Determinants into the Analysis of Fertility Levels and Trends, organized by the International Union for the Scientific Study of Population and the World Fertility Survey, London, 29 April-1 May 1984.

Lapham, Robert J. and W. Parker Mauldin (1984). Family planning program effort and birthrate decline in developing countries. *International Family Planning Perspectives* 10(4):109-118.

Lesotho (1981). Ministry of Planning and Statistics. Central Bureau of Statistics. *Lesotho Fertility Survey, 1977: First Report*. Maseru.

Lightbourne, Robert E. (1985a). Individual preferences and fertility behaviour. In John Cleland and John Hobcraft, eds., in collaboration with Betzy Dinesen, *Reproductive Change in Developing Countries: Insights from the World Fertility Survey*. Oxford: Oxford University Press, 165-198.

_____ and Susheela Singh, with Cynthia P. Green (1982). *The World Fertility Survey: Charting Global Childbearing*. Population Bulletin, vol. 37, No. 1. Washington, D.C.: Population Reference Bureau.

Liskin, Laurie and others (1985). *Minilaparotomy and Laparoscopy: Safe, Effective and Widely Used*. Population Reports, Series C, No. 9. Baltimore, Maryland: Population Information Program of the Johns Hopkins University.

Mauldin, W. Parker and Bernard Berelson (1978). Conditions of fertility decline in developing countries, 1965-75. *Studies in Family Planning* 9(5):89-147.

Nortman, Dorothy L. (1982). Measuring the unmet need for contraception to space and limit births. *International Family Planning Perspectives* 8(4):125-134.

_____, with assistance of Joanne Fisher (1982). *Population and Family Planning Programs: A Compendium of Data Through 1981*. 11th ed. New York: The Population Council.

_____ and Gary L. Lewis (1984). A time model to measure contraceptive demand. In John A. Ross and Regina McNamara, eds., *Survey Analysis for the Guidance of Family Planning Programs*. Proceedings of a seminar sponsored by the International Union for the Scientific Study of Population, in collaboration with the World Fertility Survey and the National Family Planning Board of Malaysia; held at Genting Highlands, Malaysia, December 1981. Liège: Ordina Editions, 37-73.

Ross, John A. (1983). Birth control methods and their effects on fertility. In Rodolfo A. Bulatao and Ronald D. Lee, eds., with Paula E. Hollerbach and John Bongaarts, *Determinants of Fertility in Developing Countries*, vol. 2, *Fertility Regulation and Institutional Influences*. Report of the National Research Council Committee on Population and Demography, Panel on Fertility Determinants. New York: Academic Press, 54-88.

_____, Sawon Hong and Douglas H. Huber (1985). *International Factbook on Sterilization*. New York: Association for Voluntary Sterilization.

Sathar, Zeba A. and V. C. Chidambaram (1984.) *Differentials in Contraceptive Use*. World Fertility Survey Comparative Studies, No. 36; Cross-National Summaries. Voorburg, The Netherlands: International Statistical Institute.

Schearer, Bruce S. (1983). Monetary and health costs of contraception. In Rodolfo A. Bulatao and Ronald D. Lee, eds., with Paula E. Hollerbach and John Bongaarts, *Determinants of Fertility in Developing Countries*, vol. 2, *Fertility Regulation and Institutional Influence*. Report of the National Research Council Committee on Population and Demography, Panel on Fertility Determinants. New York: Academic Press, 89-150.

Schoenmaeckers, R. and others (1981). The child-spacing tradition and the postpartum taboo in tropical Africa: anthropological evidence. In Hilary J. Page and Ron Lesthaeghe, eds., *Child-Spacing in Tropical Africa: Traditions and Change*. London and New York: Academic Press, 25-71.

Singh, Susheela (1984). *Comparability of Questionnaires: Forty-one WFS Countries*. World Fertility Survey Comparative Studies, No. 32; Cross-National Summaries. Voorburg, The Netherlands: International Statistical Institute.

Thompson, Lauralee and V. C. Chidambaram (1984). Socio-economic differentials in contraceptive use. Additional tables for World Fertility Survey Comparative Studies; Cross-National Summaries. Voorburg, The Netherlands: International Statistical Institute (unpublished).

Tietze, Christopher (1983). *Induced Abortion: A World View 1983*. 5th ed. New York: The Population Council.

United Nations (1976). Department of Economic and Social Affairs. Population Division. *Fertility and Family Planning in Europe around 1970: A Comparative Study of Twelve National Surveys*. Population Studies, No. 58. New York.
   Sales No. E.76.XIII.2.

_____ (1984). Department of International Economic and Social Affairs. Population Division. *Report of the International Conference on Population, 1984*. Mexico City, 6-14 August 1984. New York.
   Sales No. E.84.XIII.8.

_____ (1984a). *Recent Levels and Trends of Contraceptive Use as Assessed in 1983*. Population Studies, No. 92. New York.
   Sales No. E.84.XIII.5.

_____ (1986). Contraceptive practice: collected findings from the World Fertility Survey data. Working paper ESA/P/WP.93. New York.

Vaessen, Martin (1981). Knowledge of contraceptives: an assessment of World Fertility Survey data collection procedures. *Population Studies* 35(3):357-373.

_____ (1984). *Childlessness and Infecundity*. World Fertility Survey Comparative Studies, No. 31; Cross-National Summaries. Voorburg, The Netherlands: International Statistical Institute.

Westoff, Charles F. and Anne R. Pebley (1981). Alternative measures of unmet need for family planning in developing countries. *International Family Planning Perspectives* 7(4):126-136.

_____ and Anne R. Pebley (1984). "The measurement of unmet need for family planning in developing countries. In John A. Ross and Regina McNamara, eds., *Survey Analysis for the Guidance of Family Planning Programs*. Proceedings of a seminar sponsored by the International Union for the Scientific Study of Population, in collaboration with the World Fertility Survey and the National Family Planning Board of Malaysia; held at Genting Highlands, Malaysia, December 1981. Liège: Ordina Editions, 11-36.

World Fertility Survey (1975). *Core Questionnaires*. World Fertility Survey Basic Documentation, No. 1. Voorburg, The Netherlands: International Statistical Institute.

VI. THE MAJOR PROXIMATE DETERMINANTS AND THEIR CONTRIBUTION TO FERTILITY

Abstract

This chapter employs a model developed by Bongaarts to relate the level and age pattern of fertility to three major proximate determinants of fertility discussed in earlier chapters. Indices of the fertility effect of marriage, C_m; post-partum infecundability, C_i (here estimated from the duration of breast-feeding); and contraception, C_c, are presented. The indices can, in theory, range from 0.0 to 1.0, with lower values indicating a greater fertility-reducing effect.

Although all three indices range widely in value, the index of contraception varies most, indicating the great importance of birth control in producing differences in national fertility levels. At the same time, for these 38 countries, on average, marriage and breast-feeding together are estimated to be responsible for a greater reduction of fertility levels from their theoretical maximum, if all the indices equalled 1.0. Mean values and ranges of the indices are as follows: for C_m the mean is 0.72 (low = 0.56, high = 0.89); for C_i the mean is 0.74 (low = 0.52, high = 0.91); and for C_c the mean is 0.80 (low = 0.43, high = 0.99). The practice of extended breast-feeding is declining in some developing countries, and the values of C_i shown here indicate that there is a considerable potential for fertility increase if the duration of breast-feeding declines without compensating increase in contraceptive practice. On average, however, countries where breast-feeding is brief tended to have lower fertility than others because they also tended to have substantial levels of contraceptive use and relatively late marriage.

All three proximate determinants, but especially the index of contraception, varied strongly according to level of development of the country. Controlling for development, the family planning programme score is significantly related to the contraception index, but not to C_m or C_i. This is as expected, since there is no reason to suppose that family planning programmes have a strong impact on fertility determinants other than contraception.

The three indices together are more successful at explaining cross-national fertility differences for younger than older women. Although reasons for this are unclear, one factor may be incomplete measurement of fertility control, including abortion, which is likely to be least important for young married women. In most countries, age-specific potential fertility rates (hypothetical rates in the absence of fertility-reducing effects of contraception, lactation and time outside marriage) are found to decline somewhat more rapidly with advancing age than in a model schedule of natural fertility based mainly on historical European population.

The level of fertility in every society falls below its maximum potential level through the direct operation of various factors limiting exposure to intercourse and exposure to conception, and through factors affecting pregnancy outcomes and the length of the post-partum infecundable period. These have been termed "intermediate" or, more recently, "proximate" determinants of fertility in contrast to more remote influences, such as education or cultural background; the latter factors influence fertility indirectly, through one or more of the proximate fertility determinants. The intermediate factors that control fertility are in themselves a closed system: all of the variance in fertility could be accounted for, if all of these factors could be measured. Thus, differentials and trends in fertility within a country and differences in fertility levels across countries can be directly traced to differences in these proximate variables if it can be assumed that the potential level of fertility is the same in all societies and all factors directly affecting fertility have been fully accounted for.

It was nearly 30 years ago that Davis and Blake (1956) first outlined a group of 11 such direct fertility determinants, falling into three larger categories: factors affecting exposure to intercourse; exposure to conception; and gestation and successful parturition. Some of these factors are subject to individual control, while others are not. One major shortcoming of this scheme was the omission of a fourth category of factors affecting the duration of post-partum infecundability, including, in particular, the duration of breast-feeding. This omission reflects the recency with which the influence of breast-feeding on birth intervals has received general recognition. Births are followed by a period of temporary sterility, the average duration of which is well approximated by the timing of return of menses: the duration of amenorrhoea following a birth averages only from 1.5 to 2 months for women who do not breast-feed, while periods of amenorrhoea averaging from 15 to 24 months have been reported in populations where the average duration of breast-feeding is two years or more (Léridon, 1977; Bongaarts and Potter, 1983). Since the mean duration of breast-feeding in the World Fertility Survey (WFS) countries reviewed here ranges from 5 to 33 months (chapter IV), this factor clearly should be considered in any attempt to explain fertility variations.

A major contribution due to Bongaarts (1978) was the development of a model in which the main proximate determinants could be measured and their relative effects on fertility quantified. While expanding the classification to include breast-feeding, Bongaarts restricted the factors to be considered to only the four most important variables: marriage (or one aspect of exposure to intercourse); contraception (or exposure to risk of conception); abortion (one aspect of gestational outcome); and breast-feeding (the most important determinant of the duration of infecundity following a birth). Other intermediate variables (such as primary and secondary sterility or infecundity, coital frequency, temporary separations between married couples and other reasons for involuntary abstinence) were excluded, largely on the basis of the expectation that their fertility impact would not vary greatly across populations.

Empirical analyses confirmed that most of fertility variation in the majority of countries can be explained by these four factors alone (Bongaarts, 1978, 1982; Bongaarts and Kirmeyer, 1982). The Bongaarts model utilizes this assumption of a closed system to summarize the effect of each factor on reducing fertility from its potential maximum to its actual level. Unfortunately, despite the known importance of abortion in many societies, this factor is usually excluded because, even when data on legal abortion rates are available, total abortion rates are poorly reported.

One result of this model is to produce estimates of the level of "natural" and "potential" fertility in a population. "Natural" fertility, as the term is employed here, is defined as the level of marital fertility expected if no restraints are placed on reproduction either through marriage or contraception, but where the effect of breast-feeding continues at the usual duration for that population. "Potential" fertility is defined as the level of fertility that would occur if none of the intermediate variables acted in any way to limit fertility. Since the age pattern of marital fertility rates is expected to be quite similar in shape among natural fertility populations (Henry, 1961), a standard age pattern of natural marital fertility (Coale and Trussell, 1978) can be compared with the pattern of "natural" and "potential" age-specific fertility rates, derived from the model, as a test of the extent to which contraceptive use, marriage and breast-feeding are sufficient to explain cross-country variations in the age pattern as well as in the overall level of fertility.

While other models for analysing the proximate determinants have also been proposed (Hobcraft and Little, 1984; Mosley, Werner and Becker, 1982; Gaslonde and Carrasco, 1982), the Bongaarts model has been by far the most widely employed. Its relatively modest data requirements, ease of application and robustness in the face of imprecise data make it particularly suited for a comparative analysis such as the present one (see Léridon and Ferry, 1985).

In this chapter, the Bongaarts model is applied to the WFS data with the aim of providing an overview of the relative contribution of each of the three main proximate determinants to the level of fertility and to cross-country differences in fertility. While certain countries collected information on other proximate determinants when they were seen to be potentially important (i.e., data on abortion in 6 countries, contemporary spousal separations in 7, post-partum abstinence in 16, sexual intercourse in 8 (Singh, 1984)), this information was not available for all countries and is not used for this comparative analysis. Whereas other chapters in this study have looked at variations in the importance of each proximate determinant in isolation (i.e., chapter III on nuptiality, chapter IV on breast-feeding and chapter V on contraceptive use), this chapter uses the model as a means of pulling together the three factors in a comparative context to analyse variations in the importance of each determinant in relation to the others in the aggregate and for individual age groups. The analysis focuses on groups of countries,[1] classified by region, level of socio-economic development and strength of family planning programme effort, but variations within groups and interesting individual country findings are also mentioned. The adequacy of the model is evaluated by examining the extent of variation between countries in the level and age pattern of potential fertility implied by the model.

A. The Bongaarts model of proximate determinants

This multiplicative model expresses the actual level of fertility (the total fertility rate, *TFR*) as a function of the fertility-reducing effects of the proximate determinants on a maximal potential level of fertility (the total fecundity rate, *TF*). This relationship may be summarized as follows:

$$TFR = C_m \cdot C_c \cdot C_a \cdot C_i \cdot TF \qquad (1)$$

where C_m is the index of marriage; C_c, the index of contraception; C_a, the index of abortion; and C_i, the index of infecundability. The value of each index can, in principle, vary between zero and one; actual variations occur within a smaller range, as discussed below. The relationship between actual and potential fertility may be considered from both ends of the equation. *TFR* may be estimated if only C_m, C_c, C_a and C_i are known, assuming that *TF* is about 15 children per woman.[2] Alternatively, *TF* may be estimated if *TFR*, C_m, C_c, C_a and C_i are all known. This estimated *TF* can then be compared with the expected value of roughly 15 as a means of evaluating the accuracy of the measurement of the indices and *TFR*; and ultimately, the adequacy of the fit of the model in particular countries. The intermediate stages in the movement from *TFR* to *TF* can also be expressed in terms of the indices. The total marital fertility rate, *TMFR*, for which the effect of marriage alone is removed, is:

$$TMFR = TFR/C_m = TF \cdot C_c \cdot C_i \cdot C_a \qquad (2)$$

The total natural marital fertility rate, *TN*, for which the effects both of marriage and of contraception and abortion (where relevant) are removed, is:

$$TN = TFR/(C_m \cdot C_c \cdot C_a) = TF \cdot C_i \qquad (3)$$

However, abortion, C_a, is omitted in this comparative analysis because it is inadequately measured in the WFS programme.

If the indices are not calculated using age-specific data, they can be simply obtained from the total rates of fertility, contraceptive use etc. Ideally, however, the model requires age-specific inputs for all indices, which was possible in the case of WFS because the individual-level data files were available. Therefore, in this analysis, all indices were calculated with age-specific inputs and weighted by the appropriate fertility rates. A full explanation of the construction of the indices is presented in the annex to this chapter. For the few countries where samples were restricted to ages 20-49 or 15-44, some special adjustments had to be made (Casterline and others, 1984).

To interpret the meaning of the indices it must be borne in mind that the complement of each index is equal to the proportionate reduction of fertility due to that particular index. For example, a value of 0.85 for C_i means that post-partum infecundability accounts for a 15 per cent reduction in fertility below its potential level. Thus, the lower the index, the stronger the implied effect on fertility.

The model assumes an ordering of the effects of the proximate determinants, which influences the weights used to calculate the indices: post-partum infecundability modifies total fecundity and C_i is therefore weighted by estimated age-specific total fecundity rates; contraceptive use modifies natural marital fertility and C_c is similarly weighted by estimated age-specific natural marital rates; nuptiality modifies observed marital fertility and C_m is therefore an index of the proportion married among five-year age groups weighted by observed marital fertility rates. The C_c index is based on age-specific proportions currently using contraception and the average effectiveness of methods used. Although originally conceived as an index of lactational infecundability (Bongaarts, 1978), C_i can readily be generalized to include other determinants of the post-partum non-susceptible period, particularly post-partum abstinence (Bongaarts and Potter, 1983; Adegbola and Page, 1982). In the present application, however, C_i is based solely on the mean length of breast-feeding, assuming a fixed relationship between breast-feeding duration and duration of lactational amenorrhoea. To measure the fertility impact of breast-feeding, the estimated duration of amenorrhoea is related to an assumed average live-birth interval of 20 months in the absence of breast-feeding.

The rationale underlying the construction of the indices, which is given in detail elsewhere (Bongaarts and Potter, 1983), draws upon earlier research intended to describe the main features of the process of reproduction by means of simple mathematical relations (see, in particular, Henry, 1972; Sheps and Menken, 1973; Léridon, 1977). The acceptance of the Bongaarts model by demographic researchers thus rests upon its logical connections to earlier research, as well as upon empirical demonstrations of the model's ability to explain fertility variations.

A few modifications in the model in this application were made to accommodate the particular characteristics of these data. Fertility rates and proportions married (years spent married in relation to total years lived) were based on the five-year period before interview, rather than on a one-year period, as required by the current-status model.[3] This was done because of the recognized instability of single-year rates from surveys with small sample sizes and because of known date-reporting errors for births in the most recent year. This wider period should not affect results, with one small exception: in a few countries where fertility declined rapidly during the five years preceding the survey, fertility will be overestimated in relation to the two current-status proximate variables, contraception (measured at time of survey) and breast-feeding (based on the preceding 24 months). A further modification, already discussed in chapter III, was to consider informal unions equivalent to legal marriage: thus, both consensual and visiting unions were included in marital exposure. Births that occurred outside marriage, thus defined, are not included in the analysis presented in this chapter. The total fertility rates shown below are therefore somewhat lower than those given in chapter I, where all births were included. Special treatment of rates for age group 15-19, described in the annex to this chapter, also affects the total marital fertility rates presented here.

A few additional measurement problems should be noted. The completeness of reporting of contraceptive use may vary among and within countries. Secondly, the effectiveness with which particular methods are used also probably varies. Lacking any better information, it is assumed that use-effectiveness weights derived from a survey in the Philippines (Laing, 1978) apply to all countries. A further area of uncertainty is the relationship between breast-feeding and lactational amenorrhoea: it is likely that variations in the length of the full breast-feeding segments of total breast-feeding duration affect the length of amenorrhoea (see table 70 in chapter IV) and should be considered in the conversion from breast-feeding to amenorrhoeic durations. However, the average total duration of breast-feeding in a population has been found to bear a very strong relation to the average duration of amenorrhoea; one study found that 96 per cent of cross-societal variation in duration of amenorrhoea could be explained by average duration of breast-feeding (Bongaarts and Potter, 1983).

B. Aggregate indices and their components

In this section, results are presented for all 38 WFS countries and for various groups of countries with respect to the three indices, their components and the levels of fertility implied when the effect of each proximate determinant is removed. Variations in the indices among these groups and, in addition, the relationship between the indices among countries, are examined using scatter-plots and regression. Components of the C_m and C_c indices are discussed, but the C_i index, whose only component is the duration of breast-feeding (dealt with in chapter IV), is not treated in any greater detail. The fertility rates, TFR, TMFR and TN, and the total fecundity rate, TF, as previously defined, are discussed with respect to their role in providing an alternative measure of the effect of the proximate determinants on fertility.

Previous research has found that the model fitted empirical data very well. An analysis of 41 populations (developing, developed and historical) found that 96 per cent of the variation in observed TFRs was accounted for by the four proximate determinants, including induced abortion (Bongaarts and Potter, 1983). A recent application to 29 WFS surveys (all developing countries) found that 70 per cent of the variation in observed TFRs was explained by the three proximate determinants, C_m, C_c and C_i, both when the model was exactly applied and when some measures were slightly modified (Casterline and others, 1984). It is likely that omission of the abortion index contributes to the lower explained variance, but other factors, including the particular groups of populations available for analysis, are probably important as well.[4] For the 40 countries included here, the proportion of variance explained is nearly identical, 71 per cent. Although this is not as good a fit as had been reported earlier, the variance explained is, nevertheless, quite high. These findings suggest that the model gives a reasonably good fit to empirical data and support its validity and general application.

Aggregate indices

The indices and their averages by region and country, level of development and strength of family planning programme effort, presented in table 86 and figures 39 and 40, reflect the group differentials in marriage, contraception and breast-feeding observed in earlier chapters.

The ability of each proximate determinant to explain fertility differences among countries depends upon the extent of variation in the index for that determinant. Of the three major determinants considered here, the index of contraception, C_c, varies the most, as can be seen from the box-and-whisker plot of figure 39: it ranges in value from 0.99 in Mauritania, implying virtually no deliberate fertility control, to 0.43 in Costa Rica. Both the index of marriage, C_m, and the index of post-partum infecundability, C_i, have values of from roughly 0.90 to 0.55. The interquartile range (length of the "box" in figure 39) is also largest for C_c.

The amount of variation in the indices, as well as their values, depends to some extent upon the group of countries chosen for analysis, although most regional and development groups show a considerable range of values for all three indices (figure 40). The greater uniformity of C_m in Latin America and the Caribbean and of C_i in Africa are exceptions. All regions show great internal ranges in C_c, but Asia and Oceania is exceptional in having wide variation, among its constituent countries, in all three indices.

TABLE 86. THE THREE INDICES AND THE TOTAL FERTILITY RATE, BY REGION AND COUNTRY, LEVEL OF DEVELOPMENT AND STRENGTH OF FAMILY PLANNING PROGRAMME EFFORT

	Index of marriage C_m (1)	Index of contraception C_c (2)	Index of post-partum infecundability C_i (3)	$C_c \times C_i$ (4)	Total fertility rate TFR (5)
A. Region and country					
Africa					
Benin	0.840	0.884	0.645	0.570	6.80
Cameroon	0.802	0.982	0.682	0.670	5.66
Côte d'Ivoire[a]	0.841	0.978	0.656	0.642	6.75
Egypt	0.707	0.810	0.683	0.553	5.21
Ghana	0.819	0.923	0.666	0.615	6.22
Kenya	0.790	0.944	0.695	0.656	7.40
Lesotho	0.740	0.958	0.645	0.618	5.27
Mauritania	0.749	0.995	0.706	0.702	5.87
Morocco	0.723	0.840	0.732	0.615	5.82
Senegal	0.860	0.980	0.661	0.648	6.90
Sudan	0.761	0.962	0.694	0.668	5.93
Tunisia	0.655	0.747	0.742	0.554	5.83
AVERAGE	0.781	0.921	0.682	0.628[b]	6.14
Latin America and the Caribbean					
Colombia	0.602	0.633	0.846	0.536	4.27
Costa Rica	0.567	0.432	0.908	0.392	3.17
Dominican Republic	0.689	0.697	0.852	0.594	5.39
Ecuador	0.656	0.709	0.782	0.554	4.98
Guyana	0.733	0.722	0.890	0.643	4.75
Haiti	0.646	0.862	0.726	0.626	5.15
Jamaica	0.739	0.641	0.851	0.545	4.52
Mexico	0.684	0.730	0.842	0.615	5.93
Panama	0.618	0.508	0.850	0.432	3.84
Paraguay	0.626	0.711	0.811	0.577	4.56
Peru	0.629	0.755	0.769	0.581	5.35
Trinidad and Tobago	0.702	0.569	0.887	0.505	3.18
Venezuela	0.635	0.580	0.865	0.502	4.36
AVERAGE	0.656	0.658	0.837	0.551[b]	4.57
Asia and Oceania					
Bangladesh	0.888	0.930	0.524	0.487	5.96
Fiji	0.688	0.672	0.835	0.561	4.14
Indonesia	0.752	0.771	0.574	0.443	4.51
Jordan	0.755	0.797	0.807	0.643	7.63
Malaysia	0.635	0.736	0.901	0.663	4.62
Nepal	0.850	0.976	0.567	0.553	6.12
Pakistan	0.814	0.960	0.657	0.631	6.24
Philippines	0.605	0.739	0.769	0.568	5.12
Republic of Korea	0.597	0.753	0.697	0.525	4.23

TABLE 86 (continued)

	Index of marriage C_m (1)	Index of contraception C_c (2)	Index of post-partum infecundability C_i (3)	$C_c \times C_i$ (4)	Total fertility rate TFR (5)
Asia and Oceania (continued)					
Sri Lanka	0.558	0.771	0.613	0.473	3.70
Syrian Arab Republic	0.744	0.836	0.786	0.657	7.46
Thailand	0.656	0.688	0.662	0.455	4.55
Yemen	0.857	0.989	0.799	0.790	8.43
AVERAGE	0.727	0.811	0.709	0.575[b]	5.51
B. Level of development					
I. High	0.655	0.634	0.852	0.540[b]	4.27
II. Middle-high	0.669	0.745	0.757	0.564	5.37
III. Middle-low	0.782	0.908	0.666	0.605	5.89
IV. Low	0.807	0.949	0.664	0.630	6.38
C. Strength of family planning programme effort					
1. Strong	0.645	0.654	0.803	0.525	4.27
2. Moderate	0.661	0.714	0.740	0.528	4.64
3. Weak	0.746	0.818	0.728	0.596	5.56
4. Very weak/none	0.778	0.908	0.713	0.647	6.36
ALL COUNTRIES	0.721	0.796	0.741	0.590	5.41

Source: World Fertility Survey standard recode tapes.
NOTES: See annex for derivation of indices. Means for groups of countries include Nigeria and Turkey, for which values are not shown separately.
[a] Formerly called the Ivory Coast.
[b] Group average values of $C_c \times C_i$ are computed from group averages of C_c and C_i.

Figure 39. **Summary distribution of values of the three C indices**

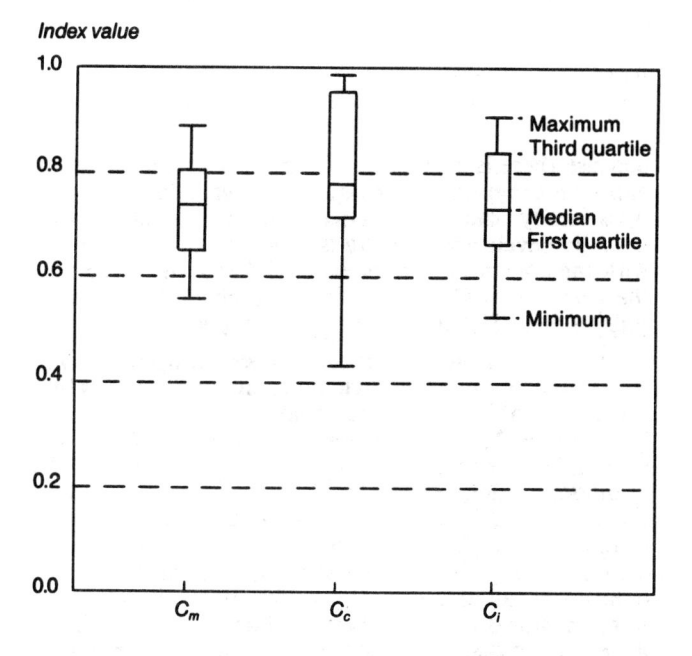

Source: Table 86.
NOTE: C_m = index of marriage; C_c = index of contraception; C_i = index of post-partum infecundability.

Turning to the average values of the indices, the reduction in sexual exposure through the timing of unions can be seen to have its strongest effect on fertility in Latin America and the Caribbean, where the C_m factor alone brings fertility roughly 35 per cent below its potential level (table 86). Both of the other two regions show a smaller effect of this proximate determinant. Interestingly, countries with a higher level of socio-economic development also show a greater effect of reduced marital exposure than the less developed countries, which may be expected with the rising age at marriage that frequently accompanies development. Instead of a steady decrease in C_m with increasing development, however, countries fall into two groups, with the two upper development groups, I and II, and the two lower groups, III and IV, showing similar effects of marriage. Groups of countries with different levels of family planning programme effort also show some variation in the importance of marital exposure, but this is probably due to the association between greater family planning effort and higher development rather than to any direct relationship between family planning effort and marriage patterns.

Over all, breast-feeding provides approximately the same degree of fertility restraint as time spent outside marriage, each factor tending to reduce fertility from its potential level by an average of 26-28 per cent. Even in the most economically advanced of these countries (development group I) breast-feeding makes a 15 per cent contribution, though the effect is substantially larger, 24 per cent, in group II and about 33 per cent in both groups III and IV. Africa and Asia and Oceania both have relatively large breast-feeding effects of roughly 30 per cent.

An interesting offsetting of the effect of contraception against the effect of post-partum infecundability can be observed in all three sets of groups: the stronger the average effect of contraception, the weaker is the effect of infecundability. However, while the extreme groups in each set exemplify this relationship, it is nevertheless worth noting that a fairly strong impact of post-partum infecundability may coexist with moderate levels of contraception, as in the case of Asian countries, the middle-high development group and countries with moderate or weak family planning programme effort.

On balance, the fertility-reducing effects of the higher levels of contraceptive use associated with higher levels of development substantially outweigh the fertility-increasing effects of declining breast-feeding duration.

Figure 40. Distribution of the three C indices within regional and development groups

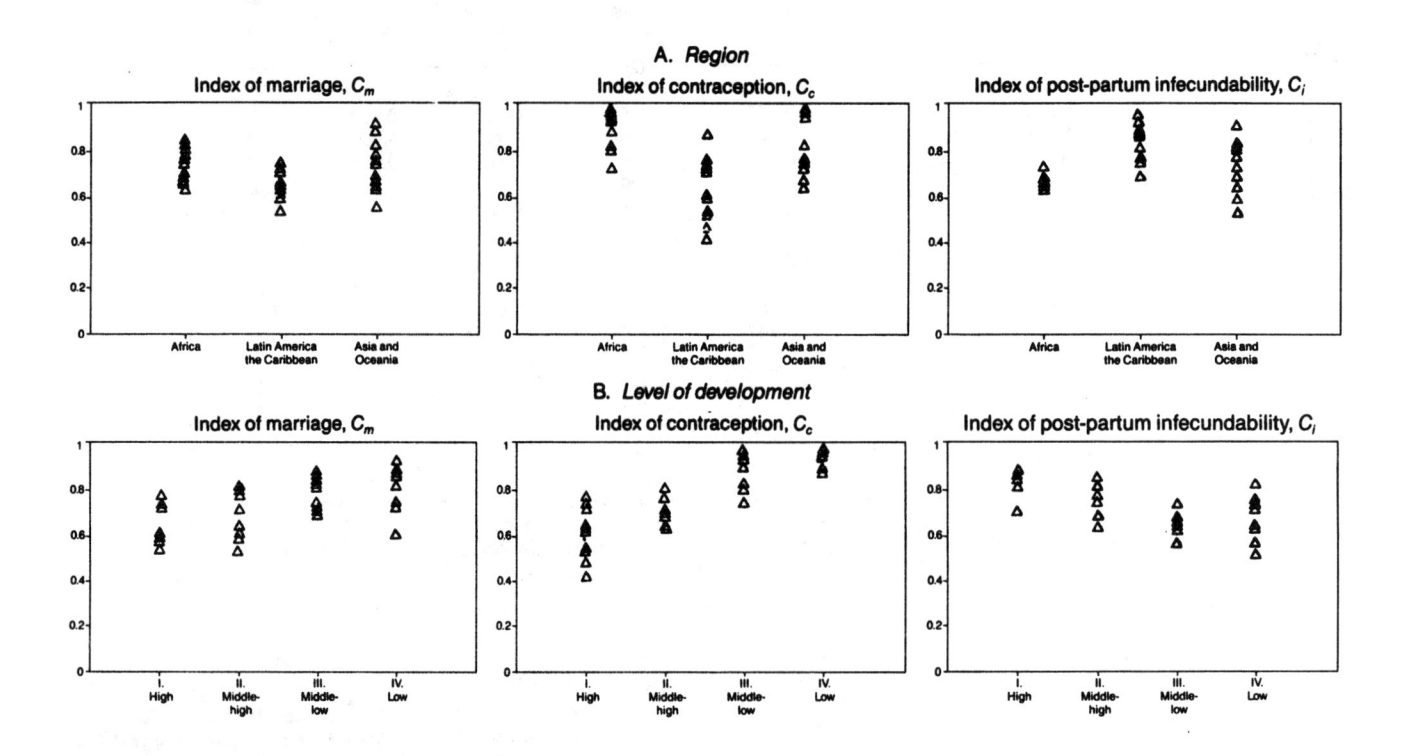

A. *Region*

B. *Level of development*

Source: Table 86.

This can be seen in table 86 from the values of $C_c \times C_i$, which represent relative levels of marital fertility as predicted by the three-factor model (see equation 2 excluding abortion).[5] For instance, the model indicates that the combined effects of breast-feeding and contraception ($C_c \times C_i$) serve to produce marital fertility that is 17 per cent higher in development group IV than in group I ($0.17 = (0.630/0.540) - 1$). None the less, the countervailing effect of lactation is quite large, since differences in contraceptive practice between the extreme development groups, acting in isolation, would produce fertility levels about 50 per cent higher in group IV than in group I ($0.48 = (0.949/0.643) - 1$). Similarly, longer lactation in countries of Asia and Oceania than in Latin America and the Caribbean greatly narrows the fertility difference that would otherwise be expected from the higher level of contraceptive practice in the latter region.

Since strong family planning programmes are more common in the upper development groups, it is not clear from table 86 whether family planning effort has a separate effect on any of the proximate determinants. To investigate this, each of the C indices was regressed on the actual development and family planning programme score values presented in the Introduction to this report. Although the development score was found to have a strong and highly statistically significant relationship with all three indices (assuming that the WFS countries can for present purposes be treated as a random sample of developing countries), the family planning score was statistically significantly related, at the 0.05 probability level, only to the contraception index when the development score was included in the analysis. This is reassuring, because there is no reason to expect an effect of family planning programmes on aspects of reproduction other than family planning practice. The analysis also shows that the development score is more strongly associated with the contraception index, explaining 76 per cent of the variance in C_c, than with the infecundity and marriage indices (57 and 43 per cent, respectively).[6]

The relationships observed between group means are also found among the individual countries. Figures 41-43 show pairs of indices plotted against each other, for the 38 countries. Where marriage has a stronger effect, post-partum infecundability has a weaker one (the twin results of modernization); similarly, where contraception is more powerful, infecundability is less so; and a strong effect of marriage is generally accompanied by a strong effect of contraception. However, within the regions (the figures indicate regional groups by different symbols), these relationships do not always hold. For example, in Latin America and the Caribbean (see figure 41), little relationship was found between marriage and contraception. This is so partially because of the mixture of the Caribbean countries, which have weaker marriage effects (C_m is from 0.65 to 0.74), with other Latin American countries with C_m from 0.56 to 0.68, while as a group these countries span a wide range of contraception effects: C_c is from 0.43 (Costa Rica) to 0.86 (Haiti) (see table 86). In Africa (see figure 42), the effect of contraception varies without much change in infecundability. This is due to the importance of contraception in the Northern African countries, Egypt, Morocco and Tunisia, compared with its very low level in sub-Saharan countries, while breast-feeding remains almost as important in these three coun-

Figure 41. **Scatter-plot of indices for marriage, C_m, and contraception, C_c, for 38 World Fertility Survey countries**

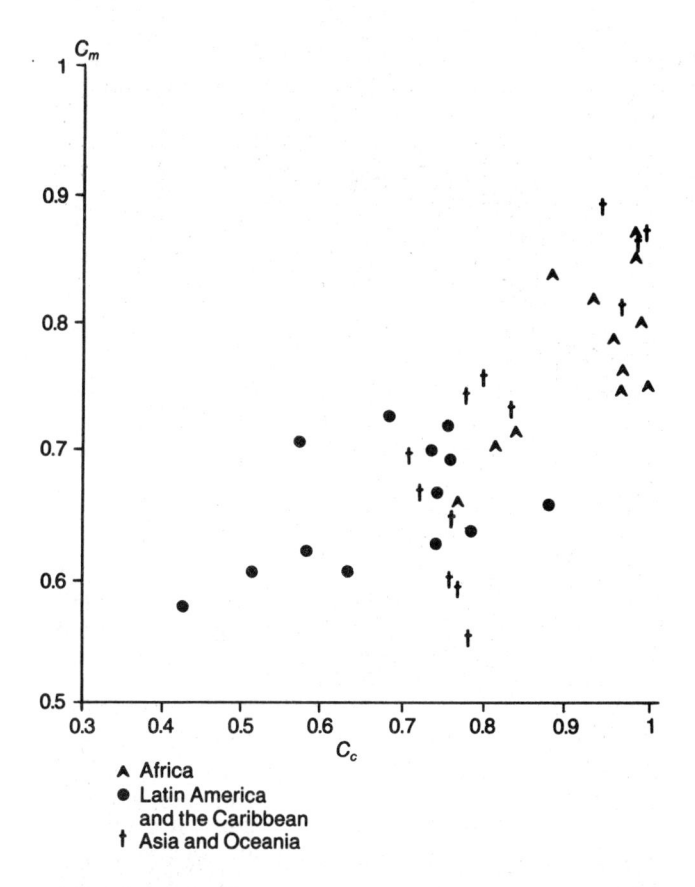

▲ Africa
● Latin America and the Caribbean
† Asia and Oceania

Source: Table 86.

Figure 42. **Scatter-plot of indices for contraception, C_c, and post-partum infecundability, C_i, for 38 World Fertility Survey countries**

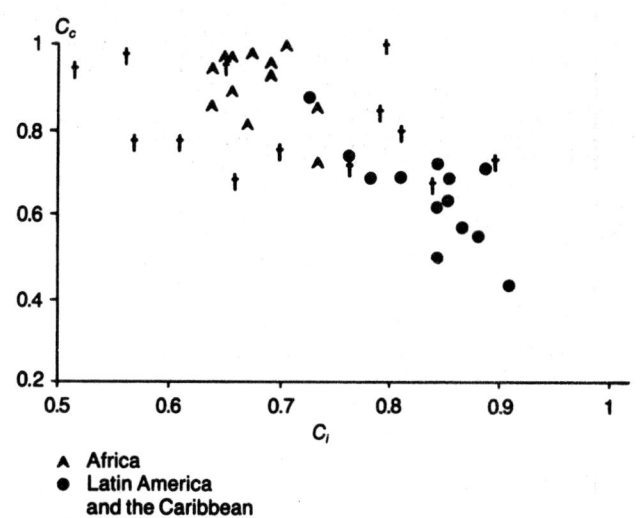

▲ Africa
● Latin America and the Caribbean
† Asia and Oceania

Source: Table 86.

Figure 43. **Scatter-plot of indices for marriage, C_m, and post-partum infecundability, C_i, for 38 World Fertility Survey countries**

▲ Africa
● Latin America and the Caribbean
† Asia and Oceania

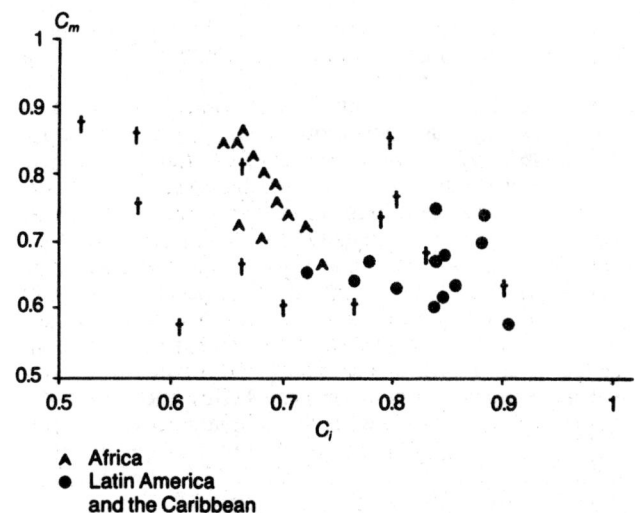

Source: Table 86.

tries (C_i is from 0.68 to 0.74) as in the sub-Saharan countries (C_i ranges from 0.65 to 0.70). On the other hand, in a fair number of countries in Asia and Oceania, a moderate level of contraception is combined with widely varying levels of infecundability. For example, in Indonesia and Sri Lanka, the contraception effect is 0.77 and breast-feeding effects are from 0.57 to 0.61. This compares with Jordan, Malaysia and the Republic of Korea, where similar contraception effects of from 0.74 to 0.80 (C_c) are combined with breast-feeding effects of only 0.70-0.90 (C_i). The examples of Indonesia and Sri Lanka are particularly interesting and suggest that some culturally based behaviour (long breast-feeding, in this case) may remain significant while other changes occur (rise in contraception and/or in the age at marriage).

The strength of these relationships is summarized in table 87 for groups of countries defined by region, level of development and strength of family planning programme effort, as well as for all countries considered together. The coefficient of determination, R^2, measures the strength of linear association between pairs of indices. The direction of the relationship, positive or negative, is also shown for each group of countries and, for all 40 countries, the regression coefficients represent the slope of the best fitting orthogonal regression line.[7]

Turning first to the strength of association between pairs of indices for all 40 countries, it can be seen that the strongest relationship is between C_m and C_c, with a little over half the variance in one index "explained" by the other ($R^2 = 0.55$). Correlations between C_c and C_i ($R^2 = 0.36$) and C_m and C_i ($R^2 = 0.29$) are notably lower, and the relationship between C_m and the composite marital-fertility factor ($C_c \cdot C_i$) is weaker still

TABLE 87. PROPORTION OF VARIANCE EXPLAINED, DIRECTION OF RELATIONSHIP AND ORTHOGONAL REGRESSION COEFFICIENTS FOR PAIRS OF INDICES, FOR ALL COUNTRIES, BY REGION, LEVEL OF DEVELOPMENT AND STRENGTH OF FAMILY PLANNING PROGRAMME EFFORT

	Number of countries	C_m regressed on C_c Coefficient (sign)	R^2	C_m regressed on C_i Coefficient (sign)	R^2	C_c regressed on C_i Coefficient (sign)	R^2	C_m regressed on $C_c \cdot C_i$ Coefficient (sign)	R^2
All countries	40[a]	0.28	0.55	−0.77	0.29	−3.55	0.36	2.07	0.21

A. Region

Africa	13	(+)	0.20	(−)	0.53	(−)	0.10	(+)	0.10
Latin America and the Caribbean	13	(+)	0.09	(+)	0.01	(−)	0.61	(+)	0.31
Asia and Oceania	14	(+)	0.60	(−)	0.11	(−)	0.06	(+)	0.08

B. Level of development

| I-II High or Middle-high | 22 | (+) | 0.11 | (+) | 0.01 | (−) | 0.32 | (+) | 0.27 |
| III-IV Middle-low or low | 18 | (+) | 0.17 | (−) | 0.12 | (+) | 0.06 | .. | 0.00 |

C. Strength of family planning programme effort

| 1-2. Strong to moderate | 15 | (+) | 0.05 | (−) | 0.01 | (−) | 0.52 | (+) | 0.03 |
| 3-4. Weak to very weak/none | 25 | (+) | 0.43 | (−) | 0.46 | (−) | 0.37 | (+) | 0.04 |

Source: Table 86.
NOTES: Regressions use logit transformation of the indices. C_m = index of marriage; C_c = index of contraception; C_i = index of post-partum infecundability.
[a] Including Nigeria and Turkey. See note 1 to this chapter.

($R^2 = 0.21$). The weaker association between the marital fertility and marriage factors than between C_m and either C_c or C_i considered separately reflects the tendency of the latter two factors to offset each other. None the less, it can be noted that the positive sign of the relationship between C_m and the marital fertility factor appears within most groups of countries, suggesting a weak but quite widespread tendency among developing countries for late marriage to occur together with relatively low marital fertility. Similarly, the direction of relationship between C_m and C_c, C_m and C_i, and C_c and C_i is usually the same within the various groups of countries as for all 40 considered together.

Weak relationships within groups might be anticipated in that the regional, development and family planning groups are likely to divide the sample of countries in ways that control to an extent some of the factors that cause the proximate determinants to co-vary. Indeed, for each pair of indices, R^2 is usually lower within groups of countries than when all 40 are considered together. This is more consistently the case for level of development than for the others, however, and some exceptions of relatively high correlations are apparent. Within Asia and Oceania, the C_m, C_c correlation is relatively strong, as is the association between C_m and C_i within Africa and within the group of countries with weak family planning effort. The correlation between C_c and C_i is pronounced in Latin America and the Caribbean and in the countries with relatively strong family planning effort.

The orthogonal regression coefficients shown at the top of table 87 indicate the average amount of change in one index expected for a one-unit change in another index.[8] For example, the coefficient of 0.28 for C_m regressed on C_c shows that a one-unit increase in C_c (rescaled using the logit transformation) is associated with a much smaller 0.28 increase in C_m (or, alternatively, that a one-unit increase in C_m is associated with a 1/0.28 = 3.5 increase in C_c). The coefficient of −3.55 for C_c regressed on C_i indicates that the higher contraceptive practice that is associated with shorter breast-feeding duration is itself sufficient to offset by roughly 3.5 times the fertility-increasing effect of longer breast-feeding. Furthermore, differences in marriage between countries with long and short breast-feeding are themselves large enough, on average, to offset about 80 per cent of the fertility-increasing effect of shorter breast-feeding.

Although the regression coefficients do indicate overcompensating differences of the other indices, and particularly C_c, when breast-feeding is short, it should be recalled that these coefficients apply only on average and that the values of R^2 indicate that the inter-country associations are only from weak to moderate in strength. For instance, as noted earlier, it is not difficult to find particular countries in which longer-than-average breast-feeding occurs in conjunction with above-average contraceptive use. More generally, figures 40-42 show many cases in which a narrow range of values of any one index is associated with a wide range of values in the others. It is of interest to note in this connection that stronger covariation between the indices (higher value of R^2) was found in a study of within-country rural/urban and education differentials in the indices (Casterline and others, 1984). The authors suggest that this is due to the implicit control, when differentials are analysed, for a variety of country-specific factors that are not held constant in the national-level analysis reported here. Both approaches find the same direction of relationships and find differences in C_c that more than compensate for opposing differences in C_i, but the precise amount of estimated "response" in one index to change in another is sensitive both to the level of analysis (national or within-country differentials) and to the group of countries chosen for analysis.

A different perspective for evaluating the relative importance of each proximate determinant is to consider its percentage contribution to the difference between the total fertility rate and the estimated total fecundity rate derived from the model. A simple decomposition of the difference between the observed total fertility rate and the estimated total fecundity rate, using a logarithmic transformation, is presented in table 88. Across all

TABLE 88. RELATIVE PERCENTAGE CONTRIBUTION OF EACH OF THE PROXIMATE DETERMINANTS TO THE DIFFERENCE BETWEEN THE TOTAL FECUNDITY RATE AND THE TOTAL FERTILITY RATE, BY REGION, LEVEL OF DEVELOPMENT AND STRENGTH OF FAMILY PLANNING PROGRAMME EFFORT

	Total	Marriage	Contraception	Post-partum infecundability	TF − TFR	TFR/TF
A. Region
Africa	100	35	12	54	6.49	0.49
Latin America and the Caribbean	100	41	41	18	8.26	0.36
Asia and Oceania	100	37	24	39	7.76	0.41
B. Level of development
I. High	100	41	44	15	7.92	0.35
II. Middle-high	100	41	30	29	8.82	0.37
III. Middle-low	100	33	13	54	6.59	0.47
IV. Low	100	32	8	61	6.24	0.51
C. Strength of family planning programme effort
1. Strong	100	40	39	20	8.70	0.33
2. Moderate	100	39	32	29	8.82	0.34
3. Weak	100	36	25	39	7.27	0.43
4. Very weak/none	100	37	14	49	6.38	0.50
ALL COUNTRIES	100	38	27	35	7.51	0.42

Source: Table 86.

NOTE: The percentage contribution of each index to the difference between the total fecundity rate and the total fertility rate is calculated as follows:

$$100 \, (\log C_x / (\log C_i + \log C_m + \log C_c))$$

where, for C_x, values of C_i, C_m and C_c are successively employed.

countries, marriage and breast-feeding are seen to be more important than contraception (38, 35 and 27 per cent, respectively) in reducing fertility below its potential level but this ranking of effects varies significantly across the groups. For Latin America and the Caribbean, and the two upper levels of development and of family planning programme effort, contraception accounts for a greater percentage of the fertility reduction than breast-feeding. In fact, in development group I, contraceptive use is the most important factor in explaining the reduction in fertility below its potential level. For all groups, marriage is an important cause of reduction in fertility —contributing from 32 to 41 per cent. In Africa, as well as in the low development group and the very weak family planning group, breast-feeding is the most important fertility-reducing factor, ranging from 9 to 61 per cent.

Components of the indices

The marriage index contains two components, the proportion of time since the first marriage, C_{em}, and the proportion of time spent between unions, C_{ds}. The first reflects the age at first marriage while the second measures the level of divorce, separation and widowhood. Table 89 shows these two components as indices themselves, the difference between C_{em} and C_{ds} being C_m.[9]

There is little variation in the dissolution component across groups, except for its greater than average importance in Latin America and the Caribbean, and less than average level in Asia and Oceania. Given the systems of marriage in these two regions (a high proportion of informal, short-duration unions in the former, compared with legal marriage being the main type of union, with generally low levels of divorce and separation, in the latter), these differences are to be expected. The differences are even more important because they are concentrated at younger ages, where fertility is concentrated, and therefore dissolution at these ages is more heavily weighted. Apart from this partial exception, however, the broad conclusion from these results is that variation in the age at marriage accounts for most of the observed differences between groups in the effect of marital exposure on fertility and that periods of dissolution are relatively unimportant.

Table 89 also shows the two main components of the contraception index, the percentage currently using any method; and the average effectiveness weight, which has a maximum of 1.0, when all users are using 100 per cent effective methods. In evaluating these indices, however, it should be kept in mind that the effectiveness index is entirely a function of the method mix reported in use; the effectiveness weights applied are specific for each method and the same for all countries. No data are available that measure variations in the effectiveness with which particular methods are used across countries. Effectiveness weights show some variation among groups, due to the greater tendency to use more efficient methods in Latin America and the Caribbean and in Asia and Oceania, compared with Africa, and in the more developed countries or those with stronger family planning effort, compared with lower-ranking groups. While average effectiveness is noticeably lower among countries with very weak or no family planning effort (0.78), it remains about the same for the other three groups (0.84-0.87) and does not show a systematic increase as family planning effort increases. It is clear that the percentage currently using is the important determinant of variation in the index of contraception, not the method mix. The percentage using is directly reflected in group differences in the C_c index discussed earlier.

Potential fertility rates

It is instructive to look at the effect of these proximate determinants from a different perspective: what would the average family size be, if all women had maximum exposure within marriage (TMFR), if in addition no one used contraception (TN) and further, if no one breast-fed

TABLE 89. COMPONENTS OF THE INDICES OF MARRIAGE AND CONTRACEPTION, BY REGION AND COUNTRY, LEVEL OF DEVELOPMENT AND STRENGTH OF FAMILY PLANNING PROGRAMME EFFORT

	Index of ever-marriage C_{em} (1)	Index of dissolution C_{ds} (2)	Percentage currently using (3)	Average contraception-effectiveness (4)
A. Region				
Africa	0.827	0.063	9.0	0.789
Latin America and the Caribbean	0.709	0.089	36.5	0.845
Asia and Oceania	0.742	0.042	21.1	0.849
B. Level of development				
I. High	0.696	0.069	39.3	0.861
II. Middle-high	0.676	0.053	29.0	0.833
III. Middle-low	0.839	0.070	10.1	0.795
IV. Low	0.859	0.069	6.2	0.817
C. Strength of family planning programme effort				
1. Strong	0.681	0.065	37.0	0.857
2. Moderate	0.680	0.061	30.6	0.870
3. Weak	0.785	0.070	20.2	0.840
4. Very weak/none	0.822	0.061	10.6	0.782
ALL COUNTRIES	0.759	0.064	22.2	0.828

Source: World Fertility Survey standard recode tapes.

NOTE: The two marriage indices, C_{em} and C_{ds}, are based on current marital status data and, therefore, are not strictly comparable with C_m presented in table 86, which is based on status during the five years preceding the survey.

(TF)? These hypothetical levels of fertility are shown for individual countries and groups of countries in table 90. The assumption that all women were married throughout their reproductive life, and bearing children at the same rate as currently married women (TMFR), is alone sufficient to smooth out group differences and even to change the ranking of development groups (see middle-high group II), as well as to raise fertility across all countries by nearly 40 per cent, from 5.4 to 7.5 children, on average. Assuming that no contraception was used (TN), the fertility of groups that currently have quite high use is, naturally, most affected—Latin America and the Caribbean, development groups I and II, and the two upper family planning effort groups. In fact, the original differentials are reversed when the fertility-reducing effects of contraception are removed.

The final assumption of no breast-feeding (TF) would be expected to produce the same level of potential fertility in all groups, barring any true differences in fecundity. The average level of estimated total fecundity derived from these data is 13, roughly two children per woman fewer than the total fecundity rate estimated by Bongaarts using data from countries where abortion was not expected to be a significant factor. The lower average level of potential fertility reported here is probably due mainly to the restriction of the present analysis to "within-union" fertility and to technical differences in construction of some of the indices, particularly the marriage index.[10] An analysis based on 29 of the WFS countries (Casterline and others, 1984) found an average level of potential fertility of 13.1 births per woman using the methods of index construction adopted here (see annex) but 14.5 births per woman using the procedures employed by Bongaarts to construct C_m, C_c and C_i.

Variation between countries in the derived total fecundity rate, on the other hand, is an indication that the three indices considered here do not completely explain national differences in fertility. Table 90 shows that TF ranges

TABLE 90. TOTAL FERTILITY RATE, TOTAL MARITAL FERTILITY RATE, TOTAL NATURAL MARITAL FERTILITY RATE AND TOTAL FECUNDITY RATE, BY REGION AND COUNTRY, LEVEL OF DEVELOPMENT AND STRENGTH OF FAMILY PLANNING PROGRAMME EFFORT

	Total fertility rate, TFR	Total marital fertility rate, TMFR	Total natural marital fertility rate, TN	Total fecundity rate, TF
A. Region and country				
Africa				
Benin	6.80	8.10	9.17	14.20
Cameroon	5.66	7.06	7.18	10.54
Côte d'Ivoire[a]	6.75	8.03	8.21	12.52
Egypt	5.21	7.37	9.10	13.32
Ghana	6.22	7.59	8.22	12.35
Kenya	7.40	9.37	9.92	14.27
Lesotho	5.27	7.12	7.43	11.52
Mauritania	5.87	7.84	7.88	11.16
Morocco	5.82	8.05	9.58	13.08
Senegal	6.90	8.02	8.19	12.39
Sudan	5.93	7.79	8.10	11.67
Tunisia	5.83	8.90	11.92	16.06
AVERAGE	6.14	7.88	8.64	12.64
Latin America and the Caribbean				
Colombia	4.27	7.09	11.20	13.24
Costa Rica	3.17	5.59	12.95	14.26
Dominican Republic	5.39	7.82	11.22	13.17
Ecuador	4.98	7.59	10.71	13.69
Guyana	4.75	6.48	8.98	10.09
Haiti	5.15	7.97	9.25	12.73
Jamaica	4.52	6.12	9.55	11.22
Mexico	5.93	8.67	11.87	14.09
Panama	3.84	6.21	11.72	14.38
Paraguay	4.56	7.29	10.26	12.65
Peru	5.35	8.51	11.27	14.66
Trinidad and Tobago	3.18	4.53	7.96	8.97
Venezuela	4.36	6.87	11.84	13.68
AVERAGE	4.57	6.98	10.67	12.83
Asia and Oceania				
Bangladesh	5.96	6.71	7.21	13.75
Fiji	4.14	6.02	8.95	10.73
Indonesia	4.51	6.00	7.77	13.54
Jordan	7.63	10.11	12.68	15.72
Malaysia	4.62	7.28	9.88	10.97
Nepal	6.12	7.20	7.38	13.03
Pakistan	6.24	7.67	7.99	12.15
Philippines	5.12	8.46	11.46	14.90
Republic of Korea	4.23	7.09	9.42	13.51
Sri Lanka	3.70	6.63	8.60	14.04
Syrian Arab Republic	7.46	10.03	12.00	15.27
Thailand	4.55	6.94	10.08	15.23
Yemen	8.43	9.84	9.96	12.46
AVERAGE	5.51	7.55	9.37	13.28
B. Level of development				
I. High	4.27	6.49	10.31	12.18
II. Middle-high	5.28	7.92	10.76	14.10
III. Middle-low	5.89	7.53	8.31	12.48
IV. Low	6.38	7.91	8.35	12.62
C. Strength of family planning programme effort				
1. Strong	4.27	6.65	10.32	12.97
2. Moderate	4.64	7.03	9.81	13.47
3. Weak	5.56	7.48	9.31	12.83
4. Very weak/none	6.36	8.18	9.14	12.73
ALL COUNTRIES	5.41	7.47	9.55	12.92

Source: World Fertility Survey standard recode tapes.
NOTE: Means for groups of countries include Nigeria and Turkey, for which values are not separately shown. For derivation of rates, see annex.
[a] Formerly called the Ivory Coast.

from approximately 9 births per woman in Trinidad and Tobago to 16 in Tunisia. Three quarters of the countries fall in the narrower range of 11-15 (and the central half between 12.2 and 14.2). The variations in total fecundity rates are probably due to a combination of factors, including omitted proximate determinants; imperfections in the underlying fertility, marriage, contraception and breast-feeding data; and approximations involved in estimating the indices from the data.

Abortion is the one factor in Bongaarts' simple model that is not measured here and that is known to be important in several countries in Latin America and the Caribbean and in Asia and Oceania, which show low levels of potential fertility (especially Guyana, Trinidad and Tobago, and the Republic of Korea, and possibly Fiji and Malaysia). Other proximate determinants not included in the simple model are likely to be important in certain countries. Above-average levels of infecundity and sterility are known to exist in some areas of Africa and may affect national levels of fertility, even though only particular regions are affected (particularly Cameroon and the Sudan). In Africa also, polygamy is thought to be associated with sexual abstinence by wives (possibly with substantial effects in Cameroon, Côte d'Ivoire,[11] Ghana and Senegal). Abstinence also adds significantly to the post-partum non-susceptible period in Haiti (Casterline and others, 1984). Lastly, spousal separation is acknowledged to be at high levels in Nepal, Lesotho and Yemen, for reasons of labour-related migration; and it appears fairly common in the Philippines as well (Casterline and others, 1984).[12]

Apart from these omitted proximate variables, measurement problems could have affected the results, particularly in the case of the contraceptive index whose construction depended upon the assumption that contraceptive use-effectiveness is constant for each method across countries and ages. In addition, breast-feeding durations do not correlate perfectly with length of amenorrhoea. It is reported that C_i estimated directly from reports of amenorrhoea differs by 0.05 or more from indirect estimates based on breast-feeding in three of eight countries with available data—Bangladesh, Haiti and Lesotho (Casterline and others, 1984). It is possible that the duration of post-partum infecundability was underestimated in countries with very long durations of unsupplemented breast-feeding. The effect of marriage could have been overestimated if periods of dissolution were underreported or if the frequency of intercourse was substantially lower within informal unions, as compared with legal unions.

C. RELATIONSHIPS FOR AGE GROUPS

Age-specific rates and indices

Table 91 presents the mean value and standard deviation of the C indices for five-year age groups. The standard deviations provide some insight into the relative explanatory power of each index across ages, since factors that themselves show little variation cannot be expected to explain much of the variability in fertility rates.

The marriage factor, C_m, represents, on average, a powerful restraint on the fertility of young women and is also highly variable for age groups under 25 years. At older ages it is surpassed, both in average importance and in standard deviation, by the contraception index. Variation in the latter index increases with age, while the mean value decreases (indicating greater effect of contraception at older ages). C_i, on the other hand, shows little change either in mean value or in variability for ages under 40; at each of these ages its standard deviation is intermediate between that observed for the other indices. The lack of age pattern in C_i is consistent with a large body of demographic work indicating a roughly constant age pattern of marital fertility (though different levels of fertility) in a variety of populations in which contraception was not practised.[13]

Since this application of the Bongaarts model is age-specific, it is also possible to look at the fertility rates resulting from the removal of each proximate determinant not only across all ages (as in table 90) but also for individual age groups. Adjustment of age-specific fertility rates (ASFR) for proportions married produces age-specific marital fertility rates (ASMFR). Adjustment of ASMFRs for proportions currently using contraception produces age-specific natural fertility rates (ASNFR). As defined in the model, ASNFRs are conceptually similar to the standard pattern of natural fertility rates estimated by Coale and Trussell (1978), using the average of 10 schedules of historical (and primarily European) populations, selected from Henry (1961) for known good quality of data and evidence of an absence of parity-specific fertility control. This standard schedule is the average expected to occur where all women are married from age 15 onward, and no voluntary use of contraception exists. However, breast-feeding duration, which affects the length of the period of amenorrhoea and anovulation following birth, is not adjusted for in this standard schedule; and variation across countries in the level of ASNFRs is to be expected, depending upon the

TABLE 91. MEANS AND STANDARD DEVIATIONS OF THE INDICES, BY AGE GROUP

	Age group						
	15-19	20-24	25-29	30-34	35-39	40-44	45-49
Index of marriage, C_m							
Mean	0.26	0.64	0.82	0.88	0.87	0.84	0.80
Standard deviation	0.16	0.15	0.09	0.06	0.05	0.06	0.08
Index of post-partum infecundability, C_i							
Mean	0.74	0.72	0.74	0.74	0.72	0.81	0.91
Standard deviation	0.10	0.11	0.10	0.10	0.10	0.08	0.04
Index of contraception, C_c							
Mean	0.91	0.84	0.79	0.74	0.73	0.72	0.74
Standard deviation	0.08	0.13	0.15	0.18	0.19	0.20	0.20

Source: World Fertility Survey standard recode tapes.

TABLE 92. AVERAGE[a] FERTILITY RATES BY AGE GROUP AND PERCENTAGE OF DIFFERENCE BETWEEN ACTUAL AND POTENTIAL FERTILITY RATES EXPLAINED BY THREE PROXIMATE DETERMINANTS

	Age group						
	15-19	20-24	25-29	30-34	35-39	40-44	45-49
Panel A							
Age-specific fertility rate, ASFR	102	247	261	215	152	80	27
Percentage of total	9.4	22.8	24.1	19.8	14.0	7.4	2.5
Age-specific marital fertility rate, ASMFR	275	367	308	244	174	94	32
Percentage of total	18.4	24.6	20.6	16.3	11.6	6.3	2.1
Age-specific natural fertility rate, ASNFR	304	445	403	338	248	131	41
Percentage of total	15.9	23.3	21.1	17.7	13.0	6.9	2.1
Age-specific fecundity rate, ASFECR	414	614	545	457	345	163	48
Percentage of total	16.0	23.7	21.1	17.7	13.3	6.3	1.9
Panel B							
Gap between ASFECR and ASFR	312	367	284	242	193	83	21
ASFR as percentage of ASFECR	24.6	40.2	47.9	47.0	44.1	49.1	56.3
Percentage of gap accounted for by:							
Marriage	70.8	43.5	22.5	16.8	16.5	22.7	29.5
Contraception	7.2	21.2	36.5	43.2	43.2	44.6	43.1
Breast-feeding	22.1	35.4	41.0	40.0	40.3	30.7	27.4
SUM	100.0	100.0	100.0	100.0	100.0	100.0	100.0

Source: World Fertility Survey standard recode tapes.
[a] All-country averages.

average length of breast-feeding in populations. Using the Bongaarts model, ASNFRs may be further adjusted, removing the effect of breast-feeding (i.e., assuming that all mothers do not breast-feed) and producing age-specific fecundity rates (here called ASFECR to distinguish them from ASFRs). Thus, four sets of age-specific rates can be derived, gradually increasing from the observed level (ASFR) to the potential level of fertility (ASFECR).

These rates, averaged over all countries, are shown in table 92. The shape of the age pattern of fertility changes as the effect of the proximate determinants are removed. Removal of the marriage factor alone results in a shift of the peak ages of childbearing from 25-29 to 20-24. This peak at ages 20-24 is maintained as other factors are adjusted for, but fertility at ages 25-49 increases proportionally more than fertility at ages 15-24 with the further removal of contraception.

The age pattern of these four sets of rates, and also of the Coale and Trussell ASNFRs based on historical populations, are shown for groups of countries in figure 44. Rates for groups show different age patterns, depending upon the relative importance of the three proximate determinants. One common pattern that characterizes Africa, development groups III and IV, and the two lower family planning effort groups, is the relatively small effect of both marriage and contraception, with the result that ASFRs, ASMFRs and observed ASNFRs are not very different in shape. For these groups, the Coale and Trussell standard pattern of ASNFRs is substantially higher than the estimated ASNFR, with the implication that breast-feeding is a much more important determinant of fertility levels in these groups of countries than was true for the historical populations on which the standard schedule was based. In contrast to this pattern, Latin America and the Caribbean, and the more developed and stronger family planning effort groups show slightly greater effects of marriage and much greater effects of contraceptive use. For these groups, the observed and standard schedules of ASNFRs are not too different in level, although estimated ASNFRs fall off more rapidly with age than the standard schedule. The implication of this similarity in level is that breast-feeding has roughly similar importance in these groups of developing countries as it does in the Coale and Trussell sample (provided the C_c indices have adequately measured the extent of fertility control in the developing countries). The region of Asia and Oceania falls in between these two more extreme types of patterns of fertility schedules, with substantial marriage and contraception contributions, but with breast-feeding being more important than in the standard schedule.

A further important point shown in these figures is the degree of similarity in the shape of ASMFRs and standard ASNFRs. The sharpness of the fall-off in marital fertility rates is an indication of the importance of contraceptive use at older ages—this is seen most clearly in Latin America and the Caribbean, the high development group and the strong family planning effort group. By comparison, ASMFRs in Africa and development group IV have much the same rounded shape as the standard schedule of natural fertility, although the levels are different. Other groups have an intermediate pattern, showing the effects of some contraceptive use at older ages, but not an extremely high level of use. These graphs also clearly show that effects of contraceptive use are substantial even at ages 20-24, in Latin America and the Caribbean, Asia and Oceania, and the upper development and stronger family planning effort groups.

Panel B of table 45 shows, by age, the percentage contribution of each factor to the gap between ASFECRs

Figure 44. Age-specific fertility rates, by region, level of development and strength of family planning programme effort

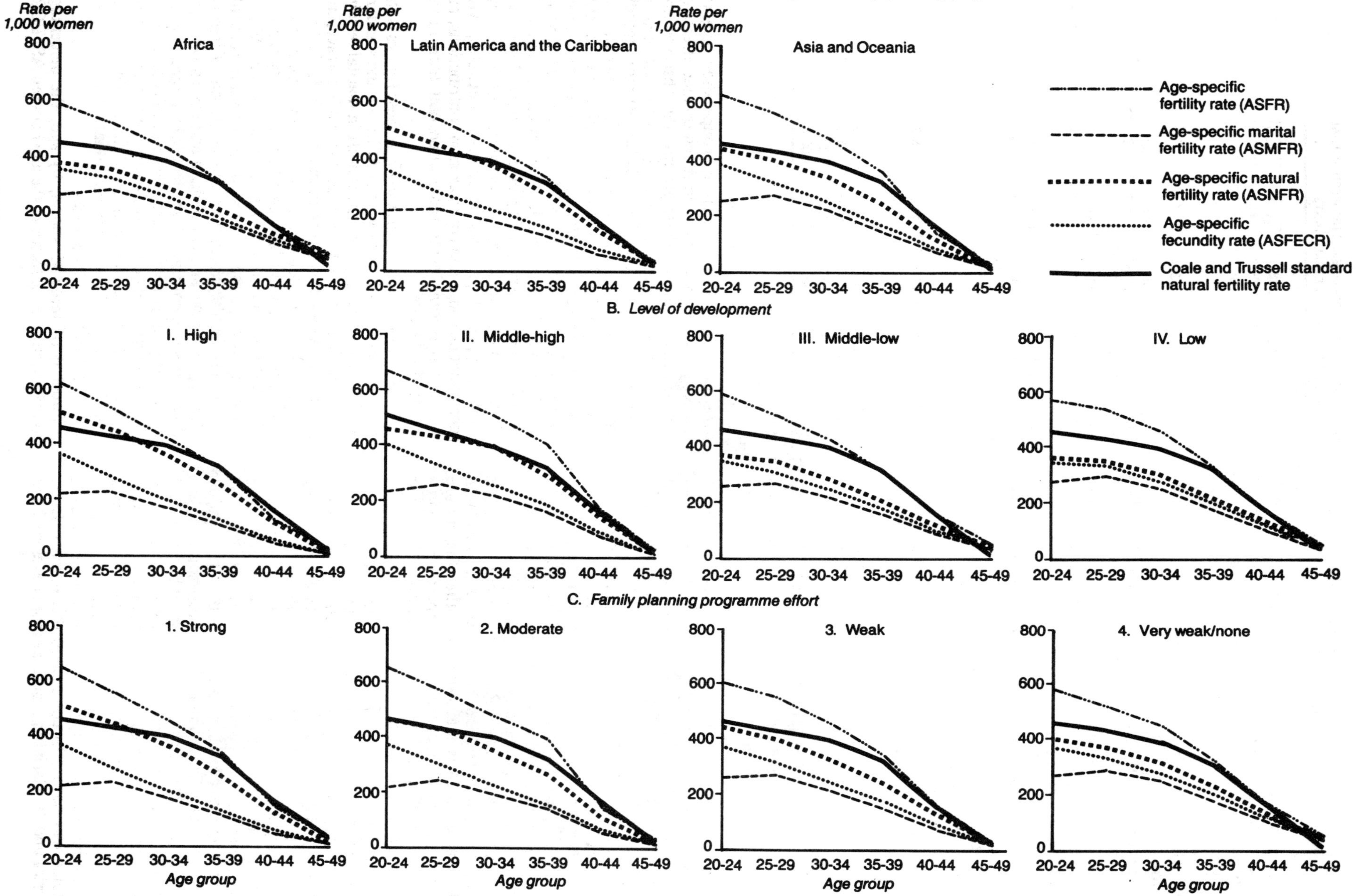
Rate per 1,000 women
Africa
Latin America and the Caribbean
Asia and Oceania
800
600
400
200
0
20-24
25-29
30-34
35-39
40-44
45-49
Age-specific fertility rate (ASFR)
Age-specific marital fertility rate (ASMFR)
Age-specific natural fertility rate (ASNFR)
Age-specific fecundity rate (ASFECR)
Coale and Trussell standard natural fertility rate
B. Level of development
I. High
II. Middle-high
III. Middle-low
IV. Low
C. Family planning programme effort
1. Strong
2. Moderate
3. Weak
4. Very weak/none
Age group

Source: World Fertility Survey standard recode tapes.

and ASFRs. On average, breast-feeding explains at least 20 per cent of the gap between the fertility rates, and roughly 40 per cent at the central reproductive ages. Contraceptive use shows an increasingly important role up to age group 35-39 and from then on contributes slightly more than 40 per cent to the fertility gap. While the importance of marital status in explaining the gap declines over all with age, its importance increases slightly at the oldest age groups, due to declines in marital exposure for reasons of widowhood and separation.

The relative importance of these three factors according to age varies across countries and groups of countries (see figure 45). The marriage patterns by age are quite similar across the regional groups, with most striking contrast being the later marriage pattern in Latin America and the Caribbean and in Asia and Oceania, and the greater impact of widowhood and separation at the oldest ages in Africa. The impact on fertility of breast-feeding in Latin America and the Caribbean is roughly half as large as its impact in the other regions and varies less

in importance with age. When comparing development groups, it is striking to note not only the increasing importance of contraception for fertility reduction with development but the steepness of its rise with age as a function of development. While this is also true when comparing strengths of family planning programme effort, the differences are less striking.

Age-specific potential fertility

While the explanatory power of the Bongaarts model has been tested for several population groups using aggregate measures, its explanatory power has not been tested for individual age groups. Among the proximate determinants excluded from the model, and which were not expected to have an important effect on the aggregate fit, it is possible that some (such as abstinence and spousal separations) may vary across countries in importance more at some ages than others, thus causing the fit of the model to vary across age groups. In addition, other

Figure 45. Percentage of difference between actual and potential fertility rates explained by three proximate determinants, by age group, according to region, level of development and strength of family planning programme effort

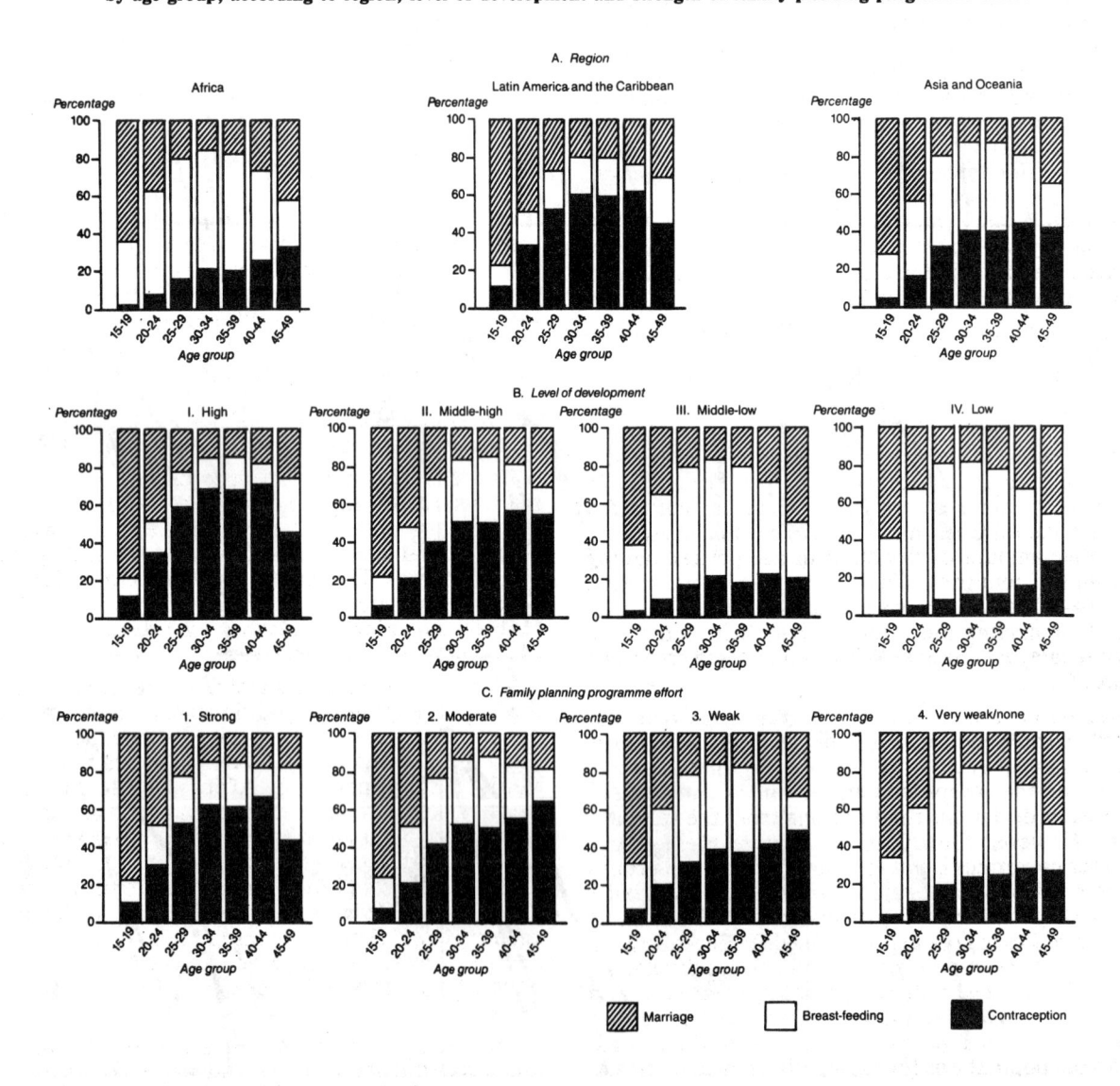

Source: World Fertility Survey standard recode tapes.

factors of known importance, such as abortion and contraceptive use-effectiveness, are likely to vary with age.

The estimates of use-effectiveness employed here reflect differences in the choice of methods between age groups, but they do not allow for possible increases with age in the efficiency with which particular methods are used. Taking account of the changing method mix alone produces only minor changes in assumed effectiveness from one age group to the next; the all-country average of effectiveness ranges from 0.81 at ages 15-19 to 0.85 at ages 45-49.

Results of another application of the Bongaarts model may have relevance for the present investigation of age-specific rates. A study of rural/urban and education differentials in fertility found that urban and educated groups had lower total fecundity rates, as derived from the model (Casterline and others, 1984). It is unlikely that these groups have genuinely lower fecundity; if anything, one might expect higher fecundity levels in the upper social groups, due to lower prevalence of disease-induced sterility and to better health and nutrition in general. The authors suggest that "greater use of induced abortion, higher efficiency of use of contraception, and possibly unreported use among the better educated and more urban strata are the most likely reasons for this pattern" (Casterline and others, 1984, p. 46). Thus, the analysis suggested that underestimation of fertility control is greatest, at least in absolute terms, in precisely those groups reporting the highest levels of contraceptive use. If so, the age pattern of derived natural fertility rates, or potential fertility rates, might be expected to decline more rapidly with age in the relatively economically advanced countries and in other groups with substantial levels of contraceptive practice.

This hypothesis can be examined by separating out differences in the age pattern from differences in level of the total fecundity schedules derived from the model. A straightforward way of doing this is to assume that differences between countries at ages 20-24 are equivalent to differences in the level of fecundity. Then if the rates for all age groups are expressed as a ratio to the 20-24 rate, these re-expressed age patterns may be compared with the standard Coale and Trussell schedule to estimate the relative amount of deviation in age pattern among the groups of countries. This comparison is restricted to ages 20-44, because the rate at ages 15-19 is partially a result of assumptions, rather than being based on observed data, and because WFS rates at 45-49 are biased upward.[14]

These results are shown for the standard Coale and Trussell schedule and for all groups (table 93). When rates are expressed in relation to ages 20-24, there is some tendency for the groups with higher contraceptive use to have greater deviations than average from the standard pattern. However, the differences between these groups and lower use groups is not very large. In fact, all groups of countries show a more rapid fall-off of fertility at older ages than expected from the standard schedule. Some of these differences may be explained by differences between historical European populations and current developing countries in the age patterns of natural fertility. In a recent review article, Knodel (1983) catalogues various reasons that the age patterns of natural fertility might vary across populations (including differences in breast-feeding duration, the importance of terminal abstinence, age of marriage etc.) but concludes that these effects should leave the age pattern convex in shape (as is in fact the case for all groups covered in table 93). One factor that is notably different between the European populations included in the Coale and Trussell schedules and those included here is the age of marriage, which is, on average, quite low in the developing countries in comparison with the historical populations. McDonald (1984) found that, in a comparison among the WFS populations, the age at last birth was younger among younger marrying groups and this could contribute to the apparent differences in age pattern shown in table 93 between the WFS countries and the historical European populations.[15] In addition, the omission of abortion and the inability to measure variation in use-effectiveness may be quite important in explaining the deviation at the older ages. Thus, it is not only possible that the age pattern of natural fertility actually falls off more sharply in currently developing countries than it did in historical Europe, but it is likely that certain aspects of the Bongaarts model that were not measurable are indeed important in explaining the gap between actual fertility and fecundity, particularly in the older age groups.

The proportion of variance in observed age-specific fertility explained by the product of the three proximate determinants is as follows:

Age	20-24	25-29	30-34	35-39	40-44	45-49
R^2	0.76	0.60	0.62	0.44	0.57	0.38

The best fit is for age group 20-24, with about three fourths of variance explained. At ages 35-39 and 45-49, the three indices explain less than half of the variance in observed rates; and for the remaining age groups, about 60 per cent. The poor fit at ages 45-49 may be due in part to unreliable measurement,[16] and in general, the sampling variability of age-specific rates is in relation to international variation, greater than for the total fertility rate. This is undoubtedly one reason that the proportion of variance explained by the three indices is lower for most age groups than for the overall rate ($R^2 = 0.71$).

At ages 20-24, where explained variance is highest, the marriage factor alone can account for about half the variability in observed fertility rates (as compared with 30 per cent at ages 25-29 and between 9 and 21 per cent at higher ages). The marital fertility factors, C_c and C_i, do make an important contribution even at ages 20-24, though, and at higher ages they are responsible for most of the total explained variance.

These results serve to direct attention, once again, to the likely importance of additional marital fertility determinants in some settings—such as abortion in parts of Latin America and the Caribbean, and Asia and Oceania, sterility and abstinence in Africa—and to the need to develop more direct measures of factors that had, in the present case, to be assumed (use-effectiveness) or inferred somewhat indirectly (infecundability) in order to calculate C_c and C_i. Errors in the underlying fertility rates are another possible source of unexplained variance (see chapter I); and simplifying assumptions about the reproductive process, incorporated into the basic model, undoubtedly contribute to unexplained variance to some degree.

Proposals for improving measurement of the proximate determinants have been advanced elsewhere (Bongaarts, 1985; Page, Léridon and Ferry, 1985; Page,

TABLE 93. AGE PATTERNS OF OBSERVED AND STANDARD FECUNDITY RATES: AGES 25-44 EXPRESSED AS A PROPORTION OF RATE FOR AGES 20-24, BY GROUPS OF COUNTRIES

Standard and observed rates	Fecundity rate at ages 20-24	Ages 20-24 = 1.00	25-29	30-34	35-39	40-44
Adjusted Coale and Trussell standard ASNFR[a]	649	1.00	0.94	0.86	0.70	0.36
Region						
Africa	586	1.00	0.89	0.75	0.55	0.30
Latin America and the Caribbean	621	1.00	0.87	0.73	0.55	0.26
Asia and Oceania	632	1.00	0.90	0.76	0.57	0.25
Level of development						
I. High	621	1.00	0.84	0.69	0.50	0.22
II. Middle-high	665	1.00	0.89	0.76	0.61	0.27
III. Middle-low	588	1.00	0.88	0.73	0.55	0.29
IV. Low	568	1.00	0.94	0.81	0.58	0.30
Strength of family planning programme effort						
1. Strong	648	1.00	0.86	0.70	0.52	0.23
2. Moderate	646	1.00	0.88	0.73	0.59	0.22
3. Weak	603	1.00	0.91	0.76	0.57	0.28
4. Very weak/none	586	1.00	0.89	0.77	0.56	0.31
Level of contraceptive use[b]						
Low	565	1.00	0.91	0.78	0.57	0.30
Moderate	648	1.00	0.89	0.75	0.59	0.26
High	629	1.00	0.86	0.69	0.51	0.23
ALL COUNTRIES	613	1.00	0.88	0.74	0.55	0.26

Source: World Fertility Survey standard recode tapes.

[a] Bongaarts and Kirmeyer (1982) adjusted the Coale and Trussell standard natural fertility schedule for lactation uniformly, with no change in the pattern of rates. Thus, the original standard rates for ages 20-44 (460, 431, 395, 322, 167) show the same age pattern as that shown here.

[b] The contraceptive use categories are formed as follows: low = less than or equal to 10 per cent of currently married women aged 15-49 currently using contraception; moderate = between 11 and 34 per cent of currently married women aged 15-49; high = greater than or equal to 35 per cent of currently married women aged 15-49. (See chapter V in the present volume.)

Cleland and Hobcraft, 1984). For the most part, these must await the collection of new data. At the same time, the role of WFS in stimulating such research should not be overlooked. The WFS data pertaining to marriage, contraception and breast-feeding made it possible to test the Bongaarts model on a wide range of contemporary populations. It is the considerable, if incomplete, success of the model that has attracted the attention of so many researchers to overcoming the problems that still remain.

D. CONCLUSION

Despite some problems with the application of the Bongaarts model to the WFS data, the model does provide a useful means of summarizing the relative importance of the three main proximate determinants among the regions, development groups and family planning effort groups, as well as across the reproductive ages. Over all, the index of contraception varies in value more than does the index of marriage or the index of infecundability, although all three factors must be considered in any attempt to account for variations in fertility among developing countries. Despite the greater variability of the contraceptive index, C_c, the amount by which it reduces fertility from its hypothetical potential level is somewhat smaller, on average, than reductions due to marriage, C_m, or lactation-induced amenorrhoea, C_i. Marital exposure is one means through which substantial reductions in potential fertility are achieved in all groups of countries covered—in most cases, 35-40 per cent of the total reduction is due to this source. In absolute terms, the index of marriage indicates that this factor is more important in some groups—Latin America and the Caribbean, development group I and the strong family planning effort group—which have an index of about 0.6, compared with 0.7-0.8 in other groups. A strong contrast is found in the relative importance of contraception and post-partum infecundability. Groups with a strong effect of contraception generally have a weak contribution by infecundability, which is seen both in the percentage of reduction due to each factor and in the absolute size of the indices. In Africa, the less developed countries and countries with weak family planning effort, infecundability contributes over 50 per cent of the total reduction from potential fertility but contraception is responsible for only about 10 per cent. At the other extreme, for Latin America and the Caribbean, development group I and the strong family planning effort group, contraception contributes roughly 40 per cent of the total fertility reduction and infecundability contributes about 20 per cent.

All three of the proximate determinants vary strongly according to level of development, with the highest correlation being that with the contraception index: the development score accounts for 76 per cent of the variance in C_c, 57 per cent of the variance in C_i and 43 per cent of the variance in C_m. All three indices also show substantial contrasts according to strength of family planning programme effort, but in the case of C_m and C_i, the association can be attributed to the fact that strong family planning programmes are found mainly in relatively economically advanced countries. The family planning score does have a statistically significant effect on the contraception index, even after control for level of development.

Regression of the indices on each other also shows that stronger effects of marriage are, on average, accompanied by greater effects of contraception. Lesser effects of breast-feeding are balanced by stronger effects of both marriage and contraception. If this cross-sectional pattern of changes indicates the typical time process of change, it suggests that when countries where fertility is now mainly restricted by breast-feeding experience declines in breast-feeding duration, this will be matched by rises in the age of marriage and in contraceptive use, possibly with a time-lag, however. Cross-nationally, the association between the indices of contraception and infecundability is only of moderate strength ($Y^2 = 0.36$). This is a weaker association, for instance, than the association between either of these indices and the development score employed in this study. Some countries with little contraceptive practice have only moderate durations of breast-feeding, while in others lengthy breast-feeding persists despite moderate levels of contraceptive use. This fact alone argues against a highly mechanistic interpretation of the relationship between contraception and breast-feeding. It is also clear that, apart from the effect on average fertility levels, the current combinations of lactation and contraception are associated in many WFS countries with a high incidence of very short birth intervals, which appear to imperil the health of children (Smith, 1985; Hobcraft, McDonald and Rutstein, 1985).

Age-specific fertility rates and indices of the proximate determinants were also examined. The derived pattern of potential fertility rates was found in general to decline somewhat more rapidly with advancing age than in a model schedule of natural fertility based primarily on historical European data. The deviation from the model schedule was slightly greater in groups of countries with high levels of contraceptive practice, suggesting that underestimation of the extent of fertility control is a contributing factor. However, even groups of countries with little evidence of deliberate fertility control showed notably more rapid decline of potential fertility with age than in the model schedule.

The three indices together were more successful at explaining fertility differences among young women, where age at marriage is an important source of variation in rates, than at older ages. At the same time, lactation and contraceptive practice have a large effect on average fertility rates and on variability in rates, even for young women. In general accord with earlier work, the average value of the C_i index was found to be nearly constant across age groups (at least until the highest ages), indicating that infecundability has little effect on the age pattern of fertility, only on its level. The average fertility-reducing effect of contraception, and its variability, increase with age, although after age 30 the contrasts between successive age groups are small in these respects.

A full explanation of cross-country differences in age-specific fertility rates would require more data to fill some of the information gaps which prevent a full application of the simple Bongaarts model. Both the practice of abortion and the use-effectiveness of contraception are expected to rise with age; and if their inter-country variability also rises with age, they should play an increasingly important role in the explanation of the inter-country fertility differences at the older ages. Without such measures, it is difficult to identify exactly how data errors and other omitted proximate determinants might also affect the observed inter-country variations in fertility. Further explorations must await more refined data.

Although the development of more precise and more complete measurements of the proximate determinants is a laudable goal, it should not be forgotten that a major strength of the Bongaarts model is its ability to yield useful estimates from the less-than-ideal data that are currently available. Nor should the great contribution of WFS to improved measurement be slighted: the simultaneous collection, on a large scale, of information about breast-feeding, contraception and marriage was crucial, among other things, for initial demonstrations of the model's empirical utility. For purposes of a broad overview, the simple model, as applied here, provides important insights into the changing relative importance of the three major proximate determinants in the course of socio-economic development as well as their changing importance over the life cycle.

NOTES

[1] In this chapter, all group averages are based on 40 countries: the 38 countries included in this publication plus Nigeria and Turkey. Data for these two countries, however, are not presented separately because, at the time the tabulations were being run, the data from these countries were not available individually for comparative analysis.

[2] In a study based on 45 societies (Bongaarts and Potter, 1983), the mean total fecundity rate was found to be 15.3.

[3] The current status model is one that relates fertility in the last year (or other brief span of time) to contemporaneously observed marital status distributions, contraceptive prevalence and breast-feeding duration.

[4] Bongaarts and Kirmeyer (1982) applied the three-factor model to 22 developing countries in which the impact of induced abortion was presumed negligible. Seventeen of the countries used in the Bongaarts and Kirmeyer (1982) study were also used for the World Fertility Survey (WFS) study (Casterline and others, 1984). For these 17 countries, the explained variance was 91 per cent using the indices and fertility rates presented by Bongaarts and Kirmeyer and 81 per cent using methods described in the annex. The lower explained variance for the 29 WFS countries analysed by Casterline and others—70 per cent—is therefore due to a considerable extent to differences in the set of countries available for analysis. The 17 countries included by Bongaarts and Kirmeyer were, generally speaking, those for which WFS data became available earliest; and the three-factor model is evidently less adequate when applied to the predominantly African and Latin American countries which conducted surveys toward the end of the WFS programme. Differences in index construction are not the only source of variant results, since some of Bongaarts and Kirmeyer's underlying data came from sources other than WFS. In addition to differences in index construction discussed in detail in Casterline and others (1984), Bongaarts and Kirmeyer treated visiting unions in Caribbean countries differently than has been done here (see Bongaarts and Potter, 1983). For the 29 countries analysed by Casterline and others (1984), exclusion of extreme cases (those with total fecundity rates outside the range of 11-15), on the grounds that omission of other relevant proximate determinants or that special data problems were distorting estimation in these outlying cases, increased the proportion of variance explained to 88 per cent.

[5] It should be noted that proportional differences in $C_c \cdot C_i$ are not precisely the same as proportional differences in the observed total marital fertility rate (shown in table 90), because the three-factor model employed here does not provide a perfect fit to the data. For instance, in the examples cited in the text, the ratio of $C_c \cdot C_i$ for development groups IV and I is 1.17, as compared with a ratio of 1.22 for the total marital fertility rate (TMFR), the ratio of $C_c \cdot C_i$ in Asia and Oceania to that in Latin America and the Caribbean is 1.04, as compared with 1.08 for TMFR. In both these cases, the observed TMFR contrast is slightly larger than predicted from C_c and C_i; failure to allow for the effects of induced abortion may be the principal reason. Comparisons

involving the composite factor $C_c \cdot C_i$ nevertheless provide a useful, if approximate, means of assessing the degree to which the fertility effects of contraception and lactation offset one another.

[6] These correlations include Nigeria and Turkey, for which separate values are not shown.

[7] In table 87, the indices have been rescaled using a logit transformation, a procedure that prevents the regression-fitted values of the indices from falling outside the allowable range of 0-1.

[8] Orthogonal regression has the advantage that since squared distances perpendicular to the fitted regression lines are minimized, rather than vertical distances, particular C indices do not need to be designated as "dependent" or "independent". For two variables A and B, the slope of the orthogonal regression line for A regressed on B is the inverse of the slope found when B is regressed on A.

[9] The marriage index derived by subtracting C_{ds} from C_{em} is not identical with the C_m presented in table 86. This is because the components of the marriage index were derived from current marital status data whereas C_m presented in table 86 is based on marital exposure for the five years preceding the survey, as explained in the annex. Note that while other indices are multiplied together to obtain the total estimated fertility effect of two or more indices, C_{ds} does not fit into the multiplicative scheme. A multiplicative index termed C_{cm} has been employed elsewhere to show the fertility effect of marital disruption (Casterline and others, 1984). C_{cm} and C_{ds} are related as follows:

$$C_{cm} = 1 - C_{ds}/C_{em}$$

[10] The most important technical features contributing to the lower average potential fertility levels reported here are, first, the exclusion from the rates reported here of births that took place outside of marital unions (including consensual unions). In most other applications of the Bongaarts model, fertility occurring outside unions has, in effect, been treated as though it took place within marriage, producing estimated marital fertility rates that are somewhat too high; this translates into higher mode-implied levels of potential fertility. It should be noted that there is often no choice in this matter open to the analyst, since age-specific fertility rates are frequently reported without any information about the mother's marital or union status at the time she gave birth. A second factor that was found by Casterline and others (1984) to have an important effect was the choice, for calculating C_m, of age-specific proportions married at the time of the survey as opposed to the average age-specific proportion of time spent within marriage during the five years preceding the survey (the period to which the fertility rates pertain); the latter proportions, which are employed in this analysis, usually resulted in lower implied levels of potential fertility. Another difference in index construction, an adjustment for overlap between contraceptive protection and post-partum infecundability, was found to have a less important effect, though it too serves to depress the implied level of potential fertility. Casterline and others (1984) also describe other aspects of index construction with potentially significant effects on analytical results; however, in these other respects the approach used here is similar between this analysis and Bongaarts' approach.

[11] Formerly called the Ivory Coast.

[12] This detailed country information on the importance of certain unmeasured proximate determinants comes from a review of the first country reports prepared upon completion of each survey. World Fertility Survey data pertaining to several determinants that were measured in a minority of countries are summarized in Singh and Ferry (1984) and in Casterline and others (1984).

[13] Although the mean duration of breast-feeding is somewhat longer for older women, this is offset, in the calculation of C_i, by the longer estimated waiting time to conception (see annex).

[14] Rates during the five years preceding the survey are mainly based on experience under age 47.5, because of the upper age-limit of 49 years at the time of the survey.

[15] Possible factors contributing to this pattern include the negative relationship between frequency of intercourse and marital duration and the negative association between age at marriage and length of exposure to the risk of sterility due to childbirth complications (Knodel, 1983; Trussell and Wilson, 1985).

[16] At ages 45-49, the sampling error of the fertility rates is larger in comparison to the total amount of inter-country variation in rates than is the case at other ages (see Little, 1982). The small number of births to women over age 45 leads to unstable estimation, and the number of woman-years in the denominator of the rates is also relatively small.

This is primarily because the count of woman-years spent at ages 45-49 is based on women no older than 49 at the survey; these women were, on average, in the 45-49 age group for only about half of the five years preceding the survey. (This exposure was, in addition, concentrated in the lower part of the 45-49 age range, producing upwardly biased rates.)

REFERENCES

Adegbola, O. and Hilary J. Page (1982). Nuptiality and Fertility in Metropolitan Lagos: components and compensating mechanism. In Lado T. Ruzicka, ed., *Nuptiality and Fertility*. Proceedings of a seminar organized by the International Union for the Scientific Study of Population, Bruges, 8-11 January 1979. Liège: Ordina Editions, 337-362.

Bongaarts, John (1978). A framework for analyzing the proximate determinants of fertility. *Population and Development Review* 4(1):105-132.

_____ (1982). The fertility-inhibiting effects of the intermediate fertility variables. *Studies in Family Planning* 13(6/7):179-189.

_____ (1985). What can future surveys tell us about the proximate determinants of fertility? *International Family Planning Perspectives* 11(3):86-90.

_____ and Sharon Kirmeyer (1982). Estimating the impact of contraceptive prevalence on fertility: aggregate and age-specific versions of a model. In Albert I. Hermalin and Barbara Entwiste, eds., *The Role of Surveys in the Analysis of Family Planning Programs*. Proceedings of the seminar organized by the International Union for the Scientific Study of Population, Bogotá, 28-31 October 1980. Liège: Ordina Editions, 381-408.

_____ and Robert G. Potter, eds. (1983). *Fertility, Biology and Behaviour: an Analysis of the Proximate Determinants*. New York: Academic Press.

Casterline, John B. and others (1984). *The Proximate Determinants of Fertility*. World Fertility Survey Comparative Studies, No. 39. Voorburg, The Netherlands: International Statistical Institute.

Coale, Ansley J. and T. James Trussell (1978). Technical note: finding the two parameters that specify a model schedule of marital fertility. *Population Index* 44(2):203-213.

Davis, Kingsley and Judith Blake (1956). Social structure and fertility: An analytic framework. *Economic Development and Cultural Change* 4(4):211-235.

Ferry, Benôit and David P. Smith (1983). *Breastfeeding Differentials*. World Fertility Survey Comparative Studies, No. 23; Cross-National Summaries. Voorburg, The Netherlands: International Statistical Institute.

Gaslonde, Santiago and Enrique Carrasco (1982). *The Impact of Some Intermediate Variables on Fertility: Evidence from the Venezuela National Fertility Survey, 1977*. World Fertility Survey Occasional Papers, No. 23. Voorburg, The Netherlands: International Statistical Institute.

Henry, Louis (1961). Some data on natural fertility. *Eugenics Quarterly* 8(2):81-91.

_____ (1972). *On the Measurement of Human Fertility; Selected Writing of Louis Henry*. M. C. Sheps and E. Lapierre-Adamcyk, eds. and trans. New York: Elsevier.

Hobcraft, John and R. J. A. Little (1984). Fertility exposure analysis: A new method for assessing the construction of proximate determinants to fertility differential. *Population Studies* 38(1):21-45.

_____, J. W. McDonald and S. O. Rutstein (1985). Demographic determinants of infant and early child mortality: a comparative analysis. *Population Studies* 39(3):363-385.

Knodel, John (1983). Natural fertility: age patterns, levels and trends. Rodolfo A. Bulatao and Ronald D. Lee, eds., with Paula E. Hollerbach and John Bongaarts, *Determinants of Fertility in Developing Countries*, vol. 1, *Supply and Demand for Children*. Report of the National Research Council Committee on Population and Demography, Panel on Fertility Determinants. New York: Academic Press, 61-102.

Laing, John E. (1978). Estimating the effects of contraceptive use on fertility: techniques and findings from the 1974 Philippines National Acceptor Survey. *Studies in Family Planning* 9(6):150-162.

Lapham, Robert J. and W. Parker Mauldin (1984). Family planning program effort and birthrate decline in developing countries. *International Family Planning Perspectives* 10(4):109-118.

Léridon, Henri (1977). *Human Fertility: the Basic Components*. Judith F. Helzner, trans. Chicago and London: University of Chicago Press.

―――― and Benôit Ferry (1985). Biological and traditional restraints on fertility. In John Cleland and John Hobcraft, eds., in collaboration with Betzy Dinesen, *Reproductive Change in Developing Countries: Insights from the World Fertility Survey*. Oxford: Oxford University Press, 139-164.

Little, Roderick J. A. (1982). *Sampling Errors of Fertility Rates from the WFS*. World Fertility Survey Technical Bulletin, No. 10. Voorburg, The Netherlands: International Statistical Institute.

McDonald, Peter (1984). *Nuptiality and Completed Fertility: A Study of Starting, Stopping and Spacing Behaviour*. World Fertility Survey Comparative Studies, No. 35. Voorburg, The Netherlands: International Statistical Institute.

Mauldin, W. Parker and Bernard Berelson (1978). Conditions of fertility decline in developing countries, 1965-75. With section by Zenas Sykes. *Studies in Family Planning* 9(5):89-147.

Mosley, W. Henry, Linda Werner and Stan Becker (1982). *The Dynamics of Birth Spacing and Marital Fertility in Kenya*. World Fertility Survey Scientific Reports, No. 30. Voorburg, The Netherlands: International Statistical Institute.

Nortman, Dorothy L. and Ellen Hofstatter (1980). *Population and Family Planning Programs: Data Through 1978*. 10th ed. New York: The Population Council.

Page, Hilary J., John Cleland and John Hobcraft (1984). The collection of data on the proximate determinants of fertility. Paper submitted to the Seminar on Integrating Proximate Determinants into the Analysis of Fertility Levels and Trends, organized by the International Union for the Scientific Study of Population and the World Fertility Survey, London, 29 April-1 May 1984.

Sheps, Mindel C. and Jane A. Menken, with assistance of Annette P. Radick (1973). *Mathematical Models of Conception and Birth*. Chicago: University of Chicago Press.

Singh, Susheela (1984). *Comparability of Questionnaires: Forty-one WFS countries*. World Fertility Survey Comparative Studies, No. 32; Cross-National Summaries. Voorburg, The Netherlands: International Statistical Institute.

―――― and Benôit Ferry (1984). *Biological and Traditional Factors That Influence Fertility: Results from WFS Surveys*. World Fertility Survey Comparative Studies, No. 40; Cross-National Summaries. Voorburg, The Netherlands: International Statistical Institute.

Smith, David P. (1985). Breast-feeding, contraception, and birth intervals in developing countries. *Studies in Family Planning* 16(3): 154-163.

Trussell, J. and C. Wilson (1985). Sterility in a population with natural fertility. *Population Studies* 39(2):269-286.

Vaessen, Martin (1984). *Childlessness and Infecundity*. World Fertility Survey Comparative Studies, No. 31: Cross-National Summaries. Voorburg, The Netherlands: International Statistical Institute.

Annex

MEASUREMENT OF COMPONENTS OF THE MODEL[a]

Measurement of components

The total fertility rate, *TFR*, is

$$TFR = 5 \Sigma f_a$$

where f_a = age-specific fertility rates for the five-year period preceding the survey.

Five-year age groups are employed ($a = 1, ..., 7$), corresponding to ages 15-19, ..., 45-49. The rates were calculated using only births occurring within a union. Unions include formal and common-law unions and, in several Caribbean countries, "visiting" unions.

The rates were calculated by the FERTRATE program developed at World Fertility Survey (WFS) headquarters.

The index of marriage, C_m, is

$$C_m = \frac{TFR}{TMFR} = \frac{\Sigma f_a}{\Sigma f_a / m_a} = \frac{\Sigma f_a}{\Sigma g_a}$$

where m_a = age-specific proportions of exposure time spent within union during the five years preceding the survey;

g_a = age-specific marital fertility rates, based on within-union births only.

Following Bongaarts, g_a for age group 15-19 is calculated as 75 per cent of g_a for age group 20-24.

In those surveys where not all women aged 15-49 were eligible for interview, household survey information was utilized in calculation of the proportion of total exposure time spent within union.

The index of contraception, C_c, is

$$C_c = \frac{\Sigma_a tn_a cc_a}{\Sigma_a tn_a} = \frac{\Sigma_a tn_a (1 - \Sigma_m u_{a,m} e_m / fec_a)}{\Sigma_a tn_a}$$

where tn_a = an age-specific schedule of natural marital fertility, obtained as g_a/cc_a;

$u_{a,m}$ = proportion of currently married women aged a who were currently using contraceptive method m;

e_m = a set of method-specific effectiveness weights;

fec_a = a schedule of age-specific proportions fecund.

Contraceptive users breast-feeding a child aged six months or less are not counted as users, under the assumption that such women are likely to be amenorrhoeic. Under Bongaarts' (1978) specification, the u_a exclude amenorrhoeic women. Only a subset of surveys in the WFS programme provide direct information on amenorrhoea, so an indirect adjustment must be employed. Tabulations for several countries indicate that the point at which roughly half of these women breast-feeding are no longer amenorrhoeic ranges from 6 to 11 months. The lowest value is chosen under the assumption that the joint status of breast-feeding and using will be selective of women no longer amenorrhoeic. The correction for overlap between use and amenorrhoea alters the value of C_c by 0.012 on average (mean absolute difference) (see Casterline and others, 1984, table 3).

The effectiveness weights are derived from Laing (1978):

Method	Use-effectiveness
Sterilization	1.00
Intra-uterine device	0.95
Pill	0.90
Other	0.70

Method "not stated" is assigned a weight of zero.

The schedule of age-specific proportions fecund, fec_a, is obtained as the simple mean of the proportions self-reported fecund in 28 WFS countries (Vaessen, 1984):

Age group	Proportion self-reported fecund
15-19	0.99
20-24	0.99
25-29	0.98
30-34	0.95
35-39	0.91
40-44	0.78
45-49	0.52

The index of post-partum infecundability, C_i, is

$$C_i = \frac{\Sigma tf_a ci_a}{\Sigma tf_a} = \frac{\Sigma tf_a (p_a/(q_a + i_a))}{\Sigma tf_a}$$

where tf_a = an age schedule of total fecundity rates, calculated as tn_a/ci_a;

i_a = an age schedule of mean durations of post-partum amenorrhoea, estimated from the mean duration of breast-feeding, B_a, as follows:

$$i_a = 1.753 \exp(0.1396 B_a - 0.001872 B_a^2)$$

B_a is estimated from current status data on breast-feeding, using the "prevalence/incidence" method (Mosley, Werner and Becker, 1982), as follows:

$$B_a = \frac{bf_a}{brth_a}$$

where bf_a = number of women aged a who were currently breast-feeding;

$brth_a$ = average number of births per month to women aged a in the two-year period preceding the survey.

To cope with small numbers of births and breast-feeding women for women classified by age, B_a and i_a are estimated for broad age groups.

The symbols p_a and q_a represent the length of the birth interval in months without the effects of lactational post-partum amenorrhoea and without the effects of lactational and non-lactational post-partum amenorrhoea, respectively. Values of p_a and q_a are set so as to reflect the variation in mean waiting-time to conception (and foetal mortality as well) with age. The schedules are derived from the Hobcraft and Little (1984) estimates of mean waiting-times to conception in the data from the 1975 fertility survey in the Dominican Republic:

Age group	p_a	q_a
15-19	18.5	17.0
20-24	17.0	15.5
25-29	20.0	18.5
30-34	20.0	18.5
35-39	23.0	21.5
40-44	38.0	36.5
45-49	94.0	92.5

NOTE

[a] For details on methods of calculation and sources of data, see Casterline and others (1984), from which this annex is directly drawn.

REFERENCES

Bongaarts, John (1978). A framework for analyzing the proximate determinants of fertility. *Population and Development Review* 4(1): 105-132.

Casterline, John B. and others (1984). *The Proximate Determinants of Fertility*. World Fertility Survey Comparative Studies, No. 39. Voorburg, The Netherlands: International Statistical Institute.

Hobcraft, John and R. J. A. Little (1984). Fertility exposure analysis: A new method for assessing the construction of proximate determinants to fertility differential. *Population Studies* 38(1):21-45

Laing, John E. (1978). Estimating the effects of contraceptive use on fertility: techniques and findings from the 1974 Philippine National Acceptor Survey. *Studies in Family Planning* 9(6):150-162.

Mosley, W. Henry, Linda Werner and Stan Becker (1982). *The Dynamics of Birth Spacing and Marital Fertility in Kenya*. World Fertility Survey Scientific Reports, No. 30. Voorburg, The Netherlands: International Statistical Institute.

Vaessen, Martin (1984). *Childlessness and Infecundity*. World Fertility Survey Comparative Studies, No. 31: Cross-National Summaries. Voorburg, The Netherlands: International Statistical Institute.

PART TWO. SOCIO-ECONOMIC FACTORS AFFECTING FERTILITY IN THE DEVELOPING COUNTRIES

VII. RURAL OR URBAN RESIDENCE AND FERTILITY

ABSTRACT

The relationship between respondents' current and childhood residence and fertility is explored in this chapter. The relationship is seen to work through two channels: (*a*) characteristics and preferences of individuals according to where they live; and (*b*) characteristics of their residential location. A woman's current place of residence is categorized as "rural", "major urban" or "other urban". In Latin America and the Caribbean, the proportion of women living in a rural area (46 per cent) was much lower than in either Africa or Asia and Oceania (70-71 per cent). Current fertility differentials are first analysed according to current residence; multivariate analysis is then used to examine long-term measures of residence, including information on both current and childhood residence, in relationship to achieved fertility.

Fertility differences between urban and rural residents are highest in the more developed countries and in Latin America and the Caribbean. Among all but the least developed countries, urban/rural fertility differentials have widened over time, due to more rapid declines in fertility in urban areas. Residence differentials according to family size desires are smaller and the patterns do not vary systematically by region or development level. While the most developed countries have higher rates of unwanted childbearing in rural than urban areas, all other countries manifest the opposite pattern.

Urban residents typically marry at later ages than rural residents, and the gap has widened as increases in the age of marriage have been greater for urban women. Differences in breast-feeding duration by residence, with longer durations in rural areas, vary widely across countries and are not related to development. At progressively higher levels of development, the proportion of women practising contraception rises and the difference in use between urban and rural areas first rises and then falls. Countries with a stronger family planning programme also have smaller differences in level of contraceptive use between urban and rural areas.

The multivariate analysis demonstrates the role of compositional effects because roughly half of observed differential in fertility between long-term rural and long-term urban residents is explained by their occupational and educational characteristics. However, the importance of these effects varies by region. For example, Latin America and the Caribbean has the largest urban/rural fertility differentials both before and after control for other factors, but 50 per cent of the differential is explained by individual socio-economic characteristics. The opposite extreme is Africa, where smaller residential differentials are essentially unaffected by socio-economic characteristics. Thus, an important part of fertility differentials by residence must be attributed to the characteristics of urban and rural settings, which affect both the cost of fertility regulation and family size desires.

Rural/urban differences are among the most widely studied socio-economic differentials in individual fertility. Prior research has established that variations in type of place of residence (whether rural or urban) are related to variations in fertility. This implies that changes in residence patterns of a population can lead to changes in fertility. Apart from this, many social trends may begin in urban areas and later spread more widely (Singh and Casterline, 1985). Thus, in predicting fertility levels and trends, it is useful to take into account the magnitude of rural/urban differences in fertility.

In addition, knowledge of rural/urban differentials in fertility is valuable for policy purposes; the design and location of development projects, which indirectly have an impact on fertility, as well as family planning programmes which directly affect contraceptive practice, can be chosen and when appropriate, adjusted to suit policy objectives.

Empirical studies have yielded various results concerning the pattern and magnitude of rural/urban fertility differences. Rural fertility has consistently been found to be higher than urban fertility in European and other developed countries (United Nations, 1977). World Fertility Survey (WFS) data for Europe indicate, for example, that achieved fertility (standardized by marriage duration only) was consistently higher among rural women, although the magnitude of the difference varied (Jones, 1982). In Belgium, the average number of births was estimated as 1.85 in rural areas, compared with 1.78 in urban areas, a difference of only 0.07 birth. In Poland, on the other hand, the corresponding figures were 2.47 and 1.82, respectively, leading to a much larger difference of 0.65 birth. Studies in Canada and the United States of America also report higher rural fertility (e.g., Johnson, Stokes and Warland, 1978; Trovato and Grindstaff, 1980).

Results for developing countries have not been as consistent. In Latin American and Caribbean countries, a pattern similar to that of the developed countries has been observed, where urban fertility is lower than rural fertility (United Nations, 1977). For example, Kogut's study (reported in Cochrane, 1983) using 1960 census data from Brazil, found that rural women had significantly higher fertility. A similar result was obtained in Costa Rica (Michielutte and others, 1975). In Africa and in Asia and Oceania, however, several patterns have been observed. In some countries, higher rural fertility has been reported; in other countries, higher urban fertility. In still other countries, no significant differences by type of place of residence have been reported. For example, studies in Kenya and the Republic of Korea (see Cochrane, 1983) and in Ghana (Gaisie, 1976) found rural fertility to be higher than urban fertility. The reverse was found, however, in Indonesia by Chernichovsky and Meesook (1980), using 1976 household data. No significant difference in adjusted fertility was found by Ketkar (1979) in Sierra Leone.

A theory that has often been suggested to explain the observed differences in unadjusted rural and urban fertility (i.e., when no socio-economic controls are taken into consideration) centres around the argument that these differences can be explained by differing compositional characteristics with respect to such factors as education, occupation, work status and income of rural and urban populations. Urban women are more likely to be better educated and to be working in the modern sector, characteristics often associated with lower fertility. According to this hypothesis, then, if the simple rural/urban differentials are adjusted for various socio-economic variables, no significant difference between rural and urban fertility should be evident. However, empirical studies have not always supported this assertion. Often, even after such adjustments are made, significant rural/urban differences in fertility remain. For example, the two Latin American studies (in Brazil and Costa Rica) cited earlier found significant differences even after controlling for various socio-economic and demographic characteristics. In contrast, in Sierra Leone, the unadjusted significant differences in fertility were reduced to statistical insignificance after standardizing for socio-economic and demographic variables (Ketkar, 1979).

Another explanation for rural/urban fertility differences, complementary to that given above, is based on the premise that "residential patterns structure the norms and beliefs of individual residents regardless of, or in addition to, their categorical memberships for other social factors" (Johnson, Stokes and Warland, 1978, p. 674). As such, the higher fertility levels of rural women are thought to be due (at least partially) to rural residence *per se*, since rural life is associated with a wide range of norms and beliefs that tend to favour larger families. Such an explanation has been referred to as the "sub-cultural hypothesis". In their study of rural/urban fertility differentials among women in the United States, Johnson, Stokes and Warland (1978) created three measures of sex-role norms and beliefs, which they considered to be determined by residence. They found that after taking into account the effects of various compositional factors (which were significant) one dimension of sex-role norms (which tapped beliefs about innate differences by gender) remained significantly related to fertility. This result is consistent with other studies which suggest that sex-role orientations may be important predictors of fertility (Stokes, 1973).

Even after controlling for various socio-economic and demographic characteristics, as well as individual level measures of norms and beliefs, significant differences between rural and urban fertility often remain. It is clear that existing studies have not been able fully to explain fertility differentials by type of place of residence. Adequately sorting out the mechanisms through which residence affects fertility is a difficult task because at least two distinct sets of factors associated with residence can influence fertility at the individual level. One set characterizes the place of residence and is often referred to as "place" or "location" factors. This set includes such characteristics as availability of educational opportunities, health facilities, job opportunities in the modern sector, communication facilities and contraceptive information and supplies; and costs of fertility regulation and of bearing and rearing children. Each of these factors is hypothesized to affect fertility. For example, in urban areas, the higher costs of rearing children and their reduced labour value can be expected to result in preferences for smaller families. The decreased costs of fertility regulation (both financial and social) mean that it is easier for urban women to realize these preferences, resulting in lower fertility.

The other set of factors associated with fertility characterizes the individual herself. These factors include such characteristics as education, occupation, work status and income, as well as individual-level measures of norms and various socio-psychological factors. The empirical studies cited earlier concentrate on these individual-level factors, which may, to some extent, be determined by the "place" factors. For example, the presence of more factories and industries in towns and cities leads to increased job opportunities in the modern sector, making it more likely for urban women to work in a modern occupation. Taken together, therefore, both "place" and individual factors are posited to influence fertility, both individually and in interaction with one another.

Multivariate analyses using individual-level data provide insight only into the individual factors that may account for the differences between rural and urban fertility. Analyses utilizing data on both individuals and residence areas (rural and urban) might provide additional insights into rural/urban fertility differentials. Such studies, using data for both rural and urban areas, have not yet been carried out, due to a lack of appropriate data. Thus, one can only speculate about the magnitude of the effects of various place factors related to urban areas. However, there have been studies based on individual- and community-level data collected in rural areas only, which can be useful in indicating which "place" variables are important in explaining rural/urban fertility differentials. Casterline (1984) provides a concise review of the findings of various studies utilizing WFS community data. Measures of industrial development, for example, have been found to be significantly associated with fertility preference measures in rural Egypt and rural

Thailand, but not in rural Bangladesh. Indices based on community indicators of modernization (electricity, piped water, mail service, telephones, paved roads, schools) have been observed to have significant effects on contraceptive use and fertility in Bangladesh, Mexico, Peru, the Philippines and the Republic of Korea. However, the presence of electricity was found to be unrelated to fertility (and related behaviour) in the Syrian Arab Republic and Thailand. In addition, a positive relationship between the accessibility or density of family planning services and contraceptive use has been established in Bangladesh, Mexico, the Philippines, the Republic of Korea and Thailand, but not in Egypt, Malaysia, and Pakistan (Casterline, 1984; Chamratrithirong and Kamnuansilpa, 1984). Taken together, these results imply that although no one factor emerges as uniquely or uniformly important, certain features of modern infrastructure and family planning programmes may account for some of the differences between rural and urban fertility. In this chapter, countries are grouped according to indices of socio-economic development and strength of family planning programme effort in order to examine this assertion.

The explanations of rural/urban differentials in fertility outlined above implicitly assume that women have been exposed to either a rural or an urban environment for a long time. This assumption is made because the effects of the environment on fertility may be manifest only after several years of exposure. For example, women who have lived in towns or cities for some time are more likely to have developed attitudes that favour lower fertility and increased acceptability of contraception as a result of exposure to the urban life-style, environment and media. On the other hand, women who recently migrated from the countryside to the city may not have had the time or opportunity to develop attitudes that favour smaller families. In addition, it takes time to become aware of all of the costs imposed and benefits provided by the community structure within an urban development. Thus, the perceived costs and benefits of children may change with the duration of residence. The weak effects of residence on fertility observed in several studies could be partially due to recency of migration for many "urban" women.

Residence (or for that matter any socio-economic variable) cannot affect fertility directly, but only indirectly through the intermediate variables. Three of the more important intermediate variables that can be investigated using the WFS data are the major proximate determinants of fertility discussed in chapter VI: age at marriage; contraceptive use; and breast-feeding. Family size preference also acts as an intervening variable between socio-economic measures and fertility. Each of these variables can be expected to vary with residence. Women in urban areas are expected to desire smaller families, to marry later, to use contraception more often and possibly to use it more efficiently, and to breast-feed less and for shorter durations. While these differences in age at marriage, contraceptive use and family size preferences are likely to result in lower urban fertility, the differences in breast-feeding behaviour may result in higher fertility (if measures to control fertility are not taken). Several studies have documented these expected residential differences in the variables.[1]

It has been theorized that the magnitude of rural/urban differences in fertility changes in the course of the demographic transition. At the initial stage, little or no rural/urban differences are expected. There is very little practice of fertility control, and fertility is high in both rural and urban areas. Under these conditions, a small fertility differential might exist, due to rural/urban differences in marriage patterns, health and other factors that have a non-intentional impact on fertility, but it is not, in general, clear what type of fertility difference to expect. During the transitional phase, larger rural/urban differences are expected to be evident. It is in the urban areas that the traditional way of life first begins to break down, due to industrialization and modernization. Couples develop preferences for smaller families, and the use of various methods of fertility control spreads among the urban population. These changes have the effect of reducing urban fertility first, so that significant differences between rural and urban fertility levels are expected. Then, at the last stage of the transition, urban attitudes and values concerning fertility and fertility-related behaviour spread to the rural areas. Fertility falls, and ultimately rural and urban fertility levels converge so that the differences are non-significant. This pattern of change and convergence has been observed in Western Europe, where residential differences widened during the period of fertility decline and then began to narrow after the Second World War (United Nations, 1973). However, data from 11 WFS countries in Europe suggest that the disappearance of rural/urban fertility differentials has not yet occurred in all the countries examined. The average difference between urban and rural fertility (measured by children ever born) varied from virtually no difference in Belgium, Italy and Spain to 0.49 child in Yugoslavia, 0.51 child in Romania and 0.65 child in Poland (Jones, 1982). The path followed by these differentials between urban and rural fertility in currently developing countries may depend upon the style of development chosen by the Government, either emphasizing the primary support of certain growth centres or the spread of infrastructure to rural areas (and agricultural development).

A similar pattern of association between the stages of the demographic transition and the magnitude of rural/urban differentials in the intermediate variables and desired family size can also be hypothesized. Take the example of contraceptive use. During the initial phase of the transition, both rural and urban levels of use are expected to be low, so that virtually no difference in use can be observed. As the transition proceeds, contraceptive use begins at first to increase rapidly in the urban areas, so that relatively large rural/urban differences occur. Then, again at the last stage, contraceptive use spreads to the rural areas; use is at relatively high levels in both urban and rural areas, resulting once more in small differences. Again, deliberate government policy to support the diffusion of family planning in rural areas can narrow these expected differentials during the transition process.[2] Therefore, it would be too simplistic to base predictions about the course of the transition in currently developing countries on the historical experience in Europe.

This chapter examines the pattern and extent of rural/urban differences in fertility and fertility-related variables for the 38 developing countries included in this study. Further, as already noted, in order to facilitate comparisons among the countries and to examine some of the hypotheses described above, these differences are examined for countries grouped according to level of socio-economic development and strength of family planning programme effort. The next section discusses the measurement of residence. Two measures are used in this study: (a) a measure of current residence; (b) a constructed measure based on information on both current and childhood residence. Sections B and C contain analyses of the relationship between residence, on the one hand, and fertility and associated factors (desired family size, unwanted fertility, age at first marriage, length of breast-feeding, current contraceptive use), on the other. In section B, which contains a more descriptive analysis, residential differentials in fertility and related variables are discussed with respect to the more commonly used residence measure, that of current residence. Since this section is exploratory and such variables as total fertility rate (TFR), length of breast-feeding and singulate mean age at marriage (SMAM) are available only for current residence, this measure is used. In section C, more detailed multivariate analyses are carried out with respect to fertility, desired family size and contraceptive use. Residence differentials are examined using the combined residence variable, which is preferable because of its ability to distinguish recent from long-term residents. The chapter concludes with a summary and discussion of the findings.

A. MEASURES OF RESIDENCE

Some information on current place of residence was obtained in all countries covered in this study. Countries differed in the combinations of questions asked to obtain this information; they also differed on whether they used a *de facto* or *de jure* definition for the sample. Regardless of these differences, however, the variable on current residence can be interpreted as the place of usual residence.

In all countries except Yemen, current residence was ultimately coded in three categories: rural; other urban; and major urban. The basic identification of rural versus urban residence was made at the discretion of the individual countries. Some countries used population-size criteria to determine the type of residence. For example, in Panama, locales with fewer than 1,500 inhabitants were classified as rural, in contrast to the Republic of Korea, where locales with fewer than 20,000 inhabitants were so classified. Other countries used socio-economic characteristics, such as the presence of sewerage, electricity and water-supply, as criteria for categorizing place of residence. Further division of urban areas into "other urban" and "major urban" was based on a set of rules (formulated later), the most important of which were: (a) cities exceeding 1 million population were classified as major urban; (b) national capital cities, regardless of population size, were classified as major urban; (c) in countries with no cities exceeding 1 million inhabitants, the one largest city was classified as major urban. The application of these rules resulted in some large cities being classified as other urban and some small cities being classified as major urban.[3] Therefore, much variation exists between countries in terms of the residence classification. The reader should keep in mind that the findings given below are in part the result of such variation and that the size of rural/urban differentials in fertility and related variables within and across countries may reflect in part the degree to which places classified here as rural or urban really differ with respect to the characteristics of each type of place that are thought to affect fertility. On the other hand, these data provide a unique opportunity to assess in a comparative context the magnitude and direction of differences in fertility by type of place of residence under a wide variety of conditions.

The percentage distribution of ever-married women aged 15-49 by current type of place of residence is shown in table 94. In each of the three regions, the largest proportion of women were living in rural areas. In Latin America and the Caribbean, the proportion living in a rural area (46 per cent) was much lower than in either Africa or Asia and Oceania, at 70-71 per cent. Within Latin America and the Caribbean, the proportion rural varied greatly, from 18 per cent in Venezuela to 68 per cent in Haiti. In Africa, the proportion of rural residents exceeded 50 per cent in every country, while the proportion living in major urban areas was greater than 20 per cent only in Egypt. In Asia, the distribution of women across residence categories was extremely variable, with over 92 per cent of women living in rural areas in Bangladesh and Nepal, while over 60 per cent lived in either minor or major urban areas in Jordan and the Republic of Korea.

Although degree of urbanization is not directly included in the index of development used here, urbanization is often designated as one component of social and economic development. It is clear from the averages by level of development shown in table 94 that, among the countries included here, distribution by residence is highly correlated with development. The proportion of respondents currently residing in rural areas increases from 47 per cent in development group I to 76 per cent in development group IV. On the other hand, 28 per cent in development group I and 13 per cent in group IV were living in major urban areas.

A further piece of information collected by most countries was the respondent's childhood place of residence. Unlike the procedure for current residence, where the name of the place was first obtained and later objectively classified as rural or urban, for childhood residence, the respondent's subjective impression of the type of place (rural or urban) where she had mainly lived during her childhood was obtained. In general, the reference period for "childhood" was up to about age 12. Although most countries used this reference period, there were a few exceptions. Pakistan used age at first marriage, the Philippines used age 15, and Côte d'Ivoire[4] and Mauritania used "during your childhood" as the reference period. In addition, three countries—Cameroon, Fiji and Senegal—obtained the name of the place of childhood residence and later objectively classified it as rural or urban. While Cameroon and Senegal applied this procedure to all women, Fiji applied it only to those women who had always lived in the same place. Further, Guyana, Jamaica, and Trinidad and Tobago did not collect any information on childhood residence, while Mauritania classified childhood residence as either nomadic or sedentary. Thus, for these four countries, information on childhood residence could not be used.[5]

Empirical studies of fertility behaviour have generally used a measure of current residence as the residence variable. As mentioned earlier, the effects of an urban or a rural environment on fertility (and related behaviour) may be manifested only after several years of exposure to that environment. Current residence, however, may not always reflect this situation. Current urban residents, for example, may include recent migrants from the rural

TABLE 94. PERCENTAGE DISTRIBUTION OF EVER-MARRIED WOMEN AGED 15-49, ACCORDING TO CURRENT TYPE OF PLACE OF RESIDENCE, BY COUNTRY, REGION AND LEVEL OF DEVELOPMENT

	Ever-married women			
	Total	Rural	Other urban	Major urban
A. Country				
Africa				
Benin	100	72	11	17
Cameroon	100	82	9	9
Côte d'Ivoire[a]	100	62	20	18
Egypt	100	58	19	24
Ghana	100	68	16	16
Kenya	100	88	7	5
Lesotho	100	92	4	3
Mauritania	100	58	23	19
Morocco	100	61	24	15
Senegal	100	69	15	15
Sudan	100	73	16	11
Tunisia	100	52	31	17
Latin America and the Caribbean				
Colombia	100	36	47	17
Costa Rica	100	48	20	31
Dominican Republic	100	44	25	31
Ecuador	100	52	23	25
Guyana	100	64	8	28
Haiti	100	68	4	28
Jamaica	100	52	15	33
Mexico	100	42	31	28
Panama	100	42	12	46
Paraguay	100	56	16	27
Peru	100	36	38	26
Trinidad and Tobago	100	40	24	36
Venezuela	100	18	54	28
Asia and Oceania				
Bangladesh	100	92	4	4
Fiji	100	64	20	16
Indonesia	100	84	7	9
Jordan	100	30	34	36
Malaysia	100	69	15	16
Nepal	100	98	1	1
Pakistan	100	73	18	9
Philippines	100	68	20	13
Republic of Korea	100	40	30	30
Sri Lanka	100	82	12	6
Syrian Arab Republic	100	49	34	17
Thailand	100	85	7	8
Yemen	100	89	11	—
B. Region				
Africa	100	70	16	14
Latin America and the Caribbean	100	46	24	30
Asia and Oceania	100	71	16	14
C. Level of development				
I. High	100	47	25	28
II. Middle-high	100	55	24	20
III. Middle-low	100	74	13	12
IV. Low	100	76	12	13
TOTAL	100	62	19	19

Source: World Fertility Survey standard recode tapes.
[a] Formerly called the Ivory Coast.

areas, who are essentially "rural" in outlook although currently experiencing the costs and benefits provided by the urban setting. Such women are likely to manifest fertility behaviour that is in some intermediate range, being closer to rural women's behaviour if they are more recent migrants, which could result in underestimating the true effects of residence on fertility behaviour. In countries with relatively large volumes of rural-urban migration, this problem is potentially serious. Problems can also occur with the reverse case of urban-rural migration.

For certain parts of this study where the data permit, it was therefore decided to combine the current place of residence (urban and rural) with childhood place of residence (urban and rural) to form a new variable. This variable is used throughout section C of this chapter. It has four categories: women with a rural childhood and rural current residence; women with an urban childhood and urban current residence; women with a rural childhood and urban current residence; and women with an urban childhood and rural current residence. For convenience, the first two categories are referred to as "long-term" rural and urban residents, respectively, while the latter two are called the "rural-urban" and "urban-rural" groups, respectively. In general, the largest differentials in fertility and related behaviour are expected to emerge between the two groups of long-term residents.

The combined measure of residence has certain advantages over the measure of current residence. As mentioned earlier, it covers a longer period of exposure to the environment. For example, women exposed to an urban setting both during childhood and currently are differentiated from women who had lived only more recently in such a setting. Thus, this detailed measure of residence may yield a more accurate estimate of the effect of individual residence on fertility and related behaviour, i.e., that aspect of residence which is embodied in a person's characteristics. In addition, the combined measure is able to utilize all available information from each respondent (that can be comparably obtained in nearly all the countries) on residence.

At the same time, the combined measure of residence has some limitations. First, this measure may be contaminated by cases of multiple moves (e.g., women who had moved from rural areas to urban and then to rural areas). It is expected, however, that the number of such cases will generally be small. Secondly, there is no information on when (or how many years ago) the respondents had moved from one type of residence to another. Thus, cross-country comparisons of differences between these longer term and more recent residence groups may be affected by country differences in the timing of rural-urban migrants which would affect the average duration of urban residence for the urban migrant group. Thirdly, there is the possibility that some women who had not moved at all may be classified as migrants. This can occur if the respondent felt that her childhood place of residence was rural in character (say), and yet the same place was currently classified as urban. This classification does not pose a severe problem conceptually, however, since the environments may actually have changed from rural to urban in character over the respondent's lifetime. A potentially more serious problem can occur when the reverse case holds, i.e., when the respondent considered her childhood place of residence to be urban in character, but the same place was classified as rural for current residence. Such cases are especially likely to occur when respondents live at the fringes of large cities. Their environment may be urban-like, yet it can be classified as rural. Nothing, however, is known about the extent of such cases.

Table 95 presents the percentage distribution of the respondents (ever-married women aged 15-49 years) in the four categories of the constructed residence variable

TABLE 95. PERCENTAGE DISTRIBUTION OF EVER-MARRIED WOMEN AGED 15-49, ACCORDING TO CATEGORY OF CONSTRUCTED RESIDENCE VARIABLE,[a] BY COUNTRY, REGION AND LEVEL OF DEVELOPMENT

	Long-term rural (1)	Urban-rural[b] (2)	Rural-urban[c] (3)	Long-term urban (4)
A. Country				
Africa				
Benin	65	7	9	19
Cameroon	78	4	8	10
Côte d'Ivoire[d]	53	9	16	23
Egypt	47	11	9	33
Ghana	53	15	6	26
Kenya	84	4	10	2
Lesotho	89	3	6	1
Morocco	59	2	15	23
Senegal	63	7	8	22
Sudan	64	9	5	22
Tunisia	46	6	11	37
Latin America and the Caribbean				
Colombia	28	8	15	49
Costa Rica	35	13	18	34
Dominican Republic	44	5	23	28
Ecuador	39	13	9	39
Haiti	60	8	10	22
Mexico	24	18	12	46
Panama	31	11	14	44
Paraguay	46	11	5	38
Peru	28	7	16	49
Venezuela	12	6	6	76
Asia and Oceania				
Bangladesh	90	2	5	3
Fiji	61	3	22	14
Indonesia	71	13	6	10
Jordan	25	5	21	49
Malaysia	58	10	15	17
Nepal	95	3	1	1
Pakistan	69	4	9	17
Philippines	58	10	13	19
Republic of Korea	35	5	40	20
Sri Lanka	77	4	8	11
Syrian Arab Republic	46	3	10	41
Thailand	82	3	8	7
Yemen	83	5	3	9
B. Region				
Africa	64	7	9	20
Latin America and the Caribbean	35	10	13	43
Asia and Oceania	70	6	13	18
C. Level of development				
I. High	36	9	18	38
II. Middle-high	49	7	12	32
III. Middle-low	67	8	10	16
IV. Low	74	6	6	14
TOTAL	56	7	11	25

Source: World Fertility Survey standard recode tapes.
[a] Data not available for Mauritania, Guyana, Jamaica, and Trinidad and Tobago.
[b] Reported urban childhood and rural current residence.
[c] Reported rural childhood and urban current residence.
[d] Formerly called the Ivory Coast.

for the 34 countries for which this measure could be constructed. Attention is first focused on the two "long-term" resident groups (columns (1) and (4)). Both Africa, and Asia and Oceania as a whole have similar proportions: in each region, 64-70 per cent were long-term rural residents, compared with 18-20 per cent long-term urban residents. As in the case of current residence, the Latin American and Caribbean region as a whole appears considerably more urbanized. Roughly 43 per cent of the respondents were long-term urban-dwellers, while 35 per cent were long-term rural residents. Not surprisingly, within each region, there is a wide range in the proportions who were either long-term rural or urban. For example, in Latin America and the Caribbean, over three fourths of the respondents in Venezuela were long-term urban residents, compared with under one fourth in Haiti. With respect to the mixed groups, in most countries the percentage with rural followed by urban residence is greater than the percentage with urban followed by rural residence, as expected. In only a few countries is the reverse observed; of these countries, in only Ghana, Indonesia, Mexico and Paraguay did the respondents with urban followed by rural residence exceed the group going from rural to urban by more than five percentage points. The Republic of Korea had the largest proportion in the rural-urban group (40 per cent), while the Dominican Republic, Fiji and Jordan had 20-23 per cent. On the other hand, Mexico had about 18 per cent in the urban-rural category, the largest proportion for any country.

From table 95, one can also obtain the proportions of current residents who had changed their type of residence. Among current rural residents (including both long-term and recent residents), a much larger proportion were long-term residents than is the case among urban residents in nearly all countries (columns (1) and (2)). The chief exception to this pattern is Mexico, where the ratio of long-term rural residents to recent residents is 4:3, i.e., of all current rural residents, 57 per cent were long term while 43 per cent reported spending their childhood in an urban setting. In contrast, the pattern among current urban residents is very different (columns (3) and (4)). In several countries, a fairly large proportion of the current urban residents had resided in rural areas as children. For example, in the Dominican Republic and Malaysia, close to half, and in Fiji, the Republic of Korea and Thailand, more than half, of the current urban residents had originated in rural areas. Whether the more recent arrivals to the cities differed from the long-term urban residents in their fertility and related behaviour is examined in later sections.

B. PRELIMINARY ANALYSIS

This section is organized into five parts, each corresponding to an important aspect of reproduction: fertility; fertility preferences; age at marriage; breast-feeding; and contraceptive use. Basic differentials in these factors with respect to type of place of residence are described. As noted earlier, "residence" in this section is measured by current residence. The threefold classification scheme (rural, other urban, major urban) is used in the study of fertility, desired family size, contraceptive use and breast-feeding. Differentials in age at marriage can only be examined with respect to the two-category scheme (rural and urban), due to data limitations.

Fertility

This subsection focuses on fertility differentials by type of place of current residence. As discussed earlier, fertility is expected to be highest in rural areas and lowest in the major urban areas. Table 96 presents two measures of fertility, one indicating recent levels, the other achieved fertility for older women. Columns (1)-(3) contain the total fertility rates for each category of current residence,

TABLE 96. TOTAL FERTILITY RATE AND MEAN NUMBER OF CHILDREN BORN TO ALL WOMEN AGED 40-49, BY CURRENT TYPE OF PLACE OF RESIDENCE, FOR COUNTRIES AND GROUPS

	Total fertility rate, all women aged 15-49				Mean children ever born to all women aged 40-49			
	Rural (1)	Other urban (2)	Major urban (3)	Difference: (1) – (3) (4)	Rural (5)	Other urban (6)	Major urban (7)	Difference: (5) – (7) (8)

A. Country

Africa
Benin	7.4	6.7	5.8	1.6	6.2	6.0	5.9	0.3
Cameroon	6.5	6.7	5.3	1.2	5.3	4.7	4.9	0.4
Côte d'Ivoire[a]	7.7	6.9	6.4	1.3	6.9	6.4	6.7	0.2
Egypt	6.1	4.9	3.8	2.3	6.9	6.7	5.7	1.2
Ghana	6.8	6.3	5.4	1.4	6.6	6.0	5.8	0.8
Kenya	8.5	6.1	5.9	2.6	7.8	5.8	7.1	0.7
Lesotho	6.2	-----4.8-----		..	5.2	-----4.6-----		..
Mauritania	6.3	6.1	6.3	0.0	5.9	6.0	5.8	0.1
Morocco	7.0	4.8	3.9	3.1	7.7	6.3	6.2	1.5
Senegal	7.5	6.3	6.8	0.7	7.0	6.6	6.9	0.1
Sudan	6.4	5.7	4.8	1.6	6.0	6.3	6.1	−0.1
Tunisia	7.0	-----4.8-----		..	6.9	-----6.5-----		..

Latin America and the Caribbean
Colombia	7.0	3.9	2.9	4.1	7.2	6.4	4.9	2.3
Costa Rica[b]	5.2	3.3	3.0	2.2	8.0	5.5	4.7	3.3
Dominican Republic	7.4	4.4	4.2	3.2	7.9	5.4	5.0	2.9
Ecuador	6.7	4.9	3.1	3.6	7.4	6.4	4.9	2.5
Guyana	5.3	5.9	4.1	1.2	7.0	6.3	4.9	2.1
Haiti	6.2	3.4	4.0	2.2	6.1	(4.5)	5.0	0.9
Jamaica	5.7	5.2	3.9	1.8	6.1	5.4	4.1	2.0
Mexico	7.6	5.7	4.8	2.8	7.6	6.2	5.8	1.8
Panama[b]	6.2	3.5	3.5	2.7	6.9	6.1	4.6	2.3
Paraguay	6.3	4.0	3.2	3.1	7.2	5.4	4.1	3.1
Peru	7.2	5.4	3.9	3.3	7.1	6.6	5.0	2.1
Trinidad and Tobago	3.7	3.3	2.9	0.8	6.1	5.4	4.9	1.2
Venezuela[c]	7.7	4.3	3.3	4.4	7.8	6.2	5.0	2.8

Asia and Oceania
Bangladesh	6.1	5.8	5.7	0.4	7.0	6.8	6.8	0.2
Fiji	4.6	3.8	3.3	1.3	6.5	6.0	5.5	1.0
Indonesia	4.9	4.3	4.6	0.3	5.2	5.1	5.6	−0.4
Jordan	9.5	7.7	6.3	3.2	8.8	8.8	8.0	0.8
Malaysia	5.0	4.5	3.5	1.5	6.3	6.0	5.4	0.9
Nepal	6.2	-----4.3-----		—	5.7	4.4	..	0.4
Pakistan	6.3	6.3	5.9	0.4	6.9	7.0	6.5	0.4
Philippines	6.0	4.0	3.5	2.5	7.0	5.7	5.1	1.9
Republic of Korea	5.0	4.2	3.3	1.7	6.1	5.1	4.5	1.6
Sri Lanka	3.9	3.2	3.1	0.8	5.7	4.9	5.0	0.7
Syrian Arab Republic	9.0	6.9	4.7	4.3	7.7	7.7	6.5	1.2
Thailand	5.0	3.6	2.5	2.5	6.4	5.0	4.8	1.6
Yemen	8.6	-----7.8-----		..	6.8	-----7.0-----		..

B. Region[d]

Africa	7.0	6.0	5.4	1.6	6.5	6.0	6.1	0.4
Latin America and the Caribbean	6.3	4.5	3.6	2.7	7.1	5.9	4.8	2.3
Asia and Oceania	6.2	4.9	4.2	2.0	6.6	6.1	5.8	0.8

C. Level of development[d]

I. High	5.7	4.3	3.5	2.2	6.9	5.9	4.9	2.0
II. Middle-high	6.8	4.9	3.8	3.0	7.2	6.2	5.4	1.8
III. Middle-low	6.7	5.7	5.1	1.6	6.5	5.7	6.0	0.5
IV. Low	6.8	5.8	5.6	1.2	6.4	6.2	6.1	0.3

D. Strength of family planning programme effort[d]

1. Strong	5.5	4.1	3.5	2.0	6.6	5.7	4.9	1.7
2. Moderate	5.5	3.9	3.3	2.2	6.7	5.6	5.1	1.6
3. Weak	6.8	5.2	4.5	2.3	7.1	6.0	5.7	1.4
4. Very weak/none	7.3	6.2	5.3	2.0	6.7	6.3	5.6	1.1
TOTAL	6.5	5.2	4.3	2.2	6.8	6.0	5.4	1.4

Source: Casterline and Ashurst (1984).
NOTE: Values in parentheses based on 10-24 cases.
[a] Formerly called the Ivory Coast.
[b] Calculated from World Fertility Survey standard recode tapes. Age-specific rate at ages 15-19 taken from the period 5-9 years before survey; other age-specific rates pertain to the period 0-4 years prior to the survey.
[c] Total fertility rate refers to ages 15-44.
[d] Averages excluding values for combined or missing categories.

based on births during the five years preceding each survey. The last three columns show the mean number of children ever born to women aged 40-49; these provide estimates of levels of completed fertility. Within each type of residence, comparisons between these two measures can be used as a crude indicator of trends in fertility differentials over time. Given the variation in the quality of the fertility data, however, such comparisons must be undertaken with considerable caution. In addition, fertility differentials for older women may be affected, to a greater extent than those for the total fertility rate, by migration between rural and urban areas—that is, some of the older women's children had been born when the mother lived in a different type of place. Information on the quality of enumeration of recent birth by country is given in chapter I (table 25). However, even in cases where the estimated levels of fertility appear to be less reliable, a comparison of recent fertility differentials and differentials derived from past levels of childbearing may be indicative of trends in differentials if errors are not thought to be more common among rural than urban respondents.

A further point that is important to note here is that there are differences in the levels of mortality experienced by children born to urban and to rural residents. These differential rates of survival have an effect on the extent to which observed rural/urban differences in number of children ever born reflect differences in the actual number of surviving children women have. As is shown in table 97, the percentage of children ever born to women aged 40-49 who were still alive at the time of the interview was highest in all regions and at all levels of development among women living in major urban areas and lowest among rural women. Averaged over all countries, the percentage surviving is nine percentage points higher among major urban than among rural women. Thus, rural/urban differences in the number of living children are smaller than these differences in children ever born. That is, the higher fertility of rural women is partially offset by the lower rate of survival among their children. For example, rural African women aged 40-49 averaged 0.4 child ever born more than major urban women. The corresponding difference in mean number of living children is 0.1 child. The rural/major urban difference is similarly reduced by differential child survival from 2.3 to 1.7 in Latin America and the Caribbean and from 0.8 to 0.3 in Asia and Oceania.

As is shown in table 96, in nearly all countries, recent fertility was highest in the rural areas, lowest in the major urban areas and in-between in the other urban areas. Relatively large differences of over three children between the rural and major urban areas were found in Morocco in Northern Africa, Jordan and the Syrian Arab Republic in Western Asia, and several countries in Latin America and the Caribbean. Venezuela had the largest such difference, over four children. The smallest differences were found in three Asian countries—Bangladesh, Indonesia and Pakistan—where the difference between the rural and major urban areas was only 0.3-0.4 child. Exceptions to this pattern of steadily lower fertility with increasing urbanism are Cameroon, Guyana, Haiti, Indonesia, Mauritania and Senegal.

Within each residence area, recent fertility (TFR) is highest, on average, in Africa. Latin America and the Caribbean had the lowest average fertility in both the urban areas; only in the rural areas was fertility roughly

TABLE 97. PERCENTAGE OF CHILDREN EVER BORN WHO WERE STILL ALIVE AT INTERVIEW AND MEAN NUMBER OF LIVING CHILDREN, FOR EVER-MARRIED WOMEN AGED 40-49, ACCORDING TO TYPE OF PLACE OF RESIDENCE: AVERAGES BY REGION AND LEVEL OF DEVELOPMENT

	Type of place of residence		
	Rural	Other urban	Major urban
A. *Percentage of children ever born who were still alive at interview*			
Region			
Africa	75	79	81
Latin America and the Caribbean	87	90	94
Asia and Oceania	81	87	89
Level of development			
I. High	89	92	99
II. Middle-high	85	90	94
III. Middle-low	75	79	79
IV. Low	71	78	81
TOTAL	81	86	90
B. *Mean number of living children*			
Region			
Africa	4.9	4.7	5.0
Latin America and the Caribbean	6.2	5.3	4.5
Asia and Oceania	5.3	5.3	5.2
Level of development			
I. High	6.1	5.4	4.7
II. Middle-high	6.1	5.6	5.1
III. Middle-low	4.9	4.5	4.8
IV. Low	4.5	4.8	5.0
TOTAL	5.5	5.1	4.9

Source: World Fertility Survey standard recode tapes.

the same as in Asia and Oceania. Although all regions show, on average, the highest recent fertility among rural women and the lowest among major urban women, the size of differential varies, being largest in Latin America and the Caribbean, and smallest in Africa. Rural women in Latin America and the Caribbean average 1.8 children more than other urban women, and 2.7 children more than major urban women. In contrast, in Africa, the corresponding differences are 1.0 and 1.6 children more than other and major urban women, respectively. In general, similar patterns with respect to completed fertility are also observed, although the differentials are smaller.

Change over time in fertility differentials can be observed by comparing the total fertility rate and the mean number of children ever born to women aged 40-49. Figure 46 plots the regional average values (given in table 96) for each residential area. A comparison of these graphs indicates that, both in Latin America and the Caribbean and in Asia and Oceania, differences between rural and major urban areas are larger for recent fertility than for completed fertility, i.e., over time, the data indicate a widening of differentials by residence. This is especially true of Asia and Oceania, where a rural/major urban difference of 0.8 child is observed for completed fertility, compared with a much larger differential of 2.0 children for recent fertility.

In Africa, the data suggest that rural/urban fertility differentials were larger in the recent period than in the past. The apparent increase observed for rural fertility is probably not a true increase, given the poor quality of data found in many countries of Africa (see chapter I for details).

To the extent that the early and intermediate phases of the fertility transition are indicated by the levels of development used in this study, differentials by residence

Figure 46. Total fertility rate and mean number of children ever born to ever-married women aged 40-49, according to current residence, by region and level of development

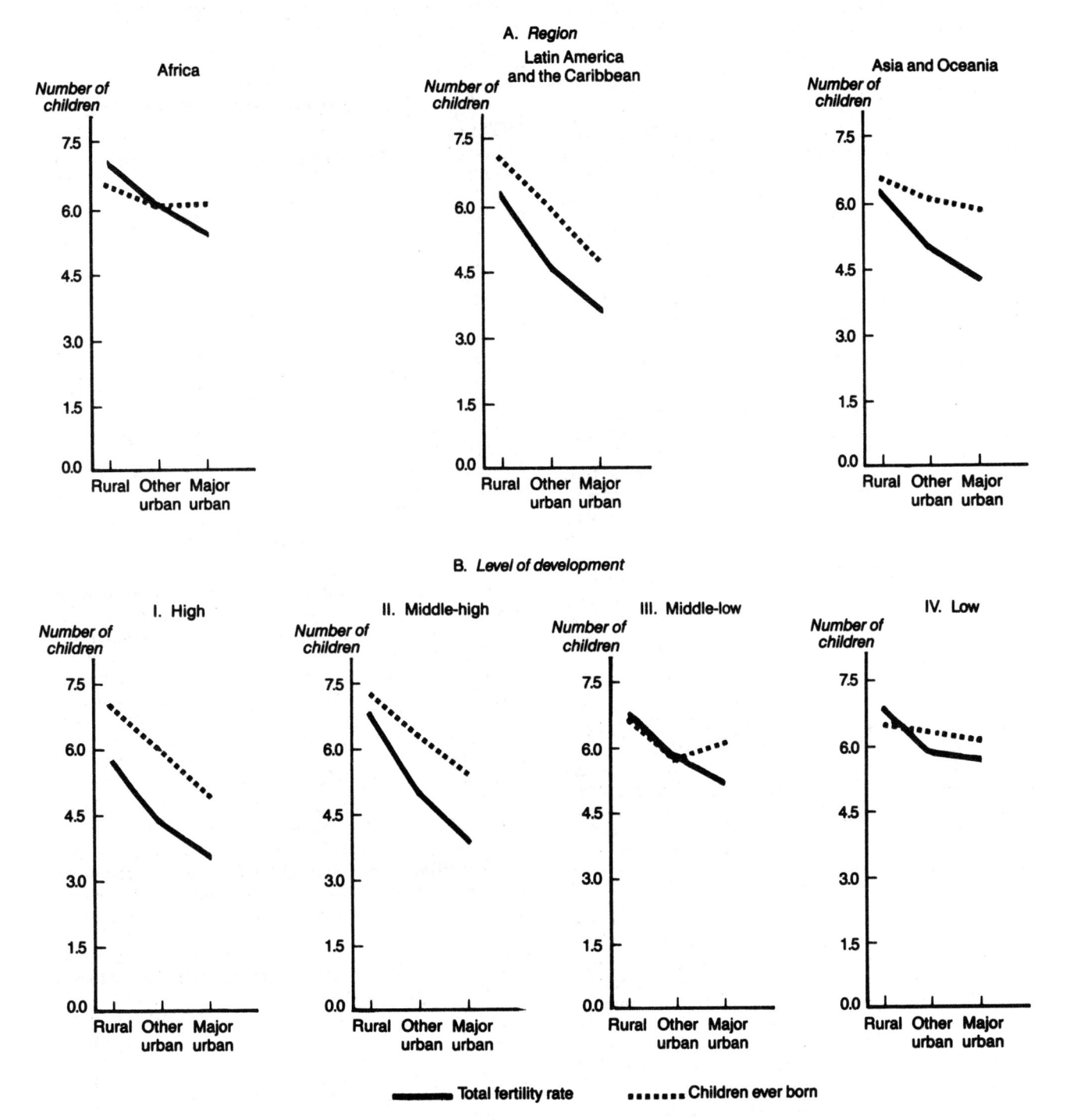

A. *Region*

[Charts for Africa, Latin America and the Caribbean, Asia and Oceania showing Number of children (0.0–7.5) by Rural / Other urban / Major urban]

B. *Level of development*

[Charts for I. High, II. Middle-high, III. Middle-low, IV. Low showing Number of children (0.0–7.5) by Rural / Other urban / Major urban]

———— Total fertility rate   ······ Children ever born

Source: Table 96.

are expected to widen with increasing levels of development. The convergence of differentials hypothesized at the later stage of the transition may not be evident here as it is not clear at precisely what level of development fertility differentials will begin to narrow.

The association between the level of development and the size of differentials by residence can be seen in figure 46. As expected, recent fertility differentials by residence increase with each increase in the development level, but only until the middle-high level. The difference between recent fertility in the rural and major urban areas increases from 1.2 children at the low development level, to 1.6 at the middle-low level and to 3.0 children at the middle-high level. This widening of differences is due mainly to the decrease of fertility in the major urban areas across development groups. Rural fertility is roughly the same, 6.7-6.8 children per woman at the lower three levels of development, while major urban fertility is almost two

195

children fewer in development group II (middle-high). These results tend to support the theory that differentials by residence widen with development. Although it is difficult to judge the significance of the observed contraction of differentials at the upper development level, it results primarily from lower rural fertility and may signify the beginning of a convergence of fertility levels among women in rural and in urban areas.

Figure 46 also shows the fertility measures by residence across development groups. Note that in development groups III and IV, recent fertility is estimated to be roughly the same as past fertility for rural and other urban women while major urban women show lower fertility in the more recent period. In development groups I and II, recent fertility was lower than past fertility in all residence groups. In the middle-high group, the largest difference between recent and past fertility (1.6 children) can be seen in the case of major urban women, while in the high development group, the largest difference, 1.6 children, is found among other urban residents.

In summary, the largest differentials between residence groups in recent fertility are in Latin America and the Caribbean and the smallest in Africa. In all regions, fertility differentials are larger for recent than for past fertility, suggesting that urban/rural fertility differentials have widened over time. On the whole, both recent and cumulative fertility differentials widen with increasing development. Although fertility differences between current and past fertility are small among urban women in countries at low levels of development, these same differences are large among women in all categories of residence in the upper development groups, with the most dramatic differences appearing among urban women.

Fertility preferences

This subsection investigates differentials in desired family size by type of place of current residence. Compared with rural areas, urban areas are generally associated with higher costs of rearing children, reduced labour value of children; and easier access to education, job opportunities and the media. These factors taken together are likely to result in preference for smaller family size among urban residents.

For this analysis, family size preferences are measured by the response to a question about desired family size. Further details on this measure, its comparability across countries and the problems associated with such a measure are discussed in chapter II. One of the more important problems relevant to this analysis is that of non-numerical responses to the question on desired family size (such as "I don't know", or "It's up to God"). As stated in chapter II, while three fourths of the countries have low rates (below 5 per cent) of non-response, several countries (mainly in sub-Saharan Africa) have very high rates of over 20 per cent. It should be noted that if there is a tendency for particular groups not to respond, the group means may be biased.

Table 98 shows the percentage who gave a non-numerical response to the question on desired family size according to the three categories of current residence. The table includes only those countries for which the overall level of non-response was greater than 10 per cent.[6] Note first that most of the countries with a high percentage of non-numerical responses are in Africa. Over all, the average proportion of women who did not give a numerical response is slightly lower in major urban areas than in either of the other two categories of residence. In 7 of 10 countries, the proportion who did not respond declines with increasing urbanism. In Côte d'Ivoire, Mauritania and Senegal, however, the pattern is reversed; the proportion who gave a non-numerical answer is higher among urban than among rural women. This pattern of non-response may be influenced by the distribution of ethnic groups across types of place of residence. Thus, although the rural and urban values for stated desired family size are presented for all countries, the reader is urged to be cautious in interpreting the results from countries having high rates of non-response.

Table 99 presents the average desired family size by current residence for ever-married women, adjusted for age differences between residence groups. The overall average for all countries grouped together shows a pattern of decreasing desired family size with increasing urbanism (i.e., from rural to other urban to major urban). This pattern is observed in all countries except Bangladesh, Guyana, Indonesia and Mauritania. In Bangladesh and Guyana, women in other urban areas desired slightly larger families than either major urban or rural women. In Indonesia, both rural and other urban women desired 4.1 children, while major urban women desired about 4.3 children. Only in Mauritania did major urban women apparently desire much larger families than either rural or other urban women: 0.6 and 1.1. more children, respectively. How much of this is due to the high level of non-response in Mauritania and how much to actual desires is unknown. Given the high level of non-response in most of Africa, it is also difficult to determine whether the expected pattern of decreasing family size desires with urbanization observed in the African countries reflects the real situation.

Among the countries with relatively low proportions of non-numerical response, there is fairly wide variation in the size of differentials by residence. The Syrian Arab Republic had the largest differential, with rural women expressing a preference for three more children than major urban women. Costa Rica, Egypt, Jordan, Paraguay and Venezuela also had differences between rural and major urban areas, averaging 1.5 children. The smallest differences (less than 0.5 child) were found in Trinidad and Tobago and in Thailand.

TABLE 98. PERCENTAGE OF EVER-MARRIED WOMEN AGED 15-49 WHO GAVE A NON-NUMERICAL RESPONSE TO THE QUESTION ON DESIRED FAMILY SIZE, BY TYPE OF PLACE OF CURRENT RESIDENCE, SELECTED COUNTRIES

Country	Current residence		
	Rural	Other urban	Major urban
Bangladesh	33	29	21
Benin	34	46	18
Côte d'Ivoire[a]	22	27	31
Ghana	12	13	5
Kenya	20	17	14
Mauritania	30	35	37
Morocco	22	10	7
Senegal	26	29	38
Sudan	20	16	11
Yemen	45	——36——	
TOTAL (EXCLUDING YEMEN)	24	25	20

Source: World Fertility Survey standard recode tapes.
NOTE: Percentages are adjusted for effects of age differences between residence groups.
[a] Formerly called the Ivory Coast.

TABLE 99. MEAN DESIRED FAMILY SIZE, EVER-MARRIED WOMEN AGED 15-49, ACCORDING TO CURRENT RESIDENCE, BY COUNTRY, REGION AND LEVEL OF DEVELOPMENT

Region and country	Rural (1)	Other urban (2)	Major urban (3)	Difference: (1) − (3) (4)
A. Country				
Africa				
Benin[a]	7.9	7.4	5.8	2.1
Cameroon[a]	8.1	8.1	7.6	0.5
Côte d'Ivoire[a,b]	8.9	7.7	7.2	1.7
Egypt	4.8	3.5	3.0	1.8
Ghana[a]	6.3	5.7	5.5	0.8
Kenya[a]	7.3	6.4	6.1	1.2
Lesotho	6.0	5.6	4.9	1.1
Mauritania[a]	8.7	8.2	9.3	−0.6
Morocco[a]	5.5	4.2	3.9	1.6
Senegal[a]	8.8	7.2	6.8	2.0
Sudan[a]	6.5	6.1	5.5	1.0
Tunisia	4.6	3.9	3.4	1.2
Latin America and the Caribbean				
Colombia	4.5	4.0	3.5	1.0
Costa Rica	5.4	4.3	4.0	1.4
Dominican Republic	5.0	4.4	4.3	0.7
Ecuador	4.4	4.0	3.4	1.0
Guyana	4.7	4.9	4.2	0.5
Haiti	3.7	3.6	3.1	0.6
Jamaica	4.4	3.8	3.6	0.8
Mexico	4.9	4.4	3.9	1.0
Panama	4.6	4.1	3.9	0.7
Paraguay	5.7	5.0	4.1	1.6
Peru	4.2	3.6	3.5	0.7
Trinidad and Tobago	3.9	3.8	3.7	0.2
Venezuela	5.0	4.2	3.6	1.4
Asia and Oceania				
Bangladesh[a]	4.1	4.2	3.7	0.4
Fiji	4.3	4.0	3.7	0.6
Indonesia	4.1	4.1	4.3	0.2
Jordan	7.2	6.2	5.6	1.6
Malaysia	4.6	4.2	3.7	0.9
Nepal	3.9	3.6	3.1	0.8
Pakistan	4.3	3.9	3.8	0.5
Philippines	4.6	4.1	3.7	0.9
Republic of Korea	3.5	3.1	2.8	0.7
Sri Lanka	3.9	3.5	3.4	0.5
Syrian Arab Republic	7.2	5.5	4.2	3.0
Thailand	3.8	3.5	3.5	0.3
Yemen[a]	5.4	-----4.8-----		..
B. Region				
Africa	7.0	6.2	5.8	1.2
Sub-Sahara[c]	7.6	6.9	6.5	1.1
Other	5.0	3.9	3.4	1.6
Latin America and the Caribbean	4.6	4.1	3.8	0.8
Asia and Oceania	4.7	4.2	3.8	0.9
C. Level of development				
I. High	4.5	4.1	3.7	0.8
II. Middle-high	5.1	4.4	3.9	1.2
III. Middle-low	6.4	5.7	5.3	1.1
IV. Low	5.9	5.5	5.1	0.8
Excluding sub-Saharan Africa[c]				
III. Middle-low	4.8	3.9	3.7	1.1
IV. Low	4.3	3.8	3.4	0.9
TOTAL	5.4	4.8	4.4	1.0

Source: World Fertility Survey standard recode tapes.

NOTES: Means are adjusted for the effects of age differences between residence groups. For Cameroon, Fiji and Pakistan, questions on desired family size are not standard (see chapter II).

[a] Non-numerical responses greater than 10 per cent.
[b] Formerly called the Ivory Coast.
[c] Including Benin, Cameroon, Côte d'Ivoire, Kenya, Lesotho, Mauritania, Senegal and Sudan.

The regions of Latin America and the Caribbean, and Asia and Oceania show very similar mean desired family sizes by residence. Rural women in each region desired 4.6-4.7 children, compared with 3.8 children for major urban women. In Africa, women in each residence group desired larger families than women in the other two regions. The averages for Africa are shown separately for sub-Saharan countries and other African countries (Egypt, Morocco and Tunisia) because, as noted in chapter II, fertility desires in the sub-Saharan countries were exceptionally high. Although sub-Saharan women desired larger families than other African women, desired family size decreases monotonically with increasing urbanism in both subregions. The rural/major urban difference was slightly smaller in the sub-Saharan countries (1.1 children) than in the other African countries (1.6 children) but, over all, this difference is larger in Africa than in either of the two other regions. The size of the rural/major urban differential tends to be somewhat larger in development groups II and III than in the other groups but no striking pattern in size of differentials by level of development is evident.

Thus, as expected, desired family size decreases with urbanism, although in general the differentials were smaller than those observed for recent fertility, especially in Latin America and the Caribbean, where the rural/major urban difference in recent fertility was 2.7 children while the difference in desired family size was less than one child. In addition, unlike recent fertility, desired family size shows only minor variation in the size of differentials by either region or level of development.

The extent to which women at the end of their childbearing years had exceeded their desired family size is addressed in table 100. The table shows the percentage of women aged 40-49 with more living children than desired averaged by region and level of development. Averages for the sub-Saharan countries are shown separately, as they differ greatly from the remaining countries of Africa. The level of excess fertility was very low in the sub-Saharan countries and was similar in all types of place of residence. The level was much higher in the other countries of Africa (Egypt, Morocco, Tunisia) and the proportion with more living children than desired was 19 percentage points higher among major urban than among rural residents. The level of unwanted childbearing was also greater among urban than rural residents in Asia and Oceania and in development groups II-IV. In Latin America and the Caribbean and in development group I, the opposite pattern is observed (i.e., more rural than urban women had a greater number of children than desired).

These differing patterns of unwanted fertility by type of place of residence may reflect a tendency for lower family-size preferences to precede the availability and use of effective contraception and for contraception to become available earlier in urban than in rural areas. The evolution of levels of unwanted fertility and urban/rural differences in unwanted childbearing may proceed along a continuum in which rural women in relatively poorly developed countries desire many children, do not use contraception and thus have a low level of unwanted fertility. At the other extreme, urban women in relatively highly developed countries prefer low family sizes and have access to family planning which enables them to achieve their desires; this situation would also result in low levels of unwanted fertility. In between these two

TABLE 100. PERCENTAGE OF EVER-MARRIED WOMEN AGED 40-49 WITH MORE LIVING CHILDREN THAN THE NUMBER DESIRED, ACCORDING TO TYPE OF PLACE OF RESIDENCE: AVERAGES BY REGION AND LEVEL OF DEVELOPMENT

	Rural (1)	Other urban (2)	Major urban (3)	Difference: (1) – (3) (4)
Region				
Africa	13	16	19	–6
Sub-Sahara[a]	6	5	8	–2
Other	33	45	52	–19
Latin America and the Caribbean	37	35	31	6
Asia and Oceania	29	31	37	–8
Level of development				
I. High	39	38	34	5
II. Middle-high	33	35	35	–2
III. Middle-low	15	14	17	–4
IV. Low	17	19	26	–9
Middle-low and low, excluding sub-Saharan Africa	25	29	39	–14
TOTAL	27	28	29	–2
TOTAL, EXCLUDING SUB-SAHARAN AFRICA	33	34	36	–3

Source: World Fertility Survey standard recode tapes.
[a] Including Benin, Cameroon, Côte d'Ivoire, Ghana, Kenya, Lesotho, Mauritania, Senegal, Sudan. (Côte d'Ivoire was formerly called the Ivory Coast.)

extremes, the extent to which contraceptive knowledge and use lag behind lower desired family size and the nature of rural/urban differences in each of these factors will determine the size and direction of rural/urban differences in unwanted fertility. This explanation is compatible with the findings of earlier studies of unwanted fertility using WFS data in which the preponderance of unwanted births were found to have shifted over time from urban to rural areas (Westoff, 1981; Blanc, 1982).

Age at marriage

Urban women are expected to marry later than rural women for a variety of reasons. First, urban areas are associated with better educational and employment opportunities for women. For example, the larger number of educational institutions in urban areas makes it more likely for urban women to be educated and to achieve higher levels of education than rural women; industries, factories, offices and other work-places provide increased opportunities for women to work, and to work in a modern occupation. Both these factors, education and employment, are thought to contribute to delayed marriage (see chapters VIII and IX). In addition, urban women are more likely to be exposed (through the media, the work-place and educational institutions) to ideas and norms that discourage early marriage.

To examine rural/urban differentials in age at entry into marriage, table 101 presents the singulate mean age at marriage for 35 countries by residence. These estimates are based on the marital status distribution at the time of the survey derived from household data. This table is based on unpublished material by Ebanks and Singh (1984), in which data for Lesotho, Nepal and Yemen are not included. These estimates of age at marriage were available only for the simple rural/urban dichotomy for type of place of current residence, i.e., the urban areas in this subsection refer to other and major urban areas combined. A box-and-whisker plot summarizing the results for all countries is shown in figure 47.

In 31 of the 35 countries included in table 101, women who were living in urban areas married later than women in rural areas. The rural/urban difference in age at marriage averaged over all countries included in table 101 is 1.7 years. Not surprisingly, substantial variation in this difference is evident among the individual countries. Small differences of less than a year were found in Côte d'Ivoire, Fiji, Haiti, Kenya and Sri Lanka, while large differences of over three years were seen in Benin, Egypt, Indonesia and Senegal. In Mauritania, there is no discernible difference in age at marriage, while in three anglophone countries in Latin America and the Caribbean—Guyana, Jamaica, and Trinidad and Tobago—the reverse situation was found: women in urban areas married earlier, on average, than women in rural areas. The difference, however, is small in each case, less than a year.

Figure 47. Singulate mean age at marriage by residence, all countries

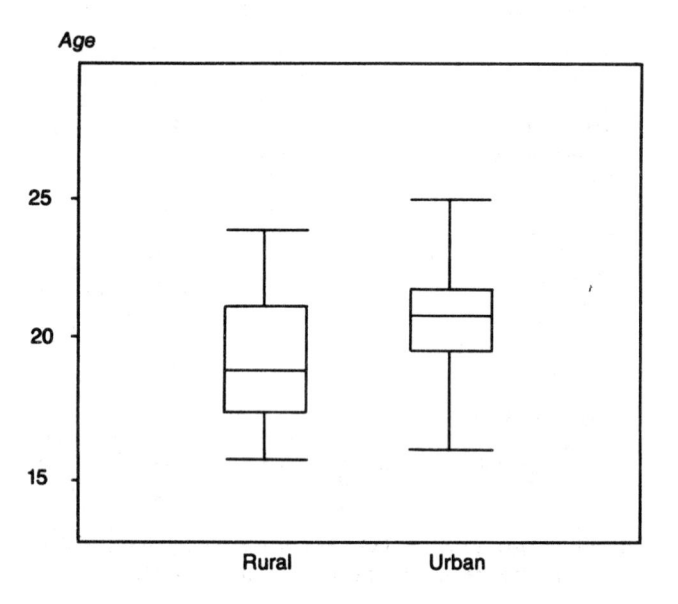

Source: Table 101

The regional averages (table 102) for Africa and for Asia and Oceania show similar rural/urban differences of 1.8-1.9 years, although, on average, women marry at different ages. Women in Asia and Oceania marry about two years later in both rural and urban areas than African women. The smallest difference of 1.3 years was found in Latin America and the Caribbean. If the three small countries of Guyana, Jamaica, and Trinidad and Tobago are excluded, this difference increases to 2.1 years.

Table 102 also shows the mean age at marriage for women aged 40-49 by residence for each region and development level. Ideally, comparisons of the mean reported age at marriage of ever-married older women

TABLE 101. SINGULATE MEAN AGE AT MARRIAGE, BY CURRENT RESIDENCE

Region and country	Rural (1)	Urban (2)	Difference: (2) − (1) (3)
Africa			
Benin	16.8	20.0	3.2
Cameroon	16.9	19.5	2.6
Côte d'Ivoire[a]	17.6	17.9	0.3
Egypt	19.8	23.0	3.2
Ghana	18.9	20.0	1.1
Kenya	19.8	20.6	0.8
Mauritania	19.1	19.1	0.0
Morocco	20.1	23.0	2.9
Senegal	16.2	19.9	3.7
Sudan	20.9	22.8	1.9
Tunisia	23.2	24.6	1.4
Latin America and the Caribbean			
Colombia	20.6	22.7	2.1
Costa Rica	20.8	23.3	2.5
Dominican Republic	19.0	20.8	1.8
Ecuador	21.1	22.9	1.8
Guyana	20.3	19.8	−0.5
Haiti	21.5	22.3	0.8
Jamaica	19.5	18.9	−0.6
Mexico	20.6	22.6	2.0
Panama	19.6	22.2	2.6
Paraguay	21.1	23.2	2.1
Peru	21.7	23.2	1.5
Trinidad and Tobago	21.5	20.7	−0.8
Venezuela	19.9	22.2	2.3
Asia and Oceania			
Bangladesh	15.5	17.2	1.7
Fiji	21.5	22.1	0.6
Indonesia	18.5	21.9	3.4
Jordan	19.8	22.1	2.3
Malaysia	22.1	25.0	2.9
Pakistan	19.2	20.7	1.5
Philippines	23.4	25.3	1.9
Republic of Korea	22.2	23.7	1.5
Sri Lanka	25.0	25.3	0.3
Syrian Arab Republic	21.5	22.6	1.1
Thailand	22.1	24.4	2.3

Sources: Ebanks and Singh (1984), and special tabulations.
[a] Formerly called the Ivory Coast.

trends in the size of rural/urban differentials in age at marriage. However, possible data errors and compositional biases have to be considered before interpreting these differences as trends. Chapter III of this volume discusses the possible sources of error in the reporting of age at first marriage (e.g., the tendency of older women to overstate their age at first marriage). An additional problem affecting the interpretation of the data is the fact that older women currently residing in urban areas may have married in rural areas before moving to urban areas, thus narrowing differentials among older women and biasing downward estimates of the real past differentials. These biases would tend to be greatest among countries experiencing the most rapid transition. SMAM may also be affected by trends in age at marriage and proportion ever marrying; and if single women are especially likely to move to urban areas, migration may contribute to the impression that urban women marry later.

It appears that mean age at marriage has increased over time in all regions (table 102). In each case, the increase in urban areas appears to be greater than that in rural areas; and, as indicated above, this may be partially due to compositional effects. For example, in Africa, rural age at marriage increased by a year (from 18 to 19 years) compared with an urban increase of almost three years (from 18.1 to 20.9 years). The Asia and Oceania region shows the most rapid increase over time in age at marriage: 4.3 years in the urban areas; 3.4 years in the rural areas. In contrast, the corresponding increases in the region of Latin America and the Caribbean are 1.4 and 1.0 years.

Residential differences in mean age at marriage appear to be widening over time. With all countries grouped together, the rural/urban differential widens from almost a year to 1.7 years. Among the regions, Africa exhibits the largest widening over time, from practically no rural/urban difference to one of almost two years. Latin America and the Caribbean, and Asia and Oceania show more modest increases over time in the size of the rural/urban differentials.

Many observers have predicted that economic development will eventually erode traditions favouring very early marriage for women. Chapter III notes that marriage age has indeed been rising in many of the WFS countries and that the average age at marriage in the more developed of these countries was currently substantially

to the corresponding SMAMs could be used to indicate not only the trends in age at marriage over time but the

TABLE 102. SINGULATE MEAN AGE AT MARRIAGE AND REPORTED MEAN AGE AT MARRIAGE AMONG WOMEN AGED 40-49, ACCORDING TO CURRENT RESIDENCE: AVERAGES BY REGION AND LEVEL OF DEVELOPMENT

	Singulate mean age at marriage			Reported mean age at marriage[a]		
	Rural (1)	Urban (2)	Difference: (2)-(1) (3)	Rural (4)	Urban (5)	Difference: (5)-(4) (6)
Region						
Africa	19.0	20.9	1.9	18.0	18.1	0.1
Latin America and the Caribbean	20.6	21.9	1.3	19.6	20.5	0.9
Asia and Oceania	21.0	22.8	1.8	17.6	18.5	0.9
Level of development						
I. High	20.8	22.1	1.3	19.0	20.0	1.0
II. Middle-high	21.8	23.4	1.6	19.4	20.3	0.9
III. Middle-low	18.8	20.8	2.0	17.7	18.1	0.6
IV. Low	18.5	20.3	1.8	17.0	17.2	0.2
TOTAL	20.2	21.9	1.7	18.5	19.4	0.9

Source: Table 101 and World Fertility Survey standard recode tapes.
[a] Calculated for ever-married women aged 40-49 years.

higher than in the lower development groups. If changes in marriage age occur rapidly, perhaps in response to a diffusion through societies of new norms with respect to appropriate marriage age, it can be expected that social differentials in age at marriage, including differentials by rural or urban residence, will widen and later contract—the same type of pattern often seen for fertility rates.

Comparisons between the measures of age at marriage within development levels indicate a widening of rural/urban differences over time at each level. The largest widening in differentials is evident in groups III and IV. Differences by residence increased over time from an average of under half a year to about two years. Smaller increases are observed in the two upper development groups, where, on average, earlier differences of about a year widened to about a year and a half.

In conclusion, Africa, and Asia and Oceania have similar rural/urban differentials; Latin America and the Caribbean shows somewhat smaller differentials. The data for all three regions imply a more rapid increase in age at marriage in urban areas compared with rural areas. No clear association is seen between size of the differentials and level of development. Over time, however, differentials in age at marriage by residence have widened, and they have done so at a more rapid pace in development groups III and IV, compared with groups I and II.

Breast-feeding

Women living in urban areas are expected to breast-feed their children for shorter durations than women in rural areas. Opportunities for working away from home in non-agricultural jobs are greater in the towns and cities. Such jobs are generally incompatible with breast-feeding. Also, in urban areas there is greater availability of infant foods, which makes it easier for mothers to substitute formulas for breast-milk. In addition, it is probably more acceptable socially for women to curtail breast-feeding earlier in the urban areas.

Table 103 presents the mean durations of breast-feeding by three categories of current residence: rural; other urban; and major urban. The difference in mean duration between the rural and major urban categories is also shown. The estimates of breast-feeding durations used in this table are based on information on current breast-feeding status and are limited to breast-feeding behaviour for recent births. Details concerning the method of calculation of these estimates can be found in chapter IV.

In every country except Mauritania, the duration of breast-feeding in the rural areas was longer than that in the major urban areas. Over all countries, the average rural/major urban difference was almost six months while the rural/other urban difference was 2.7 months (based on countries for which an estimate was available for each relevant category). Among the individual countries, rural/urban differences vary widely. At one extreme, rather small differences of less than four months were found in Mauritania and the Sudan in sub-Saharan Africa; in Jordan and the Syrian Arab Republic in Western Asia; and in Costa Rica, Guyana, Jamaica, and Trinidad and Tobago in Latin America and the Caribbean. Note, however, that these small rural/urban differences occur in countries with both long and short mean durations. While women in Mauritania and the Sudan breast-feed their children for 16-17 months, women in Guyana, Jamaica, and Trinidad and Tobago breast-feed for markedly shorter periods of 6-9 months. At the other extreme, large major rural/urban differences of over a year in breast-feeding duration were found in Indonesia and Thailand.

TABLE 103. MEAN DURATION OF BREAST-FEEDING, BY RESIDENCE

	Rural (1)	Other urban (2)	Major urban (3)	Difference: (1) − (3) (4)
A. Country				
Africa				
Benin	22.1	20.3	16.5	5.6
Cameroon	20.4	16.3	15.3	5.1
Côte d'Ivoire[a]	20.8	16.8	16.7	4.1
Egypt	21.4	16.7	13.9	7.5
Ghana	20.7	17.2	14.7	6.0
Kenya	17.3	12.4	12.9	4.4
Lesotho	21.8	..	..	..
Mauritania	17.5	16.2	17.8	−0.3
Morocco	17.6	11.6	12.7	4.9
Senegal	22.0	18.5	17.5	4.5
Sudan	17.4	15.5	16.7	0.7
Tunisia	17.7	11.6	10.0	7.7
Latin America and the Caribbean				
Colombia	11.7	8.7	5.8	5.9
Costa Rica	6.4	4.3	3.2	3.2
Dominican Republic	11.8	7.9	5.0	6.8
Ecuador	15.3	10.8	8.9	6.4
Guyana	8.3	8.0	5.2	3.1
Haiti	19.2	..	11.0	8.2
Jamaica	8.9	10.2	6.2	2.7
Mexico	12.3	8.0	6.0	6.3
Panama	10.8	5.0	4.0	6.8
Paraguay	13.6	12.6	5.7	7.9
Peru	18.9	13.0	8.3	10.6
Trinidad and Tobago	9.4	8.6	6.5	2.9
Venezuela	11.5	7.0	4.1	7.4
Asia and Oceania				
Bangladesh	33.7	29.6	..	..
Fiji	12.1	7.1	6.6	5.5
Indonesia	28.2	18.2	15.8	12.4
Jordan	13.1	11.5	10.3	2.8
Malaysia	6.9	4.6	2.1	4.8
Nepal	29.2	..	..	..
Pakistan	22.8	18.8	16.8	6.0
Philippines	15.2	10.9	7.4	7.8
Republic of Korea	20.0	15.8	14.0	6.0
Sri Lanka	23.4	18.5	..	..
Syrian Arab Republic	12.8	11.6	9.5	3.3
Thailand	21.7	..	7.5	14.2
Yemen	13.4	..	..	..
B. Region				
Africa	19.7	15.7	15.0	4.6
Latin America and the Caribbean	12.2	8.7	6.1	6.0
Asia and Oceania	19.4	14.7	10.0	7.0
C. Level of development				
I. High	10.8	7.9	5.8	5.0
II. Middle-high	16.4	12.0	8.1	7.5
III. Middle-low	21.0	15.6	14.6	6.3
IV. Low	21.9	19.8	16.1	4.1
TOTAL	17.0	12.8	10.1	5.8

Sources: Balkaran and Smith (1984); Ferry and Smith (1983).
NOTE: These estimates are current-status estimates based on surviving births, calculated using life-table methods. Averages for groups of countries should be regarded with caution when there are a large number of missing country values. For column (4), group averages are based on countries for which an estimate appears in both column (1) and column (3).
[a] Formerly called the Ivory Coast.

Figure 48. Mean duration of breast-feeding, according to residence, by region and level of development

A. Region

B. Level of development

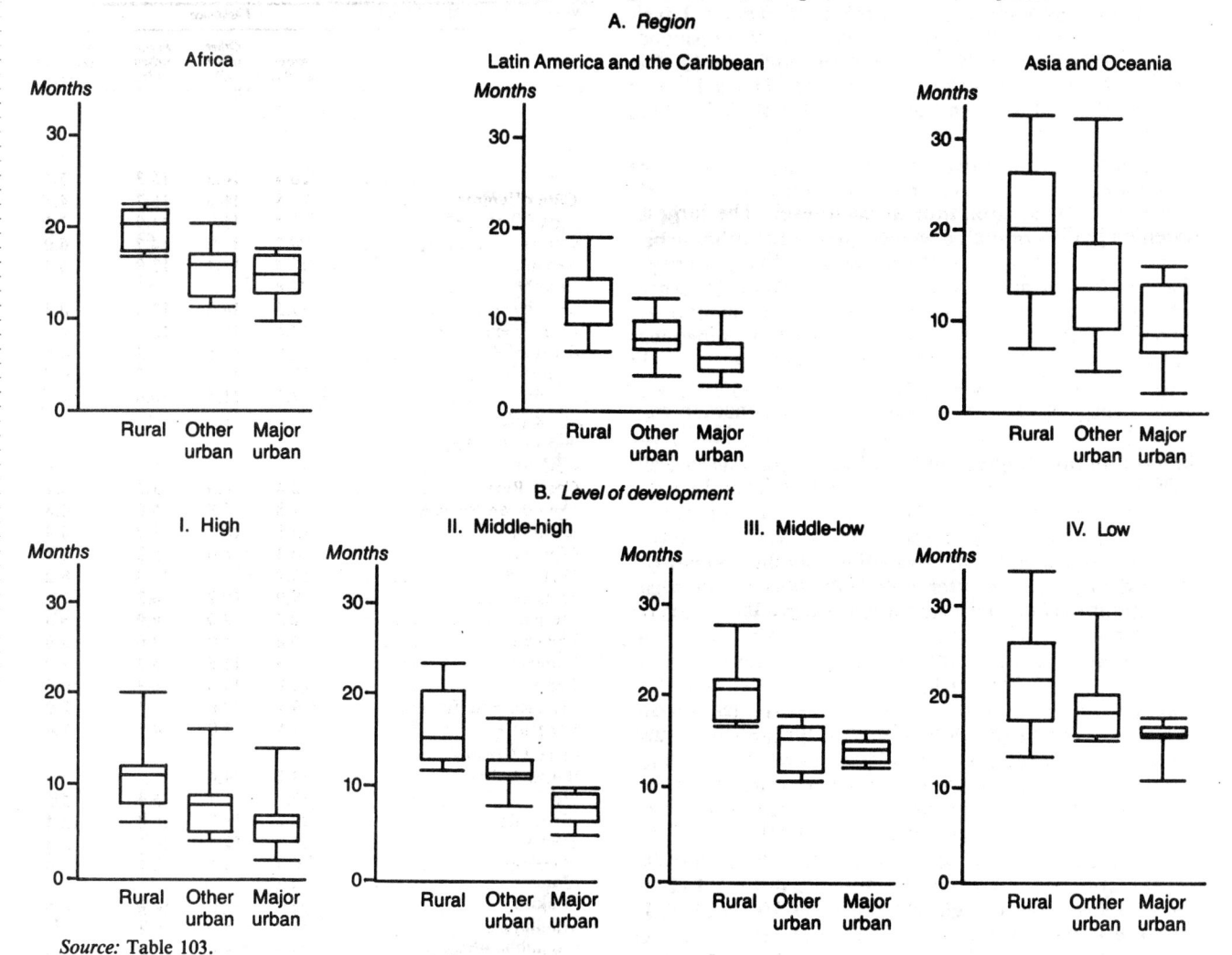

Source: Table 103.

Figure 48 summarizes the urban and rural breast-feeding durations by region and level of development. The box-and-whisker plots show the extreme values, the median and the values at the quartiles for rural, other urban and major urban women.

The variation within regions is clearly greatest in Asia and Oceania. The mean duration of breast-feeding among rural Asian women ranges from about 34 months in Bangladesh to about 7 months in Malaysia. These two countries also represent the extremes of the breast-feeding duration distribution among Asian women living in other urban areas, at 29.6 and 4.6 months, respectively. In the Latin American and Caribbean countries, breast-feeding durations were comparatively short and were (with a few exceptions) less variable within both urban and rural areas. The rural/major urban differential is, on average, somewhat smaller than in Asia and Oceania, the greatest difference (in Peru) being about 11 months.

The range of variation among the African countries is quite small, especially among rural women: the shortest breast-feeding duration, 17.3 months, was found in Kenya; and the longest, 22.1 months, in Benin, a difference of only 4.8 months. The major urban/rural differential is generally smaller in Africa than in the other two regions, averaging 4.6 months.

The largest rural/urban differences in breast-feeding duration were found in the two middle development groups (from six to eight months), although at each level, the differences averaged at least four months. Thus, the major features of the patterns of breast-feeding are the wide range in rural/urban differences across individual countries and the fact that urban women consistently breast-feed for shorter durations than rural women in the same country.

Contraceptive use

This subsection concentrates on the differentials in current contraceptive use by residence. The magnitude of these differentials and the relationship of these differentials to the degree of development and family planning programme strength form the main focus of this section.

As mentioned earlier, the level of current contraceptive practice is expected to be higher in urban areas. Compared with rural areas, the costs of rearing children are higher in towns and cities, the labour value of children is lower, parents desire smaller families, family planning services are generally more readily available and the social and financial costs of contraceptive use are often lower.

Taken together, these factors are expected to contribute to higher levels of contraceptive use in urban areas. Levels of contraceptive use by type of place of current residence are shown in table 104 and summarized in figure 49. The three-category classification of current residence is used; further, the analysis is limited to currently married women aged 15-49.

Current contraceptive use varies widely among the three residential areas. Over all, 36 per cent of currently married women in major urban areas used some type of contraception, compared with 31 per cent in other urban areas and 19 per cent in rural areas. This pattern of increasing contraceptive use with increasing urbanism is observed in most—but not all—countries. In Guyana, the proportion using contraception among rural women was five percentage points higher than that among women in other urban areas. Lightbourne (1980) attributes this higher rural contraceptive practice to differences in geographical distribution of ethnic groups. In Haiti, the "other urban" group reported the highest level of contraceptive use.

A wide variation in the size of differentials in contraceptive use across residence areas is evident. At one extreme, countries with especially large differences (of at least 25 points) between rural and major urban areas were found in Northern Africa (Egypt and Morocco), in Western Asia (Jordan and the Syrian Arab Republic), and in Latin America (Colombia, Ecuador, Mexico, Paraguay, Peru and Venezuela). At the other extreme, less than five points difference was found in Indonesia, Trinidad and Tobago, and a number of countries in Africa. In Trinidad and Tobago, contraceptive use was relatively high (50-53 per cent) for each type of residence, while in contrast, the African countries had very low levels of use in all areas.

Not unexpectedly, on a regional basis, Africa had the lowest levels of current use in each residence area. In fact, the proportion of currently married African women in major urban areas who were using contraception (18 per cent) is lower than that of either the Asian or Latin American women in rural areas (20 and 30 per cent, respectively). The widest average differential (20 percentage points) was found in Latin America and the Caribbean, followed closely by Asia and Oceania with 19 points. Africa averages only an 11 per cent difference in current use between the rural and major urban groups.

As already mentioned, differentials by residence are expected to be small (with low levels of usage) at low levels of development and then to widen as development continues. At high levels of development, differentials are again expected to be small, although at much higher levels of use. Table 104 shows rather small differences between rural and major urban areas in development groups III and IV (9-12 points). At the same time, absolute levels of use were lowest, averaging 6-9 per cent in rural areas and 15-21 per cent in major urban areas. The largest rural/major urban difference (25 percentage points) is observed in development group II. In development group I, the absolute levels of use were the highest—35 per cent in rural areas and 51 per cent in major urban areas—resulting in a slightly smaller difference of 16 percentage points.

Family planning programme strength is expected to have a similar relationship with residence differentials as levels of development. This expectation is based on the assumption that with a few exceptions, such as

TABLE 104. PERCENTAGE OF CURRENTLY MARRIED WOMEN AGED 15-49 WHO WERE CURRENTLY USING CONTRACEPTION, BY CURRENT RESIDENCE

Region and country	Rural (1)	Other urban (2)	Major urban (3)	Difference: (3) − (1) (4)
A. Country				
Africa				
Benin	8	12	12	4
Cameroon	2	1	9	7
Côte d'Ivoire[a]	2	4	5	3
Egypt	13	36	42	29
Ghana	8	12	15	7
Kenya	6	10	17	11
Lesotho	5	7	7	2
Mauritania	1	1	1	0
Morocco	10	35	40	30
Senegal	4	4	3	−1
Sudan	2	9	16	14
Tunisia	21	43	43	22
Latin America and the Caribbean				
Colombia	27	49	57	30
Costa Rica	61	65	69	8
Dominican Republic	22	38	42	20
Ecuador	22	44	49	27
Guyana	30	25	37	7
Haiti	15	40	26	11
Jamaica	34	36	47	13
Mexico	15	38	46	31
Panama	46	62	60	14
Paraguay	27	43	52	25
Peru	12	38	49	37
Trinidad and Tobago	50	51	53	3
Venezuela	29	51	60	31
Asia and Oceania				
Bangladesh	7	13	26	19
Fiji	38	47	46	8
Indonesia	26	29	29	3
Jordan	9	27	37	28
Malaysia	28	41	47	19
Pakistan	3	8	19	16
Philippines	31	45	50	19
Republic of Korea	31	36	39	8
Sri Lanka	30	35	44	14
Syrian Arab Republic	5	28	46	41
Thailand	31	43	47	16
Yemen	0	------6------		..
B. Region				
Africa	7	14	18	11
Latin America and the Caribbean	30	45	50	20
Asia and Oceania	20	32	39	19
C. Level of development				
I. High	35	46	51	16
II. Middle-high	21	38	46	25
III. Middle-low	9	17	21	12
IV. Low	6	12	15	9
D. Strength of family planning programme effort				
1. Strong	36	46	49	13
2. Moderate	28	41	36	8
3. Weak	15	29	36	21
4. Very weak/none	7	16	21	14
TOTAL	19	31	36	17

Source: World Fertility Survey standard recode tapes.
NOTE: Percentages are adjusted for the effects of age differences between residence groups.
[a] Formerly called the Ivory Coast.

Indonesia, family planning programmes are first based in urban areas where as a result, contraceptive knowledge and services are first spread, and differentials widen. As

Figure 49. **Percentage of currently married women aged 15-49 currently using contraception, by residence, all countries**

Figure 50. **Percentage currently using contraception, by residence: averages by strength of family planning programme effort within development groups**

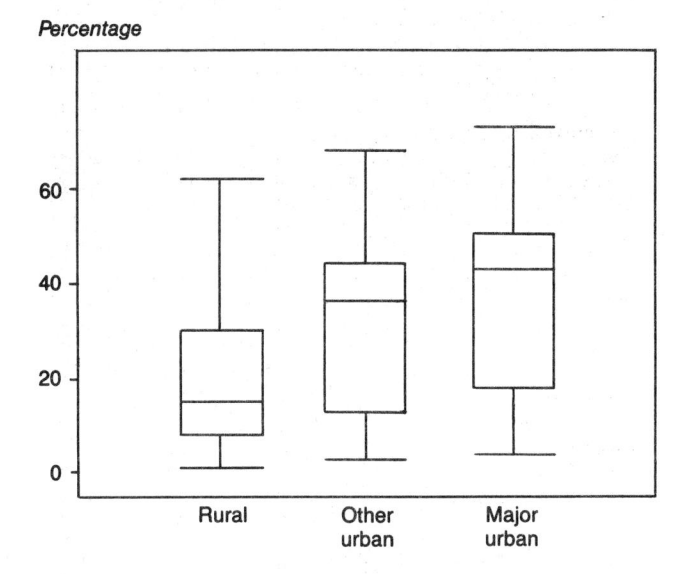

I. High

II. Middle-high

III. Middle-low

IV. Low

Source: Table 104.

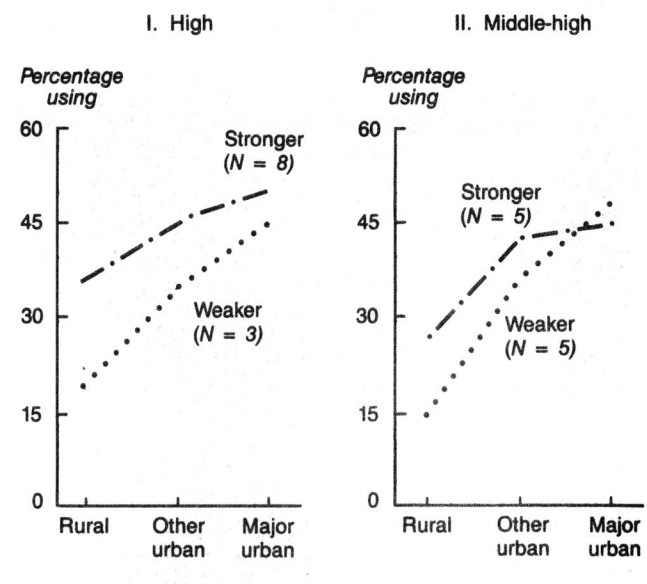

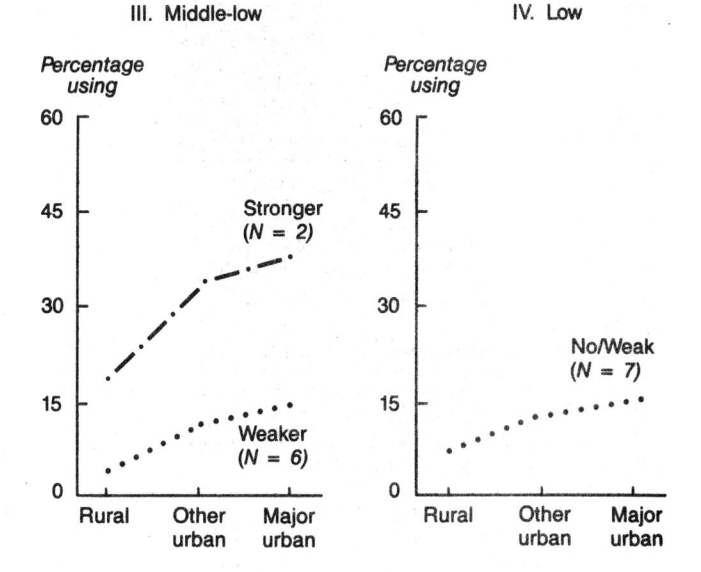

Source: Table 104.
NOTE: Figures in parentheses indicate number of countries in the group.

programmes become stronger, they extend into the rural areas, where they become effective in providing services to the rest of the population, so that differentials tend to narrow. To some extent, these expectations are supported by the results shown in table 104, where the rural/major urban differential in current contraceptive use increases at first and then steadily declines from 21 per cent at the weak level to 13 per cent at the strong level.

The discussion thus far has focused on the effects of development and family planning programme effort (taking each factor separately) on contraceptive use levels and differentials. However, these two macro factors (development and programme effort) are closely related: more developed countries are likely to have stronger programmes; less developed countries are likely to have weaker programmes. A crude way of separating the macro effects is to obtain average levels of use after grouping countries according to different programme levels within each development group. This is done in figure 50, where each level of development shows average contraceptive use at two levels of family planning programme effort: a "weaker" level obtained by combining the countries with very weak/none or weak efforts; and a "stronger" level which groups countries with moderate and strong programmes. The low level of development (IV) contains no countries with either a moderate or a strong family planning programme.

Figure 50 shows that for each type of residence within each development group, countries with a stronger programme do tend to have higher average levels of contraceptive use than those with a weaker programme. Even at the high development level, a stronger programme is associated with greater use, especially in the rural areas. At the middle-low development level, stronger programmes are also associated with much higher levels of use in both rural and urban areas, but especially in the latter. As concerns contraceptive use differentials, the following observations can be made. Small differentials in use patterns with absolute low levels of usage were found in the low and middle-low development groups with weaker programmes. At the other extreme, in the high development groups with stronger programmes, relatively small differences are again observed between the residential areas, but at much higher use levels. The in-between categories with varying combinations of development and family planning programme strength show much larger differentials. Taken together, these observations tend to support the theory outlined earlier. The reader, however, is urged to be cautious, because these results are based on small numbers of countries; and the basic groupings of countries into development and family planning programme levels are necessarily crude.

In summary, regional averages show that, with respect to contraceptive use as with recent fertility, Latin America and the Caribbean had the largest differentials, followed by Asia and Oceania, and then Africa. These differentials were larger in development groups I and II, with the largest difference observed at the middle-high level. This is very similar to the pattern observed for recent fertility. Also, after an initial widening, differentials narrow with increased family planning programme strength. Lastly, when countries are grouped by programme strength within development groups, small differentials are observed at the extremes of the combined development-programme levels, with larger differentials in between.

C. MULTIVARIATE ANALYSIS

This section presents further detailed analyses of the relationship of fertility, desired family size and current contraceptive use to type of place of residence. More specifically, these analyses attempt to examine the extent to which residence differentials in fertility (and related behaviour) are due to differences in socio-economic factors. As noted earlier, "residence" in this section is measured by the combined variable with four categories: long-term rural residence; long-term urban residence; rural-urban "migrants" (rural childhood residence and urban current residence); and urban-rural "migrants" (urban childhood residence and rural current residence). Since comparable information on residence was not collected in Guyana, Jamaica, Mauritania, and Trinidad and Tobago, they are not included in the analyses. The socio-economic factors included are respondent's education, respondent's occupation, husband's education and husband's occupation. A summary of the multivariate models presented in this section is shown in table 105.

The two long-term groups are expected to differ the most with respect to fertility and related behaviour. Also, because changes in fertility (and related behaviour) are expected to emerge first in urban areas, the comparison between the long-term urban-dwellers and the rural-urban "migrant" group is worth investigating. Thus, the discussions here centre on comparisons between the long-term residents and between the long-term urban residents and the rural-urban group.

Fertility

The fertility measure used as the dependent variable in the following regression analyses is children ever born, *CEB*, divided by years since first marriage, *D*. This variable, *CEB/D*, can be interpreted as births per year since marriage. Results are presented in terms of births per 1,000 woman-years of marriage. The sample for this analysis was restricted to ever-married women who had been married for at least three years, because inclusion of women with less than three years of marital duration would have caused statistical tests to be unreliable. Further details concerning the fertility model are discussed in the annex to part two of this volume.

TABLE 105. DESCRIPTION OF REGRESSION MODELS

Model No.	Base population	Dependent variable	Independent variables
1	First married 3+ years before survey, currently aged 15-49[a]	CEB/D	Respondent's current and childhood type of place of residence, duration since first marriage, duration squared, age at first marriage
2	First married 3+ years before survey, currently aged 15-49[a]	CEB/D	Model 1 + respondent's and husband's education, respondent's and husband's occupation
3	Ever-married women aged 15-49[a]	Number of children desired	Respondent's current and childhood type of place of residence, age, age squared, age at first marriage, number of living children
4	Ever-married women aged 15-49[a]	Number of children desired	Model 3 + respondent's and husband's education, respondent's and husband's occupation
5	Currently married women aged 15-49[a]	Current use of contraception	Respondent's current and childhood type of place of residence, age, age squared, age at first marriage, number of living children
6	Currently married women	Current use of contraception	Model 5 + respondent's and husband's education, respondent's and husband's occupation.

NOTE: *CEB/D* = children ever born/duration of marriage.
[a] For Costa Rica and Panama, aged 20-49 years; for Venezuela, 15-44 years.

The analysis in this subsection is carried out in two stages (see table 105). At the first stage, only demographic factors (i.e., duration since first marriage, duration squared and age at first marriage) are controlled. At the second stage, controls for various socio-economic factors are added. These include respondent's education and occupation, and husband's education and occupation.

Residence is entered as a set of dummy variables; long-term rural residence is the omitted category. For convenience, the models for the first and second stages are referred to as model 1 and model 2, respectively. Comparisons between the regression coefficients for residence categories calculated with (model 2) and without socio-economic controls (model 1) indicate roughly the extent to which the fertility differentials by residence groups are due to differences in socio-economic factors.

Table 106 presents the partial regression coefficients for categories of residence summarized according to region, level of development and strength of family planning programme effort. Results for the individual countries are available in United Nations (1986). Differences between the long-term resident groups are discussed first and appear in column (3). Without any socio-economic controls (i.e., model 1), the difference in cumulative fertility between long-term rural and long-term urban residents is −38 for all countries (or −0.038 per woman-year of marriage). This difference implies that long-term rural residents have approximately three quarters of a child less over 20 years of marriage than long-term urban residents (0.038 × 20 = 0.76). Of the 34 countries included in the analysis, residence is significant at the 0.01 level in model 1 in 27. The countries in which residence is not significant are Cameroon, Lesotho, Senegal, Sudan, Bangladesh, Nepal and Sri Lanka. Among the regions, Latin America and the Caribbean has the largest difference per 1,000 women-years of marriage (−87), while Africa, and Asia and Oceania show much smaller differences (−21 and −13, respectively). These regional values translate into differences of about 1.74 children in Latin America and the Caribbean, 0.42 child in Africa and 0.25 child in Asia and Oceania, per woman over 20 years of marriage.

Within regions, there is a wide variation in the long-term residence differentials (results not shown). In Africa, the difference varies from virtually none in Senegal and Sudan to almost 1.5 children at 20 years of duration in Kenya and Morocco, while differences of more than one child are found in several countries in Latin America and the Caribbean. In Asia and Oceania, three countries

TABLE 106. SUMMARY OF PARTIAL REGRESSION COEFFICIENTS ACCORDING TO RESIDENCE GROUP, BY REGION, LEVEL OF DEVELOPMENT AND STRENGTH OF FAMILY PLANNING PROGRAMME EFFORT:[a] DEPENDENT VARIABLE = CHILDREN EVER BORN/DURATION OF MARRIAGE
(Births per 1,000 women-years of marriage)

	Number of countries (1)	Model No. (2)	Urban-rural[b] (3)	Rural-urban[c] (4)	Long-term urban (5)	Number of countries in which residence is significant as a variable[d] (6)
All countries	34	1	−10	−20	−38	27
	34	2	−5	−10	−17	20
A. Region						
Africa	11	1	−6	−11	−21	7
	11	2	−7	−11	−20	6
Latin America and the Caribbean	10	1	−31	−55	−87	10
	10	2	−16	−24	−35	8
Asia and Oceania	13	1	1	−2	−13	10
	13	2	5	2	−1	6
B. Level of development						
I. High	8	1	−23	−45	−70	8
	8	2	−11	−24	−31	7
II. Middle-high	10	1	−15	−27	−48	9
	10	2	−2	−6	−11	4
III. Middle-low	8	1	5	−17	−20	6
	8	2	3	−17	−21	4
IV. Low	8	1	−7	8	−8	4
	8	2	−10	7	−7	5
C. Strength of family planning programme effort						
1. Strong	8	1	−12	−36	−52	8
	8	2	−3	−21	−25	7
2. Moderate	5	1	−18	−29	37	4
	5	2	−5	11	−9	2
3. Weak	9	1	−10	27	−47	7
	9	2	−3	−16	−25	6
4. Very weak/none	12	1	−7	−3	−21	8
	12	2	−8	2	−11	5

Source: World Fertility Survey standard recode tapes.
NOTE: Other variables in model 1 are duration, duration squared and age at marriage. In addition to these variables, model 2 includes respondent's education, respondent's occupation, husband's education and husband's occupation. In model 2 for Indonesia, the respondent's occupation variable is coded in a non-standard way. Omitted category of residence is long-term rural.
[a] Based on a sample of women married three or more years.
[b] Reported urban childhood and rural current residence.
[c] Reported rural childhood and urban current residence.
[d] Significant at the 0.01 level.

(Indonesia, Pakistan and Yemen) show a negative difference, indicating that long-term urban fertility is higher than long-term rural fertility.

The introduction of socio-economic controls (in model 2) results in a reduction of the overall difference for all countries from −38 to −17 and reduces the residence variable to non-significance in seven additional countries. A distinct regional variation in the amount of reduction is apparent. In Latin America and the Caribbean, the average difference is reduced by more than 50 per cent to −35, while in Asia and Oceania, the small difference of −13 almost disappears. In Africa, however, there is virtually no change in the size of the difference: in other words, on average, compositional differences between residence groups in educational and occupational distributions do not account for the fertility differences between long-term residence groups.

Long-term urban residents are expected to have lower fertility than the rural-urban group. This is evident in table 106, where average differences follow a regional pattern very similar to that observed for the differences between the long-term resident groups (difference between column (3) and (2) in table 106 for model 1). The differential between the long-term urban group and the rural-urban group is smaller than the differential between the two long-term resident groups, averaging −18, or 0.36 child at 20 years of duration, for all countries. Most individual countries show the expected pattern of higher fertility for more recent urban residents. Pakistan and Sri Lanka are the main exceptions, with the fertility of recent urban residents about 0.32 birth lower at 20 years of duration than that for long-term residents. As in the case of the comparison between long-term resident groups, the average regional differences are also reduced considerably with the addition of socio-economic controls in Latin America and the Caribbean and in Asia and Oceania, but not in Africa.

Table 106 also presents the average differences in the rate of childbearing (for both models) for countries grouped by level of development. Very similar patterns are noted at the lower two levels of development; the adjustment for socio-economic factors does not reduce the differences between either the long-term resident groups or between the urban groups (long-term resident and in-migrant). Differences between the long-term resident groups, for example, remain at from −7 to −8 in the lower level and from −20 to −21 at the middle-low level, both before and after the introduction of socio-economic controls. In contrast, at the upper two levels, the adjustment reduces these differentials by more than half, from −48 to −11 for the middle-high level and from −70 to −31 for the high level. Thus, at these two levels, the initial differentials are relatively large and at least half of the residence differential in the rate of childbearing can be explained by differences in the socio-economic factors. At the lower two levels, on the other hand, initial differences are relatively small and differences in factors other than the socio-economic ones included here appear to be associated with residence differentials in fertility.

Figure 51 shows the individual country coefficients (model 2) for the variable indicating long-term urban residence, grouped according to level of development. The coefficients indicate the direction and magnitude of the difference in cumulative marital fertility (per 1,000 woman-years of marriage) between long-term rural and long-term urban residents. These coefficients show a substantial amount of variation in both direction and size within all development groups. In group I, however, the range of values is somewhat less (from −7 to −55) and all of the coefficients are negative. Note also that residence has a statistically significant relationship with the rate of childbearing in seven of eight countries in the highest development group (I) after control for demographic and socio-economic variables. The proportion of countries in which residence is significant is much lower in the three lower development groups.

Figure 51. **Adjusted difference in marital fertility, *CEB/D*, between long-term rural and long-term urban residents, by level of development**

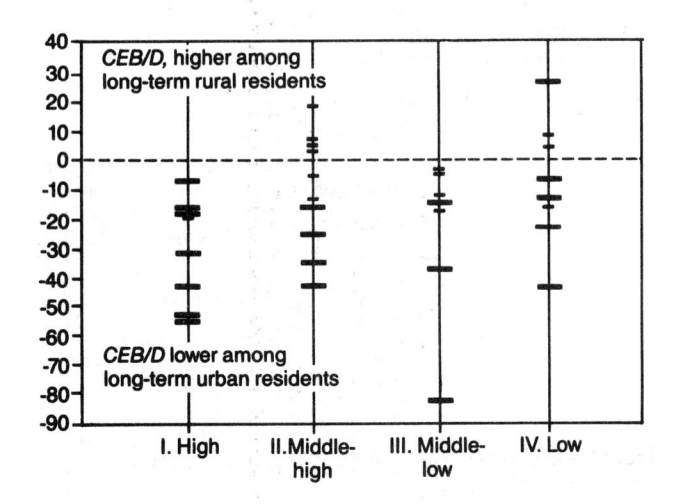

Source: Table 106, model 2.
NOTES: Shorter lines represent countries in which residence as a variable is not significant.
CEB/D = children ever born/duration of marriage.

With respect to family planning programme strength, the differentials shown in table 106 are substantially reduced with the introduction of socio-economic factors for all groups of countries. For example, differences between the long-term resident groups decrease from −21 to −11 at the very weak/none level and from −52 to −25 at the strong level of programme effort. Thus, there is little association between the proportionate reduction in differential and the strength of programme effort; socio-economic characteristics generally account for approximately half of the rural/urban differentials in the rate of childbearing.

Desired family size

As in the case of fertility, two models are estimated (with desired family size as the dependent variable) and then compared. The models, however, differ slightly from those estimated earlier, in that age, age squared, age at first marriage and number of living children[7] are used as demographic controls. The sample differs as well and

TABLE 107. SUMMARY OF PARTIAL REGRESSION COEFFICIENTS ACCORDING TO RESIDENCE GROUP, BY REGION AND LEVEL OF DEVELOPMENT:[a] DEPENDENT VARIABLE = DESIRED FAMILY SIZE

	Number of countries (1)	Model No. (2)	Urban-rural[b] (3)	Rural-urban[c] (4)	Long-term urban (5)	Number of countries in which residence is significant as a variable[d] (6)
All countries	34	3	−0.3	−0.6	−0.8	28
	34	4	−0.2	−0.3	−0.4	22
A. Region						
Africa	11	3	−0.5	−0.9	−1.3	10
	11	4	−0.3	−0.5	−0.7	9
Latin America and the Caribbean	10	3	−0.3	−0.4	−0.5	8
	10	4	−0.2	−0.2	−0.2	4
Asia and Oceania	13	3	−0.5	−0.5	−0.7	10
	13	4	−0.3	−0.3	−0.4	9
B. Level of development						
I. High	8	3	−0.2	−0.4	−0.6	6
	8	4	−0.1	−0.1	−0.2	5
II. Middle-high	10	3	−0.5	−0.6	−0.7	9
	10	4	−0.3	−0.3	−0.4	7
III. Middle-low	8	3	−0.4	−0.8	−1.0	6
	8	4	−0.2	−0.5	−0.6	6
IV. Low	8	3	−0.4	−0.6	−1.0	7
	8	4	−0.1	−0.2	−0.4	4

Source: World Fertility Survey standard recode tapes.

NOTE: Other variables in the model 3 are age, age squared, age at marriage and number of living children. In addition to these variables, model 4 includes respondent's education, respondent's occupation, husband's education and husband's occupation. In model 4 for Indonesia, the respondent's occupation is coded in a non-standard way. Omitted category of residence is long-term rural.

[a] Based on a sample of ever-married women.
[b] Reported urban childhood and rural current residence.
[c] Reported rural childhood and urban current residence.
[d] Significant at the 0.01 level.

includes ever-married women regardless of marital duration (see table 105).

Table 107 presents the estimated partial regression coefficients for residence groups for models 3 and 4, averaged over regions and development levels. As in the preliminary analysis, conclusions based on averages including countries with large non-response rates should be viewed with caution. The estimates show that the pattern of mean desired family size according to residence groups is similar across regions. Long-term rural women desire the largest families, while their urban counterparts desire the smallest. The migrant groups express preferences for family sizes that fall between these extremes, with the urban-rural group desiring, on average, either as large as or larger families than the rural-urban group. Before controls for the socio-economic factors are added, the residence effect is statistically significant in 28 of 34 countries.

Without any socio-economic controls, Latin America and the Caribbean shows the smallest difference between long-term residence groups, approximately 0.5 child. Asia and Oceania shows a slightly larger difference of 0.7 child; and in Africa, this difference is 1.3 children. It is interesting to note that this is exactly the opposite of the regional ordering of the size of the differentials observed for fertility.

As expected, adjustment for the socio-economic factors results in a reduction of the initial residence differentials. Over all countries, these differences are reduced by about half; and within each region, the differences are reduced by about the same proportion. Thus, in all three regions, about half of the observed residence differential in desired family size can be attributed to differences in other socio-economic factors. After controlling for both demographic and socio-economic differences, the variation in desired family size by residence is fairly small, less than 0.5 child difference between the two long-term residence groups averaged over all countries. However, residence remains statistically significant in 22 countries and averages roughly 0.7 child in Africa even after controls. There is no apparent association between the amount of reduction and development level; at each level, approximately half the difference is due to differences in socio-economic factors.

As shown in figure 52 and as noted in the preliminary analysis of desired family size, the differential between long-term rural and long-term urban residents does not show any clear pattern by level of development. In development group I, the variation between countries is much less than in the other three groups; and the largest difference, which occurs in Costa Rica, is −0.4 child. In the two middle groups, this difference is quite variable and is positive in two countries, Cameroon (0.5) and Thailand (0.2). Yet, residence as a variable is somewhat more likely to be statistically significant in countries in these two middle groups than in either the high or low development groups.

Contraceptive use

The two models used in this subsection to determine the extent to which differentials in contraceptive use are due to differentials in socio-economic factors, are identical to the models used in the analysis of desired family size. The sample is, however, restricted to currently

Figure 52. **Adjusted difference in desired family size between long-term rural and long-term urban residents, by level of development**

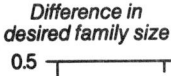

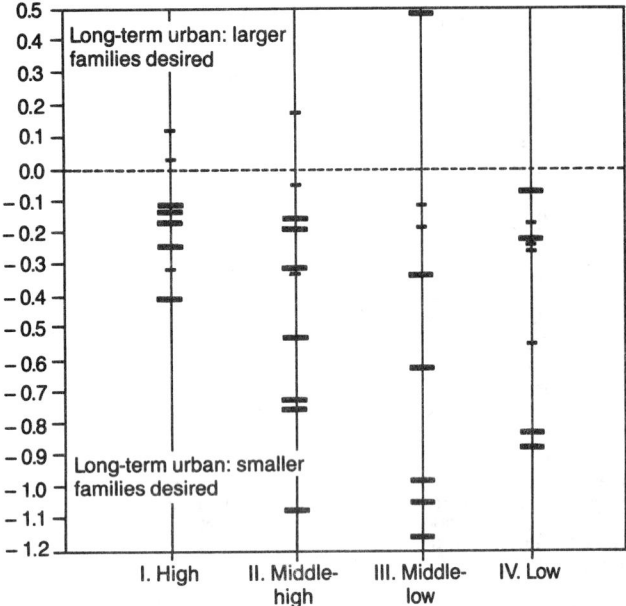

Source: Table 107, model 4.
NOTE: Shorter lines represent countries in which residence as a variable is not significant.

married women. The estimated differences in the proportion currently practising contraception between long-term rural residents and other residence groups are presented for regions, levels of development and strength of programme effort in table 108.

Results based on model 5 (which includes only demographic controls) show that despite large variations in the levels of contraceptive use across regions, the residential pattern of such use is similar within each region: long-term urban women have the largest proportion currently using contraception, while long-term rural women have the lowest. Migrant women have levels of use that are in-between, with the rural-urban group having higher levels of use than the urban-rural group. This pattern is also observed in most of the individual countries (results not shown). Further, the pattern remains the same after adjustments are made for the socio-economic factors.

In model 5, average differences between the two long-term resident groups in proportions currently using contraception are quite large. For example, when all the countries are grouped together, the percentage of long-term urban residents who use contraception is 16 percentage points higher than that of long-term rural-dwellers. Latin America and the Caribbean has the largest difference (26 points), followed by Asia and Oceania (16) and Africa (8).

The adjustment for the socio-economic factors clearly diminishes the size of these differences, resulting in a pattern that looks quite similar across regions. For example, the difference between the long-term resident groups is reduced to only eight percentage points when all countries are considered, to nine points in Latin America and the Caribbean, eight in Asia and Oceania, and six in Africa. The greatest reduction in differential size is therefore found in the first region. In spite of these relatively large reductions, however, the effects of residence remain statistically significant at the 0.01 level in about two thirds of the countries.

Table 108 also displays the results for the two models grouped by level of development and family planning programme strength. Within each level of development (and programme effort), adjustment for socio-economic factors reduces, in some cases by a substantial amount, the size of the differences between the long-term resident categories. Further, at the upper two levels of development, there is a tendency for a greater proportion of the initial residence differential in contraceptive prevalence to be explained by socio-economic factors, compared with the lower two levels of development. Differences of 22-24 percentage points (in model 5) are reduced to 10 points (after adjusting for education and occupation) in development groups I and II, compared with reductions from 11 points to 6 points in development groups III and IV. This implies that in the relatively more developed groups a larger proportion of the residence differential in contraceptive use is due to differences in the educational and occupational structure of the residence categories. None the less, the remaining differentials are larger in the more developed groups. Differences between models 5 and 6 are more uniform by strength family planning programme effort: at each level, slightly over half the residence differential in contraceptive use between the long-term resident groups, as assessed by model 5, can be attributed to differences in socio-economic factors.

The pattern of differentials (model 6) for long-term residents is shown in figure 53 for development groups. The coefficients show some tendency to be more positive in groups I and II than in groups III and IV, especially if the two countries (Egypt and Morocco) in group III with above-average differentials are removed. In groups III and IV, the proportion using contraception among long-term urban residents is less than four percentage points higher than that among long-term rural residents in 6 of 16 countries and is actually lower in two countries. In the upper two development groups, the proportion using is more than 10 percentage points higher among long-term urban residents in 10 of 18 countries. In all development groups, however, the variation in size of the differentials is quite broad.

D. SUMMARY AND CONCLUSIONS

Patterns of rural/urban differentials in fertility and related variables, including age at marriage, breast-feeding, contraceptive use and fertility preferences, are described in this chapter. While the wide variation observed at the individual country level for both urbanization and fertility complicates interpretation of the results, this same variation is one of the advantages of using WFS data for comparative analysis of rural/urban fertility patterns. Throughout the analysis, this variation allows fertility differentials to be examined in the light

TABLE 108. SUMMARY OF PARTIAL REGRESSION COEFFICIENTS ACCORDING TO RESIDENCE GROUP, BY REGION, LEVEL OF DEVELOPMENT AND STRENGTH OF FAMILY PLANNING PROGRAMME EFFORT:[a] DEPENDENT VARIABLE = PERCENTAGE WHO WERE CURRENTLY USING CONTRACEPTION

	Number of countries (1)	Model No. (2)	Urban-rural[b] (3)	Rural-urban[c] (4)	Long-term urban (5)	Number of countries in which residence is significant as a variable[d] (6)
All countries	34	5	5	9	16	32
	34	6	2	5	8	20
A. Region						
Africa	11	5	3	6	8	10
	11	6	1	3	6	5
Latin America and the Caribbean	10	5	10	17	26	10
	10	6	4	7	9	6
Asia and Oceania	13	5	8	10	16	12
	13	6	3	5	8	9
B. Level of development						
I. High	8	5	10	15	22	8
	8	6	4	7	10	4
II. Middle-high	10	5	10	16	24	10
	10	6	4	7	10	7
III. Middle-low	8	5	3	6	11	6
	8	6	2	3	6	3
IV. Low	8	5	4	5	11	8
	8	6	2	3	6	6
C. Strength of family planning programme effort						
1. Strong	8	5	8	11	17	7
	8	6	4	5	7	3
2. Moderate	5	5	10	14	20	5
	8	6	4	7	8	2
3. Weak	9	5	9	13	23	9
	9	6	4	7	11	9
4. Very weak/none	12	5	4	7	14	11
	12	6	1	3	6	6

Source: World Fertility Survey standard recode tapes.

NOTE: Other variables in model 5 are age, age squared, age at marriage and number of living children. In addition to these variables, model 6 includes respondent's education, respondent's occupation, husband's education and husband's occupation. In model 6 for Indonesia, the respondent's occupation variable is coded in a non-standard way. Omitted category of residence is long-term rural.

[a] Based on a sample of currently married women.
[b] Reported urban childhood and rural current residence.
[c] Reported rural childhood and urban current residence.
[d] Significant at the 0.01 level.

of the regional, socio-economic and family planning programme effort contexts.

On average, slightly over half of Latin American and Caribbean women were currently living in urban areas, while approximately a third of the women in Africa and in Asia and Oceania were doing so. The variation within regions was greatest in Asia and Oceania, where, for example, the proportion rural ranged from 98 per cent in Nepal to 30 per cent in Jordan. The WFS data also provide information on childhood residence. Combining this information with the data on current residence yields a crude indicator of the extent and direction of migration between rural and urban areas. Not surprisingly, these data suggest that in many countries, a substantial amount of rural-urban migration has occurred, with the result that current urban residents are less likely to be long-term residents than their counterparts in rural areas.

Rural/urban fertility differentials are addressed in this chapter from several perspectives. According to current type of place of residence (rural, other urban, major urban), both completed and recent fertility levels show that, with some exceptions, fertility is highest in rural areas and lowest in major urban areas. The rural/urban differential in recent fertility is largest in Latin America and the Caribbean, where rural women average 2.7 children more than major urban women, and smallest in Africa, where this difference is 1.6 children. In both Latin America and the Caribbean and Asia and Oceania, fertility has declined but not equally across residence groups; the larger decrease among major urban women has resulted in a widening of differentials over time. In Africa, there is no clear evidence of a similar decline, although recent fertility among major urban women may be slightly lower than past fertility in this group.

When countries are grouped according to level of development, the size of rural/urban differences in fertility increases from the low to the middle-high group. This widening is due mainly to lower fertility among women residing in major urban areas in more developed countries; rural fertility in development groups II-IV is approximately equal. In development group I, however, rural fertility is lower than in the three other groups, producing a slightly smaller differential. If the development groups are taken to represent different stages of the fertility transition, these results follow the pattern predicted by the "social-diffusion" hypothesis in which

Figure 53. Adjusted difference between percentage currently using contraception among long-term rural and long-term urban residents, by level of development

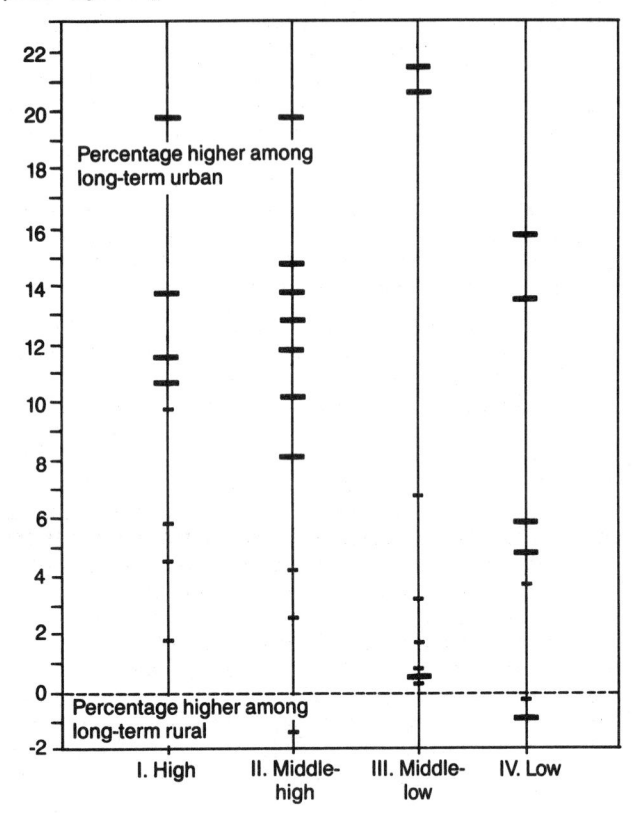

[Figure: scatter plot showing "Difference in percentage using" on the y-axis (ranging from -2 to 22) across four development categories on the x-axis: I. High, II. Middle-high, III. Middle-low, IV. Low. The upper region is labeled "Percentage higher among long-term urban" and the lower region "Percentage higher among long-term rural".]

Source: Table 108, model 6.
NOTE: Shorter lines represent countries in which residence as a variable is not significant.

fertility declines are thought to begin among the urban educated and spread to the rest of the population.

The multivariate analysis of marital fertility rates presented in this chapter provides further insights into rural/urban differences in fertility. The residence variable used in this analysis, constructed from information about current and childhood residence, permits comparisons between women who are long-term residents of rural or urban areas and those who grew up in a different type of place.

When demographic factors only are controlled, the difference over all countries between long-term residence groups implies that long-term urban residents bear approximately three quarters of a child less than long-term rural residents over 20 years of marriage. In addition, long-term urban residents average 0.36 child less than the rural-urban group over 20 years of marriage. In this model, type of place of residence is statistically significant in 27 of 34 countries. The introduction of controls for husband's and respondent's education, and for husband's and respondent's occupation, reduces the size of the overall differential between long-term residence categories by half and reduces the number of countries in which residence is significant to 20. Rodríguez and Cleland (1981) report the same proportionate reduction in their analysis of recent fertility differentials in 27 WFS populations.

By region, however, the amount of reduction in the differentials caused by the addition of socio-economic controls varies. In Latin America and the Caribbean, the difference between long-term residence groups falls from a rate that implies a difference, over 20 years, of 1.74 children to 0.70 child; in Asia and Oceania, the differential goes from 0.26 to 0.02. In Africa, however, the introduction of socio-economic factors has virtually no effect on rural/urban fertility differences. Thus, while differences in socio-economic characteristics of women and their husbands account for about half of the rural/urban differential in fertility in Latin America and the Caribbean and more than half in Asia and Oceania, this differential in Africa is attributable to other unmeasured factors. This is probably due to differences between the regions in the distribution of residents by other socio-economic characteristics and in the nature of city life. Latin America and the Caribbean has the largest differentials both before and after socio-economic controls, suggesting that certain features of city life which reduce the desirability of children and/or the costs of fertility control may be relatively important in this region.

It is also interesting to note that the difference in fertility between long-term residence groups is largest (even after the addition of socio-economic factors) and most likely to be statistically significant in the countries in development group I. The socio-economic controls reduce the size of this difference by a little more than half in development group I, by over three quarters in group II and not at all in groups III and IV.

Rural/urban fertility differentials arise from differences in intermediate factors that affect fertility, such as age at marriage, breast-feeding and contraceptive use. In this chapter, differentials in age at marriage and breast-feeding were examined for current residence groups. A clear association of current urban residence with later age at marriage and shorter breast-feeding duration is observed. In every country except Mauritania and three countries in Latin America and the Caribbean, the singulate mean age at marriage of urban women is greater than that of rural women. The rural/urban difference is smallest in Latin America and the Caribbean and in the high development group. The duration of breast-feeding was found to be consistently shorter among women in major urban areas, although the size of the difference varies from less than one month to over one year. Averaged over all countries, women in rural areas breast-feed almost six months longer than women in major urban areas. Moreover, in all residence groups, breast-feeding durations are shorter at the upper two development levels, compared with the lower two levels.

Differences in current contraceptive use according to current type of place of residence (adjusted for age) show a pattern of increasing use with increasing urbanism. This pattern is observed in the averages for all regions and levels of development. When countries are grouped according to strength of family planning effort within development groups, the results show that, within development groups, countries with a strong family planning programme tend to have higher proportions using contraception than those with a weaker programme. In addition, although relatively small rural/urban differentials in levels of use are found in countries with weaker programmes at lower levels of development and in countries with strong programmes at upper levels of development, larger differentials are found in countries that fall between these two extremes.

The multivariate analysis of contraceptive use in section C uses the constructed residence variable, which takes into account childhood residence and introduces both demographic and socio-economic controls. After addition of all the controls, the pattern of use by current and childhood residence shows the highest level of use among long-term urban residents followed by the rural-urban "migrant" group. Averaged over all countries, the proportion currently using contraception is 8 percentage points higher among long-term urban than long-term rural residents. Regional averages in residential differentials are surprisingly similar, ranging from 6 percentage points in Africa to 9 in Latin America and the Caribbean. As in the case of marital fertility, residence differentials in contraceptive use are reduced by the greatest proportionate amount with the introduction of socio-economic factors in Latin America and the Caribbean and in the upper development groups.

A recent analysis of WFS data using the Bongaarts model shows that the effect of each of intermediate variables in generating fertility differences by residence varies from country to country (Casterline, Singh and Cleland, 1983). The analysis shows that in Latin America and the Caribbean and in Western Asia, differential fertility by residence is due mainly to differential use of contraception; in Africa (and in Sri Lanka), differences in nuptiality are most important. Furthermore, the markedly shorter breast-feeding durations observed in urban areas of many countries of Africa and Asia are found to reduce although not override the impact of contraceptive use on fertility. As Cleland (1985) and others note, the erosion of traditional norms and practices, which often accompanies urbanization and modernization, may have conflicting effects on fertility.

Family size preferences are also found to vary by residence. On average, over all countries, long-term urban residents desire 0.8 child less than long-term rural residents before socio-economic characteristics are controlled. After this addition, the difference is 0.4 child. In all three regions and across all levels of development, about half of the rural/urban differential is attributable to socio-economic factors. It is worth noting that the size of urban/rural differentials in desired family size tend, in general, to be smaller than differentials in actual fertility. That is, rural and urban residents are more homogeneous with respect to their fertility desires than with respect to their actual fertility behaviour. This is not the case in Africa, however, where the participating countries show a wide range of residence differentials in family size but almost uniformly small differentials in actual fertility.

These findings clearly show that although educational and occupational differences in the composition of the population play an important role in explaining observed residence differences in fertility, fertility preferences and contraceptive use, they are not the sole cause of these differences. The characteristics of rural and urban settings in terms of infrastructure, mode of development, institutional configuration and access to services must all play a part in the differences observed. Within Latin America and the Caribbean, relatively small residence differentials in desired family size coexist with a range of relatively large residence differentials in fertility, suggesting differences within the region in accessibility of family planning services between rural and urban areas. In Asia and Oceania, fertility differentials by residence are relatively small when socio-economic factors are controlled, as are differentials in fertility preferences (except in countries of Western Asia—Jordan, the Syrian Arab Republic and Yemen), suggesting that modes of development and access to services may differ less between urban and rural areas, partially because of the greater density of settlement in Asia. In the countries of Africa, residential differentials in family size desires exceed those observed for fertility. In these countries, where services are scarce even in urban areas, certain characteristics of the place that affect fertility preferences may not yet have arisen in terms of fertility.

Throughout this chapter, rural/urban differentials in fertility and fertility-related variables have been discussed chiefly in the context of regions and development and family planning programme groups. While this approach permits some insights that are not possible with more detailed analyses, it also causes a large part of the enormous inter-country variation to be ignored. While in the large majority of countries residence differentials in fertility, family size preferences and contraceptive use are of the expected sign, the size of the coefficients varies widely both within and across regions and levels of development, suggesting that there are many aspects of the country setting as well as of the urban and rural settings that influence fertility behaviour and that have not been measured in this study. The extent to which the average differentials and trends outlined in this chapter describe differentials and predict trends on the national level depends upon a host of factors, including the nature and timing of urbanization, economic development, the development of family planning programmes, and cultural, social and religious differences between countries.

NOTES

[1] For example, in Taiwan, Province of China, Chang, Sun and Freedman (1981) for desired family size and contraceptive use; and Millman (1985) for breast-feeding; in Brazil, Anderson, Rodrigues and Thome (1983); in Thailand, Knodel and Debavalya (1980); and in several developing countries in Africa, Latin America and the Caribbean, and Asia and Oceania, United Nations (1976) for age at first marriage.

[2] Indonesia is a good example of the effect of strong government policy on rural/urban fertility differentials. The Indonesian programme has been characterized by strong political commitment and an administrative structure that appears capable of bringing information, services and supplies effectively to the village level (Freedman, Khoo and Supraptilah, 1981).

[3] To take an extreme example, Suva, the capital of Fiji (population, 118,000) was classified as major urban, while Semarang (population, 647,000), a city in Indonesia, was coded as other urban.

[4] Formerly called the Ivory Coast.

[5] Additional information on both current and childhood residence can be found in Singh (1984).

[6] Although the level of non-numerical response was also high in Cameroon, this country is excluded from the table because the information about desired size is not comparable to that obtained elsewhere. (See chapter II.)

[7] One issue that arises in the study of the determinants of fertility preferences is whether it is appropriate to control for the number of living children (Pullum, 1980, 1983). If women state a desired number of children which is biased towards agreement with their actual number of children and the number of living children is not controlled, then observed differences in desired family size between socio-economic groups will reflect differences in actual, not desired, fertility. In this case, a control for actual fertility is necessary.

If, on the other hand, the relationship between actual and desired fertility is a result of effective use of contraception, it is not appropriate to control for actual family size. In this case, desired family size is prior to, not a result of, actual family size.

The model of desired family size presented in this chapter was run both with and without the number of living children as a demographic control. Over all, the rural/urban differential in desired family size was very similar in each case. Thus, only the results from the model including the control for number of living children are presented. In contrast, the addition of this control has a somewhat larger impact on educational differentials in desired family size (see chapter VIII).

References

Anderson, John E., Walter Rodrigues and Antonio Macio Tavares Thome (1983). Analysis of breastfeeding in Northeastern Brazil: methodological and policy considerations. *Studies in Family Planning* 14(8/9):211-219.

Balkaran, Sundat and David P. Smith (1984). Socio-economic differentials in breast-feeding. Additional tables for World Fertility Comparative Studies. Voorburg, The Netherlands, International Statistical Institute (unpublished).

Blanc, Ann Klimas (1982). Unwanted fertility in Latin America and the Caribbean. *International Family Planning Perspectives* 8(4):156-162.

Casterline, John B. (1984). The collection and analysis of community data: the WFS experience. Paper submitted to World Fertility Survey Symposium, London, 24-27 April 1984.

_____ and Hazel Ashurst (1985). Socio-economic differentials in current fertility. Additional tables for World Fertility Survey Comparative Studies. Voorburg, The Netherlands, International Statistical Institute (unpublished).

_____, Susheela Singh and John G. Cleland (1983). The proximate determinants of fertility: crossnational and subnational variations. Paper submitted to the Annual Meeting of the Population Association of America, Pittsburgh, Pennsylvania, 14-16 April 1983.

Chamratrithirong, Apichat and Peerasit Kamnansilpa (1984). How family planning availability affects contraceptive use: the case of Thailand. In John A. Ross and Regina McNamara, eds., *Survey Analysis for the Guidance of Family Planning Programs*. Proceedings of a seminar organized by the International Union for the Scientific Study of Population, Genting Highlands, Malaysia, December 1981. Liège: Ordina Editions, 219-235.

Chang, Ming-cheng, R. Freedman and Te-hsung Sun (1981). Trends in fertility, family size preferences, and family planning practice: Taiwan, 1961-1980. *Studies in Family Planning* 12(5):211-228. The data in this article refer to Taiwan, Province of China.

Chernichovsky, Dov and Oey Astra Meesook (1980). *Regional Aspects of Family Planning and Fertility Behavior in Indonesia*. World Bank Staff Working Paper, No. 462. Washington, D.C.: The World Bank (mimeographed).

Cleland, John (1985). Marital fertility decline in developing countries: theories and the evidence. In John Cleland and John Hobcraft, eds., in collaboration with Betzy Dinesen, *Reproductive Change in Developing Countries: Insights from the World Fertility Survey*. Oxford: Oxford University Press, 223-252.

Cochrane, Susan H. (1983). Effects of education and urbanization on fertility. In Rodolfo A. Bulatao and Ronald D. Lee, eds., with Paula E. Hollerbach and John Bongaarts, *Determinants of Fertility in Developing Countries*, vol. 2, *Fertility Regulation and Institutional Influences*. Report of the National Research Council Committee on Population and Demography, Panel on Fertility Determinants. New York: Academic Press, 587-626.

Ebanks, G. Edward and Susheela Singh (1984). Socio-economic differentials in age at marriage. Draft and tables for World Fertility Survey Comparative Studies; Cross-National Summaries. Voorburg, The Netherlands, International Statistical Institute (unpublished).

Ferry, Benoît and David P. Smith (1983). *Breastfeeding Differentials*. World Fertility Survey Comparative Studies, No. 23: Cross-National Summaries. Voorburg, The Netherlands: International Statistical Institute.

Freedman, Ronald, Siew-Ean Khoo and Bondan Supraptilah (1981). *Modern Contraceptive Use in Indonesia: A Challenge to Conventional Wisdom*. World Fertility Survey Scientific Reports, No. 20. Voorburg, The Netherlands: International Statistical Institute.

Gaisie, S. K. (1976). Fertility trends and differentials. In John C. Caldwell and others, eds., *Population Growth and Socio-economic Change in West Africa*. New York: Columbia University Press for The Population Council, 339-345.

Johnson, Nan E., C. Shannon Stokes and Rex H. Warland (1978). Farm-nonfarm differentials in fertility: the effects of compositional and sex-role factors. *Rural Sociology* 43(4):671-690.

Jones, Elise F. (1982). *Socio-Economic Differentials in Achieved Fertility*. World Fertility Survey Comparative Studies, No. 21; ECE Analyses of WFS Surveys in Europe and USA. Voorburg, The Netherlands: International Statistical Institute.

Ketkar, Suhas L. (1979). Determinants of fertility in a developing society: The case of Sierra Leone. *Population Studies* 33(3):479-488.

Knodel, John and Nibhon Debavalya (1977). Breastfeeding in Thailand: trends and differentials, 1969-79. *Studies in Family Planning* 11(12):355-377.

Lapham, Robert J. and W. Parker Mauldin (1984). Family planning program effort and birthrate decline in developing countries. *International Family Planning Perspectives* 10(4):109-118.

Lightbourne, Robert E. (1980). *Urban-Rural Differentials in Contraceptive Use*. World Fertility Survey Comparative Studies No. 10: Cross-National Summaries. Voorburg, The Netherlands: International Statistical Institute.

_____ (1984). Quality of the WFS fertility preference data. Background paper submitted to the World Fertility Survey Symposium, London, 24-27 April 1984.

Little, Roderick J. A. (1980). *Linear Models for WFS Data*. World Fertility Survey Technical Bulletin, No. 9. Voorburg, The Netherlands: International Statistical Institute.

Mauldin, W. Parker and Bernard Berelson (1978). Conditions of fertility decline in developing countries, 1965-75. With section by Zenas Sykes. *Studies in Family Planning* 9(5):89-147.

Michielutte, R. and others (1975). Residence and fertility in Costa Rica. *Rural Sociology* 40(2):319-331.

Millman, Sara (1985). Breastfeeding and contraception: why the inverse association? *Studies in Family Planning* 16(2):61-75.

Pullum, Thomas W. (1980). *Illustrative Analysis: Fertility Preferences in Sri Lanka*. World Fertility Survey Scientific Reports, No. 9. Voorburg, The Netherlands: International Statistical Institute.

_____ (1983). "Correlates of family-size desires. in Rodolfo A. Bulatao and Ronald D. Lee, with Paula E. Hollerbach and John Bongaarts, *Determinants of Fertility in Developing Countries*, vol. I, *Supply and Demand for Children*. Report of the National Research Council Committee on Population and Demography, Panel on Fertility Determinants. New York: Academic Press, 344-368.

Rodríguez, Germán and John Cleland (1981). Socio-economic determinants of marital fertility in twenty countries: a multivariate analysis. In *World Fertility Survey Conference, 1980: Record of Proceedings*. London, 7-11 July 1980. Voorburg, The Netherlands: International Statistical Institute, vol. II, 337-414.

Singh, Susheela (1984). *Comparability of Questionnaires: Forty-one WFS Countries*. World Fertility Survey Comparative Studies, No. 32; Cross-National Summaries. Voorburg, The Netherlands: International Statistical Institute.

_____ and J. Casterline (1985). The socio-economic determinants of fertility. In John Cleland and John Hobcraft, eds., in collaboration with Betzy Dinesen, *Reproductive Change in Developing Countries: Insights from the World Fertility Survey*. Oxford: Oxford University Press, 199-222.

Stokes, C. Shannon (1973). Family structure and socio-economic differentials in fertility. *Population Studies* 27(2):295-304.

Trovato, Frank and Carl F. Grindstaff (1980). Decomposing the urban-rural fertility differential: Canada, 1971. *Rural Sociology* 45(3):448-468.

United Nations (1973). Department of Economic and Social Affairs. Population Division. *The Determinants and Consequences of Population Trends*, vol. I, *New Summary of Findings on Interaction of Demographic, Economic and Social Factors*. Population Studies, No. 50. New York. Sales No. E.71.XIII.3.

_____ (1976). Updated study of urban-rural differences in the marital status composition of the population. Working paper ESA/P/WP.59. New York.

_____ (1977). *Levels and Trends of Fertility Throughout the World, 1950-1970*. Population Studies, No. 59. New York. Sales No. E.77.XIII.2.

_____ (1986). Department of International Economic and Social Affairs. Population Division. Rural-urban residence and fertility: selected findings from the World Fertility Survey data. Working paper ESA/P/WP.95. New York.

Westoff, Charles F. (1981). Unwanted fertility in six developing countries. *International Family Planning Perspectives* 7(2):43-52.

VIII. EDUCATION AND FERTILITY

Abstract

This chapter discusses the relationships between education and fertility, desired family size, marriage, breast-feeding and contraceptive practice. Education differences in unwanted fertility and in number of surviving children are summarized. The effect of education on marital fertility, contraceptive use and desired family size after statistical control for other socio-economic variables also is examined.

Education is strongly related to fertility in most countries, but the form and size of the relationship vary considerably. At current fertility rates, averaged over all countries, women with seven or more years of education will bear 3.9 children while women with no schooling will bear nearly 80 per cent more, 6.9 on average. The differential has increased over time in many countries, due to greater fertility decline among the better educated. Although highly educated women generally have the lowest fertility, women with a few years of schooling often have slightly higher levels than those with no education. This pattern is common in the least developed countries. The contrast in number of surviving children between the most and least educated women is considerably smaller than the contrast in number of births, and in the least developed countries the number of living children is about the same for older women with seven or more years of schooling as for those with none. Fertility differentials by women's education tend to be somewhat larger and less often curvilinear, compared with differentials measured by husband's education. Education differentials are similar in rural and urban areas of most countries, but in a sizeable minority, the education effect is larger in urban areas.

Within countries, desired family size is always lower for the better educated, but actual fertility differentials do not simply reflect desires. Studies of current exposure to risk of unwanted fertility consistently show greater risk among the educated, but this may not have been universally true in the past, as indicated by patterns of excess fertility among the oldest women interviewed. In the least developed countries, where the education difference in number of living children is minimal, older women with moderate to high levels of education are the most likely to have exceeded their desired family size; in the more developed countries, the proportion with excess fertility decreases with education.

Women with seven or more years of schooling marry, on average, nearly four years later, have about 25 percentage points higher contraceptive use and breast-feed children eight months less than women with no education. Unlike fertility itself, these fertility determinants nearly always show a monotonic relation with number of years of education. Even a few years typically has a substantial effect on breast-feeding and contraceptive use.

Studies of fertility conditions and change have consistently pointed to education as an important factor in accounting for fertility differences within populations. Education, therefore, has come to occupy an important place in investigative work, both as concerns differential fertility by socio-economic status and, more fundamentally, in the search for causal explanations of fertility levels and fertility change. Knowledge of the education-fertility relationship is especially relevant for development planning because education can be directly influenced by government policy. Among national populations where high fertility is considered an obstacle to development, detailed knowledge of the education-fertility relationship would doubtlessly facilitate decisions concerning educational levels, curriculum content, the structure of the educational system and, ultimately, the division of resources between education and other competing programmes.

It is profitable to examine the conceptual significance of education, considered as an influence on fertility (see Ridker, 1976; Cochrane, 1979; Hermalin and Mason, 1980). Although attention has generally been focused on educational attainment (its quantitative aspect), it is worth noting at the outset that education is by no means a homogeneous commodity whose only important attribute is "level-reached". While educational content may not be as important as educational attainment in certain hypothesized causal paths linking education with fertility (such as postponement of marriage), it clearly is so with regard to those effects on fertility which operate "through changes in attitude, self-perception, and the productivity of human capital" (Ridker, 1976, p. 14). Education about population issues has been cited as one instance where educational content may affect fertility (Holsinger and Kasarda, 1976; Viederman, 1971). One study in the Philippines, for example, found a significant lowering in ideal family size among an experimental group subjected to a course in population education, when compared with the control group (Paik, 1973). It appears, however, that many other parts of the formal curriculum, while not dealing directly with population, are likely to exert subtle influences during the formation of attitudes and norms bearing upon fertility. The distinction has been made, for example, between religious and non-religious educational systems, especially for Muslim and Roman Catholic populations, pointing to the possibility that some religious instruction may contain a pro-natalist bias. More often, the implicit message is thought to be anti-natalist. Caldwell (1980, 1982), in particular, argues that exposure through schools to Western ideas and social values powerfully undermines traditional norms and familial relationships that favour unlimited fertility.

Besides the quantity (attainment) and content aspects of education, quality of schooling or what has been called the "hidden curriculum" has been pointed to as a likely influence on fertility and fertility ideals. Nevertheless, research in related areas has failed to find significant links between observed attitudes and features, such as size or quality of school or teaching materials available (Holsinger and Kasarda, 1976). Other aspects of education of possible importance for fertility include areas of knowledge, cognitive skills, school environment and length of school day and year (Hermalin and Mason, 1980; Wiley, 1976). But the fact remains that studies on the topic have almost exclusively relied upon the quantity aspect of education, the aspect that is easiest to measure; the present study is no exception.

The specific connections that have been theorized to exist between education and fertility can be classified in a variety of ways. To adopt the economist's terminology, individual-level effects of education can be divided into those which act on the demand for children, those which affect the supply of children and those which influence the costs, broadly defined, of fertility regulation (Easterlin, 1978).

There is some evidence from surveys preceding the World Fertility Survey (WFS) of a connection between education and desired fertility, and the WFS programme has greatly increased the amount of information available (Pullum, 1983; United Nations, 1981, 1983; Cochrane, 1979). Education may directly change attitudes, values and beliefs towards a small family norm and towards a style of child-rearing that is relatively costly to the parents in time and money (higher "child quality"). The potential for education to diffuse non-traditional values does not end in the class-room, since the educated are likely to continue to be exposed to modern or Western ideas through newspapers and books, and through ownership of radios and television sets, which they typically acquire earlier than couples of lower socio-economic status. Education also influences economic factors in ways that are thought to discourage high fertility: it reduces the economic utility of children; it creates aspirations for upward social mobility and the accumulation of wealth; and it increases the opportunity cost of women's time and enhances the likelihood of their employment outside the home (see chapter IX). Education also increases earning ability, which might, other things being equal, lead couples to want more children. This "income effect", however, is evidently usually of minor importance in relation to the fertility-decreasing effects of the other influences mentioned, since most empirical studies have found a negative relation between education and fertility or stated fertility desires (Cochrane, 1979; Pullum, 1983).

Surveys preceding WFS revealed a stong positive relasionship between education and contraceptive use (United Nations, 1979). Avenues through which education may affect fertility control include: (*a*) education facilitates the acquisition of information about family planning; (*b*) education increases husband-wife communication; (*c*) education imparts a sense of control over one's destiny, which may encourage attempts to control childbearing as well; (*d*) the higher income of educated couples makes a wide range of contraceptive methods affordable. The relationship between education and abortion, though not well studied, may be another important effect of education on fertility.

Education also affects the supply of living children through paths other than its influence on deliberate fertility control. The three most important of these influences are: (*a*) education delays entry into marital unions; (*b*) education is associated with lower prevalence and duration of breast-feeding; (*c*) education is associated with reduced child and adult mortality. In addition, in countries with a tradition of extended post-partum abstinence, educated couples tend to observe these customs less than others. The WFS data have been particularly important in documenting the pervasiveness of such relationships (McCarthy, 1982; Ferry and Smith, 1983; Ebanks and Singh, 1984; Balkaran and Smith, 1984; Hobcraft, McDonald and Rutstein, 1985; Singh, Casterline and Cleland, 1985). The breast-feeding, abstinence and mortality effects act to increase the supply of children, raising the possibility that the net effect of education on number of births or surviving children may not always be negative. Education may also be associated with increased fecundability, lower foetal loss and a longer reproductive span for women, through better nutrition and health and, in the case of fecundability, possibly through higher rates of sexual intercourse (Evidence on this point is sparse and conflicting; see Nag, 1983). It is not clear, however, that these latter factors have an important effect on aggregate fertility differences (Bongaarts and Potter, 1983; Gray 1983).

Another line of theoretical speculation concerns "spill-over effects", by which is meant the effect that others' education may have on an individual couple's fertility. One such connection involves the cost of child-care substitutes: "If women in general have very little education, an educated woman can afford massive child care substitutes and thus can combine the benefits of education with high fertility" (Cochrane, 1979, p. 76). Another spill-over effect may occur when parents with little education foresee (because the environment strongly favours education) the necessity of giving much more education to their children than they themselves received (Vlassoff, 1979). Indeed, in some ways the education given to children is probably more crucial than the parent's own schooling (Caldwell, 1982): not only does school attendance cost money and decrease the amount of productive work from children while they are young, it may also undermine children's adherence to traditional filial obligations, leading parents to expect less help from children later on, thus decreasing the incentive to have a large family.

There are theoretical reasons to expect women's education to be more strongly negatively related to fertility than men's, and earlier research tends to bear this out (Cochrane, 1979). At least in societies where well-paid jobs are open to educated women, time needed for child care has a higher opportunity cost for educated than uneducated women; this tends not to be true for men, because child care is usually the province of women, regardless of educational attainment. For men, a positive relation between education and fertility might be expected from the "income effect" mentioned earlier, at least after statistical control for other variables. Another consideration is that in most developing countries the contraceptive methods in widest use are "female methods", principally hormonal pills, female sterilization and intra-uterine devices (IUD) (see chapter V). Although the use of contraception undoubtedly depends in part upon the husband's characteristics, and upon those of other members of extended families as well, still it is the woman who must know how to obtain and use these methods, and be willing to do so. Her own education may in these respects be more important than that of her husband.

The general considerations outlined above provide no clear guidance for predicting the size of education differentials in particular populations. Some of the indirect paths through which education is thought to affect fertility ought to operate most strongly in economically advanced countries—the effect through opportunity cost of women's time, for instance (see chapter IX). Yet, the largest education differentials are not today found in the highly developed countries but in certain developing countries.

The social-diffusion or cultural-lag hypothesis, mentioned in chapter VII, is a general proposition about intrasocietal differences in the pace of demographic change. As applied to education differentials in fertility, it leads to the expectation that differentials will first widen, at the initial stages of transition to lower fertility, as the decline begins earliest among the highly educated; at a later stage, differentials are expected to narrow. In the course of the transition, the fertility of all educational groups eventually falls, as is depicted schematically in figure 54, where lines A to D represent differentials at successive stages of the transition. The cultural-lag hypothesis does not itself predict the form of the education-fertility relationship before or after the transition—in figure 54, a non-monotonic relation is shown for the pre-transition phase, on the basis of data analysis antedating WFS, as well as earlier studies based on WFS data (Cochrane, 1979; United Nations, 1983). The late-transition line, D, shows the possibility of slightly higher fertility for the best educated, particularly if indexed by male rather than female education, and especially after control for other social characteristics. The latter type of relationship is not expected to appear in the developing countries examined here, though it has been detected in some developed countries (see chapter XIV).

The data examined here represent a cross-section of countries observed at different stages of the demographic transition, rather than a history of the transition in individual countries. It can, nevertheless, be expected on the basis of the cultural-lag hypothesis that small education differentials in fertility and related variables will be found in countries where there is no evidence of recent fertility

Figure 54. Hypothesized relationship between fertility and education at different levels of development

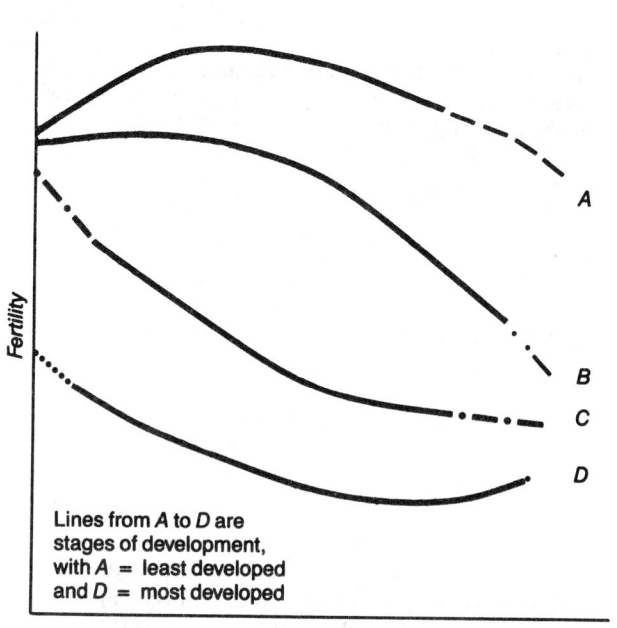

Lines from A to D are stages of development, with A = least developed and D = most developed

Source: Adapted from Cochrane (1979) and United Nations (1983).

decline, and larger differentials elsewhere. In the present volume, the differentials are examined according to level of development rather than stage of transition, but there is a strong relationship between the two (see chapter I). One consequence of the association between development and the current stage of transition should be mentioned: for pre-transition countries, A, there are relatively few highly educated persons in the sample, making it difficult to measure the form of the differential at the upper end of the educational range; for countries relatively far advanced in the transition, there are frequently few uneducated persons in the samples. This is indicated in figure 54 by the position of the solid portion of lines A-D in relation to the education axis.

From the foregoing discussion, it is obvious that the paths through which education acts on fertility are complex and intertwined. No empirical study has attempted to shed light on all of the proposed causal paths, nor does it seem possible even to conceptualize such a study. Several recent works review the copious amount of empirical research into this relationship (Cochrane, 1979, 1983; Strout, n.d.).

The present chapter takes advantage of the relative strengths of WFS data, by examining education differentials in several of the major proximate determinants of fertility as well as in fertility itself. The main focus is on differentials according to women's education, with a lesser emphasis on fertility differentials according to the husband's education. Throughout, attention is given to relationships between these differentials and macro characteristics of the countries—geographical region, which to a limited extent reflects large-scale cultural differences; relative level of socio-economic development; and, where appropriate, strength of the family planning programme effort.

The following section describes the data gathered in the individual interviews, including trends in educational attainment and the relationship between literacy and education. Section B examines education differentials in fertility, fertility preferences, entry into marriage, use of contraception and mean duration of breast-feeding. In this section, differentials are examined without statistical control for other socio-economic variables (but with control for age), in order to provide an introductory view and to take advantage of certain types of tabulations which are not available with effects of other factors controlled. Section C examines differentials in marital fertility, contraceptive use and desired family size with statistical control for other socio-economic variables gathered in WFS.

A. Measures of education

Years of schooling

Throughout this chapter, education is classified according to the number of years of schooling completed. Variations in sample design and coding of education limit comparability, though not to the same degree as for rural and urban residence. The surveys did not actually inquire about the total number of years of education but about the highest educational level attained and the number of years completed at that level. In some cases, where alternative education systems coexist or where the system has changed over time, the total number of years is known only approximately (Singh, 1984). The precise number of years is often especially difficult to determine for those with schooling beyond the intermediate or lower secondary level, because the number of years obtained before entrance into certain technical and higher academic courses can vary. An upper-limit code ("11 + years", for example) was used in a number of samples;[1] and in some cases, the number of years was not ascertained for a substantial number of respondents or, more often, of husbands.[2]

Table 109 shows the educational distribution of ever-married women and their current or most recent husband. On average, 44 per cent of the women had no formal education (unweighted mean), with the percentage in individual countries ranging from 98 per cent in Yemen to 2 per cent in Jamaica. Husbands are more likely to have received some schooling—the proportion with no education ranges from 88 per cent (Yemen) to 2 per cent (Trinidad and Tobago) and averages 34 per cent.

For those who attended school, the number of completed years is shown, divided into three-year groups, with a final category of 10 or more years. In a majority of countries, the end of primary schooling falls in the period from four to six years, as is indicated in column (1) of table 109. This group usually contains the largest number of educated men and women—an average of 22 per cent of ever-married women and 24 per cent of husbands. Only 7 per cent of respondents and 13 per cent of husbands, on average, had 10 or more years of schooling, although this figure ranges in particular countries from 0 to 42 per cent.[3]

Educational attainment of both sexes is strongly related to the national level of development; indeed, education is an integral part of socio-economic development and current educational enrolment of children is one of four main components of the development classification employed here (see the Introduction to this report). Tables 109-111 are arranged according to level of development in order to show this association clearly. Within development groups, there are particular countries with atypically high or low educational attainment, but on average the proportion of wives with no education declines from 81 per cent in group IV to 14 per cent in group I. Comparable figures for husband's education are 65 and 9 per cent, respectively. At the upper end of the educational spectrum, there is a less consistent relationship, with development groups I and II showing about the same percentage of respondents with 10 or more years of schooling. The proportion with at least seven years, however, increases strongly with level of development.

Table 109 also shows the mean number of years of education for husbands and wives; and for women, the mean based on all of those aged 15-49 (including single women) is shown for comparison, where possible. Average attainment of all women exceeds that of married women, because most single women are young and have therefore been exposed to better educational opportunities than older women, and also because among women of the same age, the highly educated are less likely than others to have married. The latter point is discussed in detail later in this chapter.

On average, ever-married women had 3.3 years of schooling and their husbands, 4.2 years. Husband/wife differences are typically small in Latin America and the Caribbean and tend to be largest in Asia and Oceania; in Bangladesh, Jordan, Kenya, Pakistan and the Republic of Korea, husbands had, on average, two years more schooling than wives. Although the difference is under one-half year in 10 countries (Philippines, Senegal and eight countries in Latin America and the Caribbean), Lesotho is the only country in which women's educational attainment exceeded that of their husbands, and it did so by nearly two years.[4]

In all countries, relatively well educated persons tend to marry each other. The correlation, r, between husband's and wife's education, measured in single years, averages 0.57 (table 109, column (19)). The weakest correlations, 0.35-0.38, are seen in Yemen, where few adults had any formal education, and in Lesotho. Latin American countries, unlike the Caribbean countries, exhibit relatively strong associations between husband's and wife's education, with maximum correlations of 0.72-0.78 in Ecuador and Peru. Another view of the association between husband's and wife's education is given by considering the proportion of couples in which both spouses fall in the same educational category (0, 1-3, 4-6, 7-9 or 10+ years). For countries in the three upper development groups (I-III) shown in table 109, an average of roughly half the spouses are in the same category of attainment; in approximately 35 per cent of couples, the husband occupies a higher educational category than the wife; and in about 15 per cent, the reverse is true (tabulation not shown). In development group IV, the proportion of couples in the same category is about 70 per cent, a consequence of the preponderance of men and women with zero education.[5]

TABLE 109. PERCENTAGE DISTRIBUTION OF EVER-MARRIED WOMEN AND THEIR HUSBANDS ACCORDING TO NUMBER OF YEARS OF EDUCATION COMPLETED, MEAN NUMBER OF YEARS FOR EVER-MARRIED WOMEN, ALL WOMEN AND HUSBANDS; AND CORRELATION BETWEEN HUSBAND'S AND WIFE'S EDUCATION

	Years to complete primary school (1)	Women							Mean number of years		Husbands							Mean number of years (18)	Correlation between husband's and wife's education [c] (19)
		Total (2)	Completed years (percentage)					Not stated[a] (8)	Ever-married (9)	All[b] (10)	Total (11)	Completed years (percentage)					Not stated[a] (17)		
			Zero (3)	1-3 (4)	4-6 (5)	7-9 (6)	10+ (7)					Zero (12)	1-3 (13)	4-6 (14)	7-9 (15)	10+ (16)			

A. Countries by level of development

I. High
Colombia	5	100	16	38	29	11	5	0	3.7	4.4	100	16	35	29	11	9	0	4.0	0.66
Costa Rica[d]	6	100	8	25	41	9	16	0	5.3	5.7	100	10	24	38	9	19	0	5.3	0.64
Fiji	8	100	19	8	29	34	10	0	5.4	...	100	8	7	28	40	14	2	6.4	0.54
Guyana	6	100	4	3	23	60	6	4	7.3	7.6	100	4	2	20	52	12	10	7.4	0.46
Jamaica	6	100	2	3	18	67	10	0	7.4	...	100	3	2	11	61	9	15	7.7	0.42
Malaysia	6	100	35	18	34	7	6	1	3.4	7.5	100	13	16	47	12	11	1	5.5	0.63
Mexico	6	100	22	33	27	13	4	0	3.7	4.0	100	18	29	29	10	10	4	4.1	0.62
Panama[d]	6	100	6	14	40	18	22	0	6.4	6.7	100	6	14	37	17	26	1	6.6	0.65
Republic of Korea	6	100	21	8	42	17	12	0	5.4	...	100	11	3	30	21	35	0	7.5	0.65
Trinidad and Tobago	7	100	4	2	12	67	15	0	7.9	8.4	100	2	1	9	64	18	6	8.4	0.52
Venezuela[e]	6	100	14	16	43	16	11	0	5.2	6.1	100	13	12	42	17	15	0	5.6	0.60

II. Middle-high
Dominican Republic	6	100	16	38	28	12	7	0	3.8	4.6	100	17	26	25	15	10	7	4.3	0.54
Ecuador	6	100	14	25	35	11	14	0	4.9	5.7	100	11	21	41	9	18	0	5.1	0.72
Jordan	6	100	50	6	21	13	9	0	3.3	...	100	22	7	30	19	22	0	5.5	0.51
Paraguay	6	100	7	31	41	9	12	0	4.8	5.5	100	5	27	42	11	15	0	5.3	0.68
Peru	6	100	31	24	23	8	14	0	3.7	...	100	11	26	30	10	23	0	5.2	0.78
Philippines	6	100	6	12	48	9	24	1	6.0	...	100	5	14	42	9	30	0	6.4	0.59
Sri Lanka	6	100	22	18	28	18	13	0	4.6	...	100	8	15	34	25	17	0	5.8	0.59
Syrian Arab Republic	7[f]	100	67	4	18	7	5	0	2.1	...	100	38	7	30	11	13	0	3.9	0.52
Thailand	7[f]	100	20	6	67	2	5	0	3.5	...	100	12	4	67	3	12	2	4.4	0.53
Tunisia	6[g]	100	77	4	13	0	6	0	1.4	...	100	62	4	20	5	10	0	2.7	0.61

III. Middle-low
Cameroon	6/7[h]	100	68	7	19	4	2	0	1.7	2.2	100	57	6	25	5	7	1	2.7	0.68
Côte d'Ivoire[i]	6	100	84	4	8	3	2	0	1.0	1.3	100	69	4	12	4	11	0	2.2	0.54
Egypt	6	100	60	11	19	3	7	0	2.1	...	100	53	6	22	5	14	0	2.9	0.53
Ghana	6	100	60	3	7	9	20	0	3.3	4.1	100	44	1	5	6	42	1	5.2	0.57
Indonesia	6	100	62	15	18	3	2	0	1.9	...	100	34	22	32	6	6	0	3.4	0.55
Kenya	7	100	53	12	18	12	4	0	2.5	3.4	100	30	8	21	27	13	2	4.7	0.58
Lesotho	7	100	8	13	55	23	2	0	5.0	...	100	39	17	28	12	4	0	3.1	0.38
Morocco	5	100	88	2	6	2	2	0	0.7	1.4	100	77	2	10	3	5	4	1.3	0.55

IV. Low
Bangladesh	5	100	78	8	11	2	1	0	1.0	...	100	57	10	15	8	8	2	2.7	0.61
Benin	7	100	88	3	6	2	1	0	0.7	1.1	100	74	3	11	2	5	6	1.3	0.50
Haiti	6	100	70	15	9	3	2	0	1.2	1.8	100	51	19	15	6	9	0	2.7	0.68
Mauritania[j]	7	100	40	56	2	2	...	0	...	...	100	42	49	3	7	0	0	...	...
Nepal	10[k]	100	95	1	2	1	1	0	0.2	...	100	71	4	6	6	5	8	1.6	0.47
Pakistan	5	100	87	2	5	2	2	2	0.6	...	100	57	5	15	9	12	0	2.9	0.45
Senegal	6	100	90	2	5	2	1	0	0.6	1.0	100	83	2	7	2	3	3	0.9	0.51
Sudan	6	100	81	7	7	2	2	2	0.9	...	100	64	10	14	5	7	0	1.9	0.57
Yemen	6	100	98	0	1	0	0	0	0.1	...	100	88	2	4	2	3	1	0.7	0.35

218

B. *Mean values for regions and development groups*

	100	66	10	14	5	4	0	1.8		58	9	15	7	10	2	2.6	0.55
Africa																	
Latin America and the Caribbean	100	17	21	28	23	10	0	5.0		13	18	28	22	15	3	5.5	0.61
	100	51	8	25	9	7	0	2.9		32	9	29	13	14	2	4.4	0.54
Asia and Oceania																	
I. High	100	14	15	31	29	11	0	5.6		9	13	29	29	16	4	6.2	0.58
II. Middle-high	100	31	16	32	9	11	0	3.8		19	15	36	11	17	1	4.9	0.61
III. Middle-low	100	60	8	19	7	5	0	2.3		50	8	19	8	13	1	3.2	0.55
IV. Low	100	81	10	5	2	1	0	0.7		65	12	10	5	6	2	1.8	0.52
TOTAL	100	44	13	22	12	7	0	3.3		34	12	24	14	13	2	4.2	0.57

Sources: World Fertility Survey standard recode tapes; and for column (1), United Nations Educational, Scientific and Cultural Organization (1981), table 3.1, pp. III-16—III-25.

NOTE: Based on ever-married women aged 15-49 and their husbands, except as noted separately.

[a] Most persons in this category have some education, but the number of years was not stated.
[b] Column (10) based on all women aged 15-49.
[c] Pearson correlation, r, between husband's and wife's education coded in single years.
[d] Based on ages 20-49.
[e] Based on ages 15-44.
[f] Lower primary equals four years.
[g] Eight years in alternative education system.
[h] Six years in Eastern Cameroon, seven years in Western Cameroon.
[i] Formerly called the Ivory Coast.
[j] Number of years not available. Education categories are: no schooling; primary incomplete or Koranic school; primary complete; more than primary.
[k] Ten years as coded in the World Fertility Survey; three years in English schools.

TABLE 110. MEAN NUMBER OF YEARS OF EDUCATION FOR ALL WOMEN INTERVIEWED, BY CURRENT AGE GROUP, AND DIFFERENCE IN MEAN EDUCATIONAL ATTAINMENT BETWEEN HUSBANDS OF WOMEN AGED 25-29 YEARS AND 45-49 YEARS

	Type of sample (1)	Mean years of education completed by age group							Education difference: ages 25-29 versus 45-49	
		15-19 (2)	20-24 (3)	25-29 (4)	30-34 (5)	35-39 (6)	40-44 (7)	45-49 (8)	Women (9)	Husbands[a] (10)

A. Countries by level of development

I. High										
Colombia	ALL	5.3	5.2	4.5	3.9	3.4	3.0	2.9	1.6	1.4
Costa Rica	ALL	..	7.2	6.2	5.5	4.9	4.3	4.3	1.9	1.6
Fiji	EM	6.7	6.8	6.2	5.4	4.6	4.0	3.3	2.9	1.8
Guyana	ALL	8.8[b]	8.5	7.7	6.9	6.6	6.4	6.0	1.7	0.9
Jamaica	ALL	9.0[b]	8.1	7.9	7.6	6.8	6.6	6.9	1.0	1.0
Malaysia	EM	5.1	5.2	4.7	3.7	2.6	1.8	1.6	3.1	2.4
Mexico	ALL	3.9[c]	5.3	4.6	3.8	3.3	2.9	2.6	2.0	1.4
Panama	ALL	..	7.9	7.2	6.6	6.0	5.4	5.1	2.1	1.5
Republic of Korea	EM	6.3	7.2	7.3	6.1	4.6	3.9	2.9	4.4	4.0
Trinidad and Tobago	ALL	9.3[b]	9.0	8.6	8.0	7.3	7.0	6.5	2.1	1.0
Venezuela	ALL	6.8	7.1	6.0	5.2	4.6	3.9	..	2.8[d]	2.2[d]
II. Middle-high										
Dominican Republic	ALL	5.3	5.4	5.0	4.0	3.4	2.9	2.6	2.4	2.0
Ecuador	ALL	6.7	6.8	5.7	5.0	4.5	4.2	3.6	2.1	1.5
Jordan	EM	5.2	5.1	4.1	3.1	2.0	1.5	1.4	2.7	3.0
Paraguay	ALL	6.1	6.3	5.5	5.1	4.8	4.4	3.6	1.9	1.5
Peru	EM	4.1	4.7	4.6	4.1	2.9	2.9	2.6	2.0	2.1
Philippines	EM	6.3	6.9	6.9	6.2	5.6	5.6	4.8	2.1	1.6
Sri Lanka	EM	5.1	5.2	5.5	5.0	4.5	3.9	3.3	2.2	1.1
Syrian Arab Republic	EM	3.3	3.0	2.3	2.3	1.8	1.0	0.7	1.6	2.6
Thailand	EM	3.7	4.0	4.1	3.7	3.3	2.9	2.6	1.5	1.1
Tunisia	EM	2.5	3.0	2.3	1.6	0.8	0.3	0.3	2.0	2.3
III. Middle-low										
Cameroon	ALL	4.2	3.5	2.4	1.3	0.8	0.4	0.3	2.1	2.0
Côte d'Ivoire[e]	ALL	2.3	1.8	1.3	0.7	0.2	0.1	0.2	1.1	2.0
Egypt	EM	1.6	2.3	2.6	2.4	1.7	1.8	1.7	0.9	1.4
Ghana	ALL	6.3	5.8	4.6	2.7	1.7	1.3	0.9	3.7	3.6
Indonesia	EM	2.6	2.8	2.6	1.8	1.2	0.9	0.7	1.9	1.6
Kenya	ALL	5.4	4.7	3.3	2.3	1.3	1.2	0.8	2.5	3.2
Lesotho	EM	5.4	5.6	5.3	5.1	4.8	4.1	4.3	1.0	0.9
Morocco	ALL	2.3	1.9	1.5	0.9	0.5	0.2	0.0	1.5	2.0
IV. Low										
Bangladesh	EM	1.5	1.3	1.0	0.7	0.6	0.6	0.5	0.5	0.7
Benin	ALL	2.7	1.4	0.8	0.9	0.5	0.4	0.3	0.5	0.8
Haiti	ALL	2.6	2.5	1.4	1.2	1.0	0.9	0.7	0.7	1.0
Nepal	EM	0.5	0.3	0.3	0.2	0.1	0.1	0.1	0.2	1.3
Pakistan	EM	0.6	0.9	0.8	0.6	0.6	0.3	0.3	0.5	1.8
Senegal	ALL	1.8	1.5	0.9	0.4	0.3	0.1	0.1	0.8	0.6
Sudan	EM	1.6	1.5	1.1	0.9	0.4	0.2	0.2	0.9	1.4
Yemen	EM	0.3	0.1	0.1	0.0	0.0	0.0	0.0	0.1	0.3

B. Mean values for regions and development groups

Africa	..	3.3	3.0	2.4	1.8	1.2	0.9	0.8	1.6	1.8
Latin America and the Caribbean	..	6.2	6.7	5.8	5.1	4.6	4.2	4.0	1.8	1.5
Asia and Oceania	..	3.6	3.8	3.5	3.0	2.4	2.0	1.7	1.8	1.8
I. High	..	6.8	7.0	6.4	5.7	5.0	4.5	4.2	2.3	1.7
II. Middle-high	..	4.8	5.0	4.6	4.0	3.4	3.0	2.6	2.0	1.9
III. Middle-low	..	3.8	3.6	3.0	2.2	1.5	1.2	1.1	1.8	2.1
IV. Low	..	1.4	1.2	0.8	0.6	0.4	0.3	0.3	0.5	1.0
TOTAL	..	4.3	4.6	4.0	3.4	2.8	2.5	2.2	1.8	1.7

Source: World Fertility Survey standard recode tapes.
NOTES: ALL = all women sample; EM = ever-married women. Mauritania excluded because of lack of data.
[a] Difference in mean years of education between husbands of women aged 25-29 and 45-49 years.
[b] Figure given for ages 15-19 assumes that women still in school had averaged 10 years of education.
[c] For ages 15-19, base population is women who had borne a child or had been in a union.
[d] Difference between age groups 40-44 and 25-29, converted to units of "change per 20 years": column (9) = column (7) − column (4) × 4/3.
[e] Formerly called the Ivory Coast.

Past trends in education for women are reflected in the mean number of years of education for successive five-year age groups, shown in table 110. The table is based on all women, where all were interviewed, and on ever-married women otherwise. Because of the association of early marriage with low education, the means for young women in the ever-married samples are biased downward, often producing the erroneous impression that educational attainment deteriorated after reaching a maximum for those currently in their twenties. Another factor to bear in mind is that in some countries an appreciable proportion of age group 15-19 had not yet completed schooling. Because of these problems, the following discussion focuses on women aged 25-29 and over; by ages 25-29, a large majority of the women had married and had completed schooling (see chapter III).[6]

On average, educational attainment increased, over the 20 years separating women aged 45-49 from those aged 25-29, by 1.8 years, or nearly one tenth of a year on an annual basis (column (9) of table 110). Countries with unusually rapid growth in attainment include the Republic of Korea (an increment of 4.4 years); Ghana (3.7); and the Dominican Republic, Fiji, Jordan, Kenya and Venezuela (2.4-2.9). For the most part, countries that were at first the most backward educationally fell even further behind over the following decades; of the 11 countries where women aged 45-49 years average less than one-half year of schooling, only Cameroon and Tunisia exhibit increases in attainment that are above 1.8 years, the average for all countries. All of the countries ranked in the low development group (IV) had experienced, in the past, much lower-than-average growth in educational attainment for women. Except in Pakistan, these countries also had below-average rates of educational advance for men, to the extent that this can be judged by comparing the attainment of men married to women aged 25-29 and 45-49 years (column (10)). The amount of difference in attainment between successive five-year groups of women is frequently smaller for older than younger pairs of cohorts (with a lower limit for comparison of 20 years for all-women samples, 25 years in the others), which suggests that the pace of change in attainment increased over time.[7]

Literacy

In addition to the questions dealing with school attendance, WFS asked about a basic product of education: literacy. A consideration of the relationship between educational attainment and literacy is important for what it indicates about the practical outcome of schooling in countries with widely differing educational systems. Knowledge of this relationship may help in interpreting the educational differentials in fertility that are examined later. It should be noted that some of the unusual patterns mentioned below (e.g., in Ghana) could be due to unidentified data problems as much as to real differences in literacy.

The WFS core questionnaire contained the question: "Can you read—say a newspaper or magazine?". In most countries, this or a similar question was asked of all respondents with fewer than six years of schooling, although other year limits were sometimes employed, as can be seen from table 111.[8] Many of the variations in question wording had to do with reading something other than a newspaper or magazine (such as a message, a letter or a book), but in a few countries, literate respondents were considered to be those who could write as well as read.[9]

Table 111 shows the percentage of women literate, by single years of education, for individual countries, regions and levels of development. Among women with five years of completed schooling, literacy is usually almost complete. Percentages below 90 are observed, however, in six countries: Benin, Cameroon, Côte d'Ivoire[10] and Indonesia, with 80-89 per cent literate; and Egypt and Ghana, with only 53 per cent literate. In Egypt, 89 per cent of women with six years of education were literate, but in Ghana, only 65 per cent were. Either the educational system in Ghana is unusually ineffective at conferring literacy, or there was confusion in the questioning or coding of literacy or educational attainment, or perhaps the amount of time spent in school during a year was not as great as in other countries.[11]

At the other end of the educational range shown in table 111, most women with zero years of completed schooling were unable to read—the median proportion literate is only 4 per cent (mean = 8 per cent). Yet, in several countries, substantial percentages of uneducated women claimed to be literate, up to 27 per cent in the Republic of Korea. In Indonesia, 21 per cent of those with zero and 79 per cent of those with one year of education were reported as literate, the latter being the highest percentage for the WFS countries. Adult literacy classes may help explain the unusually high literacy levels for women with little or no formal education in Indonesia and some other countries. The broader social context also appears to be important, since uneducated women in the more economically advanced countries have higher average levels of literacy than those in the lower development groups. In countries where most people have attended school, those without formal education have greater opportunity for informal instruction by educated friends and relatives. There may also be considerable social pressure to learn to read in societies where most others already can do so, and where an increasingly modern labour market requires literate workers. This same social pressure might also make women reluctant to admit to the interviewer that they cannot read; more objective methods of measurement would be needed to tell whether literacy has been overstated (or understated).

B. PRELIMINARY ANALYSIS

Fertility

Completed and recent fertility levels according to respondent's education

This section presents two education-specific measures of recent fertility levels: the total fertility rate (TFR) and the total marital fertility rate for the first 25 years of marriage (TMFR). Both measures summarize the level of childbearing during the five years preceding the survey. TMFRs are available for all 38 countries but because some surveys did not obtain the educational attainment of single women, TFRs are only available for 30 countries. Also shown is the mean number of children ever born to women aged 40-49 (CEB) (see table 112). Most of the discussion focuses on TFR and CEB, because, as stated later, TMFR tends to understate the size of overall fertility differentials according to education.

Comparison of the size and form of education differentials in TFR with those observed in CEB for older women indicates whether the differentials have tended to become wider or narrower over the years leading up to the survey. If both TFR and CEB are measured accurately, a comparison between them also gives information about the direction of trends in fertility levels, if it is borne

TABLE 111. PERCENTAGE OF WOMEN LITERATE, ACCORDING TO NUMBER OF YEARS OF EDUCATION, BY COUNTRY, REGION AND LEVEL OF DEVELOPMENT

Country and group	Zero	One	Two	Three	Four	Five	Six
A. Countries by level of development							
I. High							
Colombia	24	61	90	96	100	..	..
Costa Rica	23	70	88	96	98	..	..
Fiji	13	31	44	67	79	91	..
Malaysia	12	43	55	75	85	95	..
Mexico	25	71	93	98	99	99	..
Panama	11	33	73	91	95	..	..
Republic of Korea	27	47	72	73	81	90	..
Trinidad and Tobago	9	..	..	..	..	..	..
Venezuela	17	54	77	96	99	100	..
II. Middle-high							
Dominican Republic	8	38	71	93	97	..	..
Ecuador	3	39	72	93	98	100	..
Jordan	2	10	24	56	81	93	..
Paraguay	2	25	64	92	98	100	..
Peru	6	53	83	96	99	..	..
Philippines	5	28	50	75	91	..	..
Sri Lanka	8	32	60	82	94	98	..
Syrian Arab Republic	1	27	56	86	92	98	..
Thailand	22	24	53	64	..	..	..
Tunisia	1	10	13	43	65	97	..
III. Middle-low							
Cameroon	1	7	18	37	59	82	..
Côte d'Ivoire[a]	1	3	12	30	49	85	..
Egypt	1	6	10	21	34	53	89
Ghana	3	20	10	23	36	53	65
Indonesia	21	79	77	74	78	81	..
Kenya	8	19	38	65	85	94	98
Lesotho	4	56	75	92	97	99	..
Morocco	1	21	49	51	81	94	..
IV. Low							
Bangladesh	1	30	57	77	91	..	..
Benin	1	11	5	26	45	86	100
Haiti	1	45	85	91	94	100	..
Nepal	2	46	57	83	97	100	..
Pakistan	1	21	51	70	85	97	..
Senegal	3	6	35	50	51	93	99
Sudan	2	47	69	93	96	97	..
Yemen	1	----------------100----------------					..
B. Mean values for regions and development groups							
Africa[b]	2	19	30	48	64	85	..
Latin America and the Caribbean	12	49	79	94	98	100	..
Asia and Oceania[b]	10	35	54	73	87	94	..
I. High[b]	19	51	74	96	92	95	..
II. Middle-high	6	28	54	78	91	98	..
III. Middle-low	5	26	36	49	65	80	..
IV. Low[b]	2	29	51	70	85	96	..
TOTAL[b]	8	34	54	71	82	91	..

Source: World Fertility Survey standard recode tapes.
NOTE: Based on all interviewed women aged 15-49, except in Costa Rica and Panama, 20-49; and in Venezuela, 15-44. Guyana, Jamaica and Mauritania excluded because of lack of data.
[a] Formerly called the Ivory Coast.
[b] Averages excluding Trinidad and Tobago, and Yemen.

in mind that the completed fertility of women currently aged 40-49 will be slightly higher than CEB (because these women may have additional children). This trend measure does not pertain to a well-defined period, because the childbearing of older women had occurred over the 30-35 years prior to the survey and because distribution of childbearing for these women over time varies to some extent between educational groups and between countries. Nevertheless, if fertility reporting is of good quality, the TFR/CEB comparison can be expected to give a rough indication of the relative amount of trend across educational groups and across countries (see chapter I for a discussion of the biases in these fertility measures).

Even where there is reason to doubt the direction or amount of trend indicated by this comparison, it is still possible to tell whether the education differential in fertility has widened or otherwise changed over time, provided that biases in CEB or TFR affect all educational groups approximately equally. In fact, the quality of reporting is likely to be better for educated than for uneducated women, as indicated by such factors as ability to give exact birth dates of children.[12] It is unclear, however, whether this has an important effect on apparent education differentials in fertility; it is assumed here, in the absence of evidence to the contrary, that it does not.

Figure 55 serves as an introduction to cross-national ranges as well as average values of levels of recent fertility (TFR) and the nearly completed fertility of older women (CEB). The figure shows box-and-whisker plots of the fertility measures for each of four categories of respondent's education.[13] Several general observations can be drawn from figure 55. First, according to both fertility measures, women with from four to six or with seven or more years of education had substantially lower fertility, on average, than women with less education. However, the range of country values is very wide, and uneducated women in some countries had lower fertility than highly educated women in others. Within educational categories, the range between the highest and lowest values is usually on the order of from four to five children. For women with seven or more years of schooling, but not for those with less education, the values of both TFR and CEB are concentrated towards the lower end of the observed distribution. For half of the countries, TFR for the highest educational group falls in the range of 2.6 children (the lowest value, observed in Colombia and Venezuela) to 3.4 children (the median); and for CEB, the lower half of the values falls in the range from 3.1 to 4.0 children.

Figure 55. **Mean number of children ever born to women aged 40-49**[a] **and total fertility rate**[b]**: extreme values and quartiles for all countries with data available, by respondent's education**

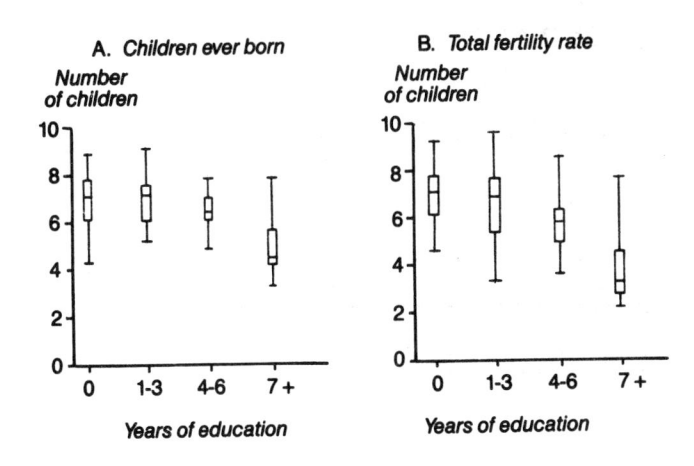

Source: Table 112.
NOTE: Each bar is based on countries for which a value is shown in table 112 for the relevant educational category. Combined and missing categories are excluded.
[a] Children ever born for ever-married or all women as in table 112.
[b] Total fertility rate for five years preceding the survey.

Figure 55 also shows that the fertility differences between educational categories tend to be larger for recent than for cumulative fertility—the difference between the highest and lowest educational categories amounts to 2.3 children for CEB and 3.0 children for TFR. The larger differential for TFR is due chiefly to lower values of TFR than of CEB for the two higher educational categories; the median TFR is nearly the same as the median CEB for women with no education, pointing to a more rapid fertility decline, on average, for educated than for uneducated women.[14]

Figure 56 compares differentials in TFR to those in CEB for countries grouped by region, level of development and strength of family planning programme effort. The figure is restricted to the 25 countries for which TFRs are available by education and for which sample size was sufficient to show CEB for all four educational categories. In Africa, only five sub-Saharan countries are included in the figure; averages based on all countries are shown in table 112. The discussion is based on both the figure and the table. Numbers mentioned in the text are from table 112.

In sub-Saharan Africa, education differentials in fertility tend to be small and non-monotonic, with the highest fertility occurring in the intermediate educational categories. In most cases, within each educational group, TFR exceeds the fertility levels reported by older women, except in Ghana, where the two measures are approximately equal. However, the quality of reporting is relatively weak in these countries (see chapter I), and the apparent increase in fertility is probably not genuine. Except in Cameroon, where a drop in the prevalence of pathological sterility may have produced a modest rise, fertility levels in the sub-Saharan countries have probably been approximately constant. However, other data sources for these countries are, in general, too weak to provide precise independent estimates of fertility trends. The fertility difference between the highest and lowest educational categories is somewhat larger according to TFR than according to CEB, suggesting some fertility decrease for highly educated women.

In Northern Africa, Latin America and the Caribbean, and Asia and Oceania, the education differential in fertility is typically larger and is more often monotonic than in sub-Saharan Africa; and on average the differential is widening. The mean TFR difference between the extreme educational categories is 3.1 children in Asia and Oceania and 3.6 in Latin America and the Caribbean; according to CEB, these differences are 1.8 and 2.9 children, respectively.

In Asia and Oceania, a large part of the overall difference between the zero and seven or more categories is due to the fertility contract between the two highest educational levels. Women with seven or more years of schooling average 1.9 fewer children than those with from four to six years, according to TFR, and 1.5 fewer according to CEB. In this region, the fertility of women with from one to three years of education is frequently as high as, or slightly higher than, the fertility of women with no education. This appears to be the case more often for CEB than TFR, but the latter measure is unavailable for many of the Asian countries. In Bangladesh and Indonesia, fertility is higher in both intermediate educational groups than for uneducated women; and in Thailand (for CEB), women with from zero to six years of schooling have nearly identical fertility. Such patterns are not found

TABLE 112. MEASURES OF CURRENT AND CUMULATIVE FERTILITY ACCORDING TO RESPONDENT'S EDUCATION:[a] TOTAL FERTILITY RATE FOR AGES 15-49;
TOTAL MARITAL FERTILITY RATE FOR DURATIONS 0-24; AND MEAN NUMBER OF CHILDREN EVER BORN TO WOMEN AGED 40-49

	Total fertility rate, by years of education					Total marital fertility rate, by years of education					Children ever born, by years of education				
	Zero (1)	One to three (2)	Four to six (3)	Seven or more (4)	Difference: (1) − (4) (5)	Zero (6)	One to three (7)	Four to six (8)	Seven or more (9)	Difference: (6) − (9) (10)	Zero (11)	One to three (12)	Four to six (13)	Seven or more (14)	Difference: (11) − (14) (15)

A. Country

Africa
Benin	7.4	8.5	5.8	4.3	3.1	6.8	7.2	5.9	5.3	1.5	6.2	...	(5.0)	(4.8)	1.4
Cameroon	6.4	7.0	6.8	5.2	1.2	5.5	6.2	6.3	5.2	0.3	5.2	5.1	4.9	(3.6)	1.6
Côte d'Ivoire[b]	7.4	8.0	6.4	5.8	1.6	6.6	7.1	5.7	6.8	−0.2	6.8	...	(6.8)	...	...
Egypt[c]	...	...	6.7	5.5	1.3	6.5	6.4	6.2	3.8	2.7	6.8	7.2	6.5	3.7	3.1
Ghana	6.8	6.7	6.7	5.5	1.3	6.2	5.7	6.0	5.3	0.9	6.4	6.4	7.0	5.5	0.9
Kenya	8.3	9.2	8.4	7.3	1.0	7.5	8.3	8.1	7.7	−0.2	7.6	8.4	7.8	7.8	−0.2
Lesotho	6.2	5.6	6.0	4.8	1.4	5.4	5.5	5.9	5.9	−0.5	4.9	5.0	5.2	5.2	−0.3
Mauritania[d]	...	...	...	...	...	6.9	...	6.0	...	...	5.9	6.0	...	...	...
Morocco	6.4	5.2	4.4	4.2	2.2	7.0	5.5	5.8	4.6	2.4	7.1	(7.3)	(6.3)	...	...
Senegal	7.3	(9.4)	6.3	4.5	2.8	7.0	(7.3)	6.8	(6.1)	0.9	6.9	...	(6.9)	...	...
Sudan	6.5	5.6	5.0	3.4	3.1	6.7	7.4	6.9	5.1	1.6	6.1	(6.9)	(5.8)	(3.9)	2.2
Tunisia[c]	...	...	...	...	...	7.3	5.9	6.0	3.9	3.4	6.8	(5.9)	6.4	(3.6)	3.2

Latin America and the Caribbean
Colombia	7.0	6.0	3.8	2.6	4.4	6.8	6.3	4.3	3.2	3.6	7.0	6.8	5.9	4.5	2.5
Costa Rica[c]	5.0	5.0	3.6	2.7	2.3	5.1	4.9	3.8	3.2	1.9	8.7	7.2	6.0	3.6	5.1
Dominican Republic	7.0	7.3	5.4	3.0	4.0	6.9	7.2	5.9	3.8	3.1	7.2	6.9	5.8	4.3	2.9
Ecuador	7.8	7.2	5.3	2.7	5.1	7.4	7.4	5.8	3.3	4.1	7.9	7.4	6.2	3.8	4.1
Guyana	6.6	7.0	5.6	4.8	1.8	(6.7)	(7.6)	5.8	5.1	1.6	7.5	6.5	6.9	5.8	1.7
Haiti	6.0	4.8	4.1	2.8	3.2	5.9	4.9	5.0	3.9	2.0	5.8	6.0	5.6	(3.5)	2.3
Jamaica	(6.2)	(5.9)	5.8	4.8	1.4	(5.6)	(4.8)	5.1	4.7	0.9	(4.4)	5.5	6.1	5.3	−0.9
Mexico	8.1	7.5	5.8	3.3	4.8	7.9	7.7	6.3	4.1	3.8	7.4	7.1	6.4	3.8	3.6
Panama[e]	7.0	6.9	5.0	3.0	4.0	6.7	6.7	5.2	3.4	3.3	7.1	7.0	5.9	4.0	3.1
Paraguay	8.2	6.6	4.6	2.9	5.3	7.7	6.6	5.0	3.3	4.4	7.4	7.2	5.4	3.1	4.3
Peru	7.3	6.8	5.1	3.3	4.0	7.6	7.1	5.6	4.2	3.4	7.4	6.6	5.8	3.9	3.5
Trinidad and Tobago	(4.6)	(3.4)	4.1	3.2	1.4	(6.1)	(2.2)	4.4	3.4	2.7	7.1	6.9	6.1	5.0	2.1
Venezuela[f]	7.0	6.4	4.6	2.6	4.4	7.4	6.6	5.1	3.6	3.8	7.9	6.9	5.3	4.0	3.9

Asia and Oceania
Bangladesh	6.1	6.4	6.7	5.0	1.1	6.1	6.3	6.9	5.9	0.2	6.9	7.0	7.6	(6.9)	0.0
Fiji[c]	...	...	...	...	...	5.0	5.1	5.2	4.6	0.4	6.9	7.1	6.1	5.6	1.3
Indonesia[c]	...	...	...	...	...	5.0	5.5	5.5	5.0	0.0	5.2	6.1	5.6	4.5	0.7
Jordan	9.3	8.6	7.0	4.9	4.4	9.7	9.3	7.7	6.2	3.5	8.9	9.0	7.2	6.2	2.7
Malaysia	5.3	5.3	4.8	3.2	2.1	6.2	6.0	5.8	4.0	2.2	6.3	6.2	5.9	3.7	2.6
Nepal[c]	...	...	...	...	...	6.0	(6.8)	(6.4)	(4.0)	2.0	5.7	(5.8)	(3.9)	(5.1)	...
Pakistan	6.5	5.4	6.1	3.1	3.4	7.0	6.2	7.0	5.1	1.9	6.9	7.4	6.5	5.2	1.8
Philippines	5.4	7.0	6.2	3.8	1.6	6.7	7.4	6.9	5.0	1.7	7.0	5.7	6.9	5.2	1.8
Republic of Korea	5.7	5.5	4.3	3.4	2.3	6.2	5.6	5.0	3.8	2.4	6.0	5.7	5.2	4.0	2.0
Sri Lanka[c]	...	...	5.6	4.1	4.7	5.6	5.3	5.3	4.3	1.3	6.4	6.0	5.8	4.4	2.0
Syrian Arab Republic	8.8	6.7	...	...	...	9.0	7.2	6.5	5.4	3.6	7.8	6.3	6.6	4.0	3.8
Thailand[c]	...	...	...	...	...	5.5	5.7	5.4	3.2	2.3	6.4	6.6	6.5	4.0	2.4
Yemen[g]	8.6	...	(5.4)	...	...	7.8	...	8.5	...	...	6.8	...	...	...	...

B. Region[h]

Africa	7.0	7.2	6.2	5.0	2.0	6.6	6.6	6.3	5.4	1.2	6.4	6.5	6.1	4.8	1.6
Latin America and the Caribbean	6.8	6.2	4.8	3.2	3.6	6.8	6.2	5.2	3.8	3.0	7.1	6.8	6.0	4.2	2.9
Asia and Oceania	7.0	6.4	5.8	3.9	3.1	6.6	6.4	6.1	4.7	1.9	6.7	6.7	6.4	4.9	1.8

224

	C. Level of development[h]														
I. High	6.2	5.9	4.8	3.4	2.8	6.3	5.8	5.1	3.9	2.4	6.9	6.6	6.0	4.5	2.4
II. Middle-high	7.7	7.2	5.6	3.5	4.2	7.3	6.9	6.0	4.3	3.0	7.3	6.9	6.3	4.2	3.1
III. Middle-low	6.9	7.0	6.4	5.5	1.4	6.2	6.3	6.2	5.5	0.7	6.2	6.5	6.2	5.0	1.2
IV. Low	6.9	6.7	5.7	3.8	3.1	6.7	6.6	6.4	5.1	1.6	6.4	6.3	6.1	4.8	1.6

	D. Strength of family planning programme effort[h]														
1. Strong	5.9	5.8	4.8	3.3	2.6	5.9	5.8	5.2	4.1	1.8	6.5	6.6	6.0	4.5	2.0
2. Moderate	7.0	6.6	5.7	4.0	3.0	6.3	5.4	5.5	3.7	2.6	6.8	6.6	6.2	4.2	2.6
3. Weak	7.5	7.2	5.9	4.4	3.1	6.9	6.7	6.2	4.7	2.2	7.1	6.9	6.5	5.1	2.0
4. Very weak/none									5.3	1.8		6.5	5.9	4.5	2.2
Total for countries with TFR available[h] (30 countries)	6.9	6.6	5.5	3.9	3.0	6.8	6.5	5.9	4.7	2.1	6.9	6.7	6.1	4.6	2.3
Total, 38 countries[h]	.	.	.	.	.	6.7	6.4	5.8	4.6	2.1	6.8	6.6	6.1	4.6	2.2

Sources: Ashurst, Balkaran and Casterline (1984); and special tabulations.

NOTE: Values enclosed in parentheses are those based on small numbers of observations: for the total fertility rate and total marital fertility rate, fertility measure based on fewer than 500 woman-years of exposure or fewer than 20 woman-years of exposure for any five-year age group under age 30 or marital duration group under 15 years; for children ever born, 10-24 cases. For children ever born, educational categories containing fewer than 10 observations are not shown or (if this would mean suppressing more than two categories) are combined with adjacent categories.

[a] Years of schooling completed.
[b] Formerly called the Ivory Coast.
[c] Children ever born based on ever married women aged 40-49, rather than on all women of these ages.
[d] Educational categories are: none; less than primary or Koranic school; primary completed; more than primary.
[e] Fertility rate at ages 15-19, used for computing the total fertility rate, is taken from the period 5-9 years before the survey.
[f] Total fertility rate refers to ages 15-44; children ever born based on ages 40-44.
[g] In Yemen, all interviewed women aged 40-49 had zero education.
[h] Averages excluding values for combined or missing categories.

Figure 56. **Average values of total fertility rate and children ever born, according to education, by region, level of development and strength of family planning programme effort**

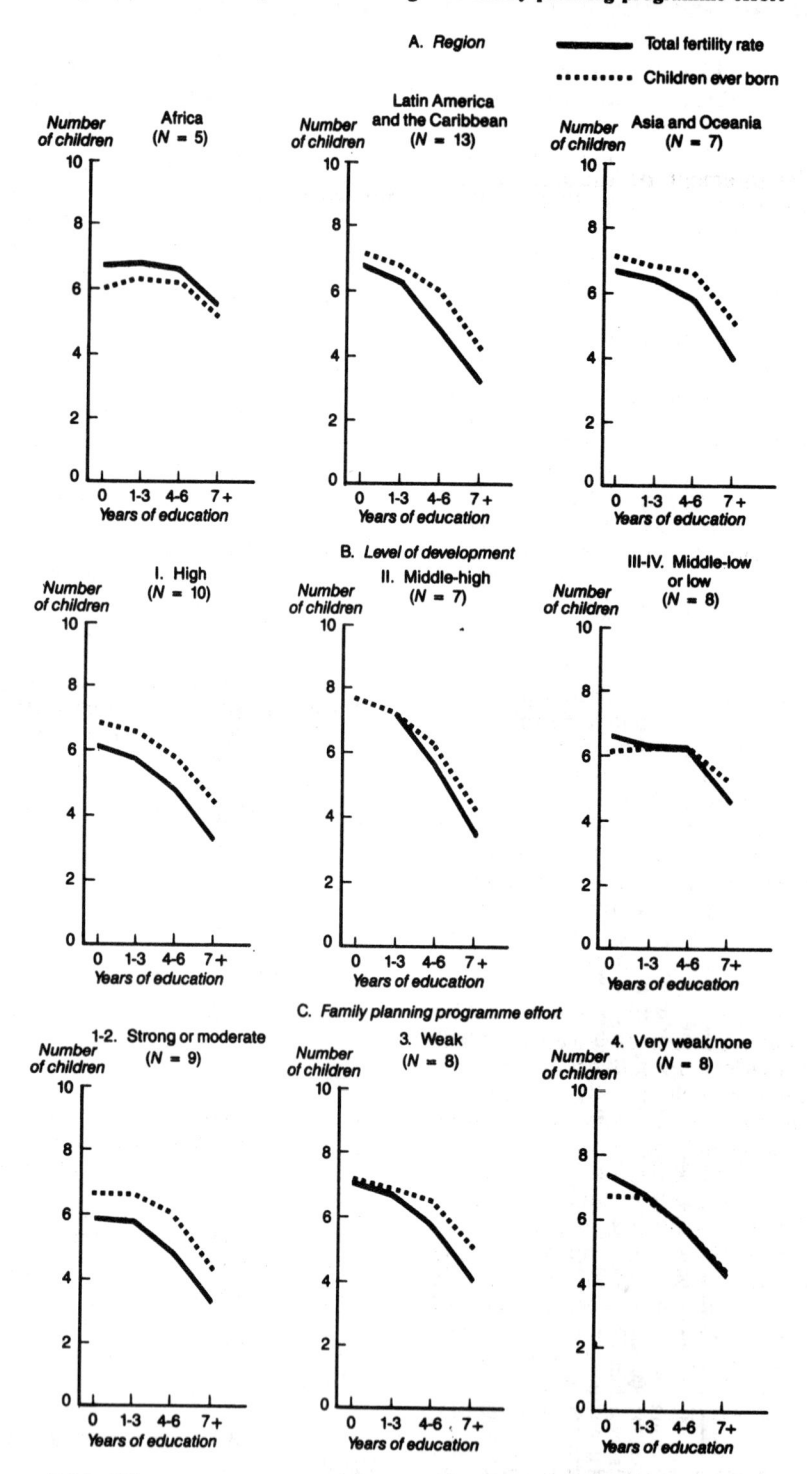

Source: Table 112.

NOTE: Based on 24 countries with total fertility rate and children ever born available for all four educational categories.

in Western Asia. Northern Africa and Western Asia together constitute a distinct subregional group characterized by large and usually monotonic fertility differentials according to education.

In Latin America and the Caribbean, the education differentials are also usually monotonic, with some exceptions evident in the Caribbean. On average, the fertility difference between the two lowest educational categories is 0.3 child for CEB, and 0.6 child for TFR, not much different from the average in Asia and Oceania. However, the differences between the two middle educational categories is distinctly larger in Latin America and the Caribbean: 0.8 child for CEB; and 1.4 for TFR. Corresponding figures for Asia and Oceania are 0.3 and 0.6 child, respectively.

Total marital fertility rates give another measure of educational differentials in recent fertility and, unlike TFRs, are available for all 38 countries. A drawback of TMFR (as calculated here) is that it suffers from biases which produce an understatement of the amount of overall fertility difference between groups, if the timing of marriage differs between the groups;[15] in effect, TMFR partially controls for the fertility effect of age-at-marriage differences between educational groups. This is doubtless the primary reason that the fertility difference between extreme educational categories averages 3.0 children as measured by TFR, but only 2.1 children (in the same 30 countries) as measured by TMFR. Even though the education differential is somewhat understated by TMFR, countries with large differentials in TFRs also show large differentials according to TMFRs. Among the countries for which TFR is unavailable by education, TMFR adds to the picture of recent fertility, showing, for instance, that Egypt and Tunisia are among the countries with very large education differentials in recent fertility, while the differential is small and non-monotonic in Fiji and Indonesia.

The nature of the education differential in fertility is expected to change with development, as discussed earlier. As hypothesized, the differentials do tend to be small and non-monotonic in the least developed countries, and they tend to be larger and monotonic in the more developed countries (figure 56 and table 112). The progression with level of development is not quite regular—the largest differentials are observed in the middle-high group (II), where uneducated women average about four children more than those with seven or more years of schooling, according to TFR. Nevertheless, there are a few countries in the upper development groups where the differential is non-monotonic, though in some cases (such as Jamaica, and Trinidad and Tobago), small sample size may be responsible for the irregular pattern observed for CEB or TFR. In the Philippines (development group II), both fertility measures indicate that women with no schooling have lower fertility than those with from one to three years, and the difference between these two groups is large (1.6 children) according to TFR. Differentials appear to be widening over time (as expected) in the lower development groups, as indicated by the larger average differentials according to TFR than CEB. In most of the countries in development groups III and IV, there is little sign that fertility has declined for the least educated women, who typically have very high levels of childbearing. In the high development group (I), fertility has clearly declined at all educational levels, and the decline has been about as large, on average, at each educational level.

The overall pattern thus provides support for the idea that differentials are relatively small before the onset of sustained fertility decline and that the differential typically widens in the early stages of decline. The hypothesized later stage of contracting differentials is seen in only a few countries, which are found (again as expected) mainly among the more developed.

Because most family planning programmes in developing countries are of recent origin, it is not clear that any relationship should be expected between current programme effort and the completed fertility of older women. Indeed, little difference is discernible for any educational group between programme effort and CEB (table 112). The pattern of fertility trends according to programme effort suggested by figure 56 is similar to that observed according to development, but weaker. Recent fertility (TFR) is lower within each educational group for the countries with stronger programmes, and the average education differential in fertility is also about 0.5 child smaller in the countries with a moderate or strong programme than in the countries with very weak or no programme effort. It is difficult to say, however, whether it is the family planning programme which is responsible for these contrasts or the associated effects of development and other factors.

One further consideration is that differences in child survival between educational groups have the effect, in most cases, of moderating differentials by education in numbers of children surviving. As is shown in table 113, on average, 79 per cent of the children born to uneducated women had survived to the interview, as opposed to 91 per cent for women with seven or more years of education. Thus, the contrast in number of living children between women with no schooling and those with seven or more years of schooling is about one child, on average, for women aged 40-49, compared with approximately two children ever born (table 112). The education differential in child survival is, furthermore, largest in absolute terms in those groups of countries where mortality levels are highest—the African region and the lower development groups, which also have relatively small differentials for children ever born. The net effect is that in some of the least economically advanced countries, and particularly in tropical Africa, even women with seven or more years

TABLE 113. PERCENTAGE OF CHILDREN EVER BORN WHO WERE STILL ALIVE AT INTERVIEW AND MEAN NUMBER OF LIVING CHILDREN, BY RESPONDENT'S EDUCATION,[a] FOR EVER-MARRIED WOMEN AGED 40-49: AVERAGES BY REGION AND LEVEL OF DEVELOPMENT

	Zero	One to three years	Four to six years	Seven or more years
A. Percentage of children ever born who were still alive at interview				
Region				
Africa	75	81	85	89
Latin America and the Caribbean	82	86	88	93
Asia and Oceania	79	83	86	91
Level of development				
I. High	85	88	89	93
II. Middle-high	81	85	88	94
III. Middle-low	75	80	83	87
IV. Low	71	79	81	90
TOTAL	79	84	86	91
B. Mean number of living children				
Region				
Africa	4.8	5.3	5.2	4.4
Latin America and the Caribbean	6.0	6.0	5.4	4.2
Asia and Oceania	5.4	5.6	5.5	4.6
Level of development				
I. High	6.0	6.0	5.5	4.4
II. Middle-high	6.1	6.0	5.6	4.2
III. Middle-low	4.7	5.2	5.2	4.5
IV. Low	4.6	5.2	5.0	4.6
TOTAL	5.4	5.7	5.4	4.4

Source: World Fertility Survey standard recode tapes.
[a] Years of schooling completed.

of education have as many surviving children, on average, as do uneducated women.

Differential fertility according to husband's education

A smaller fertility differential according to husband's than wife's education is expected both on theoretical grounds and on the basis of earlier research, as discussed in the introduction; this expectation is, in general, borne out. On average, completed fertility (CEB) is about 1.3 child lower for women whose partner had seven or more years of schooling than for those whose partner had none; the corresponding difference according to respondent's education is about two children. However, this pattern is typical only in Africa and in Asia and Oceania. In Latin America and the Caribbean, the fertility differential is approximately the same size according to either educational variable (table 114 and figure 57).

There are also more cases in which the highest fertility occurs in the middle educational groups (usually from one to three years of schooling) when fertility is classified according to husband's education. This may even be considered the typical pattern for husband's education, as it appears in the averages for Africa and for Asia and Oceania, and to a reduced degree in the average for all countries combined. In Bangladesh, Indonesia and all of sub-Saharan Africa (including the Sudan), respondents whose husband had seven or more years of schooling reported higher mean numbers of children, or at least numbers no lower than, respondents with uneducated partners.

Countries that have relatively large fertility differentials according to respondent's education also have relatively large differentials according to husband's education—hardly surprising, in view of the high degree of association between the two variables. Apart from the generally smaller size of differentials according to husband's education, patterns according to level of development and strength of family planning programme effort are similar to those already discussed (not shown). Examination of the degree of overlap in fertility effects of the two partners' education is deferred to section C of this chapter.

Fertility preferences

Table 115 shows the mean number of children desired by ever-married women, according to education, adjusted for the effects of age differences between educational groups. Women who did not give a numerical answer to the question on desired size are excluded; education differences in the proportion giving a numerical answer are considered later, and a final part of this section compares desired family size with observed fertility levels. (For a discussion of the quality of the preference data, see chapter II of this volume).

Desired family size

Within societies, mean desired family size usually decreases steadily with increasing levels of respondent's education; such monotonic relationships are much more common for desired than for achieved fertility. Women with seven or more years of schooling desired, on average, 1.3 fewer children than women with no education.

The difference in desired fertility between the two extreme education categories averages nearly two children

TABLE 114. MEAN NUMBER OF CHILDREN EVER BORN TO EVER-MARRIED WOMEN AGED 40-49, ACCORDING TO HUSBAND'S EDUCATION,[a] BY COUNTRY AND REGION

	Zero (1)	One to three years (2)	Four to six years (3)	Seven or more years (4)	Difference: (1) − (4) (5)
Africa					
Benin	6.2	(7.4)	5.6	(6.2)	0.0
Cameroon	5.1	6.1	5.5	5.1	0.0
Côte d'Ivoire[b]	6.8	7.0	6.2	6.8	0.0
Egypt	6.9	7.2	6.9	4.6	2.3
Ghana	6.4	(6.4)	6.1	6.4	0.0
Kenya	7.4	8.2	8.1	7.8	−0.4
Lesotho	4.9	5.5	5.7	5.3	−0.4
Mauritania[c]	5.6	6.3	(8.9)	..	..
Morocco	7.2	..	6.3	(6.8)	0.4
Senegal	7.0	..	(7.7)	6.3	0.7
Sudan	5.9	6.5	7.2	6.7	−0.8
Tunisia	7.0	6.4	6.3	5.4	1.6
Latin America and the Caribbean					
Colombia	7.6	7.4	6.5	5.3	2.3
Costa Rica	8.9	8.1	6.5	4.3	4.6
Dominican Republic	7.8	7.4	6.5	4.5	3.3
Ecuador	8.4	7.7	7.2	4.5	3.9
Guyana	6.2	7.8	7.3	6.1	0.1
Haiti	6.1	6.4	5.5	4.6	1.5
Jamaica	7.2	7.4	7.0	5.2	2.0
Mexico	7.8	7.6	6.6	5.0	2.8
Panama	7.7	7.2	5.9	4.4	3.3
Paraguay	8.2	7.4	6.0	3.9	4.3
Peru	7.6	7.6	6.8	4.9	2.7
Trinidad and Tobago	7.2	8.4	6.6	5.2	2.0
Venezuela	8.2	6.6	5.9	4.8	3.4
Asia and Oceania					
Bangladesh	6.8	7.2	7.1	7.6	−0.8
Fiji	6.9	6.7	6.3	6.1	0.8
Indonesia	5.0	5.6	5.7	5.5	−0.5
Jordan	8.8	9.3	9.0	7.5	1.3
Malaysia	6.1	6.8	6.3	5.0	1.1
Nepal	5.7	(5.9)	5.2	5.2	0.5
Pakistan	7.0	6.9	6.8	6.6	0.4
Philippines	7.4	7.7	7.1	6.1	1.3
Republic of Korea	6.3	6.5	5.5	4.7	1.6
Sri Lanka	6.5	6.0	6.0	5.2	1.3
Syrian Arab Republic	7.9	7.5	7.7	6.1	1.8
Thailand	6.6	6.6	6.6	5.2	1.4
Yemen	6.9	..	7.3	..	..
Africa	6.4	6.7	6.5	6.1	0.3
Latin America and the Caribbean	7.6	7.4	6.5	4.8	2.8
Asia and Oceania	6.8	6.7	6.7	5.9	0.9
TOTAL	6.9	7.0	6.6	5.6	1.3

Source: World Fertility Survey standard recode tapes.
NOTE: Values for cells containing 10-24 cases are shown in parentheses. Values for cells containing fewer than 10 cases are not shown and were excluded from computation of averages.
[a] Years of schooling completed.
[b] Formerly called the Ivory Coast.
[c] Educational categories are: none; less than primary or Koranic school; primary completed; more than primary.

in Africa, and about one child in the other two major regions. This also represents a difference from the patterns observed for fertility, since education differentials in fertility are smallest in Africa and are distinctly larger in Latin America and the Caribbean than in Asia and Oceania. Particularly large differences of from 2.0 to 3.5 children desired between the extreme educational

Figure 57. **Mean number of children ever born to ever-married women aged 40-49 years, by husband's and respondent's education: averages by region**

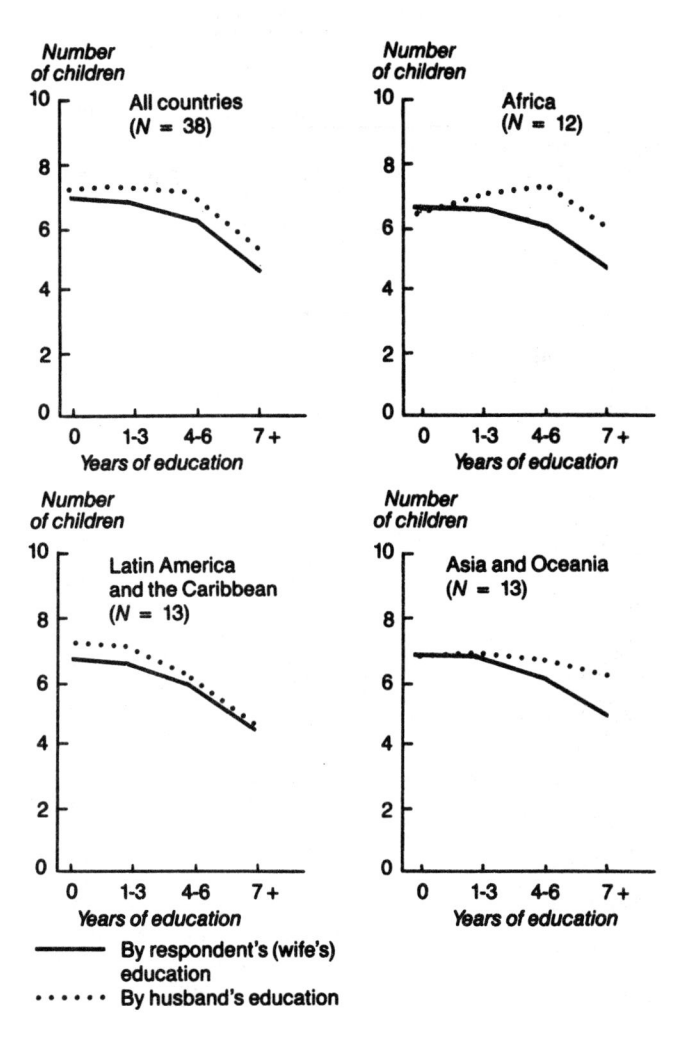

[Figure 57: Four line charts showing number of children (0-10) vs years of education (0, 1-3, 4-6, 7+) for: All countries (N=38), Africa (N=12), Latin America and the Caribbean (N=13), Asia and Oceania (N=13). Each chart has two lines: solid = By respondent's (wife's) education; dotted = By husband's education.]

Sources: Table 114 and World Fertility Survey standard recode tapes.

groups were found in four countries of sub-Saharan Africa (Benin, Côte d'Ivoire, Mauritania and Senegal), two Western Asian countries (Jordan and the Syrian Arab Republic) and only one country (Costa Rica) in Latin America. Especially small differentials, 0.5 child or less, appear in several Caribbean countries (Guyana,[16] Haiti, Trinidad and Tobago) and in Bangladesh, Fiji and Indonesia. As might be supposed from the regional patterns already mentioned, there is only a weak association at the country level between the size of differentials in desired family size and those in actual fertility.[17]

Figure 58 shows the range and distribution of values of desired family size for each educational category. The sub-Saharan countries, which were noted in chapter II as having distinctively high fertility desires, are shown separately.[18] It can be seen that sub-Saharan women tend to have high fertility desires within each educational category. Even relatively highly educated women in these

TABLE 115. MEAN DESIRED FAMILY SIZE FOR EVER-MARRIED WOMEN AGED 15-49, ACCORDING TO RESPONDENT'S EDUCATION,[a] BY COUNTRY AND AVERAGES BY REGION AND LEVEL OF DEVELOPMENT

	Zero (1)	One to three years (2)	Four to six years (3)	Seven or more years (4)	Difference: (1) − (4) (5)
A. Country					
Africa					
Benin[b]	7.7	6.5	5.6	5.1	2.6
Cameroon[c]	8.1	8.4	8.2	6.4	1.7
Côte d'Ivoire[d]	8.6	8.2	7.5	6.3	2.3
Egypt	4.5	3.9	3.5	2.6	1.9
Ghana[b]	6.6	5.8	5.9	5.2	1.4
Kenya	7.6	7.0	6.9	6.5	1.1
Lesotho	6.4	6.3	6.0	5.7	0.7
Mauritania[e]	9.0	8.6	7.1	6.0	3.0
Morocco[b]	5.1	4.0	3.9	3.4	1.7
Senegal[b]	8.5	8.3	6.7	5.0	3.5
Sudan[b]	6.5	6.1	5.4	5.0	1.5
Tunisia	4.3	4.0	3.6	3.2	1.1
Latin America and the Caribbean					
Colombia	4.7	4.2	3.8	3.5	1.2
Costa Rica	5.7	5.6	4.6	3.7	2.0
Dominican Republic	4.8	4.9	4.5	4.1	0.7
Ecuador	4.7	4.5	4.0	3.3	1.4
Guyana	5.0	4.6	4.9	4.5	0.5
Haiti	3.6	3.4	3.2	3.2	0.4
Jamaica	4.9	4.7	4.3	3.9	1.0
Mexico	5.0	4.8	4.3	3.4	1.6
Panama	4.6	4.9	4.4	3.8	0.8
Paraguay	5.9	5.8	5.0	4.1	1.8
Peru	4.1	3.9	3.7	3.4	0.7
Trinidad and Tobago	4.0	4.5	4.0	3.7	0.3
Venezuela	4.9	4.6	4.1	3.6	1.3
Asia and Oceania					
Bangladesh[b]	4.1	4.0	4.1	4.0	0.1
Fiji[c]	4.4	4.4	4.3	3.9	0.5
Indonesia	4.1	4.3	4.1	4.0	0.1
Jordan	7.2	6.3	5.9	4.7	2.5
Malaysia	4.6	4.4	4.3	3.9	0.7
Nepal	3.9	3.7	3.6	3.1	0.8
Pakistan[c]	4.2	3.7	3.6	3.3	0.9
Philippines	5.4	4.9	4.6	3.9	1.5
Republic of Korea	3.6	3.5	3.2	2.8	0.8
Sri Lanka	4.2	4.0	3.9	3.3	0.9
Syrian Arab Republic	7.0	4.7	4.7	3.9	3.1
Thailand	3.9	3.9	3.7	3.2	0.7
Yemen[b]	5.4	..	4.5	..	..
B. Averages by region and level of development					
Africa	6.9	6.4	5.9	5.0	1.9
Sub-Sahara[f]	7.7	7.2	6.6	5.7	2.0
Other	4.7	4.0	3.7	3.1	1.6
Latin America and the Caribbean	4.8	4.7	4.2	3.7	1.1
Asia and Oceania	5.4	4.3	4.2	4.0	1.4
I. High	4.7	4.6	4.2	3.7	1.0
II. Middle-high	5.2	4.7	4.3	3.7	1.5
III. Middle-low	6.4	6.0	5.8	5.0	1.4
IV. Low	5.9	5.5	4.9	4.3	1.6
Excluding Sub-Saharan Africa[f]					
III. Middle-low	4.6	4.1	3.8	3.4	1.2
IV. Low	4.2	3.7	3.6	3.4	0.8
TOTAL	5.4	5.1	4.7	4.1	1.3

Source: World Fertility Survey standard recode tapes.

NOTES: Means are adjusted for the effects of age differences between educational groups. Desired size not shown for cells containing fewer than 10 observations. Averages exclude values for such cells.

[a] Years of schooling completed.

[NOTES continued overleaf]

[b] Non-numerical responses greater than 10 per cent.
[c] Desired family size questions for Pakistan, Fiji and Cameroon are non-standard (see chapter II).
[d] Formerly called the Ivory Coast.
[e] Education categories are: none; less than primary or Koranic school; primary completed; more than primary.
[f] Benin, Cameroon, Côte d'Ivoire, Ghana, Kenya, Lesotho, Mauritania, Senegal, Sudan.

countries wanted between 5.0 and 6.5 children, while those with no schooling said they wanted from 6.5 to 9.0 children, on average. The only other subregion to show distinctly above-average desired fertility is Western Asia. The lower educational groups in Jordan and the Syrian Arab Republic report desired family sizes within the range seen in the sub-Saharan countries. Apart from these two cases, there is no overlap between the values reported in sub-Saharan Africa and those seen elsewhere.

Figure 58. **Mean desired family size,[a] by respondent's education, for sub-Saharan Africa and for other regions combined**

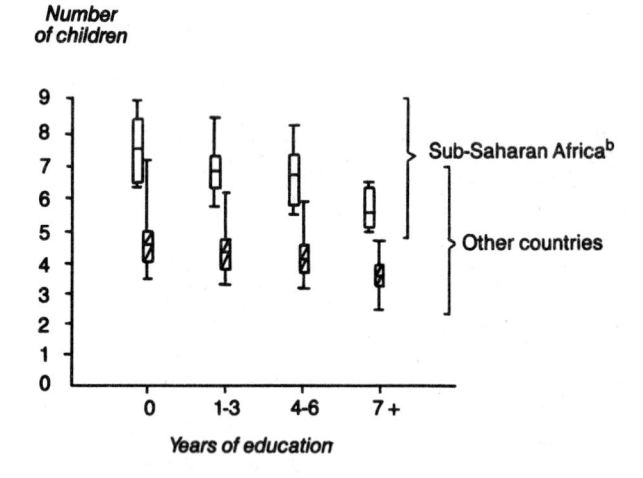

Source: Table 115.
[a] Mean number desired for ever-married women aged 15-49, adjusted for age differences between educational groups within each country.
[b] Including northern part of the Sudan.

In the countries with lower fertility desires, the desired number of children is still well above replacement level fertility, even for highly educated women. The average number of children desired by women with seven or more years of schooling is 4.1 for all countries considered together and only in Egypt and the Republic of Korea is it below 3.0 children.

The desired family sizes reported by uneducated women are more variable across countries as well as higher in average value than those reported by better-educated women (see figure 58): the standard deviation of country values is 1.6 for the lowest educational group; 1.5 for women with from one to three years of schooling; 1.3 for those with from four to six years, and 1.0 for those with seven or more years. A related observation from table 115 is that large differences in desired family size between the extreme educational categories tend to occur in the countries where uneducated women reported very high desired family sizes: the squared correlation, r^2, between columns (1) and (5) of table 115 is 0.6.[19]

Reasons were discussed earlier for expecting lower desired family size in more highly developed countries and in those with stronger family planning programme effort. Simple averaging of the country data according to level of development or family planning programme effort bears out these expectations, but a closer look shows that the relationship between development levels and desired family size is due entirely to the sub-Saharan countries. Desired family size in the least developed countries in Latin America and the Caribbean and in Asia and Oceania is no higher, on average, than in other countries outside of sub-Saharan Africa (table 115)—if anything, it is slightly lower, within each educational group. Although few would question that norms favouring high fertility will eventually be undermined by socio-economic development, current variations among developing countries in the desired family size appear to have less to do with their current levels of development than with cultural factors, as represented by regional similarities. Whatever factors tend to make desired family size higher in some countries than in others influence all educational levels similarly.

Non-numerical responses to the "desired size" question

Chapter II shows that in a number of countries, particularly those in sub-Saharan Africa, a large proportion of women did not report a desired number of children, giving instead responses such as: "It is up to God"; "As many as come"; or "I don't know". Table 116 shows, for 10 countries with high levels of non-numerical responses, that this type of answer is strongly linked to education.[20] Even the attainment of from one to three years of schooling cuts the average percentage giving non-numerical answers by eight percentage points, and only in Côte d'Ivoire, Kenya and Mauritania was the proportion of non-numerical answers for those with seven or more years of schooling above 10 per cent.

TABLE 116. PERCENTAGE OF EVER-MARRIED WOMEN AGED 15-49 WHO GAVE A NON-NUMERICAL RESPONSE TO QUESTION ON DESIRED FAMILY SIZE, BY RESPONDENT'S EDUCATION,[a] SELECTED COUNTRIES

Country	Zero	One to three years	Four to six years	Seven or more years
Bangladesh	35	26	27	6
Benin	35	24	15	7
Côte d'Ivoire[b]	27	15	14	11
Ghana	17	6	4	0
Kenya	23	19	16	11
Mauritania[c]	34	32	39	21
Morocco	19	7	2	4
Senegal	30	31	23	8
Sudan	31	12	6	6
Yemen	44	----22----		
TOTAL (EXCLUDING YEMEN)	27	19	16	8

Source: World Fertility Survey standard recode tapes.
NOTE: Percentages are adjusted for effects of age differences between education groups.
[a] Years of schooling completed.
[b] Formerly called the Ivory Coast.
[c] Educational categories are: none; less than primary or Koranic school; primary completed; more than primary.

Thus, educated women are both more likely to have an idea of the specific number of children desired, and more likely, when they give a number, to specify a small or moderate family size. It should be noted that in most of the countries where a large number of uneducated women gave non-numerical responses, many of those who gave a numerical answer mentioned a number that was higher than the aggregate fertility level.

Unwanted fertility

For older women, the lifetime incidence of unwanted childbearing can be studied by examining the proportion of women who had exceeded the desired family size. This measure may understate the amount of unwanted fertility, because some women are probably reluctant to report a desired family size smaller than the number of children they have (see chapter II). However, many women in developing countries did state that they would have preferred fewer children. (Other types of bias are also possible; see chapter II.)

Table 117 shows, for countries grouped by region and level of development, education differentials in the percentage of women for whom the number of living children exceeded the number desired. All figures are based on ever-married women aged 40-49. Averages by level of development are shown with and without the sub-Saharan countries.

TABLE 117. PERCENTAGE OF EVER-MARRIED WOMEN AGED 40-49 WITH MORE LIVING CHILDREN THAN THE NUMBER DESIRED, BY RESPONDENT'S EDUCATION:[a] AVERAGES BY REGION AND LEVEL OF DEVELOPMENT

	Zero	One to three years	Four to six years	Seven or more years
Region				
African	14	27	25	16
Sub-Sahara[b]	6	9	15	15
Other	38	62	51	28
Latin America and the Caribbean	39	36	36	26
Asia and Oceania	29	40	41	36
Level of development				
I. High	41	38	38	29
II. Middle-high	34	42	39	28
III. Middle-low	14	25	21	19
IV. Low	17	30	37	35
Low and middle-low, except Sub-Saharan Africa[b]	26	45	44	39
TOTAL	28	35	35	28
Total excluding sub-Saharan Africa	34	41	40	31

Source: World Fertility Survey standard recode tapes.
[a] Years of schooling completed.
[b] Benin, Cameroon, Côte d'Ivoire, Ghana, Kenya, Lesotho, Mauritania, Senegal, Sudan. (Côte d'Ivoire was formerly called the Ivory Coast.)

Substantial proportions of older women in each educational category—on average, between 27 and 35 per cent—had more living children than the desired number. The highest proportions are observed in the middle educational categories. When only the countries outside sub-Saharan Africa are considered, the average is higher: between 31 per cent for women with seven or more years of schooling and 41 per cent for those with from one to three years.

In sub-Saharan Africa, an average of only 6 per cent of uneducated women, and 15 per cent of those with four or more years of schooling, reported desired family sizes that were smaller than the number of living children. These relatively low percentages are mainly a consequence of the very high desired family size in sub-Saharan Africa, although it is also true that uneducated (but not highly educated) women in this region had smaller families (4.6 surviving children, on average) than uneducated women in other regions (5.4 in Asia and Oceania, 6.0 in Latin America and the Caribbean).

There is a progression with development level in the type of relationship observed between education and the prevalence of excess fertility among older women: in the least developed countries, the proportion with more children than desired tends to increase with education; in the middle development groups, the highest proportions occur in the middle educational group, with both uneducated and highly educated women showing distinctly lower values; and in the most developed countries, the proportions typically decrease with education. Even in the more economically advanced countries, nearly 30 per cent of women with seven or more years of schooling reported having more than the desired number of children. If these patterns by development can be taken to indicate transitions that frequently occur within countries over time, they suggest that one reason that the fertility transition often begins with the higher socio-economic groups is that they experience higher levels of unwanted fertility in the period immediately preceding the beginning of the transition (see Easterlin, 1983).[21]

The patterns by development level shown in table 117, coupled with the earlier consideration of fertility trends, permit some inferences about the probable evolution of education differences in unwanted fertility. The education differential in fertility had in most cases increased in the years leading up to the survey, due to lesser fertility decline for uneducated than for educated women, while there is no reason to suppose that the education differential in desired fertility had widened. (The average education differential in desired fertility for women of all ages, shown in table 115, is in fact slightly smaller than the corresponding differential for the older women.) This suggests that more and more countries will come to show the pattern already evident among older women in the more developed countries, of decreasing prevalence of unwanted fertility with increasing education. In addition, since in many developing countries the fertility of uneducated women has apparently not declined appreciably, while the risk of child death has fallen, the effective supply of surviving children has probably increased for uneducated women.

Several WFS-based studies have directly examined differentials in recent unwanted fertility and current exposure to risk of unwanted births. Westoff and Pebley (1981) found that the current risk of unwanted fertility, measured by the proportion of women who wanted no more children but were not using contraception, is greater for women with little or no education than for those with more schooling in all countries studied (see also the main reports for individual surveys). Although this has been studied in fewer countries (Westoff, 1981; Blanc, 1982; Lightbourne, 1984), the percentage of recent births that were unwanted and the projected mean number of unwanted births, based on recent rates, in most cases decrease with education. Furthermore, in most countries studied, the difference in mean number of unwanted births between the highest and lowest educational categories was larger for recent fertility than for the cumulative childbearing of women first married 20 years or more before the survey (Westoff, 1981; Blanc, 1982).

In summary, it can be said that education is everywhere negatively related to the average number of children desired; and in countries where high percentages of women did not report a number desired, education is strongly positively related to the proportion willing to state a number desired. The largest education differentials in desired family size do not tend, to any marked degree, to occur in the countries with the largest education differentials in fertility. Large differentials do tend to appear in countries where uneducated women reported unusually large numbers of children desired, as in sub-Saharan Africa, Jordan and the Syrian Arab Republic. Furthermore, women in the sub-Saharan countries reported higher desired numbers of children than women in other regions. This regional contrast in preferred family size is greater than the contrast according to development level. In fact, if the sub-Saharan countries are removed from the averages, there is no discernible relationship between level of development and mean desired family size, in any educational category.

Lastly, with respect to unwanted fertility, substantial proportions of older women have more living children than the number desired—roughly between 30 to 40 per cent, on average, depending upon the educational level, in the countries outside sub-Saharan Africa. In sub-Saharan Africa, the percentage was much smaller. The relationship between education and the proportion with more children than desired tends to be positive in the least developed countries and negative in the most developed. Differentials in the level of unwanted fertility are evolving over time, towards a situation in which uneducated women in most developing countries will experience higher levels of unwanted childbearing than more educated women.

Age at marriage

The chief significance of marriage, considered as a determinant of fertility, is that it defines, at least approximately, periods of exposure to the risk of pregnancy. Fertility analysts commonly distinguish three aspects of marriage: its universality, or the proportion who ever marry; its timing among those who marry; and the amount of the potential reproductive period spent after marital disruption and before remarriage. Marital disruption has been shown to be a minor determinant of fertility levels and of education differentials in fertility in almost all developing countries (see Singh, Casterline and Cleland, 1985), and it is not considered here.

In most but not all cases, the proportion who marry is, like marital disruption, a negligible factor in generating education differentials in fertility. Table 118 shows the average percentage of women who remained single to the end of the reproductive years for the three major regions; information was available for 29 countries.[22] In the countries of Africa and Asia and Oceania, only 1-3 per cent of women remained single, on average, regardless of educational level. Cameroon was the only country in these regions to show a substantial variation by education—defined here as a difference of at least five percentage points in the proportion remaining single between any two educational groups. Since the pattern in Cameroon is irregular and based on a small number of women, it can be concluded that there is no firm evidence that education has had more than a trivial impact on chances of ever marrying in any of the countries of Africa and Asia and Oceania.[23]

TABLE 118. PERCENTAGE OF WOMEN AGED 40-49 NEVER MARRIED, ACCORDING TO RESPONDENT'S EDUCATION,[a] BY REGIONS AND FOR SELECTED COUNTRIES

	Women never married, by education[a]			
	Zero	One to three years	Four to six years	Seven or more years
Africa (N = 9)	1	2	3	3
Latin America and the Caribbean (N = 13)	3	4	4	8
Asia and Oceania (N = 7)	3	2	2	3
Values for countries with relatively large education differentials in percentage single[b]				
Africa				
Cameroon	1	2	7	3
Latin America and the Caribbean				
Colombia	5	10	9	13
Costa Rica	8	10	8	16
Haiti	1	2	7	12
Mexico	4	3	6	15
Paraguay	5	4	5	9
Venezuela	0	1	4	10

Source: Ebanks and Singh (1984).
NOTE: Numbers are the average of the percentages single for age groups 40-44 and 45-49.
[a] Years of schooling completed.
[b] Countries shown are those for which the difference in percentage single between any two educational categories was at least five points.

In Latin America and the Caribbean, however, the average percentage single increases with education, from 3 per cent among the uneducated to 8 per cent among those with seven or more years of schooling. Six of the 13 countries in this region show differentials of five percentage points or more, with the contrast between the highest and lowest educational groups amounting to 10 points or more in Colombia, Haiti, Mexico and Venezuela. The Anglophone countries in and near the Caribbean, which counted visiting unions in the definition of marriage, do not show a sizeable differential in proportion remaining single.[24]

In contrast to the proportion who ever marry, the average age at marriage shows pronounced differences by education in all countries. The singulate mean age at marriage (SMAM) for women with seven or more years of schooling is almost four years higher, on average, than for uneducated women (table 119). Typically, SMAM increases steadily with education, with the largest difference, averaging 2.6 years, occurring between those with from four to six and those with seven or more years of education. The mean difference between the two lowest categories is only 0.2 year.

Within educational categories, there is a wide range of country values, with variability being greater for uneducated women (figure 59). Although there are some countries with quite late marriage for uneducated women, in one quarter of the countries, SMAM for this group is under 17.5 years, and in three quarters, it is below age 21.

TABLE 119. SINGULATE MEAN AGE AT MARRIAGE, ACCORDING TO RESPONDENT'S EDUCATION,[a] BY COUNTRY, REGION AND LEVEL OF DEVELOPMENT

	Singulate mean age at marriage, by respondent's education[a]				
	Zero (1)	One to three years (2)	Four to six years (3)	Seven or more years (4)	Difference: (4) – (1) (5)
A. Country					
Africa					
Benin	16.9	18.9	19.5	24.1	7.2
Cameroon	15.4	17.6	17.2	22.1	6.7
Côte d'Ivoire[b]	17.1	17.7	18.5	21.8	4.7
Ghana	17.4	18.2	19.2	20.5	3.1
Kenya	17.2	18.7	19.5	21.8	4.6
Morocco	20.3	23.6	25.1	25.9	5.6
Senegal	16.7	17.6	20.4	22.8	6.1
Sudan	21.2	21.1	22.8	24.7	3.5
Latin America and the Caribbean					
Colombia	19.5	20.2	21.1	24.7	5.2
Costa Rica	24.2	19.4	22.2	23.3	–0.9
Dominican Republic	18.0	17.4	19.4	22.7	4.7
Ecuador	19.1	20.0	20.6	24.1	5.0
Guyana	17.7	19.1	18.8	20.2	2.5
Haiti	21.5	20.9	21.0	22.6	1.1
Jamaica	..	18.3	17.7	19.1	0.8[c]
Mexico	17.4	19.4	21.7	21.9	4.5
Panama	19.1	18.6	20.2	23.1	4.0
Paraguay	18.5	20.5	21.6	23.4	4.9
Peru	21.0	20.3	21.6	25.0	4.0
Trinidad and Tobago	17.3	20.6	18.7	21.0	3.7
Venezuela	19.0	19.1	20.4	23.0	4.0
Asia and Oceania					
Bangladesh	15.0	15.1	16.5	19.5	4.5
Jordan	19.2	18.7	19.3	23.2	4.0
Malaysia	21.9	21.3	22.2	25.5	3.6
Pakistan	18.9	19.0	20.0	25.7	6.8
Philippines	24.1	21.6	22.5	25.4	1.3
Republic of Korea	21.7	21.2	22.5	24.2	2.5
Syrian Arab Republic	20.5	19.6	21.2	22.8	2.3
B. Region					
Africa	17.8	19.2	20.3	23.0	5.2
Latin America and the Caribbean	19.5[d]	19.5	20.4	22.6	3.1
Asia and Oceania	20.2	19.5	20.6	23.8	3.6
C. Level of development					
I. High	19.8[d]	19.7	20.6	22.6	2.8
II. Middle-high	20.1	19.7	20.9	23.8	3.7
III. Middle-low	17.5	19.2	19.9	22.4	4.9
IV. Low	18.4	18.8	20.0	23.2	4.8
TOTAL	19.2[d]	19.4	20.4	23.0	3.8

Sources: For Costa Rica, Guyana, Haiti, Jamaica, Panama, and Trinidad and Tobago, calculated from background tabulations for Singh, Casterline and Cleland (1985), supplied by the authors; for other countries, Ebanks and Singh (1984), tables 1 and 8.

[a] Years of schooling completed.
[b] Formerly called the Ivory Coast.
[c] Difference between columns (4) and (2).
[d] Excluding Jamaica.

At the other end of the educational scale, for women with seven or more years of schooling all of the SMAM values are greater than 19.0 (which is approximately the median value for uneducated women), and nearly three quarters of the countries have SMAM values of 22 years or more. For individual countries, the difference between extreme educational categories is rarely less than two years (this is the case in only 4 of 28 countries with information available) and amounts to four or more years in one quarter of the cases.

Figure 59. Singulate mean age at marriage, by respondent's education

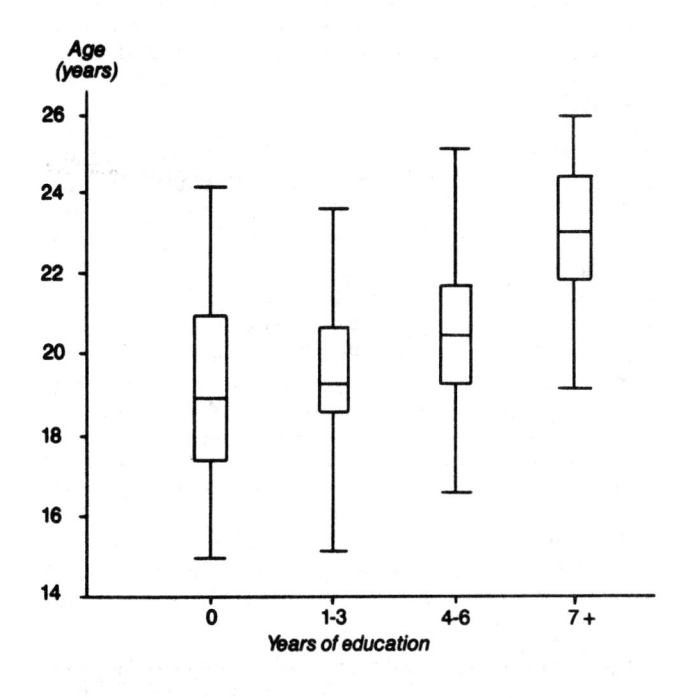

Source: Table 119.

In some cases, the marriage age for uneducated women is higher than for those with a few years of schooling. The difference is small in most countries where the pattern occurs but amounts to several years in Costa Rica and the Philippines. In Costa Rica, a related statistic—the age by which 50 per cent had married, for women currently aged 20-29 (McCarthy, 1982)—shows approximately the same average marriage age for women with no education as for those with from one to three years. The number of young women with no education is small in Costa Rica, and it is possible that SMAM gives a misleading impression for this group. In the Philippines, however, the other statistic also indicates significantly later marriage for women with no education than for those with from one to three years;[25] this undoubtedly contributes to the non-monotonic pattern of the education differential in fertility in this country, noted earlier as being unusual for a country in the middle-high development group.

In sub-Saharan Africa, the difference in SMAM between each successive pair of educational categories tends to be relatively large. The average difference between extreme educational categories is 5.2 years in Africa, 3.6 in Asia and Oceania and 3.1 in Latin America and the Caribbean. This is exactly the reverse of the ordering of regions according to the size of the education differential in fertility. A similar observation can be made about patterns according to development: SMAM differentials are largest at development levels III and IV, whereas fertility differentials are relatively small and are frequently non-monotonic in the least developed countries. However, the pattern of decreasing differentials in marriage age with increasing development is not apparent in the median age at marriage reported by women currently aged 20-29; instead, the relationship by level of development is irregular (based on statistics presented in McCarthy, 1982; and Ebanks and Singh, 1984). While the reason for the discrepant results is unclear, the lack of correspondence between these types of statistics at this level of detail dictates caution in drawing conclusions about the relationship between development and differential marriage age. The statistics based on median age also indicate a smaller difference in marriage age between extreme educational groups in Africa than that shown in table 119; correspondence is better, on average, in Latin America and the Caribbean and in Asia and Oceania.

Table 120 shows, in highly summarized form, two types of comparisons indicating trends in average age at first marriage within educational groups. The first compares the median marriage age for three cohorts of women, and the second compares the mean marriage age reported by women aged 40-49 at the interview to SMAM.[26]

Both types of comparison indicate a modest widening of the education differential in marriage age over time. The comparison based on medians shows a 3.5-year difference in typical marriage age between those with no education and those with seven or more years for women currently aged 40-49. For the 30-39 cohort, the difference is 3.9 years; and for the 20-29 cohort, it is 4.8 years. The comparison based on means shows a 3.1-year difference for older women as opposed to 3.8 years for SMAM. The median ages suggest that there was essentially no trend in age at marriage, on average, except in the highest educational group. However, as was stated in chapters I and II, recollection of marriage age was problematical in many of the countries, and trends may not always be accurately measured.[27]

Breast-feeding

Education differentials are shown in table 121 for a second major fertility determinant, mean duration of breast-feeding. The mean number of months of breast-feeding was estimated from current status data (see chapter IV) and thus refers to behaviour around the time of the surveys. Because estimates were unavailable for many of the cells due to small sample size, the averages for groups of countries, shown at the end of the table, should be treated with considerable caution.

In all countries for which the comparison can be made, breast-feeding duration decreases with increased education. The largest differences occur, in most countries, between women with from four to six years of schooling and those with seven years or more. On average, the difference in breast-feeding duration amounts to 7.5 months between the lowest and the highest educational categories. This difference is greatest, nearly nine months, in Latin America and the Caribbean, the region with the shortest average duration of breast-feeding in all educational groups. In each region, however, there are some countries with large differentials: in Egypt, Tunisia, Indonesia and Peru, the mean number of months of breast-feeding is 10-15 months greater for women with zero education than for those with seven or more years. Relatively small differences, five months or less, are seen in Lesotho, Mauritania, Fiji, Malaysia and the Syrian Arab Republic.

Figure 60 shows the inter-country range and dispersion of mean duration of breast-feeding within each educational category, by means of box-and-whisker plots arranged by region and level of development. Patterns by region and development level, described in chapter IV, tend to persist within educational categories—for instance, uneducated women in the more developed countries tend to breast-feed for a shorter period than do uneducated women in the less developed of the countries. The extremely wide inter-country variation in Asia and Oceania can be understood as being due in part to the diversity of national levels of socio-economic development. At the same time within development groups the countries with the longest breast-feeding duration tend to be in Asia: Bangladesh, Indonesia and Nepal in groups III and IV; Sri Lanka and Thailand in group II; the Republic of Korea in group I. Similarly, Yemen, one of the least developed countries, has breast-feeding behaviour more similar to that observed in the other Western Asian countries, such as Jordan and the Syrian Arab Republic, than to that seen in other countries at low levels of development.[28]

TABLE 120. SELECTED INDICATORS OF TREND IN AVERAGE AGE AT MARRIAGE, BY RESPONDENT'S EDUCATION:[a] MEAN VALUES FOR 23 COUNTRIES

	Average age at marriage, by education[a]				Difference from zero category for category:		
	Zero	One to three years	Four to six years	Seven or more years	One to three years	Four to six years	Seven or more years
Age by which 50 per cent of cohort had married:							
20-29 years at survey	17.6	18.0	19.1	22.4	0.4	1.5	4.8
30-39 years at survey	17.4	17.9	18.8	21.3	0.5	1.4	3.9
40-49 years at survey	17.5	18.1	18.9	21.0	0.6	1.4	3.5
Singulate mean age at marriage	19.3	19.5	20.4	23.1	0.2	1.1	3.8
Mean age at first marriage for ever-married women aged 40-49	18.1	18.6	19.4	21.2	0.5	1.3	3.1

Sources: McCarthy (1982); Ebanks and Singh (1984); and special tabulations.
NOTE: Based on the 23 countries for which all requisite information was available, including countries shown in table 119, except for Benin, Côte d'Ivoire, Jamaica, Morocco and Senegal. (Côte d'Ivoire was formerly called the Ivory Coast.)
[a] Years of schooling completed.

TABLE 121. MEAN DURATION OF BREAST-FEEDING, ACCORDING TO RESPONDENT'S EDUCATION,[a] BY COUNTRY, REGION AND LEVEL OF DEVELOPMENT

(Months)

	Zero (1)	One to three years (2)	Four to six years (3)	Seven or more years (4)	Difference: (1) − (4) (5)
A. Country					
Africa					
Benin	21.6	..	17.8	..	..
Cameroon	21.0	19.1	17.5	14.6	6.4
Côte d'Ivoire[b]	20.4	18.0	14.6	11.5	8.9
Egypt	21.2	19.5	16.3	10.2	11.0
Ghana	21.3	..	19.2	15.7	5.6
Kenya	19.6	17.4	15.2	12.5	7.1
Lesotho	24.0	22.2	22.0	19.9	4.1
Mauritania	17.7	17.2	15.6	15.7	2.0
Morocco	16.7	..	9.3	..	..
Senegal	21.1	..	16.8	..	..
Sudan[c]	17.3	16.1	..	..	..
Tunisia	16.8	..	8.8	6.8	10.0
Latin America and the Caribbean					
Colombia	11.9	11.4	8.3	5.3	6.6
Costa Rica	..	8.1	4.6	3.2	..
Dominican Republic	12.2	10.5	8.6	5.2	7.0
Ecuador	17.0	14.5	13.0	8.9	8.1
Guyana	..	9.2	7.7	6.6	..
Haiti	19.0	14.1	..	..	..
Jamaica	..	..	8.9	6.2	..
Mexico	12.9	10.9	8.3	3.8	9.1
Panama	..	13.0	9.2	2.4	..
Paraguay	15.7	14.6	11.4	6.1	9.6
Peru	19.3	16.6	12.0	7.0	12.3
Trinidad and Tobago	..	..	10.0	7.1	..
Venezuela	11.6	10.0	6.7	3.5	8.1
Asia and Oceania					
Bangladesh	34.4	30.4	..	..	..
Fiji	13.0	11.1	11.8	8.7	4.3
Indonesia	28.4	27.0	24.7	13.7	14.7
Jordan	13.9	13.0	10.5	7.7	6.2
Malaysia	7.6	5.7	5.7	3.8	3.8
Nepal	29.3	..	..	..	..
Pakistan	22.0	..	19.8	..	..
Philippines	18.9	17.6	14.8	9.5	9.4
Republic of Korea	21.0	17.7	18.0	13.7	7.3
Syrian Arab Republic	12.9	..	10.7	9.5	3.4
Sri Lanka	26.1	24.7	23.4	18.5	7.6
Thailand	20.9	..	20.8	..	..
Yemen	12.9	..	..	..	..
B. Region					
Africa	19.9	18.5	15.7	13.4	6.9[d]
Latin America and the Caribbean	15.0	12.1	9.1	5.4	8.7[d]
Asia and Oceania	20.1	18.4	16.0	10.6	7.1[d]
C. Level of development					
I. High	13.0	10.8	9.0	5.8	6.5[d]
II. Middle-high	17.4	15.9	13.4	8.8	8.2[d]
III. Middle-low	21.6	20.5	17.4	14.0	8.3[d]
IV. Low	21.7	19.4	17.5	..[e]	..[d]
TOTAL	18.8	15.8	13.4	9.2	7.5[d]

Sources: Balkaran and Smith (1984); Ferry and Smith (1983).

NOTE: Current status estimates based on surviving births using the life-table method. Averages for groups of countries should be regarded with caution because of the large number of missing country values, which were excluded in computing group means.

[a] Years of schooling completed.
[b] Formerly called the Ivory Coast.
[c] Northern Sudan only.
[d] Group means given in column (5) are based on available country values in column (5): countries for which breast-feeding estimates are available in both column (1) and column (4). This does not necessarily equal the difference between group averages in columns (1) and (4), which are based, in each case, on non-missing country values shown in these columns.
[e] Not shown because only one observation available (that for Mauritania).

Contraceptive use

Education differentials in contraceptive practice are generally quite large (table 122). Over all, the proportion of married women with seven or more years of education who were using contraception at the time of interview is 24 percentage points greater than for those with no education, controlling for age differences between educational groups. Even a few years of schooling usually have a marked effect on contraceptive prevalence: the mean percentage using contraception is nine points higher for women with from one to three years of education than for those with zero; the difference is five points between the two middle categories; and it is 10 points between the two highest categories. Unlike most other variables examined in this chapter, contraceptive use shows greater dispersion over countries for highly educated than for uneducated women (as indicated by the larger interquartile range shown in figure 61). For women with no education, the values are clustered towards the lower end of the range, with levels of use under 25 per cent in over three quarters of the countries. For women with seven or more years of schooling, on the other hand, the percentage is 20 or above in over three quarters of the cases and over 40 per cent in half.

Most of the countries with especially large education differentials in contraceptive practice are found in two major subregional groups: the Spanish-speaking countries of Latin America and the Caribbean (that is, excluding Guyana, Haiti, Jamaica, and Trinidad and Tobago) and in Northern Africa and Western Asia. In the former group of countries, the difference in use levels between the highest and lowest educational categories exceeds 35 percentage points in four of eight countries.[29] In the latter group, the differential is over 35 points in all cases except Yemen, where the small number of educated women precludes comparison, and the Sudan. The Philippines is the only other country to show such a large differential.

At the other extreme, in four countries—Fiji, Guyana, Lesotho and Mauritania—the percentage using contraception differs by less than 10 percentage points between women with no education and those with seven or more years. Fiji is the only case in which the level of use is lower for the better-educated women.[30] Nepal and the sub-Saharan countries (not including the Sudan) show below-average differentials because the level of use is below 20 per cent even for highly educated women; Mauritania is the extreme case, with fewer than 5 per cent of the women using contraception regardless of educational attainment. Other countries with relatively small differentials include Costa Rica, the Republic of Korea, Thailand, and Trinidad and Tobago. In Costa Rica, the educational differential in contraceptive use was once as large as in many of the other Latin American countries, according to surveys conducted in the 1960s (United Nations, 1979); and the narrowing of the differential in contraceptive use was undoubtedly a major cause, and perhaps the sole cause, of the narrowing education differential in fertility noted earlier (see Rosero B., 1981).

Figure 60. **Mean duration of breast-feeding, according to respondent's education, by region and level of development**

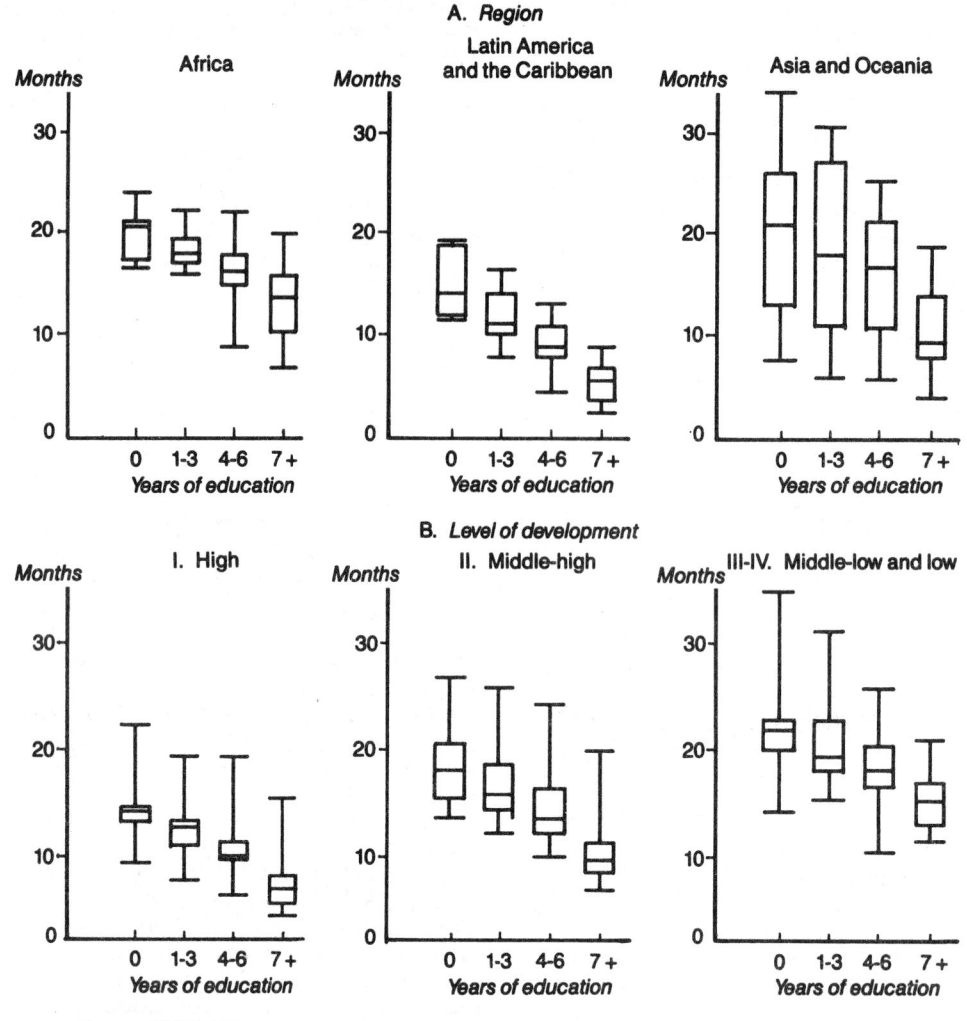

A. *Region*

B. *Level of development*

Source: Table 121.

This example shows that both differentials in contraceptive practice and the overall level of contraceptive use are capable of rapid change.

The social-diffusion, or cultural-lag, hypothesis suggests that education differentials in contraceptive use can be expected to widen at the early stages of fertility transition, because the better educated adopt birth control first. Small differentials are expected both before the transition, with use levels uniformly low, and near the end of the transition, with use levels uniformly high. To the extent that the development index divides countries according to the stage of the transition, the largest differentials might be expected to appear in the middle or upper development groups. It is less clear what relationship should be anticipated between family planning programme strength and education differentials in contraceptive practice. One hypothesis is that programmes might decrease differentials by targeting services on segments of the population who would otherwise have no access to birth control information and services. This might be more relevant to geographical than to education differentials, however. A second hypothesis is that, to the extent that programmes have an effect independent of development variables, it may be to speed up the diffusion process just described, producing first widening, later narrowing, differentials, with each stage appearing at a lower level of development than would otherwise have occurred. If large differentials during the transition are associated with especially rapid change (a point on which evidence is not clear), then active programmes might even lead to unusually large differentials at some stage of the transition.

In fact, education differentials in contraceptive use according to level of development are, on average, approximately as expected from the social-diffusion hypothesis: differentials are largest in the middle-high development category; and, within educational groups, the level of contraceptive use generally increases from one development level to the next. A similar type of relationship is seen when countries are grouped by family planning programme effort, though the contrasts are not as strong as between development groups.

Figure 62 shows average percentages using contraception for different levels of family planning programme effort within development groups. Within each level of development, the very weak/none and weak family planning groups were collapsed to "weaker" and the moderate and strong groups were combined to form the

TABLE 122. PERCENTAGE OF CURRENTLY MARRIED WOMEN AGED 15-49 CURRENTLY USING CONTRACEPTION, ACCORDING TO RESPONDENT'S EDUCATION,[a] BY COUNTRY, REGION, LEVEL OF DEVELOPMENT AND STRENGTH OF FAMILY PLANNING PROGRAMME EFFORT

	Percentage using contraception, by respondent's education[a]				
	Zero (1)	One to three years (2)	Four to six years (3)	Seven or more years (4)	Difference: (4) − (1) (5)
A. *Country*					
Africa					
Benin	8	15	12	19	11
Cameroon	0	3	5	17	17
Côte d'Ivoire[b]	2	4	6	17	15
Egypt	17	25	32	53	36
Ghana	5	12	11	17	12
Kenya	4	5	9	15	11
Lesotho	2	4	5	7	5
Mauritania[c]	0	1	4	2	2
Morocco	16	37	53	56	40
Senegal	3	5	8	20	17
Sudan	2	11	12	35	33
Tunisia	25	46	50	62	37
Latin America and the Caribbean					
Colombia	23	34	51	65	42
Costa Rica	56	60	66	68	12
Dominican Republic	17	26	37	50	33
Ecuador	10	19	37	55	45
Guyana	30	32	30	33	3
Haiti	13	28	36	39	26
Jamaica	17	27	31	41	24
Mexico	13	23	38	56	43
Panama	37	42	54	62	25
Paraguay	21	25	39	54	33
Peru	11	25	43	54	43
Trinidad and Tobago	38	46	45	53	15
Venezuela	29	39	53	60	31
Asia and Oceania					
Bangladesh	6	11	13	30	24
Fiji	46	47	39	39	−7
Indonesia	22	30	33	43	21
Jordan	10	28	36	48	38
Malaysia	22	32	39	48	26
Nepal	2	7	11	18	16
Pakistan	4	11	10	22	18
Philippines	11	22	34	48	37
Republic of Korea	28	30	35	41	13
Sri Lanka	19	26	33	42	23
Syrian Arab Republic	9	37	37	46	37
Thailand	28	32	34	42	14
Yemen	1	..	9	..	..
B. *Region*					
Africa	7	14	17	27	20
Latin America and the Caribbean	24	33	43	53	29
Asia and Oceania	16	26	28	39	23
C. *Level of development*					
I. High	31	38	44	51	20
II. Middle-high	16	29	38	50	34
III. Middle-low	8	15	19	28	20
IV. Low	4	11	13	23	19
D. *Strength of family planning programme effort*					
1. Strong	29	36	42	51	22
2. Moderate	24	33	38	50	26
3. Weak	13	21	29	38	25
4. Very weak/none	6	14	18	27	21
TOTAL	16	25	30	40	24

Source: World Fertility Survey standard recode tapes.
NOTE: Percentages are adjusted for the effects of age differences between education groups. Percentage not shown for cells containing fewer than 10 observations. Averages exclude values for such cells.
[a] Years of schooling completed.
[b] Formerly called the Ivory Coast.
[c] Educational categories are: none; less than primary or Koranic school; primary complete; more than primary.

Figure 61. **Percentage currently using contraception,[a] by respondent's education**

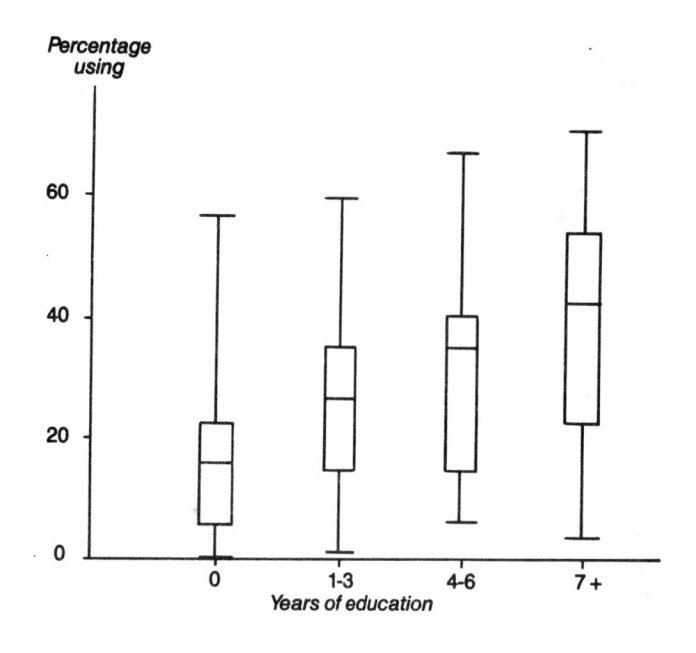

Source: Table 122.
[a] Percentages for currently married women aged 15-49, adjusted for age differences between educational groups.

"stronger" category. In development group III, countries with stronger family planning programmes have higher average levels of contraceptive practice in all educational categories, with the difference being greatest for highly educated women. Differences in use levels are large in the middle-low development group but are smaller in the upper two groups. At the upper development levels, there is some tendency for the level of contraceptive practice to be greater among uneducated women in the countries with stronger programmes, but the effect is not strong; for highly educated women, average use levels are about the same in the two family planning groups. Concerning the size of education differentials, the pattern over the four development groups gives some support to the second hypothesis mentioned above, that by speeding the process of diffusion of family planning, programme activities tend at first to lead to increased education differentials (in countries beginning the transition) and later to narrowing differentials—the same pattern observed according to development indicators. There is also some support, strongest for countries in the middle-low development group, for the idea that programmes produce these effects earlier than would otherwise have occurred through development alone. However, a need for caution and further research is indicated by the consideration that this analysis is based on a small number of countries in each of the eight groups distinguished in figure 62, that the categories employed are crude; and that the possible effects of other factors, such as region, have not been controlled.

Figure 62. Percentage using contraception, by respondent's education: averages by strength of family planning programme effort within development groups

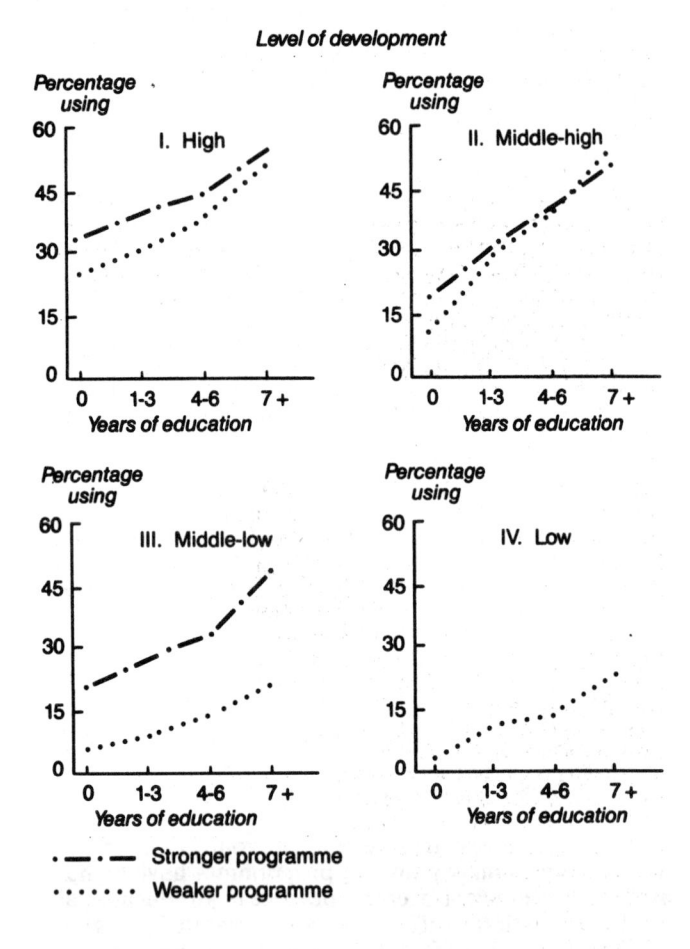

Source: Table 122.

C. MULTIVARIATE ANALYSIS

This section examines the extent to which education differentials in fertility and related variables persist when other socio-economic characteristics of the couple are controlled statistically. These characteristics are the same as those used as controls in chapter VII.[31]

Effects of respondent's education are estimated below for a number of related statistical models in which other variables are introduced in a predetermined order: first demographic controls; then residence; then spouse's education; then respondent's and husband's occupation. Of special interest are the estimated effects of education with residence controlled, because, in a causal or temporal ordering of variables, residence is prior to education. Education differentials examined without control for residence may overstate the effect that should be attributed to education itself, because such analyses fail to take into account the fact that educational attainment is influenced by residence, especially childhood residence.[32] Occupation, on the other hand, is heavily conditioned by education; and examination of education differentials before and after control for occupation may help clarify the paths through which education influences fertility. Although no clear causal ordering can be specified between husband's and wife's education, the multivariate analysis can show whether each spouse's education has an influence on fertility that is distinguishable from effects of the partner's schooling.

The dependent variables examined in the multivariate analysis are marital fertility (children ever born/duration of marriage, *CEB/D*, measured as births per 1,000 woman-years since marriage), mean number of children desired and current use of contraception. Table 123 presents an overview of the regression specifications for which results are discussed below. Ordinary least-squares regression is employed to estimate the model coefficients; and with one exception, discussed later, only linear additive effects (not interaction effects) are considered. Even with interaction effects omitted, the combination of three dependent variables and several sets of control variables yields a large number of coefficients, and only a summary of the results is given here. The tables in the text focus on average education effects for regions and development groups. Within-group variability is summarized graphically. Effects of husband's education are discussed only in relation to marital fertility, although husband's education is also included as a control variable in the analysis of contraceptive practice and desired family size.

A few other aspects of the analysis must be mentioned before turning to the results. Whereas four educational categories were distinguished in section A of this chapter, for the regression analysis the "seven or more" category is divided into two: 7-9 years of education; and 10 or more years. In most countries, each of the categories of respondent's education contains at least 50 ever-married women.[33] Because few women in the Yemen survey had any education (three of the five educational categories contain fewer than 10 respondents), this country was excluded from the multivariate analysis. The following discussion is therefore based on 37 countries.

Marital fertility

The measure of fertility used in the regression analysis, *CEB/D*, is measured as births per 1,000 woman-years of marriage, a measure that is similar to a general marital fertility rate. As explained in chapter VII and, in more detail, in the annex to part two, *CEB/D* is the number of children ever born divided by duration since first marriage, converted to a basis of 1,000 woman-years. The analysis is based on women who had married at least three years prior to the survey and who were aged 15-49 at the time of interview.

Selected results of four related regression analyses (models 1-4) are shown in table 124. The left-hand portion of the table shows the difference in *CEB/D* between women with no education (the reference category) and those with 1-3, 4-6, 7-9 and 10+ years of schooling. In the right-hand part of the table, similar results are given for marital fertility rates classified by husband's education, expressed in relation to the reference category of husbands with zero schooling completed (model 3 only). For example, it can be seen from the results for model 1, which includes controls for demographic variables only,

TABLE 123. DESCRIPTION OF REGRESSION MODELS

Model	Base population	Dependent variable	Independent variables
1	First married three or more years before survey, currently aged 15-19[a]	CEB/D[b]	Respondent's education, duration since first marriage, duration squared and age at first marriage
2	First married three or more years before survey, currently aged 15-19[a]	CEB/D[b]	Model 1 + current and childhood type of place of residence
3	First married three or more years before survey, currently aged 15-19[a]	CEB/D[b]	Model 2 + husband's education
4	First married three or more years before survey, currently aged 15-19[a]	CEB/D[b]	Model 3 + respondent's and husband's occupation
5	Ever-married women aged 15-49[a]	Number of children desired	Respondent's education, age, age squared and age at first marriage
6	Ever-married women aged 15-49[a]	Number of children desired	Model 5 + number of living children
7	Ever-married women aged 15-49[a]	Number of children desired	Model 6 + current and childhood type of place of residence
8	Ever-married women aged 15-49[a]	Number of children desired	Model 7 + husband's education, husband's occupation and respondent's occupation
9	Currently married women aged 15-49[a]	Current use of contraception	Respondent's education, age, age at first marriage and number of living children
10	Currently married women aged 15-49[a]	Current use of contraception	Model 9 + current and childhood type of place of residence
11	Currently married women aged 15-49[a]	Current use of contraception	Model 10 + husband's education, husband's occupation and respondent's occupation

[a] For Costa Rica and Panama, 20-49 years; for Venezuela, 15-44 years.
[b] CEB/D = children ever born/duration of marriage, expressed in births per 1,000 woman-years of marriage.

that the overall average difference in the marital fertility rate between women with no schooling and those with 10 or more years of education is −73 births per 1,000 woman-years spent since marriage; the negative sign denotes lower fertility for the educated women. A differential of this size implies a contrast between educational categories of approximately 1.5 child per woman after 20 years of marriage (1.5 = 20 × 73/1,000; see annex to part two of this volume).

All regions and development groups show lower average levels of marital fertility for women with 10 or more years than for the uneducated, though the amount of difference varies among groups. The very small overall average differentials for women with from one to three and those with from four to six years of schooling result from a counterbalancing of larger negative effects in some groups of countries (Latin America and the Caribbean and development groups I and II) and small positive effects in other groups.

Some note should be made of the relation between education differentials in marital fertility, examined here, and those in cumulative and recent overall fertility discussed earlier. The later marriage of educated women contributes to differentials in the total fertility rate and the mean number of children ever born to older women, discussed in section B of this chapter, whereas marriage age has been controlled statistically in model 1.[34] A detailed comparison reveals, as is to be expected, a larger number of non-monotonic relationships for CEB/D than for any of the fertility measures discussed earlier. One difference concerns the ranking of differentials in CEB/D according to region and level of development. The high development group (I) has the smallest average education differential in age at first marriage (SMAM, table 119), so that it could be anticipated that statistical control for marriage age would have less effect than in the other three development groups. With the rather minor exception of the rankings of development groups I and II, however, broad patterns of education differentials by region and development are similar for marital and overall fertility.

Statistical control for current and childhood residence diminishes the apparent fertility-lowering effect of education and, in some cases, strengthens the positive relation between a few years of education and marital fertility. In a few countries, marital fertility, as assessed by model 2, is lower for women with no education than for any other group.

On average, for all 37 countries, the contrast between the highest and lowest educational categories amounts to 56 births per 1,000 woman-years after control for residence, as compared with 73 before (compare models 1 and 2 in table 124). Control for residence reduces the size of the differential most in Latin America and the Caribbean and in development groups I and II; at the same time, the differentials for these groups of countries remain larger and more consistently negative than in other regional and development groups. The effect of respondent's education on marital fertility is statistically significant in 30 countries, the same number as before the addition of residence to the model.[35]

Figure 63 shows, for model 2, the amount of within-group variation in marital fertility differentials, measured as deviations in CEB/D from the "zero" category. Dots represent the coefficients. Within each region and development group, lines connect the dots for two example countries, representing the more strongly positive and negative differentials found within each group. Education effects are statistically significant for all the example countries. The mean values of the coefficients within each group (from table 124) are also shown.

TABLE 124. SUMMARY OF PARTIAL REGRESSION COEFFICIENTS[a] FOR CATEGORIES OF RESPONDENT'S EDUCATION, MODELS 1-4; AND FOR CATEGORIES OF HUSBAND'S EDUCATION, MODEL 3, BY REGION AND LEVEL OF DEVELOPMENT: DEPENDENT VARIABLE = CHILDREN EVER BORN/DURATION OF MARRIAGE[b]

		Difference from zero-year category								
		Respondent's education					Husband's education			
		Number of years completed				Number of countries in which education is significant as variable[c]	Number of years completed				Number of countries in which education is significant as variable[b]
Group and model No.	Number of countries	1-3	4-6	7-9	10+		1-3	4-6	7-9	10+	
Total											
1	37	−1	−8	−37	−73	30					
2	37	3	0	−24	−56	30					
3	37	4	3	−15	−39	23	8	1	−8	−24	27
4	37	3	3	−11	−26	15					

A. Region

Africa											
1	12	6	14	−4	−28	7					
2	12	10	20	4	−18	6					
3	12	7	16	0	−19	5	14	16	13	9	6
4	12	7	15	4	−7	4					
Latin America and the Caribbean											
1	13	−9	−38	−82	−132	13					
2	13	−4	−21	−53	−98	12					
3	13	0	−10	−29	−57	11	3	−15	−37	−69	13
4	13	−1	−9	−24	−40	7					
Asia and Oceania											
1	12	4	3	−21	−48	10					
2	12	3	4	−19	−45	12					
3	12	2	3	−17	−39	7	9	4	3	−7	8
4	12	3	4	−15	−29	4					

B. Level of development

I. High											
1	11	−4	−24	−65	−116	11					
2	11	1	−12	−44	−90	11					
3	11	3	−5	−27	−59	11	5	−10	−26	−55	11
4	11	3	−4	−19	−33	5					
II. Middle-high											
1	10	−3	−27	−68	−97	10					
2	10	0	−18	−51	−78	10					
3	10	0	−13	−36	−53	8	7	−5	−20	−39	8
4	10	1	−12	−34	−48	7					
III. Middle-low											
1	8	5	12	13	−10	6					
2	8	8	17	20	0	5					
3	8	5	14	16	−4	4	22	12	16	13	5
4	8	5	13	20	11	3					
IV. Low											
1	8	2	17	−10	−44	3					
2	8	7	25	−4	−36	4					
3	8	2	19	−6	−35	0	0	15	10	3	3
4	8	4	21	−5	−27	0					

Source: World Fertility Survey standard recode tapes.
Notes: For description of models 1-4, see table 123. Yemen excluded from analysis. CEB/D = births per 1,000 woman-years of marriage.

[a] Unweighted averages of regression coefficients by region and level of development.
[b] Based on a sample of women married three or more years.
[c] Significant at the 0.01 probability level.

Figure 63 shows that there are some countries even within the higher development groups where the relationship between marital fertility and education is distinctly non-monotonic, though positive coefficients are rarely large in development groups I and II. Non-monotonic or positive relations are nearly universal in the other development groups. There are four countries, all in development group III, where even women with 10 or more years of education have higher marital fertility than those with no schooling. The effect of education is statistically significant in three of these four countries (Cameroon, Indonesia and Kenya); and in Indonesia, Kenya and Lesotho, the pattern of coefficients indicates a steady increase in fertility with higher education. Africa and development group III also contain some countries with predominantly negative differentials, so that the average pattern, which indicates almost no differential, is rather misleading for these groups.

Differentials in CEB/D of 50 births per 1,000 woman-years correspond to an expected cumulative fertility difference of one child per woman 20 years after marriage, and differentials of 100 births per 1,000 woman-years to a cumulative-fertility difference of two children per woman. Employing these rather arbitrary values as cutting-points between "small", "moderate" and "large" differentials, it can be seen from figure 63 that all of the countries with large differentials between the extreme education categories (nine countries in all) are in the two upper development groups. Few of the countries in development groups III and IV have as much as

Figure 63. **Partial regression coefficients[a] for categories of respondent's education, model 2: dependent variable = *CEB/D***

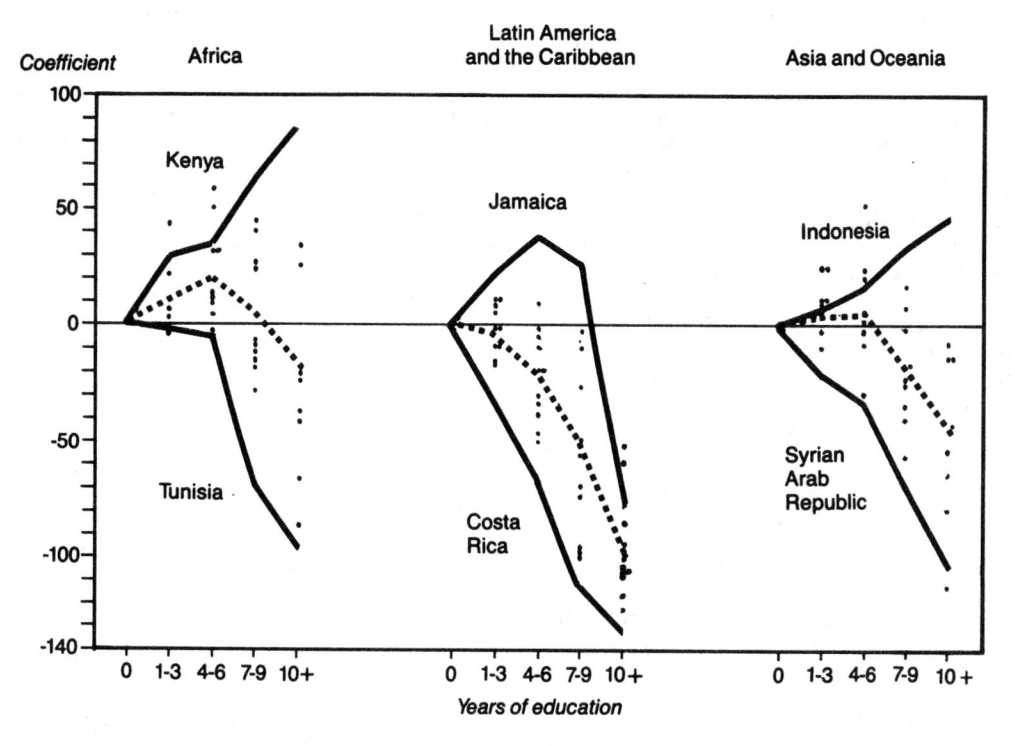

A. *Region*

B. *Level of development*

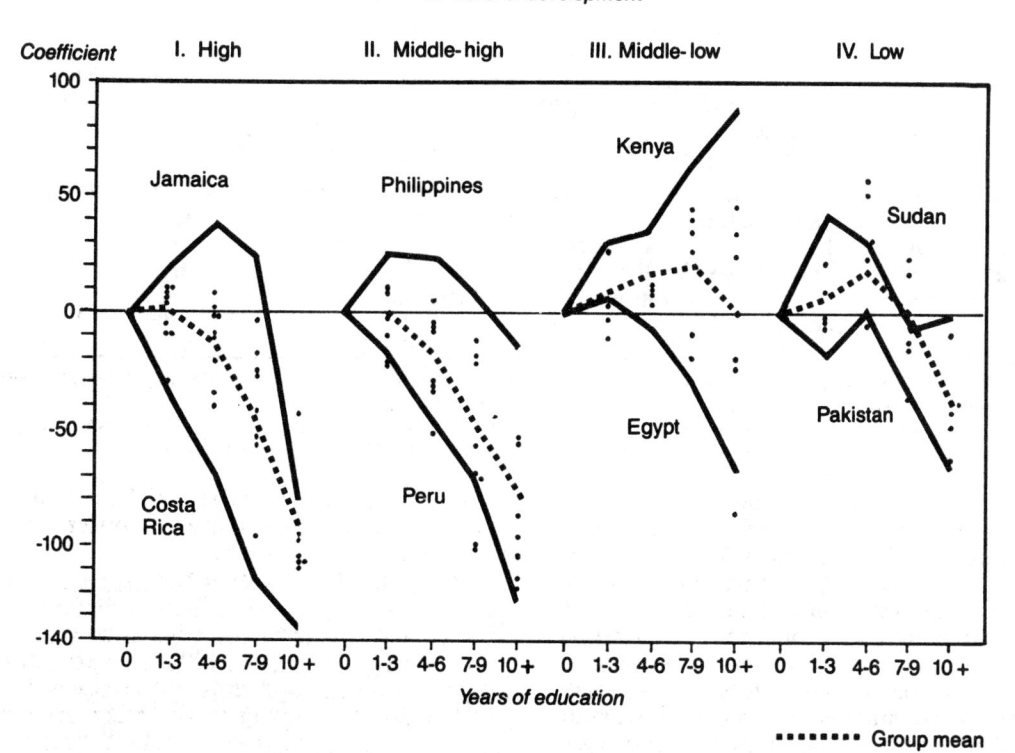

▪▪▪▪▪▪▪▪ Group mean

Source: World Fertility Survey standard recode tapes.
NOTES: Excluding Yemen. For description of model 2, see table 123.
CEB/D = children ever born/duration of marriage.
[a] Coefficients represent difference from reference category, zero education, in units of births per 1,000 woman-years since marriage.

a moderate differential. Only Pakistan in development group IV and Egypt in group III have moderate negative differentials and statistically significant education effects. All of the countries in Latin America and the Caribbean have at least moderate differentials, and over half have large ones. The only other instances of large differentials are Jordan and the Syrian Arab Republic, although one African country, Tunisia, nearly attains this level. Although control for residence usually reduces the apparent strength of the education-fertility relationship, rankings of countries according to relative size of the differential are quite similar between models 1 and 2.

Model 2 implicitly assumes that the form and magnitude of the education differential is the same in rural and urban areas—i.e., that education and residence do not interact in their effects on marital fertility. An analysis of recent marital fertility in 20 countries (Rodríguez and Cleland, 1981) found that in only a few cases were interaction effects between residence and education, or between other combinations of socio-economic characteristics, either statistically significant or of a substantively important size. Although that study gives good reason to suppose that the linear additive model does not produce seriously misleading results, the larger number of countries available for the present analysis, and differences in the variables examined, warrant some attention to the question of interaction. Space limitations preclude examination here of all possible interactions; the interaction between effects of residence and education was judged to be of special interest in the present context, and it is discussed below. In order to minimize the number of small cells produced when socio-economic variables are cross-classified, the regression analysis for examination of the interaction effect employs only a two-category classification of current residence (urban, rural) and a four-category educational classification (zero, one to three, four to six and seven or more years). The interaction effect between rural and urban residence was found to be statistically significant at the 0.01 level in eight countries.[36] In keeping with the approach throughout this study, which has emphasized generality of patterns at least as much as statistical significance, education differentials within rural and urban areas were examined in other countries as well. Figure 64 shows the differentials in all the countries in which the interaction effect was significant at the 0.05 probability level (15 countries in all, or about 40 per cent of those studied). The differentials are shown as deviations from the reference category: rural, zero schooling.

In cases where the effect of education on marital fertility differs between rural and urban areas, the education differential is usually more strongly and more consistently negative in urban than in rural areas. Frequently women with no education have about the same level of marital fertility whether they live in rural or urban areas, while highly educated urban women have lower fertility than any other group. Paraguay is the only country shown in figure 64 where the education differential is smaller in urban than rural areas. Indonesia is, once again, unusual: marital fertility increases with education in both types of place; and for the two intermediate educational categories, urban women have the higher fertility. Patterns in Mauritania, Senegal and Pakistan, which are difficult to interpret, may reflect a good deal of random variation, since the number of observations in some categories is fairly small.[37]

The finding that education effects on fertility are often stronger in urban areas can be interpreted as a result of cultural lag or diffusion, assuming that rural areas tend to enter the stages shown in figure 64 later than do urban areas. If this is the main reason for the larger effect of education in urban than rural areas, it can be anticipated that, at a later stage of the fertility transition, education differentials will become smaller in urban than in rural areas and, even later, that relatively small differentials (compared with those observed in the midst of the transition) will appear in both types of place. This interpretation, however, may not be correct. The patterns could reflect instead fairly stable rural/urban differences in social and economic structure, such that the costs and benefits of a large family differ less according to education in rural areas than is the case in cities. In that case, the pattern of larger education differentials in urban areas might be expected to persist over time. These questions cannot be resolved on the basis of fertility patterns observed at a single time or in the absence of more direct evidence as to costs and benefits of children.

For convenience in presentation, residence/education interactions are ignored when other socio-economic variables are introduced in models 3 and 4. The education differential examined in these models is in effect a weighted average of the differential in urban and rural areas. Comparison of results for models 2 and 4 shows that about half of the fertility effect of respondent's education, as assessed in model 2, is mediated by occupation or else represents the joint effects of husband's and wife's schooling. The average contrast between the zero and the 10 or more educational categories is 26 units of CEB/D in model 4, as compared with 56 in model 2; and the effect of respondent's education remains statistically significant in 15 countries, half as many as in model 2. Addition of husband's education alone (model 3) decreases the fertility contrast between extreme education categories to 39 births per 1,000 woman-years and reduces the number of countries with statistically significant relationships from 30 to 23 (table 124).

Control for the other socio-economic variables has the most impact, once again, in Latin America and the Caribbean and in the high development group. Under model 4, the differentials are only slightly larger in Latin America and the Caribbean than in Asia and Oceania, and they are slightly larger in the middle-high than in the high development group. This indicates that in the more economically advanced countries, and in Latin America and the Caribbean, the fertility effects of respondent's education are more strongly interlinked with labour force participation and with the husband's characteristics than is the case in other groups of countries.

The effect of education that remains after control for all the other variables is substantial in some individual countries. Fertility contrasts between extreme educational categories are large and negative (over 100 units of CEB/D in the Syrian Arab Republic and are moderate (over 50 units) in Benin, Tunisia, Costa Rica, Panama, Peru, Jordan and Pakistan.[38] Among countries with statistically significant education effects there are, as for model 2, some cases where even 10 or more years of schooling have a positive fertility impact: a "moderate" effect in Kenya; and a "small" effect in Cameroon.

The discussion has concentrated most heavily on the contrast between extreme educational categories, because this is usually the largest contrast and the one most

Figure 64. Partial regression coefficients[a] for categories of respondent's education, rural and urban areas of selected countries: dependent variable = CEB/D

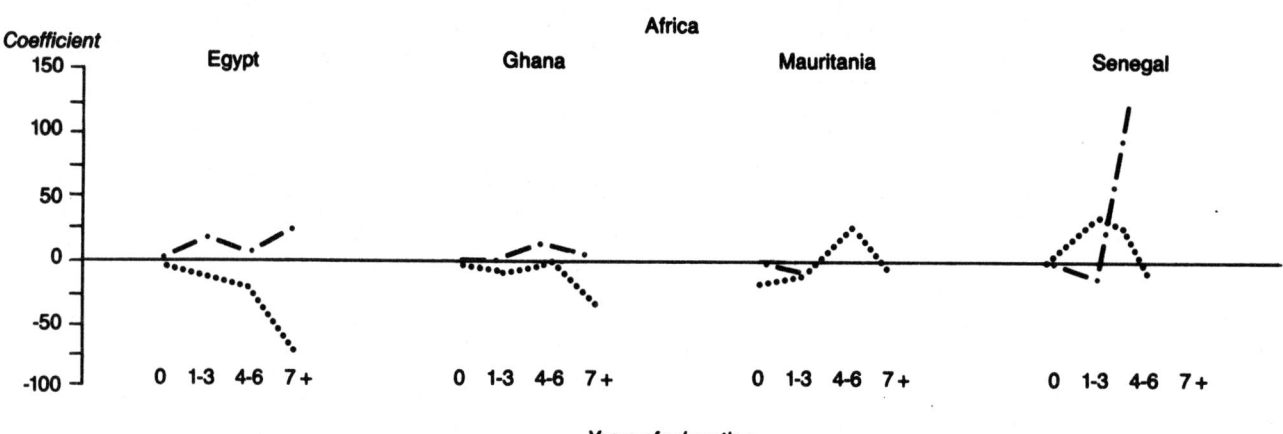

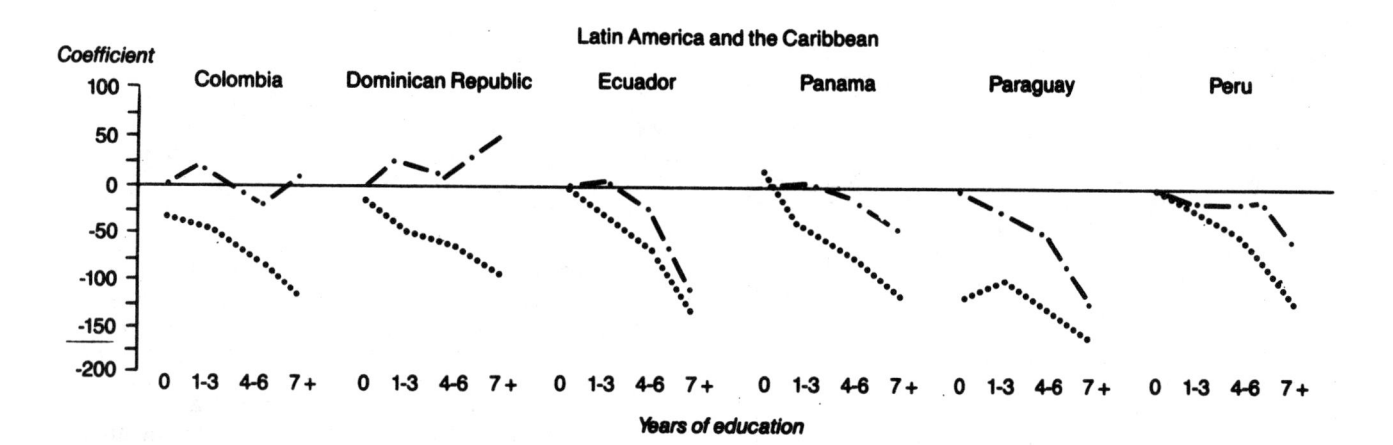

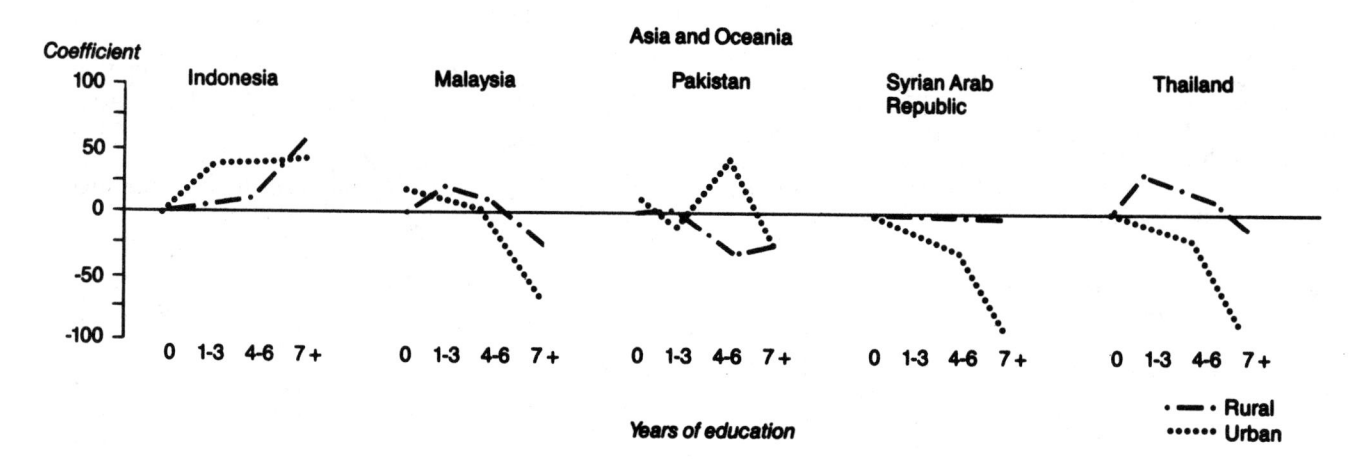

Source: World Fertility Survey standard recode tapes.

NOTES: Control variables are duration, duration squared and age at marriage. Coefficients are not shown for categories containing fewer than 10 respondents. Based on women married three or more years prior to the survey and aged 15-49 at time of survey.

CEB/D = children ever born/duration of marriage.

[a] Coefficients represent difference from reference category—rural, zero education—in units of birth per 1,000 woman-years since marriage.

strongly affected when control variables are introduced. As can be seen from the summaries for regions and levels of development given in table 124, addition of further control variables, in models 3 and 4, usually reduces the size of contrasts between the reference group and the intermediate educational categories as well, provided this contrast was negative and fairly large in model 2 (for example, in development groups I and II). In cases where the average contrast was near zero or was positive in model 2, as for the lower educational categories in the low development group (IV) and all educational categories in the middle-high group (II), there is in most instances little difference between results for models 2 and 4.

Before control for other socio-economic variables, the relationship between husband's education and fertility was found to be similar to that for wife's education, but somewhat less strongly negative on average. This tends to be the case after control for marriage age, marriage duration, residence and spouse's education as well. In model 3, the average fertility contrast between the highest and lowest education groups amounts to −39 births per 1,000 woman-years according to the respondent's education, −24 according to the husband's education. Husband's education has a statistically significant effect in more countries than does the wife's (27 countries as compared to 23), due to a larger number of significant positive associations between husband's education and fertility.

Figure 65 compares the size of the fertility contrast between extreme educational categories for husband's and wife's education, based on model 3. The longer horizontal lines represent values for countries where the set of categorical education differentials is statistically significant at the 0.01 level; shorter lines represent the countries in which the effect was not significant. Values are grouped by level of development.

In development groups III and IV, husband's education has a statistically significant effect in 8 of 16 countries: in 6 of these 8, adjusted marital fertility is no lower if the husband has 10 or more years of schooling than if he has none; usually the intermediate educational groups have the highest fertility (Cameroon, Kenya, Mauritania and the Sudan), but in Indonesia and Lesotho, adjusted marital fertility is highest for the most highly educated husbands. At these development levels, only in Haiti and Egypt does the group of husbands with 10 or more years have the lowest fertility and an education effect that is statistically significant. In model 3, by contrast, the effect of wife's education is less often significant (4 of 16 countries in development groups III and IV, but it is also more often negative in sign, at least for the highest educational category. In the upper development groups, most of the coefficients for the 10 or more category are negative; and in group I they are approximately the same size, on average, for husbands and wives. Even in the development groups I and II, however, it is not unusual for the intermediate educational categories to show higher adjusted rates than the "no education" category: for all 37 countries, the proportion of countries in which the husband's education coefficient is positive or zero (considered without respect to statistical significance) declines from 65 per cent for the category from one to three years, to about 50 per cent for the next two categories, and to about 25 per cent at the level of 10 or more years. For wife's education, the proportion of positive or zero coefficients in model 3 is also 65 per cent for those with from one to three years of education and approximately 60, 30 and 10 per cent, respectively, for the next three categories.

In most cases, the positive coefficients are small in absolute values.

In Latin America and the Caribbean, the fertility differential is slightly larger, on average, for the husband's than for the wife's education. This type of relationship is especially marked in the Dominican Republic and Haiti, where the wife's education has a statistically insignificant effect in model 3; and in Jamaica, where the wife's education has a significant effect but one that is much smaller than that estimated for the husband's education (United Nations, 1986).

Desired family size

Both before and after control for other socio-economic variables, the relationship between education and desired family size is usually monotonically negative, provided the education effect is statistically significant. Exceptions —cases in which a higher education category shows a larger desired family size than a lower category—are of minor substantive importance and may be due to sampling variation; certainly there is no suggestion in the data that a curvilinear relationship characterizes particular regions or levels of development. The discussion here focuses on what is usually the largest contrast, that between the highest and lowest educational groups. Average values for intermediate categories are, however, included in table 125, where differentials in mean desired family size are expressed in relation to the reference category: zero years of education.

One issue in the analysis of fertility preferences is whether current family size should be statistically controlled when socio-economic differentials are examined. On the one hand, reports of desired family size may be biased towards agreement with actual family size (see chapter II). If such bias is the only cause of association between actual and desired fertility, it is appropriate to introduce statistical controls for current family size; otherwise, socio-economic groups with low fertility would appear to have lower desired family size than if the reporting bias did not exist. However, an association between actual and desired family size can also arise through effective practice of birth control; in such cases, controlling for current family size would lead to underestimation of the true effect of socio-economic variables on fertility desires (Pullum, 1980, 1983). Results in models 5 and 6, summarized in table 125, show the difference that results from introduction of actual family size into the analysis of mean desired family size, when other demographic variables (age and age at marriage) are also controlled.

Addition of family size to the model reduces the contrast between the highest and lowest educational categories from an average of 1.3 children desired in model 5, to 1.1 in model 6. The number of countries with statistically significant education effects drops from 32 to 29. Control for family size makes little difference in Africa and the two lower development groups but more substantially diminishes the education differentials in other countries, especially in Latin America and the Caribbean and in the high development group: for both, the average contrast between high and low educational groups is 0.8 child in model 5 and 0.4 in model 6. These are precisely the groups of countries where practice of birth control is greatest, and where much of the association between desired and actual family size is likely to

244

Figure 65. **Adjusted difference[a] in marital fertility, *CEB/D*, at zero and at 10 or more years of respondent's and husband's education, model 3, by level of development**

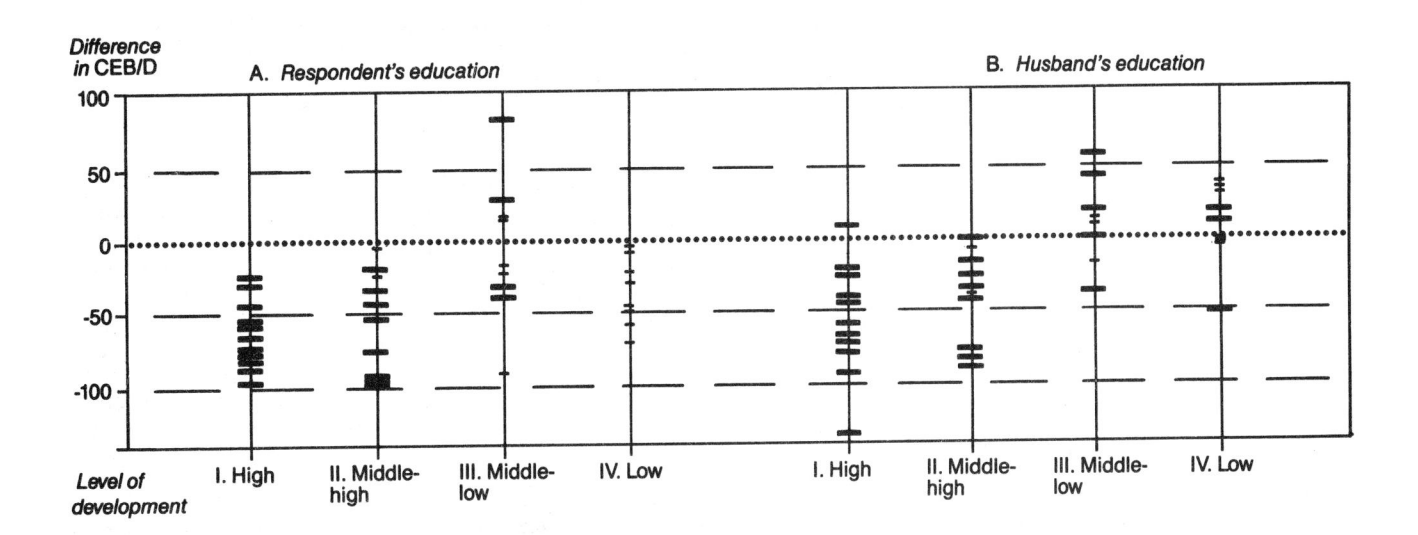

Source: World Fertility Survey standard recode tapes.
NOTES: Shorter lines represent countries in which the set of educational dummy variables was not statistically significant at the 0.01 level. A negative sign denotes lower fertility for those with 10 or more years of education.

Excluding Yemen. For Mauritania, contrast between those with "no education" and those with "greater than primary" is shown.

For base population and control variables, see table 123, model 3.
CEB/D = children ever born/duration of marriage.

[a] *CEB/D* for 10 or more years minus *CEB/D* for zero education, in units of births per 1,000 woman-years since marriage.

represent fertility control rather than reporting bias.[39] However, it should also be noted that regardless of whether family size is included in the model, differentials in desired family size are much larger in Africa and in development groups III and IV than elsewhere.

Control for type of place of residence (model 7) reduces the differential between extreme educational categories from 1.1 children to 0.8 child desired. The differential remains significant in 25 countries, about two thirds of the total number. In most groups of countries, the education differential is roughly from 60 to 80 per cent as large for model 7 as for model 6. In Latin America and the Caribbean, the differential, already small before addition of residence to the model, is statistically significant in only 4 of 13 countries, while in Africa, all the differentials remain statistically significant, and the average contrast between the highest and lowest education groups is 1.6 children.

Figure 66 shows, for model 7, the differential in desired family size between women with no schooling and those with 10 or more years of education, for individual countries (see United Nations, 1986, table A.9.5). Within group variation in the size of the differentials is somewhat smaller by region than by development, especially if subregions are distinguished: in Africa, the three smallest differentials appear in Tunisia, Morocco and Egypt; in Asia, Jordan and the Syrian Arab Republic have larger differentials than other countries. Apart from sub-Saharan Africa (including the Sudan) and Western Asia, the largest differential—1.1 children—is that for Jamaica.

While there is a relatively small range of values within the high development group, similar to that seen in Latin America and the Caribbean, the range of values in the low group is as wide as for all countries combined. These conclusions are very similar to those drawn from the simpler tabulation shown in table 115.

Model 8 adds controls for the husband's education and for both spouses' occupation. The respondent's education has a significant effect, net of all these variables, in 16 countries, only one of which is located in Latin America and the Caribbean. The net average differential in desired family size between the highest and lowest educational categories exceeds one child in Africa, is about one-half child in Asia and Oceania and is near zero in Latin America and the Caribbean. Contrasts according to region remain stronger than according to level of development.

Contraceptive use

Unlike the results discussed above for marital fertility and desired family size, education differentials in contraceptive use remain statistically significant in all but a few countries, even after all the other socio-economic variables are controlled. With only demographic variables controlled (model 9), the average proportion of currently married women who are practising contraception is 31 percentage points higher for women with 10 or more years of education than for those with zero (table 126). Control for residence (model 10) reduces this

TABLE 125. SUMMARY OF PARTIAL REGRESSION COEFFICIENTS[a] FOR CATEGORIES OF RESPONDENT'S EDUCATION, MODELS 5-8: BY REGION AND LEVEL OF DEVELOPMENT: DEPENDENT VARIABLE = DESIRED FAMILY SIZE[b]

Group and model No.	Number of countries	1-3	4-6	7-9	10+	Number of countries in which education is significant as a variable[c]
Total						
5	37	−0.3	−0.6	−1.0	−1.3	32
6	37	−0.3	−0.6	−0.9	−1.1	29
7	37	−0.2	−0.4	−0.6	−0.8	25
8	37	−0.1	−0.3	−0.4	−0.6	16

A. *Region*

Africa						
5	12	−0.5	−1.0	−1.5	−2.1	12
6	12	−0.5	−1.1	−1.5	−2.1	12
7	12	−0.3	−0.8	−1.1	−1.6	12
8	12	−0.2	−0.6	−0.7	−1.1	7
Latin America and the Caribbean						
5	13	−0.1	−0.4	−0.7	−0.8	10
6	13	−0.1	−0.3	−0.4	−0.4	8
7	13	0.0	−0.2	−0.3	−0.2	4
8	13	0.0	−0.1	−0.1	−0.1	1
Asia and Oceania						
5	12	−0.4	−0.5	−0.7	−1.0	10
6	12	−0.4	−0.5	−0.8	−0.8	9
7	12	−0.3	−0.4	−0.6	−0.6	9
8	12	−0.3	−0.3	−0.5	−0.4	8

B. *Level of development*

I. High						
5	11	−0.0	−0.3	−0.6	−0.8	9
6	11	0.0	−0.2	−0.4	−0.4	7
7	11	0.0	−0.2	−0.3	−0.3	6
8	11	0.0	−0.1	−0.2	−0.2	3
II. Middle-high						
5	10	−0.4	−0.7	−1.0	−1.1	9
6	10	−0.4	−0.6	−0.8	−0.9	7
7	10	−0.3	−0.4	−0.6	−0.6	5
8	10	−0.3	−0.3	−0.4	−0.4	5
III. Middle-low						
5	8	−0.4	−0.6	−1.0	−1.6	7
6	8	−0.4	−0.7	−1.1	−1.6	8
7	8	−0.4	−0.5	−0.8	−1.2	8
8	8	−0.3	−0.4	−0.5	−0.8	6
IV. Low						
5	8	−0.4	−1.0	−1.3	−1.9	7
6	8	−0.4	−1.0	−1.4	−1.8	7
7	8	−0.3	−0.8	−1.0	−1.3	6
8	8	−0.1	−0.5	−0.6	−0.9	2

Source: World Fertility Survey standard recode tapes.
NOTES: For description of models 5-8, see table 123. Yemen excluded from analysis.
[a] Unweighted averages of regression coefficients.
[b] Based on ever-married women aged 15-49.
[c] Significant at the 0.01 probability level.

contrast to 25 percentage points. After control for other socio-economic variables (model 11), the average difference between the extreme education groups amounts to 16 percentage points and is statistically significant in 32 countries.[40] This indicates that a substantial part, but by no means all, of the education-contraception relationship can be viewed as operating in conjunction with the effects of the spouse's education, or through occupation, which is in itself partially determined by education. In each group of countries shown in table 126, the differential between women with no education and those with 10 or more years is roughly from 50 to 75 per cent as large with all socio-economic variables controlled as when only residence and the demographic variables were controlled.

Figure 67 shows, for individual countries, the size of the differential in percentage using contraception between the highest and lowest educational groups, based on model 10 (see also United Nations, 1986, table A.9.6). For purposes of discussion, differentials of 10, 20 and 30 percentage points are taken as dividing points between "small", "moderate", "large" and "very large" differentials. Eleven countries have very large differentials of 30 or more points even after control for residence and demographic variables: 2 of the 12 in Africa (the Sudan and Tunisia); 6 of 13 in Latin America and the Caribbean (Ecuador, Colombia, the Dominican Republic, Jamaica, Mexico and Peru); and 3 of 12 in Asia and Oceania (Jordan, the Philippines and Sri Lanka). Countries with

Figure 66. Adjusted difference in number of children desired at zero and at 10 or more years of education, model 7, by region and level of development

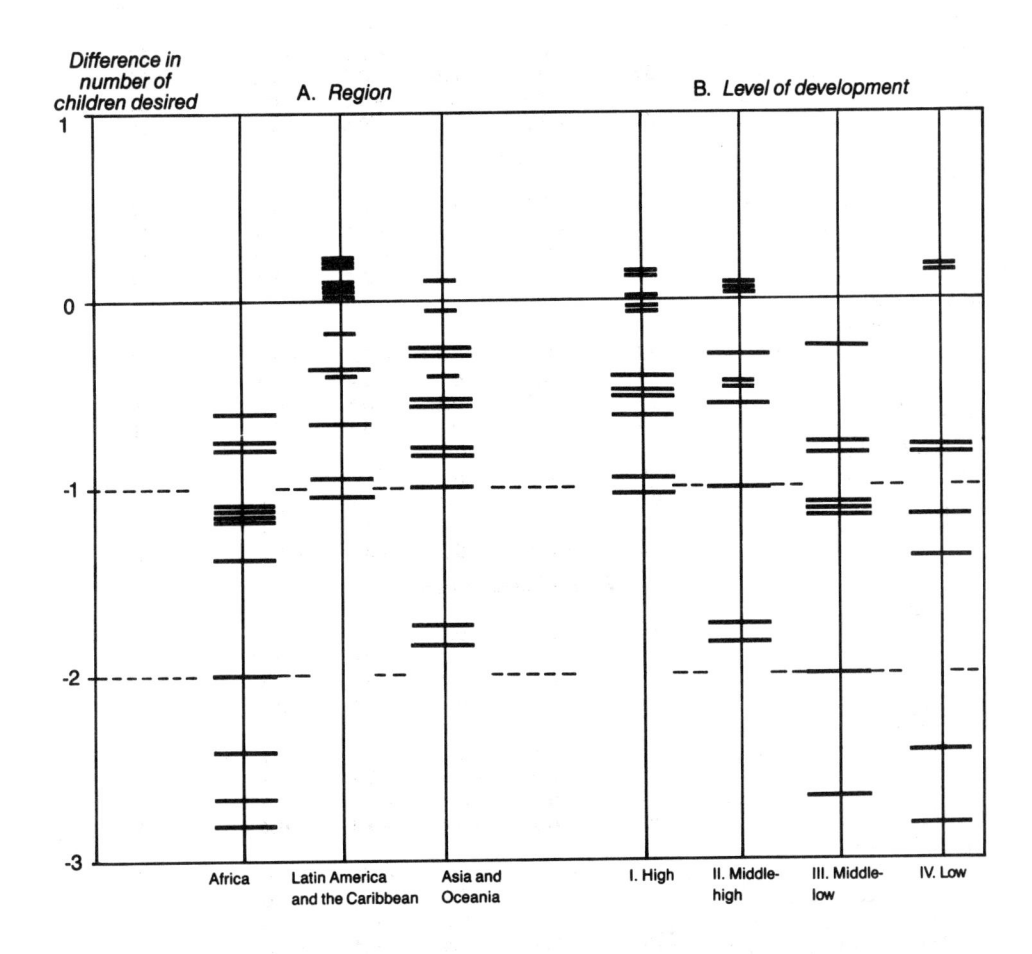

Source: United Nations (1986), table 9.A.5.

NOTES: Shorter lines represent countries in which the set of educational dummy variables was not statistically significant at the 0.01 level. Negative sign denotes lower fertility for women with 10 or more years of education.

Excluding Yemen. For Mauritania, contrast between those with "no education" and those with "greater than primary" is shown.

For base population and control variables, see table 123, model 7.

small differentials are Fiji, Lesotho and Mauritania; the education effect is statistically insignificant in Fiji and Thailand. Neither region nor level of development can be said to capture very well the inter-country variability in size of the differential, since there is a wide range of values within all groups. Yet large or very large differentials are certainly more typical of development groups I and II (18 of 21 countries have at least a large differential) than of groups III and IV (6 of 16 countries). Moderate or large differentials are also more characteristic of Latin America and the Caribbean (12 of 13 countries) than other regions, although 7 of 12 countries in Asia and Oceania and 5 of 12 in Africa also have differentials of at least 20 percentage points.

As in the preceding discussion, attention has focused here on the contrast between the extreme educational groups. With minor and infrequent exceptions, contraceptive use increases monotonically with increasing education, after as well as before addition of socio-economic variables to the regression model.

D. SUMMARY AND CONCLUSIONS

The World Fertility Survey furnishes an opportunity to explore the education-fertility relationship using comparable data from a wide variety of settings:[41] in countries with both high and low levels of educational attainment and varying levels of fertility. The proportion of

TABLE 126. SUMMARY OF PARTIAL REGRESSION COEFFICIENTS[a] FOR CATEGORIES OF RESPONDENT'S EDUCATION, MODELS 9-11, BY REGION AND LEVEL OF DEVELOPMENT: DEPENDENT VARIABLE = CURRENT USE OF CONTRACEPTION[b]

Group of countries	Number of countries	1-3	4-6	7-9	10+	Number of countries in which education is significant as a variable[c]
Total						
9	37	8	14	23	31	36
10	37	6	11	18	25	35
11	37	5	8	12	16	32

A. *Region*

Africa						
9	12	7	10	19	26	11
10	12	5	7	15	22	11
11	12	4	6	10	12	10
Latin America and the Caribbean						
9	13	8	20	30	37	13
10	13	7	15	23	29	13
11	13	5	11	17	20	11
Asia and Oceania						
9	12	9	13	19	29	12
10	12	7	10	15	23	11
11	12	5	8	9	15	11

B. *Level of development*

I. High						
9	11	7	14	23	31	11
10	11	5	11	18	25	11
11	11	3	7	12	15	9
II. Middle-high						
9	10	12	22	34	40	10
10	10	9	17	25	30	9
11	10	7	13	18	20	9
III. Middle-low						
9	8	6	10	17	24	7
10	8	5	8	13	20	7
11	8	3	5	8	10	7
IV. Low						
9	8	6	9	16	26	8
10	8	6	7	13	22	8
11	8	4	5	10	16	7

Source: World Fertility Survey standard recode tapes.
NOTES: For description of models 9-11, see table 123. Yemen excluded from analysis.
[a] Unweighted averages of regression coefficients.
[b] Based on currently married women aged 15-49.
[c] Significant at the 0.01 probability level.

women with no schooling ranged from 2 to 98 per cent in the 38 countries included in this study, while the proportion with 10 or more years of schooling ranged from 0 to 42 per cent. Husbands usually had received more education than wives. Educational attainment has been increasing in all countries, though rates of increase differ. On average, women aged 25-29 years had received about two years more schooling than those aged 45-49; the average difference in attainment is similar in size for husbands of these two groups of women.

Education differentials in both current and completed fertility show an overall pattern of decreasing fertility with increasing education. Both the size of the differentials and their direction varies dramatically across countries, however. For example, in the countries of sub-Saharan Africa, differences in fertility tend to be small, and women with a few years of education usually have the highest fertility. By contrast, fertility differentials in most countries of Northern Africa, Latin America and the Caribbean, and Western Asia are large and fertility decreases consistently with increasing education. In roughly 40 per cent of the countries with available information, women with seven or more years of schooling will have under half as many children as women with no education at current rates of childbearing.

In most countries, the fertility difference between uneducated and highly educated women appears to have increased over time. As compared with differentials in completed fertility for the oldest women interviewed, contrasts between extreme education groups tend to be larger for recent fertility (TFR), and the pattern is more often one of steadily decreasing fertility as successively higher educational groups are examined. On average, the fertility difference between women with no education and those with seven or more years of schooling is 2.2 children for older women and 3.0 children for total fertility rate. This widening of differentials should be viewed in the context of the recent declines in overall fertility; while there may be societies where, from the beginning, fertility decline proceeds more or less at the same pace for all socio-economic groups, decline more typically begins among the most highly educated, and those with lesser attainment follow later. In a few cases, the widening of the education differential may have been accomplished

Figure 67. Adjusted difference in percentage of currently married women currently using contraception at zero and at 10 or more years of respondent's education, model 10 by region and level of development

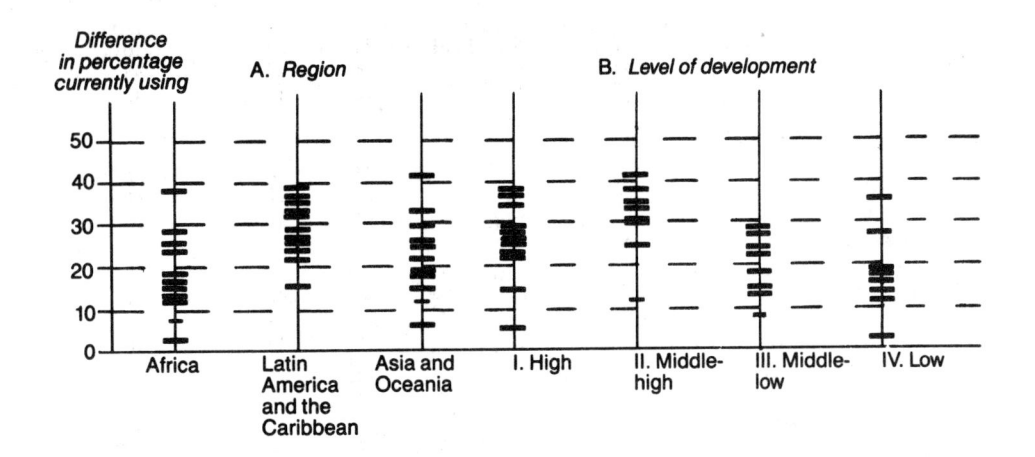

Source: World Fertility Survey standard recode tapes.

NOTES: Shorter lines represent countries in which the set of education dummy variables was not statistically significant at the 0.01 level.

Excluding Yemen. For Mauritania, the contrast between those with "No education" and those with "Greater than primary" is shown.

For base population and control variables, see table 123, model 10.

in part through small fertility increases among those with little or no education. The predominant trend, however, has clearly been towards lower fertility; and in most of the relatively economically advanced developing countries, all education groups have experienced substantial recent fertility declines. In most of the less economically developed countries, declines (if any) have occurred primarily among those with at least several years of education.

The number of living children shows a weaker relation with education than does the number of children ever born, because of differential child mortality. Among women aged 40-49, those with seven or more years of schooling average 2.2 fewer children ever born than women with no education, but the difference in number of children living is only 1.0. In many countries, especially among the least developed, the average number of children living is highest for women with a few years of education.

The multivariate analysis of marital fertility presented in section C provides a way of assessing the extent to which the observed education differentials in marital fertility are due to other demographic and socio-economic factors which are related to education and through which education may affect fertility. On average, in all regional and development groups, when only demographic variables are controlled, the fertility of women with 10 or more years of education is lower than that of uneducated women, although often women with a few years of schooling have slightly higher marital fertility than those with none. In this model, the overall difference in marital fertility between women with no education and those with 10 years of schooling amounts to approximately 1.5 children over the course of 20 years of marriage. The addition of a statistical control for type of place of residence tends to reduce the magnitude of the fertility differential (to approximately 1.1 children over 20 years between the highest and lowest educational categories); nevertheless, the effect of education is statistically significant in 30 of 37 countries after the effect of residence has been taken into account. The model probably provides the best indication of the overall effect of respondent's education on marital fertility; the other socio-economic variables mentioned below are themselves influenced by education or, in the case of husband's education, can be assigned no clear causal order with respect to respondent's education. The analysis also shows that educational differentials in marital fertility are usually similar within rural and urban areas. In a sizeable minority of countries, though, the education differential is larger in the urban areas. In a number of cases, the fertility of uneducated women is similar in rural and urban areas, while highly educated women in urban areas have much lower fertility than any other group. It is unclear whether such relationships will continue over the longer term or whether they merely reflect a tendency for large education differentials to emerge during a transition to lower fertility, coupled with a tendency for these changes to begin earlier in urban than in rural areas.

In the majority of countries, each spouse's schooling has some independent effect on fertility. Except in Latin America and the Caribbean, the fertility-depressing effect of high education tends to be smaller for the husband's than for the wife's schooling, and it is more common for intermediate categories of husband's education to exhibit the highest fertility. In several countries, fertility increases steadily with increasing education of the husband, especially once the effect of the wife's education is controlled.

Part of the fertility effect of education operates indirectly, through the influence of education on labour force status and occupation. In about 40 per cent of the countries, however, there is a residual, statistically significant effect of respondent's education that remains after control for these mediating variables and the other socio-economic characteristics. On average, this residual effect is not large, amounting to an estimated 0.5-child difference between the extreme educational categories after 20 years of marriage, but in some individual countries the "direct" education effect is much more substantial.

Control for the socio-economic variables diminishes the size of the education differential in fertility by the greatest amount in Latin America and the Caribbean and in the high development group, indicating that in these countries the effect of education on the fertility behaviour of women is mediated to a greater extent by employment and the husband's characteristics than in other countries. This finding is compatible with the findings of both the previous and the following chapters in which fertility differentials by type of place of residence and women's occupation are found to decrease most dramatically in the above-mentioned region and development group when other socio-economic factors are controlled. Nevertheless, the size of the fertility differentials according to socio-economic variables remains, in general, greatest in Latin America and the Caribbean and among the most economically advanced countries. For example, after all socio-economic controls, the difference in marital fertility between extreme educational categories after 20 years of marriage is 0.14 child in Africa, 0.58 in Asia and Oceania, and 0.80 in Latin America and the Caribbean.

The relationship of education and selected intermediate fertility variables is also addressed in this chapter. Examination of education differentials in these intermediate factors can provide clues to the paths through which educational attainment affects fertility behaviour. For example, differences in contraceptive use by education are likely to have a substantial impact on education differentials in fertility. With few exceptions, contraceptive use increases monotonically with increasing education, with even a few years of schooling making an appreciable difference. The overall proportion of women who were using contraception at the time of the interview, controlling for demographic factors only, is 31 percentage points higher for married women with 10 or more years of schooling than for those with no schooling. The all-country average difference between women in extreme educational categories is 25 percentage points after addition of a control for residence and 16 percentage points after control for other and socio-economic variables. Even with all the other socio-economic variables controlled, the effect of education is statistically significant in 32 of 37 countries.

Age at marriage also shows pronounced differences by education. Over all countries, the singulate mean age at marriage for women with seven or more years of education is almost four years higher than for women with no education. Typically, SMAM increases steadily with increasing education. Since age at marriage is linked to the duration of exposure to the risk of pregnancy, the late age at marriage among relatively well-educated women is consistent with lower fertility.

Education differentials in the duration of breast-feeding, however, tend to counter effects of marriage age and contraception, because breast-feeding duration is found to decrease with increasing education. Averaged over all countries, those with no schooling breast-feed 7.5 months longer than those with seven or more years of schooling. In the absence of contraceptive use, the ovulation-suppressing effect of breast-feeding would cause those who breast-feed longer to have a shorter period of exposure to the risk of pregnancy and, consequently, lower fertility. There is also evidence from WFS and other sources which suggests that where a period of post-partum abstinence is traditionally observed, its length is often less among educated than among uneducated couples (Léridon and Ferry, 1985).

A recent study estimated the effects of nuptiality, contraceptive use and breast-feeding in generating education differences in fertility for 24 WFS countries (Casterline and others, 1984). The findings indicate that most of the observed differentials in fertility by education result from a combination of the opposing effects of contraception and delayed marriage, on the one hand, and shortened breast-feeding durations, on the other, and that the relative contribution of each factor varies by country. They also note that the combined effects of later marriage and greater use of contraception among highly educated women more than compensates for the effect of shorter breast-feeding duration in every country examined.

An important question is whether, or to what degree, observed differentials in fertility reflect education differences in the number of children desired. In general, the magnitude and form of the relationship between desired family size and education does not correspond well with fertility differentials in the same country, even though both actual and desired fertility are usually lowest for the women with the greatest education. Fertility desires are consistently negatively associated with educational attainment both before and after appropriate statistical controls, and education is positively related to the likelihood that a woman will give a numerical answer when asked to state her desired family size. On average, women with seven or more years of schooling desire 1.3 fewer children than those with no schooling. The countries of sub-Saharan Africa and, to a lesser extent, those of Western Asia, exhibit both a desire for large families and large differences in desired family size according to education. On average for the major regions, differentials are largest in Africa and smallest in Latin America and the Caribbean, the reverse of the regional pattern observed for education differentials in fertility. Furthermore, in sub-Saharan Africa, fertility differences between the highest and lowest educational groups are frequently smaller than difference in desired family size; and actual fertility, but not desired fertility, is often highest at intermediate levels of education. In Latin America and the Caribbean, on the other hand, differentials in desired family size tend to be much smaller than differentials in fertility. Given that the regional pattern of contraceptive-use differentials is consistent with the pattern of fertility differentials, one might conclude that fertility differences are less reflective of stated desires than they are of a differential propensity to translate desires into behaviour (i.e., to use contraception) (see Cleland, 1985).

Some further evidence on this point is provided by examining education differentials in unwanted or excess fertility. In sub-Saharan Africa, while the overall level of unwanted childbearing is low (as a result of large desired family sizes), the proportion of women aged

40-49 years with more living children than desired tends to increase with education. By contrast, in Latin America and the Caribbean, this proportion decreases with education. When countries are grouped by level of development, there is a progression from a positive relation between education and excess fertility in the least developed countries to a negative one in the more developed. These varying patterns for older women appear to have changed recently, as fertility has declined most rapidly within the upper educational groups—studies of exposure to risk of unwanted fertility at the time of the surveys have found that the risk nearly always decreases consistently and sharply with increased education. This in itself suggests that current fertility differentials do not simply reflect patterns of fertility preferences, but are determined to an important extent by differential success at controlling fertility.

The evidence presented in this chapter regarding the association between education, fertility and fertility-related variables is, in general, consistent with the findings of previous research. However, if most of these results confirm hypotheses that can be found in studies predating WFS (e.g. Cochrane, 1979; United Nations, 1977), even a brief examination of earlier reviews shows how difficult it was, before WFS, to make comparisons from one setting to another. Different ways of classifying education and widely varying analytical approaches often made it impossible to tell how much of the apparent variability in results was in fact due to variations in study design. It is now possible to discuss comparative education-fertility relationships much more precisely and with more confidence.

It is important to note that while the emphasis here has been on overall patterns and average effects, the relationship of education to the variables under study varies widely and is in some countries opposite to that hypothesized. The advantage of a broad comparative approach, however, is that it enables one to examine the strength and direction of these relationships under a variety of conditions. The comparative overview given here is not a substitute for more intensive country studies which may clarify the reasons for typical relationships, but the comparative approach can help guide country studies by helping to determine which aspects of a country's population dynamics are in fact unusual. The present study shows that relationships between education and fertility are indeed complex and that they tend to vary by region, with the relative level of socio-economic development and over time. Yet, changes in these relationships themselves exhibit a degree of regularity, in that the early stages of fertility decline usually involve a widening of social differentials in fertility and at least some of its proximate determinants.

Increased education is among the aims of development planning in all countries, and policies that call for the increased integration of women into the development process specifically require that increased educational opportunities be provided for women. The extent to which education affects not only fertility levels but other factors that may be targets of development policy, such as maternal and child health, breast-feeding, contraceptive use, familial relationships and labour force participation, can have important implications for the achievement of population policy goals. Certainly the survey data examined here cannot in themselves resolve many of the questions that policy-makers confront when attempting to estimate the long-run effects of alternative strategies of investment in education. Although the World Fertility Survey has led to great advances in documenting the nature of education-fertility relationships and in tracing their major proximate causes in differential marriage, contraceptive and breast-feeding behaviour, the particular features of formal education that influence demographic variables remain largely a matter for speculation. Furthermore, the cross-sectional nature of these data makes it difficult to distinguish what may be persistent fertility effects of education, associated perhaps with stable differences by education in costs and benefits of children, from a transient widening of socio-economic differentials during the demographic transition. Yet, for many developing countries, the ability to describe existing relationships, using data of good quality, itself represents a considerable advance, without which effective formulation and implementation of policy would be rendered more difficult.

NOTES

[1] Open-ended categories were used in Bangladesh (11+ years), Nepal (11+ years), Thailand (13+ years), Peru (14+ years), Jamaica (15+ years), Kenya (post-university) and Côte d'Ivoire (20+ years). For the sake of uniformity and to avoid the distorting effect of outliers, in tables showing the mean number of years of education (tables 109 and 110), educational attainment of 11 or more years is recoded as exactly 12 years, which, for countries that did not employ an upper-limit code, approximated the average for the 11+ group as a whole. In countries that did not employ an upper-limit code, this recoding made only a trivial difference to the mean.

[2] Exclusion of these cases is likely to bias downward the estimate of mean educational attainment shown in tables 109 and 110, because most persons for whom the number of years was not ascertained did have some education.

[3] Ghana is unusual among countries containing a large percentage of respondents who did not attend school, in that a large proportion is also coded as having reached 10 or more years. Most of the latter persons had completed the intermediate level, which in Ghana requires 10 years, but had not gone beyond.

[4] "Until very recently most boys in Lesotho aged from seven to about thirteen years were regarded as economically useful in that they participated in livestock farming", while labour of girls was regarded as less valuable, so that they were more apt to be sent to school (Lesotho, 1981, vol. I, p. 11). By comparison with other countries at a similar level of socio-economic development, however, it is the high educational attainment of women in Lesotho, not the low attainment of men, that is remarkable.

[5] It should be noted that husband/wife comparisons understate the educational advantage of men over women of the same age, because educational attainment has been increasing (see below), and husbands tend to be older than wives (Casterline and McDonald, 1985).

[6] On average, 12 per cent of women aged 25-29 were single. In some countries with ever-married samples, however, the proportion was over 20 per cent, indicating the potential for a non-negligible bias in the mean education estimate for this age group: Tunisia (20 per cent); Peru (23 per cent); Philippines (29 per cent); Sri Lanka (32 per cent). Other sources of education data, not confined to ever-married women, are available for most of the countries and can be consulted for a more complete picture of educational levels and trends than is feasible in this brief survey of data from the World Fertility Survey individual interviews (United Nations, 1985; United Nations Educational, Scientific and Cultural Organization, 1981).

[7] Caution is required here, because, especially in the least developed countries, higher mortality of less educated women may cause cohort education differences to be understated towards the upper end of the age range; the distortions in age reporting noted in chapter I are probably related to education and the reporting of education may also be worse for older women.

[8] Guyana and Jamaica did not ask about literacy.

[9] In the Syrian Arab Republic, the Sudan and Yemen, the literacy variable apparently refers to women who can both read and write a letter or message. Several other countries asked about writing ability (Singh, 1984), but the information transferred to the standard recode tape and employed in table 111 refers to reading.

[10] Formerly called the Ivory Coast.

[11] Ghana, it may be noted from table 109, had a very high proportion of respondents with 10 or more years of schooling, especially for a country where a large proportion did not attend school at all. The highly educated respondents in Ghana should probably not be assumed to have acquired as much formal knowledge from schooling as those in other countries.

[12] Educational variations in reporting are examined in the country data evaluations published in the World Fertility Survey Scientific Reports series. See also Goldman, Rutstein and Singh (1985).

[13] The distance between the ends of the lines extending from each box shows the range of values observed across all countries with the relevant data available; the box itself spans the 25th to the 75th percentile values (the interquartile range), a measure of dispersion. The median or 50th percentile value is shown by a line through the box.

[14] This probably does not mean that there has been no overall decline in the fertility of uneducated women, because older women in some countries may have understated the number of children ever born. However, some of the values for children ever born (CEB) pertain to ever-married women rather than to all women, a circumstance that increases CEB by a small amount.

[15] The bias referred to in the text derives from the nature of the sample and the method of calculating the estimate of total marital fertility (TMFR) rather than from reporting errors, which may also be present. The bias results from the restriction of the sample to women currently aged under 50 years and may not apply to other TMFRs calculated differently from those presented here. TMFRs shown in table 112 are constructed as follows:

$$TMFR = 5\Sigma B_i / W_i$$

where i = successive five-year periods since first marriage (0-4, ..., 20-24);

B_i = number of births in the five years before the survey to interviewed women who, at the time of birth, were in duration group i;

W_i = number of years lived by surveyed women, in the five years before the survey, while those women were in duration group i.

For further details concerning calculation, see Alam and Casterline (1984). TMFR, as calculated for this report, is biased in the sense that it does not possess one of the main desirable attributes of a "synthetic cohort" measure—specifically, it would not, in general, correctly reproduce the mean completed parity of a genuine marriage cohort of women under (idealized) conditions of a stationary demographic régime: constant duration-specific fertility rates over time such that period duration-specific fertility rates are identical to cohort rates for the same duration; no pre-marital fertility; and no mortality of women before the end of the reproductive years. TMFRs shown in table 112 are biased in this special sense, first, because they exclude some births that occur after duration 25 years (a downward bias); and, secondly, because the duration-specific rates for the higher durations are based disproportionately on the experience of women who married at younger than average ages (an upward bias). The latter effect derives from the age limit of 49 years imposed on the individual-interview samples. Women who married at age 30, for example, cannot contribute to the rates at durations over 20 years; the effect is to bias the rates for higher durations upward, because the remaining women are younger and hence more likely to be fecund at longer durations than those who are excluded. Since better-educated women marry relatively late, TMFR for the highly educated is most seriously affected by this source of upward bias, which usually has the effect of making their fertility level appear closer to that of less educated women than would otherwise be the case. The downward bias due to exclusion of births at durations over 25 years, on the other hand, is greatest for less-educated women, because they tend to marry relatively early and are therefore more likely to be capable of bearing children at durations over 25 years. This source of bias also usually leads to the understatement of education differentials in relation to those which would be observed if high-duration births were included.

[16] Guyana, which is in South America, is included with the Caribbean countries because it has similar marriage patterns.

[17] Differentials in desired family size, measured as the arithmetical difference between means for the zero and seven or more years educational categories, are positively but weakly correlated for similarly defined differentials in the fertility measures shown in table 112. For example, for the differentials in children ever born (CEB) and desired family size, $r^2 = 0.2$ ($N = 32$).

[18] For statistical convenience in discussion of this topic, the Sudan is grouped with the sub-Saharan countries; elsewhere, it is grouped in Northern Africa with Egypt, Morocco and Tunisia.

[19] Based on 37 countries, excluding Yemen.

[20] Table 116 includes all of the countries in which at least 10 per cent of ever-married respondents gave non-numerical answers, except Cameroon, where some women were not asked the question. In table 116, all non-numerical answers are shown, including "no response".

[21] Table 117, which presents only averages for groups of countries, somewhat overstates the regularity of the relationship between development and the nature of the education differential in unwanted fertility; not all individual countries have patterns resembling the average. For instance, in two of the countries in development groups III and IV, Cameroon and Haiti, the percentage with more children than desired decreases steadily with increasing education (not shown). However, in all other countries in these groups where sample size permits the comparison, the percentage is at least as great for women with seven or more years of education as for those with no schooling. This type of pattern appears in four of nine countries in development group II (Jordan, the Philippines, Sri Lanka and the Syrian Arab Republic) but in only 2 of 11 in the high development group (Colombia and Jamaica). Thus, the relationship of development to the pattern of differentials, though not perfect, is strong.

[22] The percentage remaining single at the end of the reproductive years is often estimated by averaging the percentages single at ages 45-49, and 50-54. Table 118 shows instead the average for ages 40-44 and 45-49, because the percentage single at ages 50-54 was not available by education in most cases. Average figures for the two age groups were preferred to the percentage for ages 45-49 alone because of the very small sample size in some educational categories. In these developing countries, very few first marriages occur after age 40, so that the figures do represent, to a close approximation, the percentage single at the end of the childbearing years.

[23] It should be noted that this information was unavailable for some countries in Africa and in Asia and Oceania: Fiji, Egypt, Indonesia, Mauritania, Nepal, Sri Lanka, Thailand, Tunisia and Yemen.

[24] Haiti, which also included visiting unions, shows a substantial differential, but one that is not reliably measured, because there were few highly educated women in the sample.

[25] For the Philippines, the median or 50th percentile age at marriage for women aged 20-29 at interview for the zero, one to three, four to six and seven or more educational categories are 20.6, 18.3, 20.4 and 24.9 years, respectively. In Costa Rica, the corresponding values were 19.6, 19.3, 20.7 and 23.6. While it is common for the median age among women aged 20-29 to be somewhat lower than the singulate mean age at marriage (SMAM) because of differences in the nature of the two statistics and because of trends in marriage age, the difference between these statistics is usually smaller than for uneducated women in Costa Rica: 24.2 years for SMAM; 19.6 years for the median age. Based on McCarthy (1982).

[26] All statistics are based on the 23 countries for which all items of information were available. Detailed statistics for countries are presented elsewhere (McCarthy, 1982; Ebanks and Singh, 1984). In addition to the countries for which the singulate mean age at marriage was unavailable by education (see table 119), several were excluded because very small numbers of women were available in some of the categories shown in the table.

[27] Another factor contributing the impression of little or no trend on average within educational groups is that these measures were unavailable for a number of the Asian countries, where overall trends in marriage age have been large. There is also considerable variation in apparent trends from country to country. See McCarthy (1982), and Ebanks and Singh (1984).

[28] Here, the comparison can be made only for uneducated women.

[29] Colombia, Ecuador, Mexico and Peru.

[30] Another study has found that addition of more demographic control variables reverses the direction of relationship in Fiji, although the differential remains relatively small (United Nations, 1981a).

[31] Current and childhood type of place of residence, coded as in chapter VII (always urban; rural childhood, currently urban; urban childhood, currently rural); and respondent's and husband's current or most recent occupation since marriage, coded, for both spouses, as in chapter IX (no work; modern = professional and clerical; transitional = domestic household employee, service; mixed = sales, skilled and unskilled; traditional = agriculture). All countries asked about occupation, but the questions and coding varied somewhat. For Indonesia, the occupational categories are: no work; professional and clerical; sales and service; skilled and unskilled labour; agriculture; and a small category coded "other". Other variations are discussed in chapter IX.

[32] The causal ordering of the socio-economic variables is not completely straightforward—prior education can affect migration to urban areas, for example. However, the predominant reason for the association between education and type of place of residence is the effect of residence on educational attainment. In path-analytical terms, the "total effect" of a variable, x, is determined by examining the effect of x on the dependent variable after controlling for all variables that are causally prior to x but not those variables which themselves depend upon x (Duncan, 1975; Kendall and O'Muircheartaigh, 1977). The situation is clearest when variables can be assigned an unambiguous recursive causal order. The closest approximation to the idea of "total effect" of respondent's education, given the measures considered here, is provided by models that control for the influence of residence and the demographic control variables, but not the other socio-economic variables.

[33] Countries with 30-49 ever-married respondents in a category are: Nepal (7-9 and 10+ years); Benin, Haiti, and Senegal (10+ years); and Jamaica (zero years). For Mauritania, the educational categories were not comparable to those in other countries. For the purposes of presenting averages, the following educational categories were included for Mauritania: no education; less than primary completed or Koranic schooling; primary completed; more than primary. These were included with categories zero, one to three, four to six and seven or more respectively. Average values for the 10 or more educational category exclude Mauritania.

[34] The total marital fertility rate (table 112) is in effect partially, but only partially, standardized for age-at-marriage differences between education groups. See note 9 above.

[35] Addition of the control for residence causes the effect to become statistically insignificant in Haiti and Morocco, but in Nepal and Pakistan, effects that appeared insignificant in model 1 become significant in model 2.

[36] The countries where the interaction effect was significant at the 0.01 level are: Dominican Republic; Egypt; Ghana; Mauritania; Malaysia; Peru; Pakistan; and the Syrian Arab Republic.

[37] For the 15 countries included in figure 64, the following countries have small (unweighted) numbers of observations in particular categories of the residence-education interaction variable: (a) fewer than 10 observations: Mauritania (rural, 4-6 and 7+ years), Senegal (rural, 7+ years); (b) 10-24 observations: Pakistan (rural, 7+), Senegal (rural, 1-3 and 4-6); (c) 25-49 observations: Colombia (rural, 7+), Ghana (urban, 1-3), Mauritania (urban, 7+), Pakistan (rural, 1-3), Panama and Paraguay (urban, 0), Senegal and Thailand (urban, 1-3) and the Syrian Arab Republic (rural, 1-3 and 7+).

[38] The education effect is not statistically significant in two of the countries mentioned in the text—Benin and Pakistan.

[39] The small difference between results for models 5 and 6 in Africa and in the least developed countries does not necessarily imply a lack of bias in these countries towards agreement between actual and desired family size: in order for the added control for family size to have a pronounced effect on the education differential, there must be substantial education differentials in desired and actual family size, as well as a substantial correlation between actual and desired family size. Africa and the lower development groups have relatively small differentials in fertility, on average. A country-by-country examination of differences between models 5 and 6 does show, however, that control for family size has little impact in some countries with large education differentials in both actual and desired fertility, particularly the Northern African countries, plus Jordan and the Syrian Arab Republic. The control for family size makes the most difference to the education differential in Paraguay, where a difference of 1.1 children in desired fertility between extreme educational categories in model 5 is reduced to near zero (and to statistical insignificance) in model 6. Other countries with relatively large substantive differences between models 5 and 6 are Costa Rica, Panama, Venezuela and Ecuador.

[40] Countries in which the education differential in contraceptive practice is not statistically significant in one or more of the models are: Benin, Jamaica and Panama (model 11); Lesotho and Thailand (models 9-11).

[41] The World Fertility Survey data allow researchers to calculate estimates of fertility (and related quantities) by education that are reasonably comparable across countries. This is a distinct improvement over earlier cross-national studies in which data were collected from a variety of surveys and from vital statistics yielding estimates that were difficult to compare (see, for example, United Nations, 1965 and 1977).

REFERENCES

Alam, Iqbal and John Casterline (1984). *Socio-Economic Differentials in Recent Fertility*. World Fertility Survey Comparative Studies, No. 33; Cross-National Summaries. Voorburg, The Netherlands: International Statistical Institute.

Ashurst, Hazel, Sundat Balkaran and J. B. Casterline (1984). *Socio-Economic Differentials in Recent Fertility*. World Fertility Survey Comparative Studies, No. 42; Cross-National Summaries. Rev. ed. Voorburg, The Netherlands: International Statistical Institute.

Balkaran, Sundat and David P. Smith (1984). Socio-economic differentials in breast-feeding. Additional tables for World Fertility Survey Comparative Studies. Voorburg, The Netherlands: International Statistical Institute (unpublished).

Blanc, Ann K. (1982). Unwanted fertility in Latin America and the Caribbean. *International Family Planning Perspectives* 8(4):156-162.

Bongaarts, John and Robert G. Potter, eds. (1983). *Fertility, Biology and Behaviour: an Analysis of the Proximate Determinants*. New York: Academic Press.

Caldwell, John C. (1980). Mass education as a determinant of the timing of the fertility decline. *Population and Development Review* 6(2): 225-255.

_____ (1982). *Theory of Fertility Decline*. London: Academic Press.

Casterline, John B. and Peter F. McDonald (1983). The age difference between union partners. World Fertility Survey Technical Bulletin 2070. London, unpublished.

_____ and others (1984). *The Proximate Determinants of Fertility*. World Fertility Survey Comparative Studies, No. 39. Voorburg, The Netherlands: International Statistical Institute.

Cleland, John (1985). Marital fertility decline in developing countries: theories and the evidence. In John Cleland and John Hobcraft, eds., in collaboration with Betzy Dinesen. *Reproductive Change in Developing Countries: Insights from the World Fertility Survey*. Oxford: Oxford University Press, 223-252.

Cochrane, Susan H. (1979). *Fertility and Education: What Do We Really Know?* Baltimore, Maryland: The Johns Hopkins University Press.

_____ (1983). Effects of education and urbanization on fertility. In R. A. Bulatao and Ronald D. Lee, eds., with Paula E. Hollerbach and John Bongaarts, *Determinants of Fertility in Developing Countries*, vol. 2, *Fertility Regulation and Institutional Influences*. Report of the National Research Council Committee on Population and Demography, Panel on Fertility Determinants. New York: Academic Press, pp. 587-626.

Duncan, Otis Dudley (1975). *Introduction to Structural Equation Models*. New York: Academic Press.

Easterlin, Richard A. (1978). The economics and sociology of fertility: a synthesis. In Charles Tilley, ed., *Historical Studies of Changing Fertility*. Princeton, New Jersey: Princeton University Press, 57-133.

_____ (1983). Modernization and fertility: a critical essay. In Rodolfo A. Bulatao and Ronald D. Lee, eds., with Paula E. Hollerbach and John Bongaarts, *Determinants of Fertility in Developing Countries*, vol. 2, *Fertility Regulation and Institutional Influences*. Report of the National Research Council Committee on Population and Demography, Panel on Fertility Determinants. New York: Academic Press, 562-586.

Ebanks, G. Edward and Susheela Singh (1984). Socio-economic differentials in age at marriage. Preliminary tables for World Fertility Survey Comparative Studies; Cross-National Summaries. Voorburg, The Netherlands, International Statistical Institute (unpublished).

Ferry, Benoît and David P. Smith (1983). *Breastfeeding Differentials*. World Fertility Survey Comparative Studies, No. 23; Cross-National Summaries. Voorburg, The Netherlands: International Statistical Institute.

Freedman, Ronald, ed. (1975). *The Sociology of Human Fertility: An Annotated Bibliography*. A Population Council Book. New York: Irvington Publishers.

Goldman, Noreen, Shea Oscar Rutstein and Susheela Singh (1985). *Assessment of the Quality of Data in 41 WFS Surveys: A Comparative Approach*. World Fertility Survey Comparative Studies, No. 44. Voorburg, The Netherlands: International Statistical Institute.

Gray, Ronald (1983). The impact of health and nutrition on natural fertility. In Rodolfo A. Bulatao and Ronald D. Lee, eds., with Paula E. Hollerbach and John Bongaarts, *Determinants of Fertility in Developing Countries*, vol. I, *Supply and Demand for Children*. Report of the National Research Council Committee on Population and Demography, Panel on Fertility Determinants. New York: Academic Press, 139-162.

Hermalin, Albert I. and William M. Mason (1980). A strategy for the comparative analysis of WFS data, with illustrative examples. In *The United Nations Programme for Comparative Analysis of World Fertility Survey Data*. New York: United Nations Fund for Population Activities, 90-168.

Hobcraft, J. N., J. W. McDonald and S. O. Rutstein (1985). Demographic determinants of infant and early child mortality: a comparative analysis. *Population Studies* 39(3):363-385.

Holsinger, Donald B. and John Kasarda (1976). Education and human fertility: sociological perspectives. In Ronald G. Ridker, ed., *Population and Development: The Search for Selective Interventions*. Baltimore, Maryland: The Johns Hopkins University Press for Resources for the Future, 154-181.

Kendall, M. G. and C. A. O'Muircheartaigh 1977. *Path Analysis and Model Building*. World Fertility Survey Technical Bulletins, No. 2/Tech.414. Voorburg, The Netherlands: International Statistical Institute.

Léridon, Henri and Benôit Ferry (1985). Biological and traditional restraints on fertility. In John Cleland and John Hobcraft, eds., in collaboration with Betzy Dinesen, *Reproductive Change in Developing Countries: Insights from the World Fertility Survey*. Oxford: Oxford University Press, 139-164.

Lesotho (1981). Ministry of Planning and Statistics. Central Bureau of Statistics. *Lesotho Fertility Survey, 1977: First Report*. Maseru.

Lightbourne, Robert E. (1984). *Fertility Preferences in Guyana, Jamaica and Trinidad and Tobago, from World Fertility Survey, 1975-77: A Multiple Indicator Approach*. World Fertility Survey Scientific Reports, No. 68. Voorburg, The Netherlands: International Statistical Institute.

McCarthy, James (1982). *Differentials in Age at First Marriage*. World Fertility Survey Comparative Studies, No. 19; Cross-National Summaries. Voorburg, The Netherlands: International Statistical Institute.

Nag, Moni (1983). The impact of socio-cultural factors on breastfeeding and sexual behaviour. In Rodolfo A. Bulatao and Ronald D. Lee, eds., with Paula E. Hollerbach and John Bongaarts, *Determinants of Fertility in Developing Countries*, vol. I, *Supply and Demand for Children*. Report of the National Research Council Committee on Population and Demography, Panel on Fertility Determinants. New York: Academic Press, 163-198.

Paik Hyun Ki (1973). A field try-out of population education curriculum materials for teacher education programmes—an experimental study: a case of the Philippines. Bangkok, Asia Regional Office of the United Nations Educational, Scientific and Cultural Organization.

Pullum, Thomas W. (1980). *Illustrative Analysis: Fertility Preferences in Sri Lanka*. World Fertility Survey Scientific Reports, No. 9. Voorburg, The Netherlands: International Statistical Institute.

_____ (1983). Correlates of family-size desires. In Rodolfo A. Bulatao and Ronald D. Lee, eds., with Paula E. Hollerbach and John Bongaarts, *Determinants of Fertility in Developing Countries*, vol. I, *Supply and Demand for Children*. Report of the National Research Council Committee on Population and Demography, Panel on Fertility Determinants. New York: Academic Press, 344-368.

Ridker, Ronald G. (1976). Perspectives on population policy and research. In Ronald G. Ridker, ed., *Population and Development: The Search for Selective Interventions*. Baltimore, Maryland: The Johns Hopkins University Press for Resources for the Future, 1-35.

Rodríguez, Germán and John Cleland (1981). Socio-economic determinants of marital fertility in twenty countries: a multivariate analysis. In *World Fertility Survey Conference 1980: Record of Proceedings*. London, 7-11 July 1980. Voorburg, The Netherlands: International Statistical Institute, vol. 2, 337-414.

Rosero Bixby, Luis (1981). *Fecundidad y anticoncepción en Costa Rica, 1981*. San José: Asociación Demográfica Costarricense and Westinghouse Health Systems.

Singh, Susheela (1984). *Comparability of Questionnaires: Forty-one WFS Countries*. World Fertility Survey Comparative Studies, No. 32; Cross-National Summaries. Voorburg, The Netherlands: International Statistical Institute.

_____ and Benôit Ferry (1984). *Biological and Traditional Factors That Influence Fertility: Results from WFS Surveys*. World Fertility Survey Comparative Studies, No. 40; Cross-National Summaries. Voorburg, The Netherlands: International Statistical Institute.

_____, J. B. Casterline and J. G. Cleland (1985). The proximate determinants of fertility: sub-national variations. *Population Studies* 39(1):113-135.

Strout, Toby (n.d.) Some relations between educational attainment and fertility in the developing world: a review of the literature. Project paper prepared for the Fertility Determinants Group, Bloomington, Indiana State University.

United Nations (1965). Department of Economic and Social Affairs. Population Division. Rural-urban and education differences in fertility. In *Population Bulletin of the United Nations, No. 7-1963, with special reference to conditions and trends of fertility in the world*. New York, 122-133.
  Sales No. E.64.XIII.4.

_____ (1977). *Levels and Trends of Fertility throughout the World, 1950-1970*. Population Studies, No. 59. New York.
  Sales No. E.77.XIII.2.

_____ (1979). Department of International Economic and Social Affairs. Population Division. *Factors Affecting the Use and Non-Use of Contraception: Findings from a Comparative Analysis of Selected KAP Surveys*. Population Studies, No. 69. New York.
  Sales No. E.79.XIII.6.

_____ (1981). *Selected Factors Affecting Fertility and Fertility Preferences in Developing Countries*. Non-sales publication ST/ESA/SER.R/37. New York.

_____ (1981a). *Variations in the Incidence of Knowledge and Use of Contraception: A Comparative Analysis of World Fertility Survey Results for Twenty Developing Countries*. Non-sales publication ST/ESA/SER.R/40. New York.

_____ (1983). *Relationships between Fertility and Education: A Comparative Analysis of World Fertility Survey Data for Twenty-Two Developing Countries*. Non-sales publication ST/ESA/SER.R/48. New York.

_____ (1986). Education and fertility: selected findings from the World Fertility Survey data. Working paper ESA/P/WP.96. New York.

_____ (1985). Department of International Economic and Social Affairs. Statistical Office. *Demographic Yearbook, 1983*. New York.
  Sales No. E/F.84.XIII.1.

United Nations Educational, Scientific and Cultural Organization (1981). *UNESCO Statistical Yearbook 1981*. Paris.

Viederman, Stephen (1971). Population education in the United States. In *Report to the Commission on Population Growth and the American Future*. Washington, D.C.: United States Government Printing Office.

Vlassoff, M. (1979). Labour demand and economic utility of children: a case study in rural India. *Population Studies* 33(3):415-528.

Westoff, Charles F. (1981). Unwanted fertility in six developing countries. *International Family Planning Perspectives* 7(2):43-52.

_____ and Anne R. Pebley (1981). Alternative measures of unmet need for family planning in developing countries. *International Family Planning Perspectives* 7(4):126-136.

Wiley, David (1976). Another hour, another day, quantity of schooling, a potent path for policy. In W. H. Sewell and others, eds., *Schooling and Achievement in American Society*. New York: Academic Press.

IX. WOMEN'S EMPLOYMENT AND FERTILITY

ABSTRACT

The World Fertility Survey data on women's employment are used to explore variations in women's work patterns and in the relationship between women's work and fertility. The broad definition of work used in the survey resulted in higher recorded levels of work in most countries than estimated by the International Labour Organization. In general, work rates increased with age. In Africa and in Asia and Oceania, rural women were more likely to work, whereas the opposite was found in Latin America and the Caribbean. These patterns are clearly linked to different work-opportunity structures. As a rule, the most educated and the least educated were most likely to work, whereas respondents in the middle educational categories were least likely.

Four occupational groups were distinguished: modern (professional, clerical); transitional (domestic household employee, service); mixed (sales, skilled and unskilled); and traditional (agricultural). In Africa and most of Asia and Oceania, the majority of women worked in traditional agricultural occupations. In Latin America and the Caribbean, the occupational distribution was less skewed: larger proportions were found in the modern sector among countries at upper development levels.

A multivariate analysis of the relationship between women's work and fertility concluded that in many countries of Asia and of Latin America and the Caribbean, women in modern occupations bore somewhat fewer children on average than women with no recorded economic activity. In Africa, however, no such relationship is observed. The existence and strength of the relationship between occupation and fertility are clearly linked to level of socio-economic development. While a strong and consistent negative relationship was observed between employment in modern occupations and fertility in the more developed countries, that was not the case among the poorer countries. Similar findings emerged with respect to work in "transitional" and "mixed" occupations, although the coefficients are usually smaller. In contrast, women in agriculture generally showed remarkably similar fertility patterns to women with no recorded economic activity. Others factor found to be important in the relationship included status of women and strength of family planning programmes.

Lastly, the relationships between women's work and four intermediate fertility variables (desired family size, contraceptive use, breast-feeding and fecundity) are discussed. Occupation was less often significant in explaining variations in family size desires or contraceptive use than in fertility. Also, no consistent pattern emerged with respect to level of development. The measured work-fertility relationship may be partially explained by the influence of fertility experience on subsequent work patterns. Fecundity differences between working and non-working women were not found to be significant; breast-feeding was slightly less frequent and shorter in duration among women working away from home.

Increased labour force participation of women has been proposed repeatedly in both the demographic literature and population policy statements as a means of promoting development and reducing fertility in developing countries. The World Population Plan of Action formulated at Bucharest in 1974 stresses the need to eliminate discrimination against women in the spheres of education and employment and to provide for their full integration into the economic sector, as one way to "moderate" fertility levels and achieve development goals (United Nations, 1979, pp. 43-45). At the International Conference on Population, held at Mexico City in 1984, these recommendations were further strengthened in order to place women's active participation in a more central position with respect to development and fertility decline, thus underscoring the fact that women's full integration can make a major contribution to further progress (United Nations, 1984, recommendations 5-10). In addition, the population policies of many Governments include strategies directed to improving the "status of women", which often includes encouraging women's employment (United Nations, 1984). A multitude of empirical studies have been conducted which attempt to document both the direction and the strength of the relationship between women's work and fertility. These studies not only contribute to the more general understanding of the determinants of fertility in developing countries but may be useful for policy-makers in shedding light on the potential implications of women's increased labour force participation.

The aim of this chapter is to add to the understanding of the work-fertility relationship. The level and pattern both of women's labour force participation and of fertility vary widely across the countries that participated in the World Fertility Survey (WFS). This variation allows for an examination of the work-fertility interrelationship under a broad spectrum of conditions.

The remainder of this introduction is devoted to a review of the theoretical issues addressed and the analytical frameworks that have been advanced in research on the topic of women's work and fertility. A review of some of the empirical research conducted to date is also included. Section A of this chapter outlines some of the data and measurement problems encountered in attempting to measure women's economic activity in developing countries. In addition, the WFS data on women's work are described, and a simple assessment of the quality of the data with respect to its overall coverage is performed. The second section describes and summarizes the level and pattern of female economic activity in the 38 developing countries included in the study. The patterns of current work by age, education, residence and marital status of the respondent are considered along with data on occupation. The variations in these micro-level variables are summarized using macro-level characteristics of countries, including region, level of socio-economic development and family planning programme strength. Section C contains a multiple regression analysis of the work-fertility relationship, in which the relationship of work to fertility net of other important factors is examined. Again, macro-level country characteristics are used to provide insight into variations in this relationship across countries. The last section examines intermediate variables, such as family size preferences, contraceptive use, breast-feeding and fecundity, and their relationship to women's employment.

The theoretical framework for analysing the relationship between women's employment and fertility emerges from complementary economic and sociological perspectives. These two perspectives make similar predictions concerning the relationship between the employment of women and fertility; one uses a primarily sociological orientation while the other phrases the argument in economic terms. The first, a "sociological" perspective, is the role-incompatibility hypothesis. Here, emphasis is placed on the diverse roles that women play in daily life. Two of these roles are mother and worker. It is hypothesized that the more incompatible these two roles are, the more negative the employment-fertility relationship will become. In other words, if economic and social life are structured such that it is difficult to combine both child-rearing and employment, an inverse relationship between fertility and work will emerge. When no such constraints are present, there will be no relationship.

The second perspective relating women's work to fertility focuses primarily on the opportunity cost of children and is based on the well-developed micro-economic theories of household decision-making. The concept of opportunity costs derives from the economic theory of time allocation in which the value or cost of time allocated to a particular activity is determined by the value of its best alternative use, which in many cases can be approximated by determining the relevant market wage. This perspective hypothesizes that as the opportunity cost of children increases due to increased labour market opportunities for women, fertility will decrease.[1] That is, under conditions where the decision to have a child involves cost or trade-offs (both time and financial), women will have fewer children. As it would appear that role incompatibility increases with rising opportunity costs, these two approaches are entirely consistent.

In recent work in this area, however, these perspectives are criticized as inadequate explanations for what seems to be a more complex relationship. In addition, their applicability to developing countries is uncertain (Standing, 1978). One study points out that the role-incompatibility hypothesis is incomplete in that it does not offer any explanation for a positive relationship between work and fertility and does not take into account variations in child-care practices and standards (Mason and Palan, 1981). An alternative framework has been proposed based on "household opportunity structure". According to this framework, a household's opportunity structure is posited to be the determinant of its child-care standards, fertility and internal division of labour, which, in turn, determine the employment-fertility relationship. The three important facets of opportunity structures are mother versus child contributions to household income, the importance of individual wage-earning versus joint economic enterprise and the emphasis placed on the formal schooling of children.

In another effort to expand and improve the role-incompatibility and opportunity-cost hypotheses, the concept of women's roles has been expanded to include seven roles women play in social life—the maternal, conjugal, domestic, occupational, kin, community and individual roles (Oppong, 1983; see also Oppong and Abu, 1984). Both the behaviour and the expectations associated with each of these roles is hypothesized to have an impact on the opportunity costs of children and hence on fertility.

A great deal of empirical work has been carried out which examines the connection between women's employment and fertility in developing countries. The assertion that women's employment is negatively related to fertility receives support from most empirical studies. Nevertheless, the claim that work is causally related to fertility is, as yet, premature. With a few recent exceptions, these studies are rarely able to use measures that adequately capture the concept of role incompatibility or opportunity costs. Other factors, such as education and age at marriage, that may moderate the relationship between work and fertility are not always controlled. The importance of examining intervening factors was demonstrated by a study conducted in central Java (Hull, 1977). The lower fertility of working women was found to result from the fact that poor women were more likely to work out of economic necessity and also to be more likely to experience conditions associated with low fertility, such as a high incidence of divorce, long periods of post-partum abstinence and secondary sterility. A further problem for empirical analysis is that adequate historical or longitudinal data for appropriate testing of hypotheses have not been available to researchers.

A variety of work-related factors have been identified which are thought to determine the extent and nature of women's role incompatibility and the opportunity costs of children. The type, location and amount of work women perform may all have an effect on the employment-fertility relationship. Women who perform work for wages or salary outside of the home are thought to experience greater role incompatibility than women who work on a family or other farm or who work without pay. It is often argued that combining family work with childbearing presents women with few difficulties (see Miró and Mertens, 1968; Stycos and Weller, 1967; Goldstein, 1972; Hass, 1972; Kasarda, 1971). Women who work outside the home, on the other hand, may find it difficult to combine bearing and rearing children with the demands of a job requiring that long periods of time be spent away from home each day. Wage or salary employment may also be more likely to offer the opportunity for career development and rising real income over time, thereby raising the cost of interrupting or ceasing employment. Those employed in the modern sector are more likely to be exposed to modern methods of fertility control and lower family size values. Women who have employment of this type are also less likely to enjoy flexible work schedules and may have longer workdays than farm or home industry workers.

In a comparative study using data from 20 World Fertility Survey countries (Rodríguez and Cleland, 1980), the nature of the work women do and its relationship to fertility were investigated. Work status of women was classified into three categories: women employed by a non-relative; women who were self-employed, family farm workers or family employees; and non-workers. The relationship between wife's work status and fertility was found to be significant in 19 of 27 study populations,[2] even after adjusting for socio-economic and demographic factors. The sign of the relationship for each of the three categories of work status, however, varied across countries. In some countries, a negative relationship between fertility and any type of work was found. In several other countries, the largest differences in fertility were between non-family workers and all others. In general, however, in practically every country women engaged in non-family work were found to have the lowest fertility.

Additional factors often cited as major determinants of both labour force participation and fertility are childcare practices and beliefs. Prevailing attitudes concerning the amount and type of care children require regulate the proportion of their time that mothers feel they should devote to children. One study using data from Malaysia (Mason and Palan, 1981) shows that women who perceived normatively based conflict between working and child-rearing exhibited a more negative employment-fertility relationship than other women. The existence of readily available child-care substitutes can reduce the amount of time mothers invest in this activity. In many developing countries, child-care responsibilities are often delegated to kin, such as grandparents or younger siblings, although this may be changing (Oppong, 1983). In addition, low-cost domestic help is available in many urban areas (Chahil, 1977; Hull, 1977; Standing, 1978). If child-care substitutes are available and are considered acceptable alternatives to maternal care, women who are employed may not feel pressured by time constraints to limit fertility.

Parents' desire for schooling of children may also play a role. If formal schooling of children becomes important to parents, particularly if they see it as a means of social mobility, they are more likely to keep their children in school, rendering them unavailable for the care of younger children or productive labour. This may increase the amount of time mothers allocate to child care and, in turn, increase the costs of children and the degree of role incompatibility.

An additional set of factors considered important in the determination of the work-fertility interrelationship is the group of norms and beliefs governing family life. Particularly important are attitudes towards women as mothers and as workers. When motherhood is highly valued in relation to employment, women may be discriminated against in the labour market and the status of working women will be low. This situation would encourage women to have large families (Ware, 1977; Oppong, 1983). Conversely, if working brings status and economic independence to women, they may avoid having large families.

Increased employment of women may also alter the nature of the relationship between husbands and wives. It has been argued that women who work may be more independent and enjoy a more egalitarian marital relationship, which allows them to exercise more control over fertility decisions (Oppong, 1983). In addition, some evidence indicates that with increasing education and greater participation of women in the labour force, domestic labour becomes more equally divided between husband and wife. Although women still perform the majority of domestic labour, this change may precipitate a shift to lower desired family sizes among men.

Fertility may also be related to the timing of work. Women who work prior to marriage may marry later than women with no pre-marital work experience (Standing, 1978). They may also develop greater work commitment and motivation to work, thereby raising the opportunity cost of children during marriage.

A. DATA AND MEASUREMENT

Measuring women's labour force participation in developing countries

Data on female labour force participation in developing countries are notorious for poor quality and non-comparability across countries. Collecting information on women's employment in developing countries presents many problems,[3] and surveys and censuses are generally criticized for undercounting female workers (Recchini de Lattes and Wainerman, 1982). First, it is important to recognize that cultural definitions and perceptions of women's work vary widely. While wage or salary employment constitutes most of what is considered "work" in developed countries, women in developing countries often work in agriculture, where they may be unpaid or paid in kind or services (Boserup, 1970). Trading in the market-place (Ware, 1977), seasonal work (Hull, 1977) and home industry (Recchini de Lattes and Wainerman, 1982) are also important components of women's employment in developing countries.[4] Thus, when Western concepts of work, which imply regular wage or salary employment away from home, are applied in non-Western settings, the majority of the work women perform may be neglected (Dixon, 1982).

Underreporting of female labour force participation may also be a result of the reluctance of some respondents to report women's work when the employment of female members of a household is considered a sign of low social status (Anker, 1983; Chahil, 1977). In addition, the wording of questions has been shown to have a great influence on responses (Standing, 1978). For example, in a survey in Kenya in 1974, the proportion of women aged 20-49 in the labour force varied from 20 to 90 per cent, depending upon whether the respondents were asked about a "job" or "work" (Anker, 1983).

Whether work in a particular reference period is specified (e.g., last week, last year) and whether work is self-reported or reported by proxy can substantially alter reported levels of activity. In addition, questions that include specific examples of the type of economic activity meant to be included as work may yield responses that are less subject to diverse interpretation by respondents and thus are more comparable. The sex and social class of both the respondent and the interviewer may also affect reported rates of labour force activity. There is some evidence, for example, that male respondents are less likely to report female economic activity than female respondents. Male interviewers may be more likely to make assumptions about female respondents (e.g., to assume that they are housewives) than female interviewers.

The presence of other family or household members, such as parents, grandparents or in-laws, during an interview, the translation of questions into local languages and the level of training of interviewers are all thought to influence the reporting of female labour force participation. The nature of these effects, however, is unknown.[5]

Concept of women's work in the World Fertility Survey

The core questionnaire for the World Fertility Survey recommends a standard question intended to determine whether the respondent was currently working. The question contains a fairly long introductory statement which mentions several types of activities the respondent is meant to consider to be work. The standard question is:

> "As you know, many women work—I mean aside from doing their own housework. Some take up jobs for which they are paid in cash or kind. Others sell things, or have a small business or work on the family farm. Are you doing any such work at the present time?"[6]

Several countries elected to use variations of the standard question (Singh, 1984). In fact, the work variables have been called the major source of non-comparability in the WFS data (Cleland, Johnson-Acsádi and Marckwardt, 1984). These variations are outlined in the notes to table 127 and are discussed in detail in Singh (1984).

In addition to the questions on women's current work, the WFS core questionnaire contains several questions concerning work both before and since marriage. Women were asked to supply information on their occupation, work status (i.e., employed by family, self-employed etc.), mode of payment and number of years worked before marriage. Questions on employment since marriage include those mentioned above, plus a question on the location of work. Most countries included a question on whether the respondent also worked during the first birth interval. The surveys in Guyana, Jamaica, and Trinidad and Tobago asked about the period before and since the first birth instead of the first marriage. Some of the countries with samples that included both married and unmarried women asked never-married women the questions on employment but since there was no marriage, data on the current or most recent job only were obtained.[7]

Table 127 shows the percentage of women who reported that they were currently working in each of the 38 countries included in this study. In order to make a rough assessment of the quality of these data, the International Labour Organisation (ILO) estimates of women's labour force participation are also presented in table 127. The ILO used a variety of national sources, including censuses and labour force surveys, as well as United Nations population estimates, in order to calculate economic activity rates by sex and age; these estimates were adjusted to conform to a standard definition of labour force[8] and to apply to mid-1975.

Unfortunately, the two sets of estimates are not exactly comparable, because the WFS data include only ever-married women while the ILO data are for all women.[9] In order to increase comparability, both sets of estimates have been restricted to women aged 25-49. Since the large majority of women in the countries included here have been married by age 25 (Smith, 1980),[10] the WFS estimates for ever-married women aged 25-49 should be roughly comparable to the ILO estimates for all women in that age group.

The WFS estimates are expected to be higher, in general, than the ILO estimates for a variety of reasons (Anker, 1983). First, most WFS questionnaires mentioned particular types of activities which respondents were meant to consider work activities. Notably, work on the family farm was specifically mentioned. In addition, many of the interviewers' instructions stressed that all work activities, except housework, were to be counted as work. Furthermore, most of the WFS interviewers were female and relatively well trained (interviewer training courses averaged about three weeks) (Scott and Singh, 1981).

As table 127 shows, most of the WFS estimates of economic activity are, in fact, higher than the ILO estimates, despite the fact that the ILO estimates are likely to include the unemployed in the labour force as well as the employed, whereas WFS focused only on the employed. There are 13 countries for which the WFS estimates are more than 10 percentage points higher than the ILO estimates. Of these, six are Arab countries—Egypt, Tunisia, Mauritania, the Sudan, the Syrian Arab Republic and Yemen. It has recently been noted that the ILO estimates are generally conservative in their inclusion of female agricultural workers in these countries (Dixon, 1982). The fact that the World Fertility Survey stressed the inclusion of family farm workers probably accounts for the higher WFS estimates for these countries.

Among the other countries where the WFS estimates were significantly higher, the following facts are interesting to note. In Peru, the WFS interviewers were women who had previously been interviewers for labour force surveys. These interviewers may have been more likely to include unpaid family labour as work than WFS interviewers in other countries. Even though the Pakistan survey omitted work on the family farm from its definition of work, the WFS estimate of 18.4 per cent of women in the labour force is still higher than the ILO estimate of 11.3 per cent. Similarly, despite the fact that only work for pay or profit in Ghana and for money in Fiji was specified, the WFS estimates are higher than the ILO data.[11]

In Bangladesh, the omission of all work except employment for cash has yielded an estimate of labour force participation that is probably too low. In Kenya and

TABLE 127. PERCENTAGE OF WOMEN AGED 25-49 WHO WERE CURRENTLY WORKING: ESTIMATES OF THE WORLD FERTILITY SURVEY AND THE INTERNATIONAL LABOUR ORGANISATION

Region and country	WFS estimates Year of survey (1)	WFS estimates Ever-married women (2)	ILO estimates, all women, 1975 (3)	Difference (2) − (3) (4)
Africa				
Benin	1982	76.8	77.6	−0.8
Cameroon	1978	69.8[a]	67.7	2.1
Côte d'Ivoire[b]	1980	79.6	81.3	−1.7
Egypt	1980	18.0	6.1	11.9
Ghana	1979/80	91.5[c]	63.0	28.5
Kenya	1977/78	7.4[d]	47.2	−39.8
Lesotho	1977	18.5[d]	84.3	−65.8
Mauritania	1981	29.0	4.1	24.9
Morocco	1980	18.1	12.3	5.8
Senegal	1978	68.9[e]	59.6	9.3
Sudan	1979	35.4	10.7	24.7
Tunisia	1978	18.9	5.1	13.8
Latin America and the Caribbean				
Colombia	1976	28.3[f]	27.9	0.4
Costa Rica	1976	28.5[f]	22.5	6.0
Dominican Republic	1975	25.1	13.4	11.7
Ecuador	1979	33.7	22.6	11.1
Guyana	1975	35.4	30.3	5.1
Haiti	1977	67.6[g]	74.4	−6.8
Jamaica	1975/76	49.2	60.3	−11.1
Mexico	1978	22.6	17.5	5.1
Panama	1977	34.0	33.6	0.4
Paraguay	1979	49.8	26.2	23.6
Peru	1977/78	52.9[f]	23.3	29.6
Trinidad and Tobago	1977	35.5	41.5	−6.0
Venezuela	1977	25.0[h]	27.2	−2.2
Asia and Oceania				
Bangladesh	1975	15.3[i]	20.9	−5.6
Fiji	1974	18.9[j]	12.5	6.4
Indonesia	1976	70.3	37.0	33.3
Jordan	1976	10.8	5.4	5.4
Malaysia	1974	49.5	40.5	9.0
Nepal	1976	67.3[k]	58.3	9.0
Pakistan	1975	18.4[l]	11.3	7.1
Philippines	1978	48.1	43.5	4.6
Republic of Korea	1974	51.6[m]	40.0	11.6
Sri Lanka	1975	38.5	31.1	7.4
Syrian Arab Republic	1978	21.0	9.1	11.9
Thailand	1975	84.9	77.5	7.4
Yemen	1979	48.4	4.0	44.4

Sources: For columns (1) and (2), World Fertility Survey standard recode tapes; for column (3), International Labour Office. Special table, pp. 16-47.

[a] Asked about employment "at certain times of the year".
[b] Formerly called the Ivory Coast.
[c] Only employment for pay or profit.
[d] Only work for wage or salary.
[e] Added phrase "to meet their needs".
[f] Left out last sentence of introductory statement.
[g] Asked only, "Are you working?"
[h] Women aged 25-44.
[i] Only work for cash.
[j] Only work for money, in the past 12 months.
[k] Asked only, "Aside from housework, are you doing any other work?"
[l] Work on family farm omitted.
[m] Asked about employment "these days".

Lesotho, including only wage and salary work clearly eliminated a large percentage of the work women perform and resulted in estimates far below the ILO data and other sources (see, for example, Anker and Knowles, 1980; Kenya, 1980). In Haiti, where women were simply asked if they were working, without any introductory statement defining work, the percentage of women who reported that they were working is about seven percentage points lower in the WFS estimate than in the ILO estimate. Also, women in Jamaica and in Trinidad and Tobago, both of which used introductory statements omitting the reference to work for cash or kind, reported less economic activity than was estimated by the ILO.

Over all, the WFS labour force participation data appear to have captured more working women than the censuses and surveys used by the ILO in making its estimates. Use of a broad and fairly explicit definition of work intended to include many types of activities and careful training of interviewers are reflected in the higher WFS estimates. If the claim that women's labour force participation in developing countries is often underestimated is accurate, then these higher estimates provide a more realistic picture of women's economic activity in the less developed regions. Thus, the labour force data collected in WFS make possible a more complete description of the economic contribution of women than previous data have allowed.

B. LEVEL AND PATTERN OF WOMEN'S WORK

The World Fertility Survey provides a great deal of reasonably comparable data which can be used to examine the structure and pattern of female labour force participation in the developing countries. The descriptive data given in this section provides an indication of the level of economic activity among women with particular characteristics. These data are used to guide the choice of variables for the multivariate analysis of work and fertility and to provide useful background information about various aspects of women's employment for the countries included here.[12]

It should be noted that Kenya and Lesotho are not included in this analysis because it is clear from the discussion in the previous section that the restrictive definition of work used in these two countries seriously limits the use of these data for comparative analysis. The remaining countries in which non-standard definitions were used are retained for most analyses, although careful interpretation of the results is required.

Current work patterns

The reported level of labour force participation among ever-married women aged 25-49, as shown in table 127, ranges from very high to very low. In Latin America and the Caribbean, the approximate range of women currently working was from 23 to 68 per cent, but most values were between 25 and 50 per cent. In Asia and Oceania, the range is wider, from 11 per cent in Jordan to almost 85 per cent in Thailand; and the average is somewhat higher at about 45 per cent. In the countries of Africa, the variation in labour force participation is also very broad; the percentage currently working ranges from 18 in Egypt to over 90 in Ghana. In addition, the level of women's work was consistently low in countries with a predominantly Muslim population, such as Bangladesh, Egypt, Jordan, Pakistan and the Syrian Arab Republic, where cultural restrictions that discourage women from doing most types of work are common.

Three general patterns of current work by age are found in the data. These patterns are represented in figure 68 by: (a) Ecuador and Sri Lanka; (b) Nepal; and (c) Tunisia. In most of the countries, participation increases with age. The percentage of ever-married women currently working generally peaks between the ages of 35 and 45, and then is either stable or declines at later ages. For example, in Ecuador, 37.5 per cent of women aged 40-44 worked, compared with 14.2 per cent of women aged 15-19, a difference of 23 percentage points. Similarly, in Sri Lanka, while 43.8 per cent of women aged 35-39 worked, only 18.8 per cent of women aged 15-19 did so. Since these are countries in which most women begin childbearing soon after marriage, the increasing rate of participation with age may be a result of the easing of restrictions imposed by child care as children grow older. Cautious interpretation of these age patterns in a life-cycle context is necessary, however. If work levels and patterns have been changing, the age-specific work rates will not accurately represent the experience of any individual cohort.[13]

In such countries as Tunisia, where few women work, the age pattern of participation in the labour force tends to be almost flat: the highest level of participation was 20.5 per cent among women aged 40-44; the lowest level, 13.4 per cent, was found in age group 20-24. Thus, there is a difference of approximately seven percentage points between the highest group and the lowest group. Similarly, the difference between the highest and the lowest groups in Pakistan is only 9 per cent; in Jordan, it is 5 per cent. In Bangladesh, Egypt, Fiji and the Syrian Arab Republic, a similar pattern appears; few women were working and the level of participation varied little across age groups.

Figure 68. Age patterns of current work, selected countries

In Benin, Cameroon, Ghana, Haiti, Indonesia, Nepal, Senegal and Thailand, a somewhat different pattern emerges. This pattern is represented by Nepal in figure 68. In these countries also, the level of participation across age groups does not vary greatly. In Nepal, for example, age group 15-19, with the lowest level of participation, had a level of 59.8 per cent; the group with the highest level had 70.4 per cent, a difference of approximately 11 percentage points. The difference between this group of countries and the previous group is that the level of participation among all age groups is very high. In each of these countries, more than 50 per cent of all ever-married women in almost every age group were currently working.

The pattern of labour force participation by type of place of residence is summarized graphically in figure 69. Box-and-whisker plots are used to show the distribution of the percentage of ever-married women aged 15-49 currently working in each of the three regions. The plots are constructed in the following manner. The percentage of women currently working by type of place of residence is computed for each country. For figure 69, within regions and categories of residence, the percentages are ranked from lowest value to highest value. The horizontal lines shown on the plots correspond, from top to bottom, to the highest value, the value at the level of the third quartile, the median, the value at the level of the first quartile and the lowest value.[14] Thus, in the major urban category for Latin America and the Caribbean, the topmost horizontal line corresponds to the percentage of women in major urban areas who were currently working in Jamaica, the country with the highest value. The third horizontal line from the top corresponds to the median value for the category, which occurs in Peru. The "whiskers" represent the extreme end-points of the distribution, and the "box" represents the range of values encompassed by the central 50 per cent of the countries.

In Africa, rural women are more likely to be working than urban women. The variation in the percentage of rural women working is great, however, from 17.8 per cent in Morocco to 88 per cent in Ghana. In Latin America and the Caribbean, the variation across countries is less (note the shorter boxes). Over all, rural women in this region are less likely to be currently working than urban women. In addition, women living in "other urban" areas are less likely to work than women living in major urban areas, although the difference is small. In Haiti, however, this pattern is reversed.

The pattern in Asia and Oceania is similar to that found in Africa. Urban women are, on average, less likely to be working than rural women. Two exceptions to this pattern are Fiji and the Philippines. In Fiji, only 16 per cent of rural women were currently working, but 24 per cent of urban women worked. In the Philippines, the proportion of women who were working is approximately equal (about 43 per cent) in each residence group. The variation in the percentage of women working in rural areas is large, similar to Africa, ranging from 12 per cent in Bangladesh to 86 per cent in Thailand.

The education of women is also related to female labour force participation. Increased education for women is often suggested as one way to raise their status and to promote their participation in the labour force. Three typical patterns of labour force participation by level of education are shown in figure 70. The most typical pattern is represented by Senegal. In most countries,

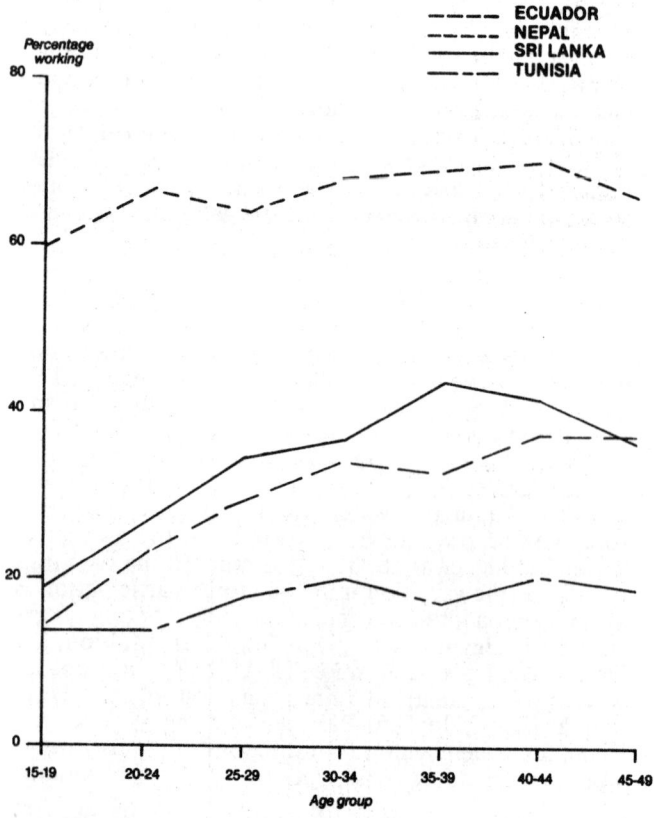

Source: World Fertility Survey standard recode tapes.

Figure 69. **Percentage of ever-married women currently working, by region and type of place of residence**

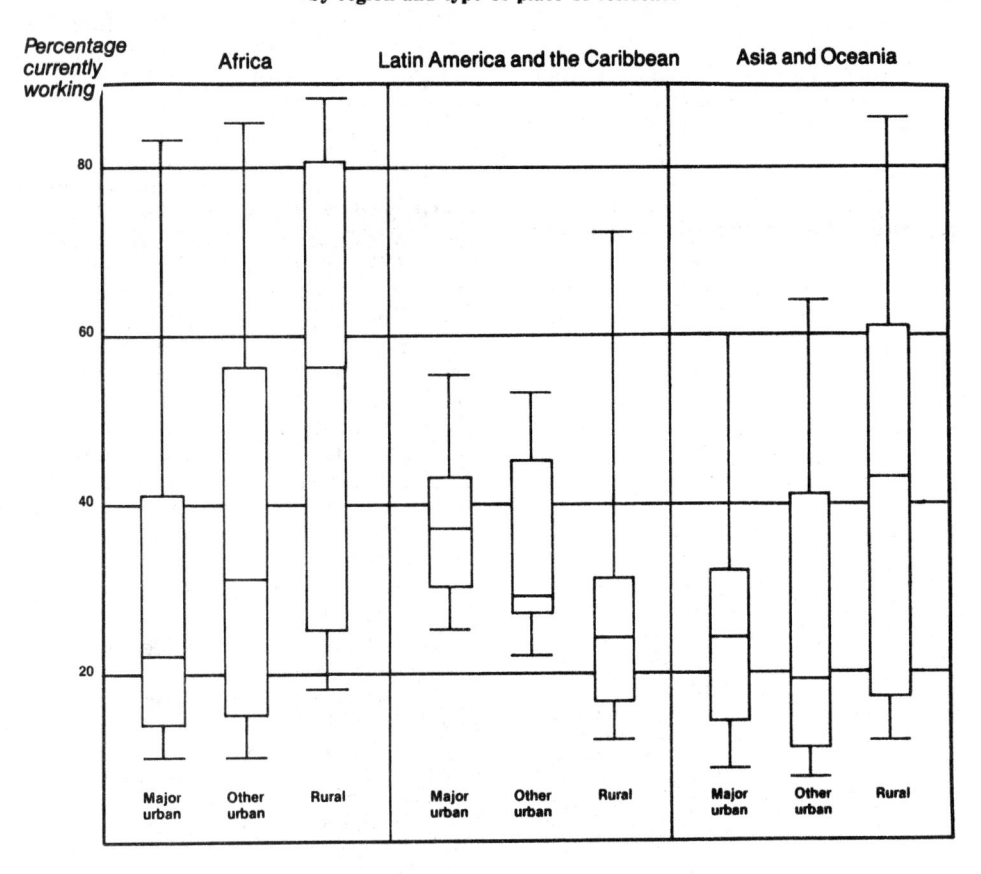

Source: World Fertility Survey standard recode tapes.

the most highly educated women and those with no education are most likely to work. Women in the middle categories are generally the least likely to work. A slightly different pattern, which appears in a number of countries, is represented by the Dominican Republic and Jordan in figure 70. Here, the most educated women are by far the most likely to work: the percentage of women with no education who work is only slightly higher than that of women in the middle categories. Some exceptions to these two patterns are Cameroon, Nepal and the Republic of Korea, where participation declines with increasing years of education.

A plausible explanation for the typical U-shaped pattern of participation by education is offered by Standing (1978, p. 153):

"The relatively high participation rates of the least educated, whether they be men or women, can be explained simply by the tendency for the least educated to belong to households in which incomes are very low, making labour force participation a necessary condition for survival. Since the poor often rely on subsistence, informal sector, or non-wage forms of economic activities all family members, including both the very young and the elderly, are liable to do some work. Thus, a large proportion of the least educated can be expected to be in the labour force. But those with somewhat higher levels of education are less likely to belong to such households and are also likely to be at a competitive disadvantage in the wage-labour market.

As such many can be expected to be discouraged from labour force activity. Finally, those with higher levels of education have the necessary competitive advantage and correspondingly are most likely to have opportunities for high-paying wage or salary employment."

The data strongly suggest that labour force participation among women is highly correlated with education. Since it is also known that fertility is correlated with education, it is important to consider education in the analysis of work and fertility.

It has been suggested that one reason working women are often observed to have lower fertility than non-working women is that those who work are less likely to be currently married than women who do not work. If one assumes that women who are not married are less exposed to the risk of pregnancy than married women and that formerly married women are more likely to work, attributing the lower fertility of working women to "work" (rather than marital status) may be misleading.

The ratio of the proportion of formerly married women (i.e., divorced, widowed or separated) who work to the proportion of currently married women who work is shown in figure 71. This ratio is greater than or equal to one (i.e., the proportion of formerly married working women is greater than the proportion of currently married working women) in every country except Benin, Jamaica, Mauritania and Senegal. Furthermore, figure 71 also shows that the lower the overall level of female labour force participation, the higher the ratio.

Figure 70. **Current work, by years of education, selected countries**

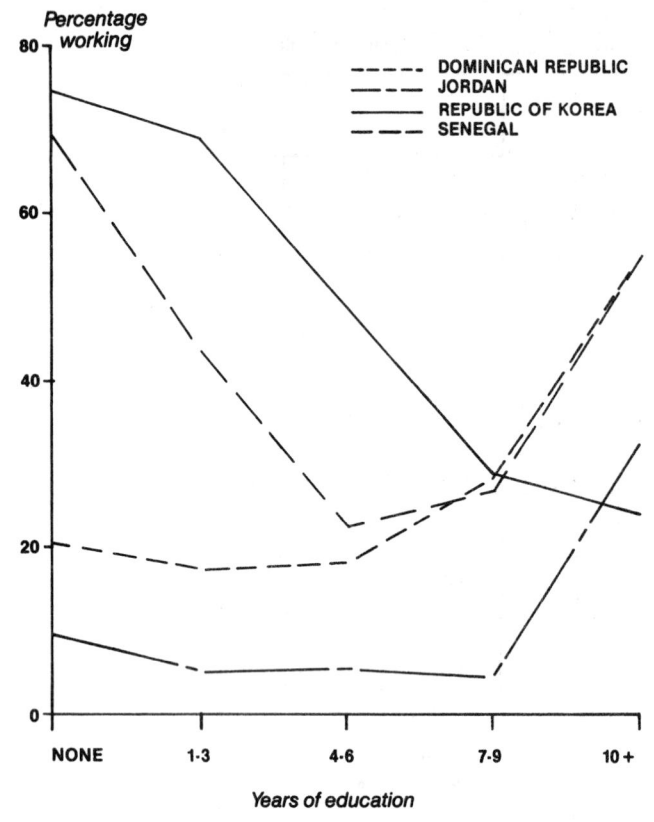

Source: World Fertility Survey standard recode tapes.

Conversely, with high levels of overall participation, married women are almost as likely to work as unmarried women. For example, in Bangladesh, where approximately 13 per cent of all ever-married women were currently working, formerly married women are more than 3.5 times as likely to be working as currently married women. In Ghana and Thailand, where over 80 per cent of all ever-married women were working, approximately equal percentages of currently married and formerly married women worked. It may be that in places where working is associated with low social status for women, few women work and most who work do so because of economic need. Women who are not married are less likely to be supported economically and more likely to need to work. Thus, a low overall level of participation would be associated with a high proportion of formerly married women compared with currently married women working.

Occupation

In the World Fertility Survey, women who reported that they were currently working or had worked since marriage were asked about their occupation. These responses were then coded, in most countries, into a nine-category scheme. The United Nations has further simplified that scheme into a four-category coding scheme (United Nations, 1981a). The four categories were chosen on the basis of data constraints and criteria that are theoretically relevant for the study of fertility. These categories are intended to combine occupations based on the type of work a woman does and the conditions under which she does it.[15] An additional factor guiding the combination of occupations is the concept of modernism; occupations are grouped according to their relationship to a developing economy.

The four occupational categories are: modern, transitional, mixed and traditional.[16] The modern occupational group includes women who were coded as professional or clerical workers by WFS. These women are generally employed by someone other than a family member and work away from home for a wage or salary. The transitional group (domestic household employees and service workers in WFS) also generally work away from home for someone other than a family member but use traditional skills requiring little education (such as cleaning and washing clothes). Women in the mixed group (WFS codes for sales, skilled and unskilled workers) may work at home or away. They are often self-employed and perform jobs that require some level of training or skill (e.g., growing or making items for sale, trading in the market-place). The traditional group is comprised of women who work in agriculture. These women are often employed by a family member, have little education and live in rural areas.

The distribution of women by occupation is shown in table 128 for all ever-married women and for women who had worked since marriage. Indonesia is excluded because the occupational variable was coded in a way that made it impossible to create categories comparable to those used here. Although the occupational distributions have undoubtedly been affected in some cases by the non-standard definitions of work mentioned previously, some broad regional patterns are revealed. In the African countries studied, the majority of women who had worked since marriage were engaged in traditional agricultural occupations. A considerable proportion of women had also worked in occupations that fall into the mixed group; and very few women had been employed in modern occupations, except in Egypt, where 25 per cent of the women who had worked since marriage were in a modern occupation. It seems likely that many women actually engage in more than one type of occupation (although this cannot be determined with these data). This pattern of labour force participation of African women has been observed by Boserup (1970). She notes that when women are actively engaged in producing crops, as they are in many of the non-Arab countries of Africa, they also tend to sell their crops and other items in the market and to be heavily involved in trade.

In Latin America and the Caribbean, working women are more evenly distributed across occupational groups. The fairly high proportion of women with work experience since marriage who had been involved in transitional occupations is probably a reflection of the tendency for Latin American women to engage in paid domestic service. Of all women who had been employed since marriage, the proportion who had been employed in modern occupations was also higher in Latin America than in Africa, reaching 45 per cent in Venezuela, 36 per cent in Panama and 30 per cent in Costa Rica. In most of the Latin American and Caribbean countries, under 25 per cent of those who had worked since marriage were engaged in traditional occupations. The exceptions are Haiti, Peru and Venezuela, where the proportion is over 30 per cent.

In Asia and Oceania, the majority of women who had worked since marriage in Malaysia, Nepal, the Republic

Figure 71. Ratio of proportion of women formerly married and currently working to proportion currently married and currently working, by overall level of female labour force participation

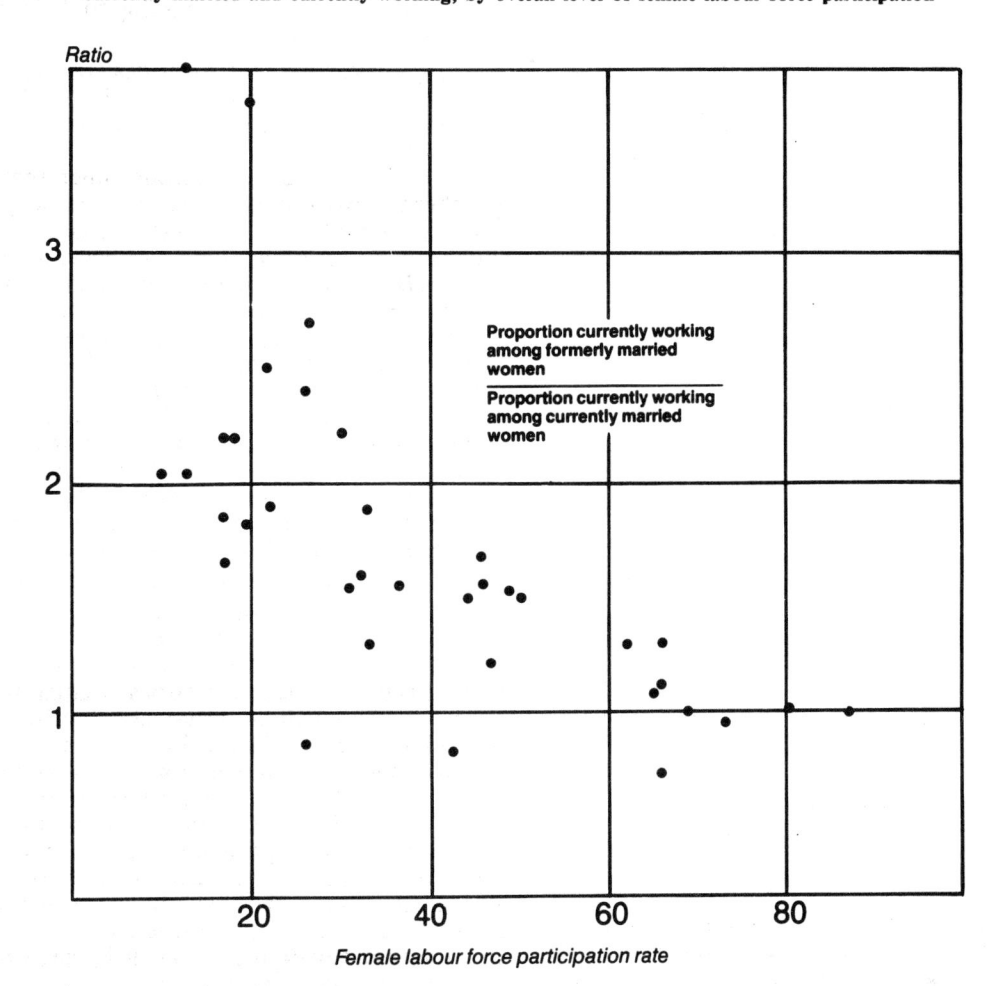

Source: World Fertility Survey standard recode tapes.

of Korea, Sri Lanka, the Syrian Arab Republic, Thailand and Yemen, had worked in traditional occupations. The proportion reported in traditional occupations in Bangladesh, Fiji and Pakistan is much lower and was probably influenced by the non-standard definitions of work (emphasizing work for cash) used in those surveys. The overall percentage of women who had worked in occupations in the mixed category is approximately the same in Asia and Oceania as it is in Africa. In most Asian countries, this percentage is between 25 and 60 per cent. Only in Nepal, the Syrian Arab Republic and Yemen, where the overwhelming majority of women with work experience since marriage had worked in traditional occupations, is the proportion under 20 per cent. The percentage of Asian women with experience in a modern occupation ranges from virtually none in Nepal to over 30 per cent of women who had ever worked in Jordan.

As would be expected, the distribution of women across occupations (but not the overall proportion who had ever worked) is associated with levels of socio-economic development. The proportion of women who had worked in a modern occupation increases from the low to the high development group. Conversely, the proportion with experience in a traditional occupation is only 22 per cent in the high group and greater than 55 per cent in the middle-low and low groups. Women in countries at the two lower levels of development (III and IV) are also less likely to have worked in transitional occupations. The proportion of women in mixed occupations does not vary much across development levels, ranging from about 26 per cent at the middle-low level to about 31 per cent at the low level.

Over all, the data presented above indicate that large differentials exist between countries in both the level and pattern of women's work. Further, while these differentials have been affected by some definitional inconsistencies, they appear to be linked fairly consistently to macro-level characteristics of countries, such as region and the socio-economic context.

Age at marriage

It has already been noted that the timing of work may be related to fertility in a variety of ways. One way is by delaying marriage among women who work before they marry. The relatively better financial situation of never-married women who work compared with non-working women may contribute to the working woman's ability and desire to extend single life. In addition, particular

TABLE 128. PERCENTAGE DISTRIBUTION ACCORDING TO CURRENT OR MOST RECENT OCCUPATION SINCE MARRIAGE, EVER-MARRIED WOMEN AGED 15-49 AND WOMEN WHO HAD WORKED SINCE MARRIAGE, BY COUNTRY, REGION AND LEVEL OF DEVELOPMENT

Region and country	Ever-married[a] Modern	Transitional	Mixed	Traditional	Had worked since marriage Modern	Transitional	Mixed	Traditional
A. Country								
Africa								
Benin	1.1	0.6	48.6	27.5	1.5	0.6	62.4	35.3
Cameroon	1.7	0.8	6.7	58.9	2.5	1.1	9.8	86.5
Côte d'Ivoire[b]	1.8	1.2	24.7	48.0	2.4	1.6	32.7	63.4
Egypt	4.9	1.4	3.5	9.5	25.3	7.1	18.0	49.6
Ghana	4.3	1.7	40.9	42.9	4.7	1.9	45.6	47.7
Mauritania	2.0	4.0	10.7	12.5	6.9	13.5	36.7	42.9
Morocco	1.6	2.2	4.3	11.1	8.3	11.3	22.2	57.3
Senegal	1.1	2.7	9.9	58.4	1.6	3.7	13.7	81.0
Sudan	1.7	1.0	8.4	23.0	4.9	2.8	24.6	67.6
Tunisia	2.4	1.4	3.2	13.3	12.1	6.7	15.8	65.4
Latin America and the Caribbean								
Colombia	7.4	15.3	16.4	4.5	16.9	35.1	37.6	10.3
Costa Rica	13.1	15.0	11.7	4.6	29.5	33.8	26.3	10.4
Dominican Republic	5.6	22.0	12.8	4.4	12.5	49.1	28.6	9.9
Ecuador	6.9	7.8	18.5	9.3	16.2	18.4	43.5	21.9
Guyana[c]	8.2	15.4	15.0	8.6	17.3	32.6	31.8	18.3
Haiti	1.7	7.5	23.6	42.1	2.2	10.0	31.6	56.2
Jamaica[c]	14.0	29.8	23.9	7.0	18.7	40.0	31.9	9.3
Mexico	6.7	10.6	10.9	4.4	20.7	32.5	33.3	13.6
Panama	19.3	20.5	11.5	1.8	36.3	38.5	21.7	3.5
Paraguay	7.5	10.4	26.0	14.5	12.9	17.8	44.5	24.9
Peru	7.3	7.9	24.3	22.6	11.8	12.7	39.1	36.3
Trinidad and Tobago[c]	14.1	17.9	17.4	4.8	26.1	33.0	32.1	8.8
Venezuela	17.8	0.3	6.3	15.6	44.5	0.8	15.6	39.1
Asia and Oceania								
Bangladesh	0.5	6.1	6.0	1.3	3.6	43.5	43.2	9.1
Fiji	6.2	7.5	7.6	3.3	25.2	30.5	30.8	13.4
Jordan	4.3	0.7	3.7	5.5	30.4	4.7	26.3	38.6
Malaysia	4.7	4.9	12.1	34.5	8.4	8.8	21.4	61.4
Nepal	0.0[d]	0.1	4.1	63.7	0.0[d]	0.1	6.1	93.7
Pakistan	0.7	1.9	11.0	5.4	3.5	10.0	58.0	28.4
Philippines	9.2	4.5	22.4	19.2	16.7	8.1	40.5	34.7
Republic of Korea	2.3	4.4	20.9	32.8	3.8	7.3	34.6	54.3
Sri Lanka	4.0	1.2	9.9	27.2	9.4	2.9	23.4	64.2
Syrian Arab Republic	2.9	0.2	3.3	16.7	12.5	1.1	14.4	72.0
Thailand	3.9	1.9	18.6	66.2	4.3	2.1	20.5	73.1
Yemen	0.2	0.4	2.8	45.6	0.4	0.7	5.7	93.1
B. Region								
Africa	2.3	1.7	16.1	30.5	7.0	5.0	28.2	59.7
Latin America and the Caribbean	10.0	13.8	16.8	11.1	20.4	27.3	32.1	20.2
Asia and Oceania	3.2	2.8	10.2	26.8	9.9	10.0	27.1	53.0
C. Level of development								
I. High	10.3	12.9	14.0	11.1	22.5	26.6	28.8	22.0
II. Middle-high	5.4	5.8	14.3	19.9	13.9	11.2	29.7	44.1
III. Middle-low	2.9	1.5	16.0	34.1	8.6	4.6	25.7	60.9
IV. Low	1.0	2.7	13.9	31.1	2.7	9.4	31.3	56.4
TOTAL	5.5	6.6	14.3	22.0	13.0	15.0	29.3	42.7

Source: World Fertility Survey standard recode tapes.
[a] Percentages for occupational categories do not sum up to 100 because some ever-married women did not work.
[b] Formerly called the Ivory Coast.
[c] For Guyana, Jamaica, and Trinidad and Tobago, percentage of women aged 15-49 with one birth or more, by current or most recent occupation since first birth.
[d] Less than 0.1.

types of occupations may provide exposure to ideas and norms that discourage early marriage. It may also be true that the parents of single working women who contribute to household income have some influence on women's decisions to postpone marriage.[17]

Some of the WFS data may shed some light on this question. It should be recognized, however, that a problem exists in the interpretation of these data. Although the reasons outlined above lead one to expect that women who work before marriage marry later than women who do not work, it is also the case that the longer a woman stays single, the more likely it is that she will work. That is, women who marry later are exposed to the "risk" of working for a longer period of time than women who marry early.[18] If this is the case, however, one would not expect to find differences in age at marriage between women who were engaged in different occupations before marriage; a longer period of exposure would not necessarily dispose women to chose one occupation more often than any other.

In table 129, mean age at marriage by occupation before marriage, controlling for education using multiple classification analysis, is shown for ever-married women aged 23 or older at the time of the survey. Only ever-married women are included to maximize the number of countries, because many of the surveys used samples of ever-married women. The age restriction is necessary because an ever-married sample that includes women under about 23 years of age contains an unusually high proportion of women married at early ages; this would cause the mean age at marriage to be biased downward. Since education is known to be highly correlated with age at marriage, level of education is controlled. Guyana, Jamaica, and Trinidad and Tobago are excluded because the surveys have no information on work before marriage. Fiji and Indonesia are excluded for reasons of non-comparability. Unweighted arithmetical averages for regional and developmental groups are shown in order to facilitate comparisons between occupational groups.

The results show that, in general, women who had worked at all before marriage married somewhat later than women who had never worked before marriage. For example, averaged over all the countries in the table, women who had worked in a modern occupation married about three years later than women who had not worked before marriage. Similarly, women who had worked in transitional, mixed and traditional occupations married, respectively, about 1.4 years, 1.6 years and 0.7 year later than women with no pre-marital work experience.

Among women who had been employed before marriage, age at marriage differed between occupations. In 23 of 30 countries, women with experience working in a modern occupation before marriage had the highest mean age at marriage. The lowest mean age at marriage generally appears among women in traditional occupations, although in a number of cases, women in transitional occupations married earliest. On average, women in traditional occupations married 2.3 years earlier than women in modern occupations. There are no striking regional differences.

On the basis of the data examined here, it appears that work of any type before marriage is associated with a later age at marriage, thus providing some evidence that the longer "exposure to risk" among women who marry late is partially responsible for this difference. In addition, however, one finds consistent differences in age at marriage between women in different occupations, net of the effect of education. This finding suggests that work, particularly work in the modern sector, has an effect on the age at which women marry. The implication for fertility is that because later ages at marriage are associated with lower fertility, work before marriage may contribute indirectly to lower fertility during marriage.

C. WOMEN'S WORK AND FERTILITY

This section presents an analysis of the relationship of women's work after marriage to fertility. In chapters VII and VIII, current fertility rates according to respondent's residence and education were presented to provide an introduction to the discussion of fertility differentials before more complex statistical models were introduced. This is not possible in the case of respondents' work status because such data were not collected in the household interview and thus estimates of woman-years of exposure according to occupation cannot be made for samples based on ever-married women. None the less, data on children ever born to older women who have largely completed their childbearing can be examined for crude evidence of the pattern of fertility differentials by women's work. Therefore, before presenting the multivariate analysis of women's work and fertility, fertility differentials among older women are discussed. This introduction to the material is followed by a detailed discussion of some of the problems involved in measuring this relationship with the WFS data and the measures used in the analysis.

TABLE 129. MEAN AGE AT MARRIAGE, ACCORDING TO OCCUPATION BEFORE MARRIAGE, ADJUSTED FOR EDUCATION, BY COUNTRY, REGION AND LEVEL OF DEVELOPMENT
(Ever-married women aged 23 or older)

	\multicolumn{5}{c}{Mean age at marriage for:}
	No work	Modern	Transitional	Mixed	Traditional

A. Country

Africa

Benin	19.0	22.2[a]	18.2	18.7	18.6
Cameroon	17.5	19.5	19.4	17.5	18.2
Côte d'Ivoire[b]	17.5	20.3	19.6	17.9	18.6
Egypt	17.7	22.0	19.4	20.1	17.7
Ghana	18.2	21.2	19.5	18.7	18.7
Mauritania	15.6	17.2[a]	17.3	18.2	15.8
Morocco	16.9	19.7	18.1	16.9	17.3
Senegal	16.4	19.7	17.6	17.9	16.4
Sudan	16.5	20.5	18.0[a]	17.3	16.8
Tunisia	19.4	22.3	20.4	21.3	19.3

Latin America and the Caribbean

Colombia	19.1	21.8	20.7	21.2	20.7
Costa Rica	19.4	22.8	21.3	21.8	21.0
Dominican Republic	17.9	20.3	18.4	19.7	18.6
Ecuador	18.8	21.3	20.1	20.7	20.2
Haiti	19.1	21.6	20.0	20.5	20.9
Mexico	18.6	21.2	19.6	20.4	18.3
Panama	18.5	21.7	19.8	20.4	18.9
Paraguay	19.2	23.1	20.7	21.6	19.7
Peru	18.9	22.1	19.9	20.7	20.0
Venezuela	18.3	21.1	19.4	21.3	19.4

Asia and Oceania

Bangladesh	12.5	17.4[a]	12.3	13.6	15.0
Jordan	17.4	21.1	21.2[a]	20.0	18.1
Malaysia	17.9	21.5	21.4	21.1	18.6
Nepal	15.6	14.8[a]	15.7[a]	16.6	17.4
Pakistan	16.6	19.4	16.5	17.1	16.5
Philippines	19.9	23.9	21.7	21.8	19.9
Republic of Korea	20.1	21.4	21.8	21.7	20.4
Sri Lanka	19.3	23.1	22.2	21.4	19.7
Syrian Arab Republic	18.7	21.8	23.0[a]	20.6	19.3
Thailand	19.0	21.3	21.1	20.6	19.7
Yemen	16.3	[a]	14.5[a]	18.4	16.6

B. Region

Africa	17.5	20.5	18.8	18.5	17.7
Latin America and the Caribbean	18.8	21.7	20.0	20.8	19.8
Asia and Oceania	17.6	20.6	19.2	19.4	18.3

C. Level of development

I. High	18.8	21.6	20.6	21.1	19.6
II. Middle-high	18.9	22.0	20.8	20.8	19.5
III. Middle-low	17.6	20.5	19.2	18.2	18.1
IV. Low	16.4	19.1	16.7	17.6	17.1
TOTAL	17.9	20.9	19.3	19.5	18.6

Source: World Fertility Survey standard recode tapes.
[a] Fewer than 20 cases.
[b] Formerly called the Ivory Coast.

Children ever born by occupation

The data on occupation have been selected for use in the present analysis. There are several reasons for using these occupational data instead of other data on work. First, each of the four broad occupational categories provides a simple way of representing a set of job characteristics as described above in the section on occupation. Secondly, the question on occupation was asked in every country with very little variation in wording.[19] Thus, using these data permits inclusion of the maximum number of countries in the analysis and maintains a broad comparative perspective. Thirdly, because the question on occupation was open-ended and interviewers were instructed to obtain detailed information on this topic, it seems likely that those who coded the data had enough information to make a reasonably accurate judgement about which occupational code to assign. A fourth factor is that since occupation was coded at the country level, coders presumably were aware of country or region-specific job names or descriptions and were able to code them consistently and accurately. One disadvantage of this factor, however, is that specific categories of occupation may not be completely comparable across countries.

In order for the data on occupation to be useful for this analysis, it must be assumed that the characteristics of a woman's most recent or current job are similar to the characteristics of any previous job(s) she may have held. If women are likely to move between very different types of jobs, then the data on the most recent job will not accurately represent women's job or work experience since marriage. Previous analyses of these data show a fairly high degree of occupational continuity (with respect to the period before and after marriage), so this assumption is probably not a bad one (see United Nations, 1985).[20]

Table 130 presents a summary of the fertility of women aged 40-49 at the time of the survey according to occupation since marriage. This table provides an indication of the direction and magnitude of the differences in fertility among older women at the end of their reproductive span in different occupations. In every region, women in modern occupations had the smallest number of children ever born and women in traditional occupations the greatest. Those who had never worked had, on average, slightly fewer children than women in traditional occupations but more than women in any of the other occupation groups. The size of the differences is largest in Latin America and the Caribbean, where, for example, women who have never worked average 2.7 children more than women who have worked in a modern occupation. This difference is 2.2 children in Asia and Oceania and 1.4 children in Africa.

At each level of development except group IV, the same pattern of differences emerges, with women in modern occupations having borne the fewest children and women in traditional occupations the most. In development group IV, it is women in transitional occupations who had the lowest fertility and those who had never worked the highest. The magnitude of the differences between occupational groups tends to increase with increasing development. For example, while in development groups III and IV, women in modern occupations had 1.6 and 1 children fewer than women who had not worked

TABLE 130. MEAN NUMBER OF CHILDREN EVER BORN TO EVER-MARRIED WOMEN AGED 40-49,[a] ACCORDING TO RESPONDENT'S OCCUPATION SINCE MARRIAGE, BY REGION AND LEVEL OF DEVELOPMENT

	Mean number of children ever born for:				
	No work	Modern	Transitional	Mixed	Traditional
Region					
Africa	6.3	4.9	5.5	5.9	6.6
Latin America and the Caribbean	6.9	4.2	6.2	6.0	7.4
Asia and Oceania . . .	6.7	4.5	5.1	6.1	6.8
Level of development					
I. High	6.7	4.0	5.9	5.8	7.2
II. Middle-high	7.1	4.3	6.3	6.3	7.6
III. Middle-low	6.2	4.6	5.4	5.7	6.7
IV. Low	6.4	5.4	4.6	6.1	6.3

Source: World Fertility Survey standard recode tapes.
[a] For Guyana, Jamaica, and Trinidad and Tobago, sample is ever-married women aged 40-49 with one or more births.

since marriage, this difference in groups I and II was 2.7 and 2.8 children, respectively.

While these figures present only a summary of differences in fertility by occupation they indicate that the relationship between women's work and fertility is related to the type of work. In addition, table 130 suggests that the relationship between work and fertility may vary between regions and according to the social and economic context. These observations are explored further in the discussion of results of the multivariate analysis.

Data and methods

The WFS data on women's work are not ideally suited to the analysis of the determinants of fertility. Many pieces of information that are theoretically important in the analysis of the work-fertility relationship, such as child-care management, number of hours worked, wages and work commitment, were not collected. Furthermore, in addition to the measurement and definitional problems already reviewed, the most difficult problem is that most of the work variables refer to a woman's current or most recent work activity since her first marriage. For a woman who was not currently working but who had worked since marriage, the period during which she worked most recently may have been before she had any children, between births or after she had completed childbearing, or it may have spanned all or some of these intervals. Although the total number of years each woman had worked since she was first married is known, there are no data on the duration of her current or most recent job. It is not possible, then, to link particular periods of work to subsequent births. A further problem for comparative analysis involves differences in the selection of work questions that were asked in each country and various changes individual countries incorporated into the core questionnaire and the coding process.

Because of the absence of detailed work histories, it is not possible to estimate models in which work in a particular period is related to the number of births or the probability of having a birth in that or a later period. As a result, this analysis is limited to estimation of the relationship of the type of work experience each woman had had since marriage (her occupation) to her fertility cumulated up to the date of the interview, or the number of children ever born. The actual dependent variable used in the regression models is children ever born/duration of marriage, *CEB/D*; this variable may be interpreted as the number of children per year of marriage or the yearly rate of marital childbearing. Details of the method used to estimate the relationship between work experience and fertility are discussed in the annex to part two of this publication. Because the relationship of work and fertility is of primary concern here, the discussion focuses on the magnitude and direction of the coefficients of the set of occupation variables. Occupation is coded as a set of dummy variables, one for each of the four occupational categories—modern, transitional, mixed and traditional. No work since marriage is the reference category. For convenience of presentation, the regression coefficients are multiplied by 1,000. Thus, they may be interpreted as the difference in the number of children per 1,000 woman-years of marriage between women in each occupational category and women who do not work.

The relationship between work in a modern occupation and the rate of childbearing, *CEB/D*, is expected to be negative. Since women who have jobs in the modern sector are likely to work relatively long hours away from home for a wage or salary, both the role-incompatibility hypothesis and the opportunity-cost perspective predict that this type of work will have a negative impact on fertility. Women in modern occupations are also more likely than other women to be exposed to modern family planning methods and to have lower family size ideals.

Work in a traditional occupation, compared with the reference category of no work since marriage, is expected to be weakly related to fertility because this type of work is generally performed at or near home and is highly compatible with childbearing and child-rearing. Also, while the conceptual distinction between work in a traditional occupation and no work may be clear, in practice the distinction may be more a matter of the way in which traditional, agricultural work is viewed by the respondent than any real difference in the activities of the two groups.

A negative relationship is expected between work in a transitional occupation and fertility, but this relationship may be weaker than that between work in a modern occupation and fertility. Women in transitional occupations generally work away from home and may be exposed to the development process; yet, the opportunity costs of leaving the work-force are less for this group than for the modern group because fewer investments in the job are required and returns to experience are generally lower.

The relationship between fertility and work in a mixed occupation is also expected to be negative. Again, however, this type of work should be less strongly related to fertility (i.e., the coefficient of this variable should be smaller) than work in a modern occupation. Many women in this group are self-employed. Although they may have some exposure to modernizing influences (e.g., buying and selling in a modernizing economy), they often work in or near home and are relatively flexible with respect to entering and leaving the labour market.

The purpose of using a multivariate model is to determine whether the relationship between work and fertility persists when other casually prior factors are controlled. The factors used as controls here are: marital duration and marital duration squared in years; age at marriage in years; dummy variables representing whether the respondent's first marriage is still intact; type of place of residence (urban or rural, as provided in the standard recode tapes); respondent's education and husband's occupation in categorical variables as developed by the United Nations as part of its WFS research programme.[21]

As already discussed in chapters VII and VIII, a reasonable causal ordering of the factors that are hypothesized to influence marital fertility places demographic variables first, followed by type of place of residence, education and then occupation. (These results are not shown.) The set of occupation variables is then added to the model. The coefficients of the control variables were examined to see if and how they are changed by the addition of occupation. The addition of the set of occupation variables to the equation generally changes the coefficients of the demographic variables very little. Among the other variables, education, type of place of residence and husband's occupation, the magnitude of the coefficients is generally reduced somewhat, although usually not significantly, by the addition of the occupation variables. Some of the coefficients, however, increase slightly. Over all, the dummy variable indicating that the respondent had more than 10 years of schooling and the variable indicating that the respondent's husband worked in a modern occupation tend to show the largest reduction in magnitude when the occupation variables are added.

Multivariate analysis

The results of the multivariate analysis are shown in tables 131 and 132. Since only the coefficients of the occupation variables are of interest here, they are the only ones shown. Nepal, the Syrian Arab Republic, Venezuela and Yemen are excluded from the multivariate analysis because in each of these countries, there are fewer than 20 cases in one or more of the occupational categories. Again, Indonesia is excluded because of non-comparability in coding of occupation. In all of the countries included, except Guyana, Jamaica, and Trinidad and Tobago, the sample is restricted to women who had first married three or more years prior to the survey. For Guyana, Jamaica, and Trinidad and Tobago, it was necessary to restrict the sample further to women with at least one birth because the data on occupation in these three countries refer to the respondent's occupation since her first birth. The results for these three countries, then, are not strictly comparable to the results for the rest of the countries.

Table 131 shows that, as expected, the coefficient of the variable that indicates experience in a modern occupation is negative in 26 of 31 countries and significant at the 0.01 level in 11 countries. This coefficient is positive but not statistically significant in Egypt, Mauritania and the Sudan. It is somewhat larger and positive in Benin and the Dominican Republic. Among the Latin American and Caribbean countries with negative coefficients on this variable (excluding Guyana, Jamaica, and Trinidad and Tobago), these coefficients imply that women in modern occupations would have, on average, a little over 0.5 child less after 20 years of marriage than women who had not worked since marriage. If Guyana, Jamaica, and Trinidad and Tobago are included, this difference would be approximately 0.75 child after 20 years of marriage. In Asia and Oceania, the average size of the negative coefficients is approximately 24, a rate that yields an expected difference of roughly 0.5 child over 20 years of marriage. None of the coefficients for the countries of Africa is

TABLE 131. PARTIAL REGRESSION COEFFICIENTS FOR OCCUPATION VARIABLES, WOMEN MARRIED THREE OR MORE YEARS: DEPENDENT VARIABLE = CHILDREN EVER BORN/DURATION OF MARRIAGE
(Births per 1,000 woman-years of marriage)

Region and country	Modern	Transitional	Mixed	Traditional	R^2	Percentage contributed to R^2 by occupation	Significance of occupation as a variable[a]
Africa							
Benin	46	−40	16	23[a]	0.140	3	X
Cameroon	−1	−5	−20	42[a]	0.173	8	X
Côte d'Ivoire[b]	−1	16	12	0	0.151	<1	−
Egypt	11	0	20[a]	4	0.201	<1	−
Ghana	−4	−8	21[a]	36[a]	0.086	9	X
Mauritania	7	14	46[a]	3	0.130	8	X
Morocco	−69	−56[a]	−20	−11	0.240	2	X
Senegal	−34	−5	−12	−15	0.146	1	−
Sudan	1	−22	−30[a]	−11	0.207	2	−
Tunisia	−20	−24	−8	5	0.187	<1	−
Latin America and the Caribbean							
Colombia	−45[a]	−21	−29[a]	1	0.177	4	X
Costa Rica	−37[a]	−3	−31[a]	6	0.196	3	X
Dominican Republic	31	−8	−30[a]	−2	0.220	3	X
Ecuador	−28	−9	−24[a]	−17	0.232	2	X
Guyana	−51[a]	−9	−6	2	0.171	3	X
Haiti	−4	−50	6	−1	0.097	9	X
Jamaica	−92[a]	−35[a]	−49[a]	−22	0.193	11	X
Mexico	−34[a]	−12	−23[a]	−12	0.222	2	X
Panama	−30[a]	−3	−23[a]	11	0.231	2	X
Paraguay	−42[a]	−38[a]	−30[a]	−4[a]	0.235	4	X
Peru	−11	−14	−13[a]	−18[a]	0.230	1	X
Trinidad and Tobago	−51[a]	−9	−24[a]	11	0.135	9	X
Asia and Oceania							
Bangladesh	−26	1	−15[a]	−26	0.198	1	X
Fiji	−24	−46[a]	−17	−19	0.145	5	X
Jordan	−10	−27	−28	17	0.241	1	−
Malaysia	−34[a]	−22[a]	−15[a]	1	0.250	1	X
Pakistan	−13	17	−2	4	0.154	<1	−
Philippines	−24[a]	−27[a]	−20[a]	−9	0.173	3	X
Republic of Korea	−39[a]	−20[a]	−10[a]	13[a]	0.399	2	X
Sri Lanka	−22	−29	−7	−13[a]	0.160	2	X
Thailand	−23	−43[a]	−22	−3	0.150	2	X

Source: World Fertility Survey standard recode tapes.
NOTE: Other variables in the equation are duration, duration squared, age at marriage, marital dissolution, type of place of residence, respondent's education and husband's occupation. Omitted category is no work since marriage.
[a] Statistically significant at the 0.01 level.
[b] Formerly called the Ivory Coast.

statistically significant; and they are quite variable, ranging from 46 in Benin to −69 in Morocco.

The coefficients of the variable that indicates participation in a traditional occupation also generally conform to expectations. In the majority of countries, women in traditional occupations bear children at a rate that is very similar to that of women who have not worked since marriage. Most of the coefficients are very close to zero and only seven are statistically significant; of these, four are positive and three are negative. The positive coefficients in Cameroon and Ghana, however, are relatively large, at 42 and 36, respectively.

The coefficients of the variables for the transitional and mixed categories are mostly negative, although their magnitude is somewhat less than that of the coefficients for the modern category. For the transitional category, 27 out of 31 coefficients are negative; eight of these are statistically significant at the 0.01 level. For the mixed category, 25 coefficients are negative and 15 of these are significant. In the Latin American and Caribbean countries, these coefficients imply that women in transitional occupations would have about 0.36 child less after 20 years of marriage than women with no work experience; the comparable number for women in mixed occupations would be 0.46. In Asia and Oceania, women in transitional occupations would have approximately 0.44 child less than women who have never worked and those in mixed occupations would have 0.30 child less. There is no consistent pattern in the African countries.

Although the overall signs of the coefficients are quite uniform across countries, except for the traditional category, their magnitude is rather small. The largest of the coefficients (for modern work in Jamaica) suggests a rate of childbearing that differs from that of women with no work experience since marriage by about 92 children per 1,000 woman-years, or almost two children over the course of 20 years. Most of the coefficients indicate much smaller differences. Nevertheless, when the statistical significance of the set of occupation variables was tested, they were significant in 24 countries. That is, occupation was significantly associated with fertility in over three quarters of the countries in the analysis. The seven

TABLE 132. PARTIAL REGRESSION COEFFICIENTS FOR OCCUPATION VARIABLES, WOMEN MARRIED THREE OR MORE YEARS, BY REGION AND LEVEL OF DEVELOPMENT: DEPENDENT VARIABLE = CHILDREN EVER BORN/ DURATION OF MARRIAGE

	Number of countries	Modern	Transitional	Mixed	Traditional	Number of countries in which occupation is significant[a] as a variable
Region						
Africa	10	−6	−13	3	8	5
Latin America and the Caribbean	12	−33	−18	−23	−4	12
Asia and Oceania	9	−24	−22	−15	−4	7
Level of development						
I. High	10	−44	−18	−23	−1	10
II. Middle-high	9	−17	−24	−20	−5	7
III and IV. Middle-low and low	12	−7	−12	2	4	7

Source: World Fertility Survey standard recode tapes.

NOTES: Other variables in the equation are duration, duration squared, age at marriage, marital dissolution, type of place of residence, respondent's education and husband's occupation. Omitted category is no work since marriage.

[a] Statistically significant at the 0.01 level.

countries in which the occupation variables were not significant are Côte d'Ivoire,[22] Egypt, Jordan, Pakistan, Senegal, the Sudan and Tunisia, all countries with significant Muslim populations. It may be the case that the high value placed on bearing children in such countries outweighs any effect that work has on fertility decisions. Nevertheless, in other countries with large Muslim populations, such as Malaysia, the relationship of work and fertility seems to be significant. More detailed ethnographic type studies may be needed to understand the relationship between work, religion and fertility. The contribution of the set of occupation variables to the total explained variance, R^2, is quite small, ranging from less than 1 per cent in Côte d'Ivoire, Egypt and Tunisia to 11 per cent in Jamaica.

Variation by macro-level characteristics

It may be possible to gain some insight into the sources of variation in the relationship between work and fertility by examining how the coefficients of the occupation variables vary with the macro-level characteristics of countries (Hermalin and Mason, 1980). Many previous studies have suggested that the negative relationship between work and fertility only appears, or at least is stronger, in more developed countries; but few, if any, studies have actually been able to investigate this assertion (see, for example, Stycos and Weller, 1967; Goldstein, 1972; Standing, 1978; Hass, 1972). This suggests that if countries are grouped according to their general level of socio-economic development, the coefficients should be larger in countries at higher levels of development than in countries at lower levels.

In figure 72, the coefficients of each of the occupation variables are plotted with the countries grouped according to their overall level of socio-economic development. For reasons of sample size, the countries at middle-low and low levels of development have been grouped together. The coefficients for those countries in which the set of occupation variables is not significant—Côte d'Ivoire, Egypt, Jordan, Pakistan, Senegal, the Sudan and Tunisia—are indicated by using shorter lines than those used for the rest of the countries.[23]

Examining first the variation across development groups within occupations, the coefficients of the variable indicating participation in a modern occupation are clearly more consistently negative and larger in absolute size in the countries at the upper levels of development than in countries at the lower development levels. In other words, in countries at relatively high levels of development, women in modern occupations consistently have fewer children than women with no work experience. There are several possible reasons for this pattern across levels of development. The types of jobs open to women that are classified as modern in relatively more developed countries may be somewhat different from modern jobs in relatively less developed countries. For example, women in modern jobs in countries in development group I may be more likely to work for large firms in offices where inflexible work-hours and no maternity benefits are the norm. In addition, they are likely to earn higher wages. It may also be true that increasing wages of domestic household employees and decreasing availability of traditional child-care substitutes in a developing economy reduce the ability of women in modern-sector jobs to combine employment and childbearing. In addition, discrimination against women in the modern-sector labour force may be less severe in these countries. As a result, career mobility, wages and, consequently, the opportunity costs of leaving a job are greater.

The coefficients of the variable indicating work in a transitional occupation show no strong pattern across levels of development. For the countries in development groups I and II, however, all of the coefficients are negative. In the low development group, five of the coefficients are positive or zero and seven negative.

The coefficients for the mixed occupation category are also all negative in development groups I and II. The variation in the magnitude of these coefficients is generally somewhat smaller than the variation in the transitional category coefficients, ranging from about −6 to −31, except for Jamaica, which has a coefficient of −49. The coefficients for the countries in development groups III and IV are extremely variable; 7 of the 12 are positive. They range from 46 in Mauritania to −30 in the Sudan. The lack of a clear pattern of an increasingly strong

Figure 72. **Partial regression coefficients of occupation variables, by level of socio-economic development**

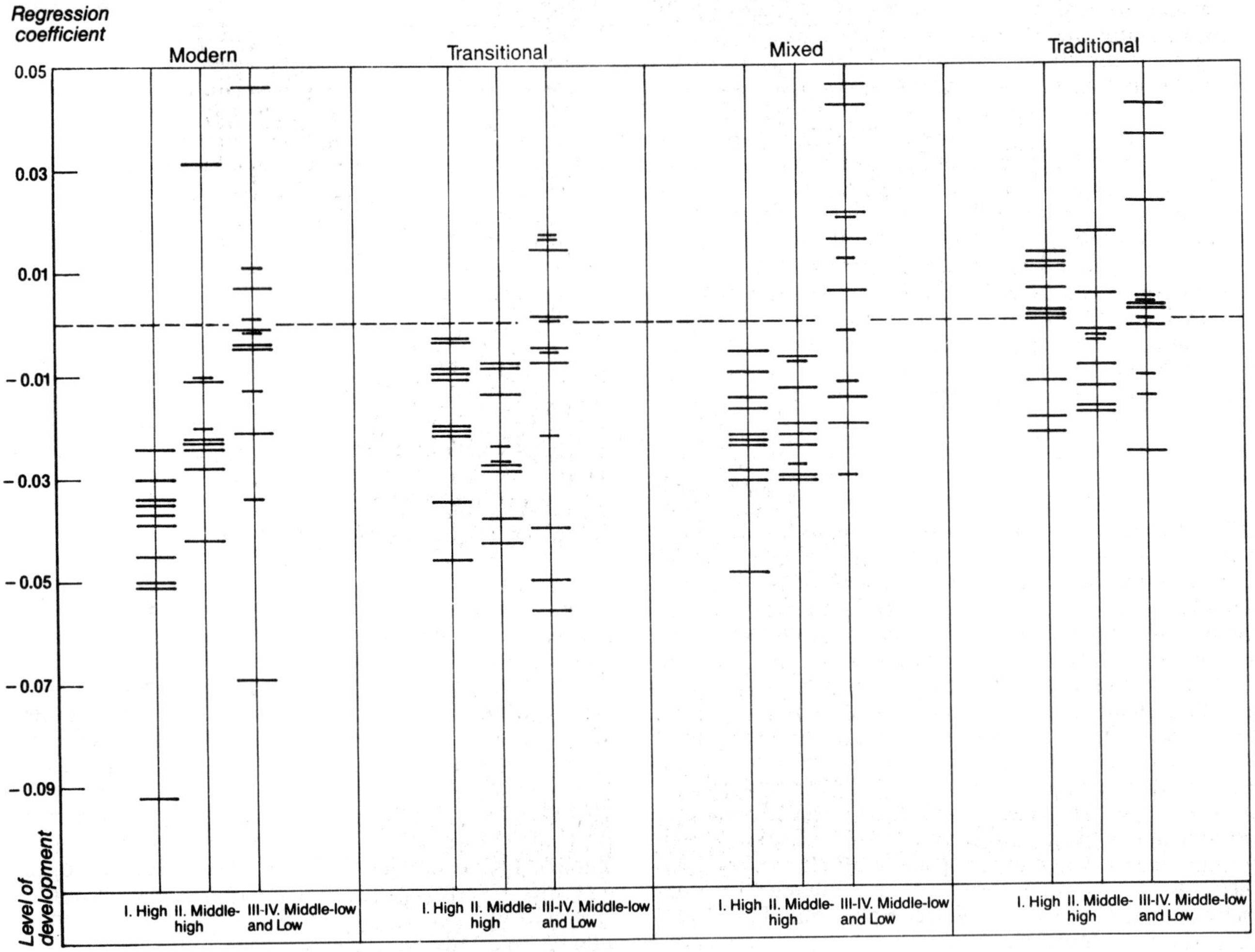

Source: World Fertility Survey standard recode tapes.
NOTE: Shorter lines are for coefficients that were not significant at 1 per cent level.

relationship with increasing development in these two middle categories of occupation is perhaps not surprising in the light of the wide range of activities included in these categories. Nevertheless, the relationship appears to be negative in the large majority of countries and somewhat more consistently negative in countries at higher levels of development than in countries at lower levels.

The coefficients of the variable indicating work in a traditional occupation appear to be independent of the level of development. In development group IV, the coefficients have a wide range, from 42 in Cameroon to −26 in Bangladesh. In group II, all but two of the coefficients are negative but the magnitude of the largest is less than 20. In the high development group, seven coefficients are positive and three are negative.

Comparing the coefficients across occupational categories within development groups, figure 72 suggests that, holding other factors associated with fertility constant, women in modern occupations in countries at relatively high levels of development bear children at a significantly lower rate than that for women in those same countries who do not work. The relationship between work in transitional and mixed occupations and the rate of childbearing is also negative but weaker. The rate of childbearing for women who have worked in a traditional occupation is approximately the same as the rate for non-working women.

In the middle-high development group, all of the coefficients (except three) for all of the occupational categories are negative, although the coefficients of the modern category are larger (more negative) than the coefficients of the other categories. This suggests that work of any type in these countries is associated with lower fertility. For the countries in groups III and IV, the coefficients are both positive and negative for all occupational categories and are rarely statistically significant. No type of work experience appears to be consistently related to the rate of childbearing in these countries.

The hypothesis that it is not likely, in general, that an association between work and fertility will appear unless a moderate to high level of socio-economic development has been achieved is supported by the foregoing observations. Where a large proportion of women are educated, live in urban areas, are working in modern settings, are receiving reasonable compensation for their work and are exposed to lower family size ideals and contraceptive information, childbearing is more likely to be assessed in terms of its opportunity costs. Moreover, it seems plausible that the social significance of women's work and the extent to which work confers or detracts from women's status and domestic autonomy may affect the strength and direction of the work-fertility relationship. An additional factor of importance may include how much control women are able to exercise over fertility decisions. In fact, the observation of statistically significant positive relationships between work in a traditional occupation and achieved fertility in countries at all levels of development suggests that the effect of achieved fertility on the likelihood of working is an important phenomenon in those environments where women are less likely to have full and effective control over their fertility. In the rest of the discussion, some of these more specific macro-level characteristics are considered. Since the variable that indicates experience in a modern occupation has proved, over all, to be the most strongly related to the rate of childbearing, this variable is the focus of the discussion.

The status of women in different cultural contexts is one factor that appears particularly likely to have some effect on the way in which work is related to fertility. The issue of how the status of women should be measured and exactly what it should measure is complex, and it is not addressed here. The term "status" is used to indicate the overall position of women in society, including the amount of control women exercise over economic, social, domestic and political spheres, the esteem accorded them and the amount of personal autonomy they enjoy (Curtin, 1982). Where the status of women in relation to men is high, work in a modern occupation may be more strongly associated with low fertility than where the status of women is low. The reason is that some of the mechanisms through which work experience is thought to affect fertility operate only in situations in which women have relatively high status. For example, unless women are free to leave their homes to travel to work, it is unlikely that they will be employed in the types of jobs that are associated with low fertility. If women are not permitted to hold certain jobs or if it is thought improper for them to work, this may also serve to discourage their participation in modern-sector employment. It is likely that the amount of control women have over personal and household decisions, such as fertility decisions, may also affect the extent to which work is related to childbearing. In addition, where the overall educational level of women is low and where women are not encouraged to continue their education, there will not be a supply of educated women available to fill modern-sector jobs.

In figure 73, the coefficients of the variable indicating work in a modern occupation from table 131 are plotted against a frequently used indicator of women's status, the gross enrolment ratio for females. A large proportion of the eligible female population enrolled in school is often considered indicative of relatively high status for women. Figure 73 shows that, in general, where a large proportion of females are in school, the relationship between modern-sector work and the rate of childbearing is more strongly negative than in countries where the school enrolment of females is low. An equivalent plot (not shown) of the regression coefficients against the singulate mean age at marriage for females suggests that in countries where women marry relatively late (a sign of relatively high female status), work in a modern occupation has a stronger negative association with fertility than in countries where women marry early.

Figure 73. Partial regression coefficients of variable indicating work in a modern occupation, by gross enrolment ratio for females, 1975

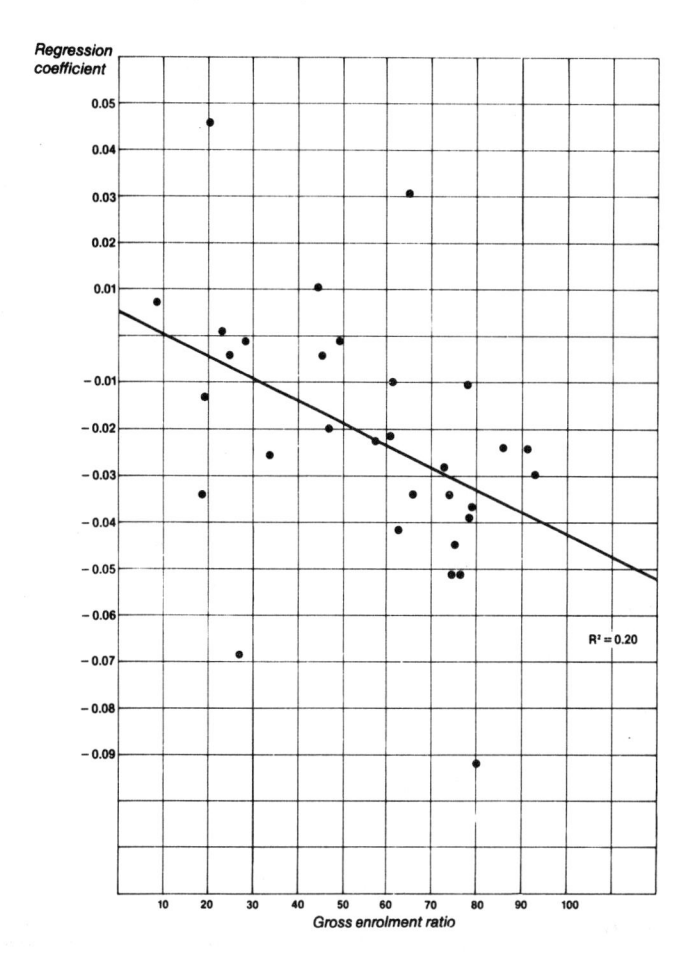

Sources: For gross enrolment ratio, United Nations Educational, Scientific and Cultural Organization (1980); for regression coefficients, table 131 based on World Fertility Survey standard recode tapes.
NOTE: Enrolment ratios for the Dominican Republic and Haiti are for 1974 and 1970, respectively.

Another factor that may be related to the strength and direction of the work-fertility relationship is women's access to family planning information and services. The theoretical arguments linking work in the modern sector with lower fertility imply that when work and childbearing are viewed as incompatible, women will voluntarily control their fertility. This seems more likely to occur in countries in which contraception is readily available. This hypothesis is generally supported by the pattern of coefficients shown in figure 74. The coefficients are grouped according to their score on the index of family planning programme strength, and the moderate and weak categories have been grouped together because of problems of sample size. Again, the seven countries for which the set of occupation variables are not significant are indicated with shorter lines. They are clearly more consistently negative and of greater magnitude (one exception is the Dominican Republic) in countries with strong programme effort than in countries with weak or no programme effort.

The results of the multivariate analysis presented above may be summarized as follows. A statistically significant

Figure 74. **Partial regression coefficients of variable indicating work in a modern occupation, by family planning programme effort**

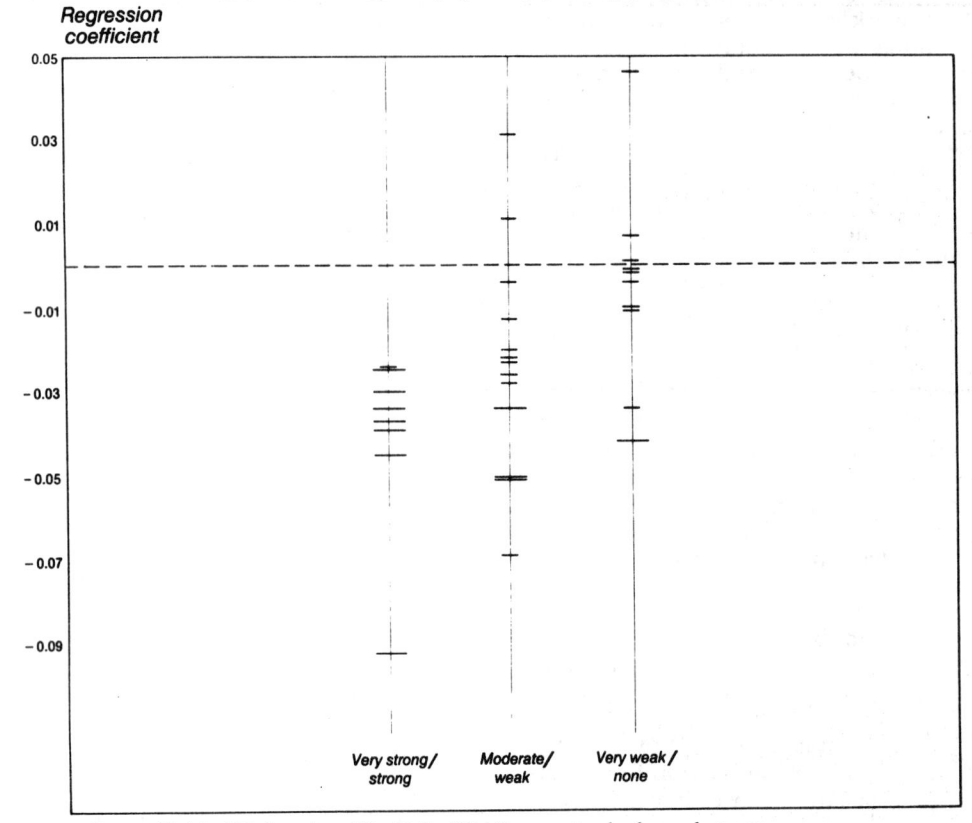

Source: Table 131, based on World Fertility Survey standard recode tapes.
NOTES: For derivation of index of family planning programme effort, see annex. Coefficients not significant at the 1 per cent level, in relation to the "no work" category, are indicated by shorter lines.

relationship between occupation and the rate of childbearing was found in 24 of 31 countries. The seven countries in which the relationship was not significant are Côte d'Ivoire, Egypt, Jordan, Pakistan, Senegal, the Sudan and Tunisia. The relationship between fertility and work in a modern occupation (in relation to no work experience) is generally negative. In every country in which this coefficient is statistically significant, it is negative. The relationship between experience in a transitional or mixed occupation and fertility is also overwhelmingly negative but this relationship is somewhat weaker. The association between work in a traditional occupation and fertility appears to be negligible in most countries. The results suggest that the strength of the relationship between work, particularly work in the modern sector, and childbearing depends upon the overall level of development, upon the availability of family planning information and services and upon the status of women in each country.

D. WOMEN'S WORK AND INTERMEDIATE VARIABLES

In this section, the relationship between women's work and four intermediate fertility variables, desired family size, contraceptive use, breast-feeding and fecundity, are discussed. These variables merit attention because differences in fertility are achieved through differences in the levels of these intermediate factors. Other such factors include abortion and foetal death, for which data are unavailable or are of poor quality; and age at marriage, which was discussed previously.

It should be noted that although the fertility differentials observed above refer to fertility since marriage, which is a cumulative measure, the differentials discussed here, which relate to the intermediate variables, are in most cases based on "current status" data. Thus, the evidence in this section cannot be directly related to the results of the fertility analysis. It should, however, provide an indication of the direction of the differentials and whether they are compatible with observed fertility differentials.

Desired family size

Consistent with the findings already presented in chapters VII and VIII, differences in desired family size between occupational groups are most pronounced in Africa, where occupational differentials in fertility are relatively small. Table 133 shows the results of the multivariate analysis with socio-economic controls for the 31 countries which had comparable occupational data with sufficient observations in each occupational group. Occupation as a variable was significant in explaining variation in family size desires in slightly less than one half of the countries, whereas it had been significant in more than three quarters of the countries when applied to fertility differentials. The observed differences in desired family size are negligible in most cases, in particular in Latin America and the Caribbean, in Asia and Oceania, and in development groups I and II. In Africa and in particular in sub-Saharan Africa, the differentials reach roughly 0.5 child, with women in modern

TABLE 133. SUMMARY OF PARTIAL REGRESSION COEFFICIENTS ACCORDING TO RESPONDENT'S OCCUPATIONAL GROUP, BY REGION AND LEVEL OF DEVELOPMENT: DEPENDENT VARIABLE = DESIRED FAMILY SIZE[a]

	Number of countries	Modern	Transitional	Mixed	Traditional	Number of countries in which occupation is significant[b] as a variable
Region						
Africa	10	−0.36	−0.29	−0.09	0.33	5
Latin America and the Caribbean	12	0.05	−0.07	−0.11	0.06	5
Asia and Oceania	9	−0.11	−0.21	−0.07	0.02	4
Level of development						
I. High	10	0.01	−0.03	−0.10	0.15	5
II. Middle-high	9	−0.11	−0.23	−0.12	−0.01	3
III and IV. Middle-low and low	12	−0.25	−0.26	−0.06	0.24	6
Sub-Saharan Africa	7	−0.51	−0.29	−0.09	0.46	3
Other	5	0.10	−0.23	−0.03	−0.07	3

Source: World Fertility Survey standard recode tapes.
NOTES: Other variables in model 3 are age, age squared, age at marriage, number of living children. In addition to these variables, model 4 includes respondent's education, residence, husband's education, husband's occupation. Omitted category is no work.
[a] Based on a sample of ever-married women.
[b] Statistically significant at the 0.01 level.

occupations desiring 0.5 child less than women who did not work and women in traditional occupations desiring roughly 0.5 child more. In a few African countries (Mauritania and Senegal), these differences approach one child. The pattern of these preference differentials is consistent with expectations and suggests that fertility differentials in Africa will become more apparent as contraceptive use becomes more widespread.

Contraceptive use

As stated above, it seems likely that the differences in fertility between women in different occupations are at least partially a result of differential contraceptive use. In particular, one expects that women working in those occupations which are most strongly associated with lower fertility, namely, modern-sector occupations, are more likely to use contraception than women in more traditional occupations or women who do not work.

A number of previous studies utilizing WFS data, however, have shown only small differences in contraceptive use between women with various types of work experience. In several recent United Nations studies (1981, 1985), the wife's occupation was strongly related to contraceptive use before education was controlled. Once the effect of education was accounted for, however, occupation was statistically significant in less than one half the countries covered in each case and differentials between occupational groups were significantly narrowed.

The analysis presented here includes data from countries that were not available when the previous study was conducted. In addition, the sample and variables are somewhat different. (They are comparable to the contraceptive use analysis utilized in chapters VII and VIII.) Differential use of contraception by occupation is examined using multiple classification analysis. This procedure allows calculation of the percentage of women currently using contraception in each category of current occupation after adjustment for other factors associated with contraceptive use. The countries included are the same as those included in the analysis of fertility, except for Pakistan.[24] Due to very small numbers of women working (i.e., fewer than 20) in some occupations, some categories have been combined.

The results of the analysis, given in figure 75 and table 134, show some puzzling findings. In the case of education and residence, differences in current contraceptive practice are consistent with patterns observed in achieved marital fertility, as would be expected. In the case of occupation, this is not so clear. In fact, in only 11 out of 30 countries is the occupation variable statistically significant in explaining variations in current contraceptive use. In 8 of the 30 countries, the proportion of women using contraceptives is less in modern occupations than in the "no work" category, when other factors are controlled. Among subgroup averages, the only differentials larger than five percentage points (which were defined as small differences in chapter VIII) are 10 percentage points higher use among women in modern occupations in Africa (compared with the "no work" category) and nine percentage points higher use in transitional occupations (e.g., services and domestic employment) in development group II. In the Latin American and Caribbean region, where fertility differentials by occupation were consistently large and statistically significant, only two countries (Jamaica and Haiti) show a statistically significant effect; and in the case of Haiti, the pattern is perverse although consistent with the fertility differentials for that country.

It appears, then, that differential contraceptive use by occupation is largely a reflection of the correlation of other socio-economic factors with occupation. Nevertheless, even after adjustment for these other factors in many countries, women who work in non-agricultural occupations have a higher level of use, on average, than both women who work in traditional agricultural occupations and those who do not work.

Since differences in fertility were shown to be greatest in countries at the highest levels of socio-economic development, differences in contraceptive use might also be

Figure 75. **Differential in contraceptive use between designated occupational group and "no work" category, by level of development**

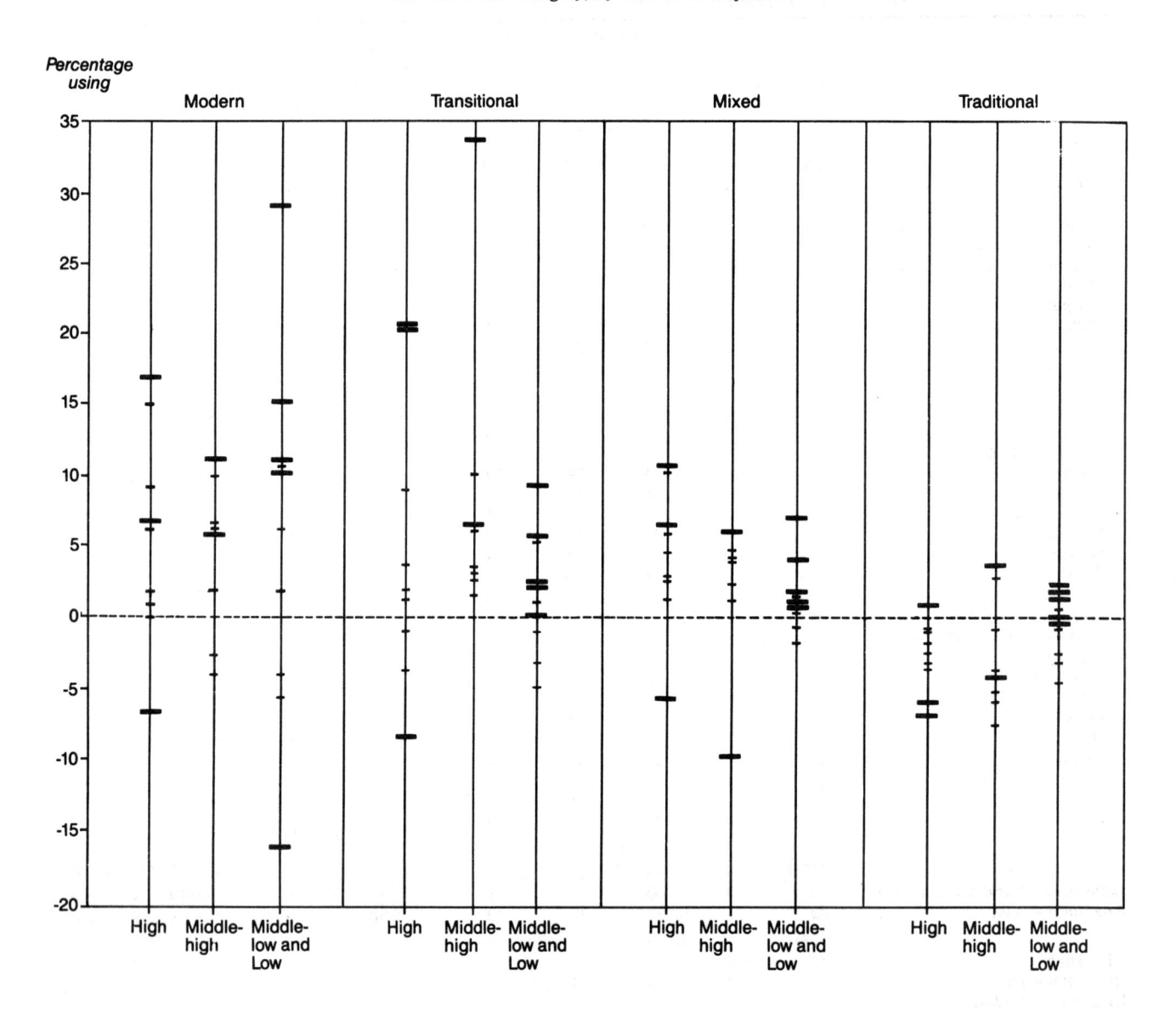

Source: Table 134.

expected to be greatest in such countries. In figure 75, the difference between the adjusted percentage of those in each of the four occupational categories who are currently using contraception and the percentage not working who are currently using contraception is shown with the countries grouped according to level of socio-economic development. Figure 75 shows no consistent pattern in contraceptive use differentials by development in terms of either the signs of the differences or the significance levels. This is largely because most of the countries showing significant and consistent findings are the least developed countries of Africa. It must be remembered that in this analysis, current work status is being related to current contraceptive practice. In countries where overall levels of use are low, current work status appears to be an important factor related to the use of contraception. In countries where current use levels are higher,

this is not as consistently the case. While this may be partially explained by the importance of other factors, such as education, and their interactions (which have not been measured here), it cannot provide a complete explanation because, when these other factors are controlled, contraceptive patterns by work status do not reflect the relationship with stage of development shown by fertility differentials in figure 72. This suggests the possibility that the work-fertility relationship is largely due to the effect of fertility on work, with women with larger families being less likely to work in occupations that are incompatible with child-rearing. In more developed countries, this relationship would be expected to be stronger because the process of modernization changes the nature of work in ways that would increase incompatibility with child-rearing. It could also be that unmeasured proximate variables are more important

TABLE 134. PERCENTAGE OF CURRENTLY MARRIED WOMEN WHO WERE CURRENTLY USING ANY CONTRACEPTIVE METHOD,
ACCORDING TO CURRENT OCCUPATION, BY COUNTRY, REGION AND LEVEL OF DEVELOPMENT

	Percentage using contraception[a]					Significance of occupation as a variable[b]	Differences from "no work" category			
	Modern	Transitional	Mixed	Traditional	No work		Modern	Transitional	Mixed	Traditional
A. Country										
Africa										
Benin	26	-----19-----		28	12	X	14	7	7	16
Cameroon	12	2	3	2	2	X	10	0	1	0
Côte d'Ivoire[c]	13	4	3	3	2	X	11	2	1	1
Egypt	19	30	26	22	25	–	–6	5	1	–3
Ghana	22	9	10	8	7	X	15	2	3	1
Mauritania	3	0	1	1	1	–	2	–1	0	0
Morocco	30	17	18	15	20	–	10	–3	–2	–5
Senegal	31	7	3	4	2	X	29	5	1	2
Sudan	11	0	4	4	5	–	6	–5	–1	–1
Tunisia	43	65	22	28	32	X	11	33	–10	–4
Latin America and the Caribbean										
Colombia	42	46	44	38	42	–	0	4	2	–4
Costa Rica	64	70	73	61	63	–	1	7	10	–2
Dominican Republic	28	35	35	24	32	–	–4	3	3	–8
Ecuador	40	36	34	29	34	–	6	2	0	–5
Guyana	41	31	36	28	32	–	9	–1	4	–4
Haiti	0	28	24	16	17	X	–17	9	7	–1
Jamaica	51	54	44	28	34	X	17	20	10	–6
Mexico	33	33	33	28	31	–	2	2	2	–3
Panama	59	54	59	52	53	–	6	1	6	–1
Paraguay	42	42	39	30	36	–	6	6	3	–6
Peru	30	35	34	28	32	–	–2	3	2	–4
Trinidad and Tobago	53	54	53	55	51	–	2	3	2	4
Asia and Oceania										
Bangladesh	4	9	8	6	8	–	–4	1	0	–2
Fiji	49	34	36	35	42	X	7	–8	–6	–7
Jordan	15	-----27-----		27	25	–	–10	2	2	2
Malaysia	25	52	38	33	32	X	–7	20	6	1
Philippines	40	40	40	37	34	X	6	6	6	3
Republic of Korea	50	31	36	34	35	–	15	–4	1	–1
Sri Lanka	33	34	32	33	31	–	2	3	1	2
Thailand	43	43	37	32	33	–	10	10	4	–1
B. Region[d]										
Africa	21	15	10	13	11		10	4	–1	2
Latin America and the Caribbean	40	43	42	32	38		2	5	4	–6
Asia and Oceania	32	35	32	30	30		2	5	2	0
C. Level of development[d]										
I. High	47	46	45	39	42		5	4	3	–3
II. Middle-high	35	41	34	30	32		3	9	2	–2
III and IV. Middle-low and low	16	11	10	10	9		7	2	1	1
TOTAL[d]	32	32	29	25	27		5	5	2	–2

Source: World Fertility Survey standard recode tapes.
[a] Adjusted for age, age squared, age at marriage, number of living children, residence, respondent's and husband's education and husband's occupation.
[b] Significant at the 0.01 level.
[c] Formerly called the Ivory Coast.
[d] Averages excluding combined categories.

here, such as the incidence of abortion as well as contraceptive use-effectiveness. While education is strongly related to the use of contraception, current work status may be more strongly related to the effectiveness of use, with working women adopting more effective methods, using them more effectively and possibly seeking abortion more frequently than non-working women. These patterns could also be related to development. Unfortunately, these hypotheses cannot be explained here at this point; it can only be concluded that the path through which the occupation-fertility relationship develops may differ from the path through which education and residence effects are manifested largely because education and residence characteristics are largely set before family-building begins, whereas work experience and fertility patterns develop after marriage and chance factors influencing early fertility can affect the course of a woman's working life in ways that cannot be measured with the WFS data.

Breast-feeding

Breast-feeding is another intermediate variable which is known to have a negative effect on fertility through its positive effect on the duration of post-partum amenorrhoea. Women who work in jobs associated with lower fertility (i.e., jobs in the modern sector) are expected to be less likely to breast-feed and to do so for shorter periods as a result of constraints imposed by such employment on the ability and desire to breast-feed. Thus, in the absence of contraceptive use, breast-feeding patterns according to type of occupation may actually serve to moderate fertility differences.

The particular aspect of work that is most often mentioned with regard to breast-feeding is its location. It may be the case that women who work away from home find it difficult to combine such work with breast-feeding a child. Most studies predict, therefore, that women who work away from home will be less likely to breast-feed and that those who do breast-feed will do so for a shorter period of time than women who do not work away from home.

A number of studies using WFS data have examined the relationship between various aspects of women's employment and breast-feeding. Again, however, the fact that the women's work variables in the WFS standard recode tapes refer to the entire period since marriage rather than to particular birth intervals causes difficulty in interpreting the results.

Jain and Bongaarts (1981) conducted a study in which they used breast-feeding data on currently married women from eight countries (Bangladesh, Colombia, Guyana, Indonesia, Jordan, Peru, Paraguay and Sri Lanka) whose penultimate birth had occurred between 3 and 15 years prior to the survey. The mean duration of breast-feeding in the last closed interval by place of work was estimated after adjustments for respondent's age, parity, education, place of residence and husband's occupation. They expected that since modernization usually implies a decrease in the duration of breast-feeding, women who worked on a family farm would have the longest average duration and women who worked away from home (not on a farm) would have the shortest duration. Although this particular pattern was not found, the results did show that in every country the breast-feeding duration for family farm workers was longer than the duration for women who worked away from home. This difference, however, was small, ranging from about six months in Bangladesh and five months in Panama to less than half a month in Colombia and Peru. These rather weak results are not very surprising in the light of the fact that the location-of-work variable refers to the current or most recent job since marriage and not to work in the birth interval in question. It seems likely that any effect of work away from home would appear only if the work was performed during the period immediately following a birth. The variable used by Jain and Bongaarts is intended only as an indicator of the "modernity" of a woman and is apparently not as useful as other such indicators, like education.

A more detailed study was conducted by Akin and colleagues (1981), using the Sri Lankan WFS data. The advantage of using the Sri Lankan data was that information was collected on work in specific birth intervals. A probit model was used to estimate the effect of various factors on the probability of breast-feeding at particular durations. Two dummy variables related to work were used; the first simply indicated whether the woman worked in the interval and the second indicated whether the woman worked away from home. The results suggested that, net of other factors associated with breast-feeding, work by itself did not have a substantively important effect on the probability of breast-feeding. Work away from home, however, had a significant negative effect on this probability at all durations. The magnitude of this effect varied across durations. For example, work away from home decreased the probability that a woman breast-fed for at least three months by about 4 per cent; the probability of breast-feeding for at least six months was reduced by 8 per cent and, at 12 months, by about 7 per cent.

In a comparative analysis of 28 WFS countries, Ferry and Smith (1983) use currrent status data on breast-feeding to estimate the mean duration of breast-feeding by work status (no work, self-employed, employed by others) and by work-place since marriage. They did not find any consistent pattern of differences by work status but did find that, without any control variables, women who worked away from home breast-fed for a shorter average period of time than women who worked at home.

Overall available evidence appears to indicate that work away from home is associated with lower prevalence and duration of breast-feeding. In the absence of contraceptive use, one would expect that the shorter duration of breast-feeding among women who work away from home would cause these women to have at least somewhat higher fertility than other women, not lower. It seems likely, therefore, that although the higher prevalence of breast-feeding among women who work at home may have some "contraceptive effect", this effect is outweighed by the deliberate limitation of fertility through contraception by women who work in the modern sector.

Fecundity

It has been suggested that the differential fertility of working and non-working women may result from a process whereby women who are subfecund are more likely to work because they do not have the constraints of childbearing and child-rearing which could prevent them from doing so. Thus, while it may be true that work has a negative effect on fertility, it may also be the case that the direction of causation runs in the opposite direction. It is exceedingly difficult, however, to bring to bear any conclusive evidence from the World Fertility Survey on this point.

In their analysis of recent marital fertility, Rodríguez and Cleland (1981) attempt to provide some evidence by examining differential fertility at short marital durations. They suggest that if subfecundity is randomly distributed across both work status groups and other socio-economic groupings, fertility differences by work status and, say, education at short marital durations, when the level of contraceptive use is quite low, should be of about the same magnitude. They found, in fact, that differences in fertility with respect to employment were no larger than differences by other socio-economic factors and concluded that fecundity was not the prior cause of both lower fertility and employment. It was later noted (Lloyd and Weinberger, 1981), however, that these results do not rule out the possibility that either higher subfecundity or a chance absence of births in the recent past among working women may have contributed to the strong relationship that Rodríguez and Cleland found between work and recent fertility.

Another, albeit crude, way to examine the issue of fecundity and work is to look at differences in self-reported fecundity[25] by work status. If subfecund women are more likely to work than other women, one would expect that the proportion who report that they are infecund of all women who have worked would be consistently higher than this proportion for women who have never worked. One might also expect to find differences between women in different occupations because infecund women may be more likely to pursue career-type jobs as a result of long periods of availability for work.

In table 135, the percentage of women who reported that they were infecund (i.e., thought at the time of the survey that they would be unable to have a(nother) child but had not been sterilized for contraceptive reasons) has been calculated for the same countries used in the analysis of fertility differentials. This percentage has been adjusted for age, education, husband's occupation and type of place of residence; it is averaged within regions by occupational groups. As shown in table 135, there are no consistent differences in self-reported fecundity between women by occupation since marriage.

TABLE 135. PERCENTAGE WHO REPORTED THEMSELVES INFECUND, BY TYPE OF OCCUPATION SINCE MARRIAGE AND BY REGION

Region	Modern	Transitional	Mixed	Traditional	No work
Africa	12.7	12.1	14.3	10.8	11.8
Latin America and the Caribbean	9.8	8.4	8.4	8.2	8.0
Asia and Oceania	9.2	15.2	13.5	11.4	11.1

Source: World Fertility standard recode tapes.

Among the countries studied in Latin America and the Caribbean, women with no work since marriage have the lowest reported infecundity and women in modern occupations the highest, but the difference is less than two percentage points. In the countries of Africa and of Asia and Oceania, it was found that women who had not worked since marriage were not consistently more or less likely to report themselves infecund than women who had worked; and among women who had worked since marriage, no occupational group was consistently more likely to report infecundity than another. Although these findings do not provide conclusive evidence on this point, they do suggest that observed fertility differentials between occupational groups are not likely to be explained to any significant degree by systematic differences in fecundity.

E. CONCLUSION

In this chapter, some evidence on the topic of women's work and its relationship to fertility has been presented for selected developing countries. The data presented here, however, perhaps do more to provoke questions than to provide answers. Two recent reviews of the evidence provided by WFS on this topic conclude that this relationship is "elusive" (Cleland, 1985) and "ambiguous" (Singh and Casterline, 1985). The large variation between countries in the proportion of women who work and the disparate distributions of women across different types of work invite questions about why women enter particular types of jobs in different settings. Certainly, the economy of each country determines to some extent the types of jobs available to women, but it may also be important to look at social, political and religious factors which influence the roles women play in different settings.

It has also been shown that the issue of how best to obtain information from women about their work is complex. Even small variations in the wording of questions appear to cause differences in interpretation and response.

A major part of this chapter was devoted to the analysis of fertility differentials according to occupation among ever-married women. As predicted by a number of hypotheses proposed in the demographic literature, the analysis revealed that women who work in the modern sector tend to have lower fertility than women who work in the traditional, agricultural sector and women who do not work. The fertility differentials were often small, however, despite the fact that occupation was statistically significantly related to fertility in 24 of 31 countries. After control for other socio-economic variables, women in modern occupations were found to bear children at a rate that would result in fertility about 0.5 child lower, on average, after 20 years of marriage, than that of women who did not work. Perhaps the most important finding is that the relationship between occupation and fertility appears to be strongest in countries at higher levels of socio-economic development. More specifically, the difference in fertility between women who work in the modern sector and women who work in the traditional sector or do not work is greatest in countries in development group I; and among the countries in development groups III and IV, no type of work activity appears to be consistently related to the rate of childbearing. This finding indicates that both the type of job a woman performs and the setting in which she performs it may have some impact on the extent to which work affects childbearing. Further evidence of this link is shown by the fact that the relationship between occupation and fertility is strongest where women's status is relatively high, as measured by educational attainment and age of marriage, and where strong family planning programmes operate.

The mechanisms through which these differences in fertility are achieved, however, is not clear. To the extent that one can measure them, differentials in fecundity and breast-feeding do not help to explain observed fertility differentials. Work before marriage appears to be associated with later age at marriage and may contribute to lower fertility not only through its effects on the age of marriage but through the likelihood of continued work after marriage. Levels of contraceptive use appear to be higher among women in modern-sector occupations than among women in traditional occupations and those who do not work. But the differentials are small and infrequently statistically significant, and the pattern of differentials does not show the same relationship with development that was apparent in the case of fertility. To date, the causal paths through which fertility and work are related have not been disentangled but the results with respect to contraceptive use suggest strongly that the effect of achieved fertility on subsequent work plays an important role in the measured relationship. That is, the number of children a woman has and when she has them determines in part whether she works, when she works and the type of work she does.

The relationship between work and fertility is clearly a complex one. A proper investigation of this relationship would require more detailed data than are currently available. In addition, further evidence obtained from ethnographic studies in which women are observed during the course of everyday life would provide valuable insights which could aid in both the formulation and the testing of more refined hypotheses.

Notes

[1] The increased economic activity of women will also lead to an increase in household income, which could in certain circumstances (depending upon trade-offs between preferences for number of children versus child quality) lead to a countervailing increase in family size desires. Empirically, however, the substitution effect or opportunity-cost effect has always been found to dominate the income effect when women's work is concerned.

[2] In the case of Fiji, Guyana and Malaysia, ethnic subgroups were examined as separate populations, so the number of units of analysis exceeded the number of countries.

[3] Most of the discussion of the measurement of women's labour force participation is taken from Anker (1983).

[4] Safilios-Rothschild (1977, p. 362) points out that a considerable number of women in developing countries are also involved in remunerative "illegal activities such as prostitution, brewing alcohol, or black market trading".

[5] Anker (1983a) describes a controlled survey experiment being conducted by the International Labour Organisation in Egypt and India. This experiment attempts to assess the effects on reported levels of labour force participation of questionnaire design, definition of labour force participation, sex of interviewer and whether the responses are by self or by proxy.

[6] It should be noted that the definition of work used in the World Fertility Survey did not include housework. In fact, respondents were specifically asked about any work other than their own housework, although the meaning of the word "housework" was not defined and is likely to have had different meanings in different contexts. In view of the fact that housework in developing countries is likely to include much productive work, such as fetching water and firewood, grinding corn, weaving cloth, making clothing, tending the vegetable garden and feeding poultry, it is important to point out that the respondents referred to in this study as "not working" or "never worked" are those who responded negatively to the questions about current or past work other than housework.

[7] A variety of other questions related to employment were included by a few countries. For example, in about half of the countries, questions were asked about the seasonality of work and about part- or full-time employment. Child care, family approval of women working and unemployment were topics that also received some attention.

[8] The labour force is defined as all employed and unemployed persons, which includes "employers, own account workers, employees, unpaid family workers, members of producers' cooperatives and members of the armed forces". (International Labour Office, 1978).

[9] In addition, the International Labour Organisation estimates include unemployed persons, while the World Fertility Survey estimates do not (at least not explicitly).

[10] The proportion of women aged 25-49 ever married calculated from available World Fertility Survey data is over 0.85 for every country except Colombia and Costa Rica.

[11] In Ghana, the interviewers' instructions were very explicit about the types of activities that were to be included. For example, the instructions state that women on leave without pay, seasonal workers and women who are not currently working because they are temporarily ill, laid-off or involved in a labour dispute were to be counted as working. Interestingly, although the World Fertility Survey argued that female interviewers should be used as much as possible, about three quarters of the interviewers in Ghana were male. It was asserted that Ghanaian women would be more likely to speak openly to male interviewers because they would be afraid of gossip from female interviewers (Scott and Singh, 1981).

[12] All of the findings discussed in this section are discussed more fully and detailed tables are presented in United Nations (1985).

[13] For a fuller discussion of age patterns of work, see United Nations (1982).

[14] For a more detailed explanation and examples of box and whisker plots, see Turkey (1977).

[15] For a full discussion of work status, stability and timing, see United Nations (1985).

[16] The World Fertility Survey standard recode tape codes for these occupations are: (a) modern, 1 and 2; (b) transitional, 6 and 7; (c) mixed, 3, 8 and 9; (d) traditional, 4 and 5.

[17] Another way in which work experience may affect fertility is through its effect on a woman's chances of further employment subsequent to marriage, as previously discussed (see United Nations, 1985, chap. III).

[18] A life-table type of analysis, which would control for exposure to risk, is not possible with the limited data available in most of these surveys.

[19] The question was worded as follows: "What (is, was) your occupation—that is, what kind of work (do, did) you do?".

[20] A comparison of women's occupations before and after marriage indicates that the majority of women who work in both periods continue in the same occupation. Of women who worked both before and after they were married, the percentage who fall into the same occupational category in both periods is over 65 in every country; in 12 countries, this figure is over 90 per cent.

[21] The results shown here are those given in United Nations (1985). These control variables differ somewhat from those used in the multivariate analysis of marital fertility given in chapters VII and VIII. This model was developed for United Nations (1985) before the models for chapters VII and VIII were finalized. However, coefficients estimated from a model consistent with chapters VII and VIII show substantially the same pattern of results with, if anything, slightly larger and more significant occupation effects.

[22] Formerly called the Ivory Coast.

[23] The significance level for the individual coefficients can be found in table 131. They are not shown in the figure because the individual coefficients were very volatile. Therefore, the statistical significance of the whole group of variables seemed to be a better measure of the relative weight to give the individual country findings.

[24] Pakistan was excluded because there were too few women in modern occupations currently using contraception.

[25] A number of problems are associated with measuring fecundity based on self-reports. Because the intent here is to examine not the actual levels of infecundity but only the differentials between occupations, and the factors that might be associated with differential accuracy of reporting are controlled, these biases should not be very important.

References

Akin, John and others (1981). The determinants of breast-feeding in Sri Lanka. *Demography* 18(3):287-308.

Anker, Richard (1983). Female labour force activity in developing countries: a critique of current data collection techniques. *International Labour Review* 122(6):709-723.

_____ (1983a). Effect on reported level of female labour force participation in developing countries of questionnaire design, sex of interviewer and sex/proxy status of respondent: description of a methodological field experiment. World Employment Programme, Research, Population and Labour Policies Programme working paper, No. 137. Geneva: International Labour Organisation.

_____ and James C. Knowles (1980). *Population Growth, Employment and Economic-Demographic Interactions in Kenya: Bachue-Kenya.* An International Labour Office report. New York: St. Martin's Press.

Boserup, Ester (1970). *Women's Role in Economic Development.* New York: St. Martin's Press.

Casterline, John B., Susheela Singh and John G. Cleland (1983). The proximate determinants of fertility: crossnational and subnational variations. Paper submitted to the Annual Meeting of the Population Association of America, Pittsburgh, Pennsylvania, 14-16 April 1983.

Chahil, Renu (1977). The status of women, work and fertility in India. In Stanley Kupinsky, ed., *The Fertility of Working Women: A Synthesis of International Research.* New York: Praeger Publishers, 146-171.

Cleland, John (1985). Marital fertility decline in developing countries: theories and the evidence. In John Cleland and John Hobcraft, eds., in collaboration with Betzy Dinesen, *Reproductive Change in Developing Countries: Insights from the World Fertility Survey.* Oxford: Oxford University Press, 223-252.

_____ G. Johnson-Acsádi and A. M. Marckwardt (1984). Towards a new core questionnaire for fertility surveys. Paper submitted to the World Fertility Survey Symposium, London, 24-27 April 1984.

Curtin, Leslie B. (1982). *Status of Women: A Comparative Analysis of Twenty Developing Countries*. Population Reference Bureau Reports on the World Fertility Survey, No. 5. Washington, D.C.: Population Reference Bureau.

Dixon, Ruth B. (1982) Women in agriculture: counting the labour force in developing countries. *Population and Development Review* 8(3):539-566.

Ferry, Benôit and David P. Smith (1983). *Breast-feeding Differentials*. World Fertility Survey Comparative Studies, No. 23: Cross-National Summaries. Voorburg, The Netherlands: International Statistical Institute.

Goldstein, Sidney (1972). The influence of labour force participation and education on fertility in Thailand. *Population Studies* 26(3):419-436.

Hass, Paula H. (1972). Maternal role incompatibility and fertility in urban Latin America. *Journal of Social Issues* 28(2):111-127.

Hermalin, Albert I. and William M. Mason (1980). A strategy for the comparative analysis of WFS data, with illustrative examples. In *The United Nations Programme for Comparative Analysis of World Fertility Survey Data*. New York: United Nations Fund for Population activities, 90-168.

Hull, Valerie J. (1977). Fertility, women's work and economic class: a case study from Southeast Asia. In Stanley Kupinsky, ed., *The Fertility of Working Women: A Synthesis of International Research*. New York: Praeger Publishers, 35-80.

International Labour Office (1978). *Yearbook of Labour Statistics 1978*. Geneva: International Labour Organisation.

Jain, Anrudh K. and John Bongaarts (1981). Breast-feeding: patterns, correlates, and fertility effects. *Studies in Family Planning* 12(3):79-99.

Kasarda, John D. (1971). Economic structure and fertility: A comparative analysis. *Demography* 8(3):307-317.

Kenya (1980). Ministry of Economic Planning and Development. Central Bureau of Statistics. *Kenya Fertility Survey 1977-1978, First Report*. Vol. 1. Nairobi.

Little, Roderick J. A. (1980). *Linear Models for WFS Data*. World Fertility Survey Technical Bulletin, No. 9 Tech./1282P. Voorburg, The Netherlands: International Statistical Institute.

Lloyd, Cynthia B. and Mary Beth Weinberger (1981). Letter captioned "Fertility and working women", in Letters to Editor. *People* 8(2).

Mason, Karen Oppenheim and V. T. Palan (1981). Female employment and fertility in Peninsular Malaysia: the maternal role incompatibility hypothesis reconsidered. *Demography* 18(4):549-575.

Miró, Carmen A. and Walter Mertens (1982). Influences affecting fertility in urban and rural Latin America. *The Milbank Memorial Fund Quarterly* 46(3), part 2:89-117.

Oppong, Christine (1983). Women's roles, opportunity costs and fertility. In Rodolfo A. Bulatao and Ronald D. Lee, eds., with Paula E. Hollerbach and John Bongaarts, *Determinants of Fertility in Developing Countries*, vol. 1, *Supply and Demand for Children*. Report of the National Research Council Committee on Population and Demography, Panel on Fertility Determinants. New York: Academic Press, 547-589.

_____ and Katherine Abu (1984). The changing maternal role of Ghanaian women: impacts of education, migration, and employment. World Employment Programme, Research, Population and Labour Policies Programme working paper, No. 143. Geneva, International Labour Organisation.

Recchini de Lattes, Zulma and Catalina H. Wainerman (1982). Female workers undercounted: the case of Latin America and Caribbean censuses. Working papers of the Latin American and Caribbean Regional Office of The Population Council.

Rodríguez, Germán and John Cleland (1981). Socio-economic determinants of marital fertility in twenty countries: a multivariate analysis. In *World Fertility Survey Conference 1980: Record of Proceedings*. London, 7-11 July 1980. Voorburg, The Netherlands: International Statistical Institute, vol. II, 337-414.

Safilios-Rothschild, Constantina (1977). The relationship between women's work and fertility: some methodological and theoretical issues. In Stanley Kupinsky, ed., *The Fertility of Working Women: A Synthesis of International Research*. New York: Praeger Publishers, 354-368.

Scott, Chris and Susheela Singh (1981). Problems of data collection in the World Fertility Survey. In *World Fertility Survey Conference, 1980: Record of Proceedings*. London, 7-11 July 1980. Voorburg, The Netherlands: International Statistical Institute, vol. 3, 17-94.

Singh, Susheela (1984). *Comparability of Questionnaires: Forty-one WFS Countries*. World Fertility Survey Comparative Studies, No. 32: Cross-National Summaries. Voorburg, The Netherlands: International Statistical Institute.

_____ and John Casterline (1985). The socio-economic determinants of fertility. In John Cleland and John Hobcraft, eds., in collaboration with Betzy Dinesen, *Reproductive Change in Developing Countries: Insights from the World Fertility Survey*. Oxford: Oxford University Press, 199-222.

Smith, David P. (1980). *Age at First Marriage*. World Fertility Survey Comparative Studies, No. 7: Cross-National Summaries. Voorburg, The Netherlands: International Statistical Institute.

Standing, Guy (1978). *Labour Force Participation and Development*. Geneva: International Labour Organisation.

Stycos, J. Mayone and Robert Weller (1967). Female working roles and fertility. *Demography* 4(1):210-217.

Tukey, John W. (1977). *Exploratory Data Analysis*. Reading, Massachusetts: Addison-Wesley Publishing Co.

United Nations, 1979. Department of International Economic and Social Affairs. Population Division. *Review and Appraisal of the World Population Plan of Action*. Population Studies, No. 71. New York. Sales No. E.79.XIII.7.

_____ (1980). Some implications of variations in type and duration of work for the analysis of WFS data. Paper prepared for the Fourth Meeting of the United Nations Working Group on Comparative Analysis of World Fertility Survey Data, Geneva, 18-21 November 1980. UN/UNFPA/WFS.IV/16. New York.

_____ (1981). *Variations in the Incidence of Knowledge and Use of Contraception: A Comparative Analysis of World Fertility Survey Results for Twenty Developing Countries*. Non-sales publication ST/ESA/SER.R/40. New York.

_____ (1981a). Occupational classification systems constructed for application in the United Nations programme of international comparative analysis of the World Fertility Survey data. Working paper ESA/P/WP/70. New York.

_____ (1982). Some demographic characteristics of women's work patterns and rates in ten World Fertility Survey countries, In *World Population Trends and Policies, 1981 Monitoring Report*, vol. I, *Population Trends*. Population Studies, No. 79. New York: 207-215. Sales No. E.82.XIII.2.

_____ (1984). *Report of the International Conference on Population, 1984*, Mexico City, 6-14 August 1984. New York. Sales No. E.84.XIII.8.

_____ (1985). *World Population Trends, Population and Development Interrelations and Policies, 1983 Monitoring Report*, vol. I, *Population Trends*. Population Studies, No. 93. New York. Sales No. E.84.XIII.10.

_____ (1985a). *Women's Employment and Fertility: Comparative Analysis of World Fertility Survey Results for 38 Developing Countries*. Population Studies, No. 96. New York. Sales No. E.85.XIII.5.

United Nations Educational, Scientific and Cultural Organisation (1980). *UNESCO Statistical Yearbook 1980*. Paris.

Ware, Helen (1977). Women's work and fertility in Africa. In Stanley Kupinsky, ed. *The Fertility of Working Women: A Synthesis of International Research*. New York: Praeger Publishers, 1-34.

Annex to Part Two

THE MULTIVARIATE MARITAL FERTILITY MODEL

The purpose of this annex is to provide a detailed discussion of the procedure followed for the estimation of fertility differentials in chapters VII-IX. The discussion includes an overall description of the fertility model used, its implications and its interpretation. Details concerning specific explanatory and control variables included in the models presented in each chapter are addressed in the appropriate chapter.

The basic fertility measure, which measures fertility cumulated up to the date of the interview, is children ever born, CEB. Two problems arise, however, when CEB is used as a dependent variable in an additive regression model (Little, 1980). The first problem is that in an additive model, differences in CEB between categories of an independent variable are assumed to be the same for all marriage durations. This is probably an inaccurate specification because CEB increases as duration increases, and differences in the number of children ever born appear likely to become larger with increasing duration of marriage as well. A more plausible assumption is that differences in CEB between categories of a variable are proportional to duration of marriage. In other words, differences in the rate of childbearing per year of marriage between categories of an independent variable are constant. Therefore, the dependent variable used here is children ever born (CEB) divided by years since first marriage, D. For purposes of clarity of presentation, CEB/D is multiplied by 1,000. Thus, this variable may be interpreted as births per 1,000 woman-years since first marriage.

A second problem with using CEB or CEB/D as the dependent variable is that the linear regression assumption of constant variance in the error term for all observations (homoscedasticity) is violated. The variance of CEB/D when D is small is likely to be larger than the variance of CEB/D when D is large. This causes statistical tests to be unreliable. To correct this problem, the observations are commonly weighted, using weights that are inversely proportional to the variance. An inspection of the variance of CEB/D for several countries revealed that its variance is generally very high in the first two or three years of duration; and, thereafter, it declines more or less linearly. This pattern is especially strong in countries in which pre-marital births are common. For this reason, women with under three years of marital duration have been removed from each sample for the regression analysis. For the remaining cases the procedure suggested by Little (1980) is adopted, in which it is assumed that the variance of CEB/D is inversely proportional to D and that the weights are therefore proportional to D. Each observation is thus given a weight equal to the respondent's marital duration. For samples that were not self-weighting, sampling weights were also employed in the analysis: the weighting factor was the sampling weight times marital duration. The weights are then scaled so that the observations sum to the correct total number of cases.

In chapters VII-IX of part two, the explanatory variables of interest (type of place of residence, years of education, woman's occupation) were entered into the fertility model as a set of dummy variables. Thus, in each case, the coefficients presented are correctly interpreted as the difference in number of children born per 1,000 woman-years of marriage between each category of the explanatory variable and the omitted category, net of other factors. A more intuitively appealing result is obtained by dividing the coefficient by 100 or by 50, yielding the difference in number of children born after 10 and 20 years of marriage, respectively.

It should also be noted that the results reported in part two are evaluated at the 0.01 level of significance rather than the more conventional 0.05 level. This more conservative test has been used because violation of the homoscedasticity assumption, while partially corrected by the weighting procedure, makes statistical testing less reliable than would be the case if the statistical assumption had been met. In addition, the statistical tests assume that a simple random sample was used.

REFERENCE

Little, Roderick J. A. (1980). *Linear Models for WFS Data*. World Fertility Survey Technical Bulletin, No. 9/Tech. 1282P. Voorburg, The Netherlands: International Statistical Institute.

PART THREE. REGIONAL PERSPECTIVES FROM THE DEVELOPING COUNTRIES

X. A REVIEW OF THE FERTILITY SITUATION IN COUNTRIES IN THE REGION OF THE ECONOMIC AND SOCIAL COMMISSION FOR ASIA AND THE PACIFIC

*Economic and Social Commission for Asia and the Pacific**

ABSTRACT

The World Fertility Survey findings from 10 countries in the region of the Economic and Social Commission for Asia and the Pacific (ESCAP)—Bangladesh, Fiji, Indonesia, Malaysia, Nepal, Pakistan, the Philippines, the Republic of Korea, Sri Lanka and Thailand—canvassed mostly around the mid-1970s, are presented in this chapter. The major similarities and differences between these countries in fertility behaviour are highlighted and policy implications of the findings are discussed.

Estimates of total fertility rates for the five years before the survey ranged from 6.3 children per woman in Pakistan to 3.8 per woman in Sri Lanka, while fertility rates among married women for the same period ranged from 8.8 children in the Philippines to 6.3 in Fiji. The parity distribution of women shows that the majority of women in the ESCAP countries had given birth to six or more children by the time they reached their thirties. For the six countries with reliable trend information, declines in total fertility rates over a 10-year period before the survey ranged from 23 per cent in the Republic of Korea to 38 per cent in Fiji, with the rate of decline being higher in the more recent five-year period. For the most part, larger declines occurred in the two extreme age groups—among women under 20 years and those 30 years or over. Small declines in marital fertility were observed but declines were confined mostly to the older age groups.

Analysis of the determinants of fertility change showed that rising age at marriage and increases in contraceptive prevalence were the primary factors responsible for fertility change in those ESCAP countries in the process of transition. The proportion of women using contraception varied substantially between countries, from only 2 per cent of currently married women reported currently using in Nepal to 37 per cent in Fiji. The impact on fertility change of contraceptive use is negligible in Bangladesh, Nepal and Pakistan but is greater in Fiji and Thailand. Residence had a strong relationship with fertility, and although factors such as education and work status were found to be associated with fertility, the relationship was not entirely straightforward. Total marital fertility rates were systematically lower at higher levels of education in all countries except Indonesia and Sri Lanka, where women with no education had lower fertility than those with some education.

Over the past two decades, the rapid growth of population has been a matter of great concern for most of the countries in the region of the Economic and Social Commission for Asia and the Pacific (ESCAP). As attempts were made to solve the problem of population growth through fertility reduction, analysis of fertility behaviour of the population became the focus of attention of policy-makers and scholars. Analysis of fertility behaviour is also essential in order to monitor and evaluate the impact of national family planning programmes, to ascertain the population situation in the countries of the region and to prepare population projections needed for development plans. A comparative analysis of fertility behaviour among the countries of the ESCAP region is a meaningful approach which can contribute to understanding of such behaviour.

The absence of a reliable vital registration system has seriously limited the study of fertility behaviour in most of these countries. Although periodic surveys have been conducted to overcome this deficiency, the data had not been readily usable for inter-country comparative analysis owing to great variations in quality, coverage and timing of the survey. Therefore, in the early 1970s the World Fertility Survey (WFS) programme was initiated to assist a large number of countries to carry out nationally representative and internationally comparable surveys of human fertility behaviour. The WFS data thus collected provide a rare opportunity for comparative analysis of fertility behaviour in the countries of the ESCAP region. This comparative analysis is intended to draw a clear

---

*Population Division.

picture of the fertility situation by presenting estimates of fertility levels and taking note of the changes occurring along with the factors associated with these changes.

A. THE DATA

In the comparative analysis of fertility, questions are often raised about the validity and reliability of the data, which are a function not only of sampling design but of non-sampling factors, such as respondents' and interviewers' errors, which affect the quality of the data differentially from country to country. These problems are compounded by socio-cultural differences between the countries, which further limit the generalizations that can be drawn from the data. The main source of data for this analysis is the individual maternity histories obtained in the surveys of the participating countries. The limitation for fertility analysis of this approach is well documented in the demographic literature. Although the quality of the WFS data stands out quite remarkably compared with other surveys and censuses, the data are not free of three main sources of error: misreporting of respondent's age and omission of and displacement of events over time. Evaluation of the WFS data is a separate issue and has been studied quite intensively (Chidambaram, Cleland and Verma, 1980; United Nations, 1983, 1986). A summary of findings on data quality can be found in the annex to chapter I. Only the relevant parts of the findings are mentioned below to provide the necessary caution in interpreting the results of this analysis of the ESCAP region.

In terms of coverage of live births, the surveys in the ESCAP countries achieved major improvement, giving consistently higher means for older age groups than other sources (United Nations, 1983). The detailed country evaluation reports indicated that many of the maternity histories were characterized by some omissions of births, but for the majority of the countries, the level of omission is not high and seemed to occur for only the oldest cohorts.[1] Displacement of dates of birth was found to be more prevalent (or detectable) than omission of births. Older women tend to have displaced their early births towards the survey date, which resulted for some countries in the overreporting of births in the periods from 5 to 14 years prior to the survey. For the period five years prior to the survey, comparisons of the WFS data with reliable data from other sources show that they appear to agree closely in most cases (see chapter I for exceptions). The WFS data could therefore be used without much difficulty to establish the level and pattern of fertility but greater caution needs to be exercised in analysing trends over the 15-year period prior to the survey.

The measure of the current level of fertility is mainly based on current parity and the total fertility rate. Age-specific fertility rates for the period five years prior to the survey are considered to establish the pattern and the current level of fertility.[2] The analysis of trends is limited to the period 5-10 years prior to the survey by comparing the period 0-4 years with the period 5-9 years prior to the survey.

This chapter presents findings from 10 countries in the region—Bangladesh, Fiji, Indonesia, Malaysia, Nepal, Pakistan, the Philippines, the Republic of Korea, Sri Lanka and Thailand.

B. LEVELS AND PATTERNS OF FERTILITY

In this section, the number of children ever born— i.e., current parity—is used to measure the level of fertility and the tempo of childbearing among various cohorts of women. The percentage distribution of women by number of children and the age-specific fertility rates are examined to determine the childbearing patterns and the current or recent fertility levels.

Current parity and early marital fertility parity distribution: patterns of childbearing

The percentage distribution of all ever-married women according to the number of children ever born is given in table 136. Childlessness[3] (by ages 45-49) among women in the ESCAP countries varies quite considerably; those in the Republic of Korea appear to have the lowest proportion (1.6 per cent), while the largest proportion was found among Indonesian women (9 per cent). The next most striking feature of the parity distribution is that many women had given birth to six or more children by the time they reached their thirties: more than 40 per cent of the women aged 35-39 (except in the Republic of Korea); and more than 50 per cent of age group 45-49 (except in Indonesia). These proportions clearly indicate the prevalence of high fertility among older women in the region. Table 137 shows that, on average, Asian women of reproductive ages had borne about four children, with little variation among countries. It is important to take note that by ages 30-34, women in all countries except the Republic of Korea had borne nearly four children, and among older cohorts the number was higher.

Table 138 shows that in all countries except Nepal women in their first marriage for a duration of from five to nine years had at least two children. Childbearing appears to slow (meaning a difference of less than one child between each successive marriage cohort) at different marriage durations in different countries. In the Republic of Korea, women married for more than 10 years had less than one child difference between each of the older five-year marriage duration groups. The same is true in Bangladesh, Indonesia, Malaysia and Nepal, among women married for more than 15 years; and in Pakistan, the Philippines, Sri Lanka and Thailand, the tempo of childbearing is slower among women married more than 20 years. In Fiji, no pattern is observed. The data presented above represent a cross-section of marriage cohorts; therefore, no conclusive remarks can be made on the pace of childbearing among the various marriage cohorts.

Current fertility

The current level of fertility is more precisely measured by the total fertility rate (TFR), which, as a summary measure, has several advantages over alternative summary measures of fertility. In the analysis of current fertility, the total fertility rate of the most recent year would have been ideal. Owing to the relatively large sampling errors found for the annual estimates, however, an average rate based on the past five years which could be used with reasonable confidence for estimating the current level of fertility is recommended (Chidambaram, Cleland and Verma, 1980; United Nations, 1983). The following analysis of the current level of fertility is based on the total fertility rates for the period 0-4 years prior to the survey.

TABLE 136. PERCENTAGE DISTRIBUTION OF EVER-MARRIED WOMEN AGED 30-49, BY NUMBER OF CHILDREN EVER BORN, FOR FIVE-YEAR AGE GROUPS, COUNTRIES IN THE ESCAP REGION

Percentage distribution by children ever born for age group

Country	30-34 Zero	30-34 One to two	30-34 Three to five	30-34 Six or more	35-39 Zero	35-39 One to two	35-39 Three to five	35-39 Six or more	40-44 Zero	40-44 One to two	40-44 Three to five	40-44 Six or more	45-49 Zero	45-49 One to two	45-49 Three to five	45-49 Six or more	All ages Zero	All ages One to two	All ages Three to five	All ages Six or more
Bangladesh	2.5	6.1	35.3	56.1	1.6	4.1	22.3	72.1	2.7	6.0	17.6	73.5	2.7	7.9	21.8	67.7	14.3	24.8	30.1	30.8
Fiji	5.2	14.8	53.9	26.1	4.2	12.5	36.7	46.6	3.9	9.9	27.3	59.0	6.8	9.3	19.3	64.7	11.4	27.9	34.6	26.1
Indonesia	6.3	21.8	44.2	27.7	5.9	17.2	34.5	42.4	4.8	15.8	30.8	48.6	9.0	18.1	25.2	48.2	13.4	32.0	31.1	23.6
Malaysia	2.7	19.1	50.3	27.7	2.0	12.6	36.8	48.7	2.6	11.1	30.5	55.9	3.1	12.7	27.2	56.9	7.5	26.3	35.5	30.6
Nepal	4.7	17.3	52.9	25.2	3.1	13.0	38.3	45.6	4.4	11.1	33.6	50.8	4.5	11.1	31.4	53.1	17.8	27.6	33.2	21.3
Pakistan	4.5	12.7	38.5	44.4	4.5	8.0	26.0	61.5	4.2	5.5	18.5	71.8	2.9	7.5	20.7	68.7	14.1	22.7	29.2	33.9
Philippines	2.4	18.5	50.9	28.0	2.4	9.8	34.7	53.2	2.3	7.8	25.3	64.6	2.6	7.2	21.5	68.9	4.9	24.4	35.9	34.7
Republic of Korea	2.8	21.3	70.1	5.8	1.3	10.0	63.9	24.8	1.5	9.7	45.8	42.9	1.6	7.5	35.0	55.9	6.5	28.4	45.4	19.7
Sri Lanka	5.2	23.4	49.7	21.7	3.9	16.8	38.9	40.3	4.2	12.8	32.0	51.1	3.2	13.2	26.7	57.0	8.4	28.6	35.2	27.8
Thailand	2.5	24.9	50.2	22.3	1.5	15.0	53.2	40.3	2.5	11.0	28.2	58.3	2.6	8.2	25.7	63.5	8.0	30.9	34.2	26.8

Source: Hodgson and Gibbs (1980), table 1.

TABLE 137. MEAN NUMBER OF CHILDREN EVER BORN TO EVER-MARRIED WOMEN, BY CURRENT AGE GROUP, COUNTRIES IN THE ESCAP REGION

Country	Under 20	20-24	25-29	30-34	35-39	40-44	45-49	All ages	Sample population
Bangladesh	0.7	2.4	4.2	5.7	6.7	7.1	6.7	4.0	6 515
Fiji	0.5	1.5	2.7	4.2	5.2	6.2	6.6	3.8	4 928
Indonesia	0.6	1.7	2.8	4.0	4.8	5.3	5.2	3.5	9 155
Malaysia	0.8	1.7	2.8	4.2	5.5	6.1	6.2	4.2	6 321
Nepal	0.3	1.4	2.9	4.1	5.1	5.6	5.8	3.3	5 941
Pakistan	0.6	1.9	3.4	5.0	6.0	7.0	6.9	4.2	4 952
Philippines	0.8	1.9	3.0	4.3	5.7	6.7	7.0	4.6	9 268
Republic of Korea	0.5	1.0	2.0	3.4	4.4	5.1	5.8	3.6	5 430
Sri Lanka	0.7	1.5	2.5	3.8	4.9	5.5	6.0	3.9	6 810
Thailand	0.7	1.5	2.6	3.9	4.9	6.1	6.8	3.9	3 820

Source: Hodgson and Gibbs (1980), table 5.

TABLE 138. MEAN NUMBER OF CHILDREN EVER BORN TO ALL EVER-MARRIED WOMEN, BY NUMBER OF YEARS SINCE FIRST MARRIAGE, COUNTRIES IN THE ESCAP REGION

Country	Under 5	5-9	10-14	15-19	20-24	25-29	30+	All durations	Sample population
Bangladesh	0.6	2.1	3.5	5.0	6.1	6.9	6.8	4.0	6 515
Fiji	1.0	2.6	3.9	5.0	5.7	6.7	7.4	3.8	4 928
Indonesia	0.7	2.1	3.3	4.3	5.0	5.4	5.4	3.5	9 155
Malaysia	1.1	2.8	4.1	5.3	6.2	6.8	6.2	4.2	6 321
Nepal	0.5	1.7	3.1	4.4	5.3	5.8	6.1	3.3	5 941
Pakistan	0.6	2.5	4.1	5.4	6.5	6.9	7.2	4.2	4 952
Philippines	1.2	2.9	4.4	5.8	7.1	7.9	8.5	4.6	9 268
Republic of Korea	1.1	2.7	3.7	4.4	5.1	5.5	6.3	3.6	5 430
Sri Lanka	0.9	2.4	3.8	4.8	5.8	6.5	7.0	3.9	6 810
Thailand	0.9	2.5	3.8	5.0	6.1	7.2	7.5	3.9	3 820

Source: Hodgson and Gibbs (1980), table 7.

Total fertility rate

From table 139 it is quite evident that in terms of the total fertility rate, there is a wide variation in levels of current fertility among countries of the ESCAP region. According to these estimates, Pakistani women, who are likely to have roughly 6.3 children in their lifetimes, seem to have the highest fertility; the lowest was found among Sri Lankan women, 3.8 births per woman. These estimates indicate that even in such countries as Sri Lanka, where fertility is known to have declined in recent years, the fertility levels were almost twice as high as the replacement level of fertility.

Total marital fertility rate

The total fertility rate is determined by a set of factors, such as age at marriage, nuptiality patterns, breast-feeding, sterility and subnormal fecundity, and contraceptive use. The difference between populations can be understood in terms of differences in these factors. It is therefore necessary to consider the total marital fertility rates (TMFR) from which the effects of age at marriage and the nuptiality pattern on fertility have been removed. The total marital fertility rates for within-union fertility after age 30, as presented in column (2) of table 139, show very clearly that the older women in the region still bear children during the later reproductive ages. However, the variations observed in the fertility of this group reflect mainly differences in the prevalence of contraception, induced abortion or prolonged sexual abstinence.

Total marital fertility, which includes all births since first marriage, ranged from 6.26 in Fiji to 8.85 in the Philippines, which certainly reflects the high level of fertility among married women. The range of variations in marital fertility among countries is narrower, as compared with the range of variations in total fertility rates. The relationship between the two rates is primarily a function of the proportion ever married and indicates the effect of different nuptiality patterns on the fertility level.

Fertility pattern

The frequency of childbearing varies markedly from one age group to another within a population. The age pattern of fertility found among women in countries of the ESCAP region can be seen in table 140. For the purpose of this analysis, age-specific fertility rates for the period 0-4 years prior to the survey are considered. Five-year period rates are considered to describe better the current fertility pattern, for the reasons stated earlier.

The women in Bangladesh, Fiji and Indonesia reach their peak period of fertility at ages 20-24, while women in Malaysia, Nepal, Pakistan, the Philippines, the Republic of Korea, Sri Lanka and Thailand reach their peak period at 25-29 years. In this respect, there are two distinct groups of countries, with Nepal and Thailand showing a relatively broad peak across the twenties.

Some interesting inter-country differences that are revealed by the age pattern of fertility were not so evident from looking at the total fertility rates. In all countries, except in the Republic of Korea, the births occurred in

TABLE 139. TOTAL FERTILITY RATE AND TOTAL MARITAL FERTILITY RATE FOR THE FIVE YEARS PRECEDING THE SURVEY, COUNTRIES IN THE ESCAP REGION

Country	Total fertility, rate, ages 15-49 (1)	Total marital fertility rate, ages 30-44 [a] (2)	Total marital fertility rate, ages 15-49 (3)
Bangladesh	6.08	2.40	6.43
Fiji	4.22	1.62	6.26
Indonesia	4.73	1.88	5.78
Malaysia	4.66	2.08	7.65
Nepal	6.01	2.75	6.97
Pakistan	6.26	2.84	7.52
Philippines	5.25	2.85	8.85
Republic of Korea	4.28	1.75	7.26
Sri Lanka	3.75	1.99	6.89
Thailand	4.63	2.32	7.22

Sources: For columns (1) and (3), chapter I, tables 12 and 13, respectively, in the present volume; for column (2), Alam and Casterline (1984).

[a] Within a reunion.

fairly widespread fashion among different age groups and a substantial number of births occurred to older women. In the Republic of Korea, births appear to be squeezed in the age range 20-34, after which there was an abrupt drop in fertility rates. Although Bangladesh and the Republic of Korea have very different total fertility rates, they have almost similar (319 against 340 per 1,000) age-specific fertility rates at ages of peak fertility (25-29 and 20-24, respectively).

Marital age-specific fertility rates can be contrasted with age-specific rates by comparing tables 140 and 141. The major differences between these two sets of rates can be seen at the younger ages (15-19 and 20-24), where marital fertility rates are much higher than age-specific rates. The higher the proportion single at ages 15-19 and 20-24, the higher the marital fertility rate is in relation to the age-specific fertility rate.

In Malaysia, Sri Lanka and Thailand, the age-specific marital fertility rate declines continuously with successively older age groups from the youngest age group (15-19). On the other hand, in Bangladesh, Fiji, Indonesia, Nepal, Pakistan, the Philippines and the Republic of Korea, the marital fertility rate peaks, instead, at ages 20-24, as does the natural fertility rate. The marital fertility schedules of Bangladesh, Indonesia, Nepal and Pakistan conform relatively closely to the natural fertility schedule, in view of the fact that in these countries, few young women practised family planning at the time of the survey and a relatively large number of those aged 15-19 were married. The cases of Fiji, the Philippines and the Republic of Korea are very different, however, because relatively few women aged 15-19 years were married. Among the countries of the ESCAP region, the estimated marital fertility rate for women aged 15-19 varied from 0.213 in Nepal to 0.432 in Malaysia, which is closely followed by the Philippines with 0.429. Variations in marital fertility in this age group cannot be fully explained by variations in contraceptive practice but depend also upon the characteristics of the women who marry in this age group and the distribution of marriage ages within this group.

C. ANALYSIS OF FERTILITY CHANGE

An important limitation of the WFS data is that they mostly refer to the mid-1970s and hence do not reflect the current situation; they are, however, the most recent comparable data available for most countries. For the purposes of this analysis, the changes in fertility are measured by the changes in age-specific fertility rates (ASFR) and total fertility rates. Owing to the fact that the oldest women interviewed were aged 49 at the time of the survey, the comparisons are limited to three periods: 0-4; 5-9; and 10-14 years prior to the survey. Due to the relatively poor quality of the data (as assessed in chapter I of this publication and in United Nations, 1986), Bangladesh, Indonesia, Nepal and Pakistan are not included in this part of the analysis. The calculation of rates was limited to the age groups from 15-19 to 40-44 years because age-specific rates are not available for women aged 45-49 years for the period 10-14 years prior to the survey.

Trends in age-specific fertility rates and total fertility rates for three periods are presented in table 142. The rates of decline in TFR over roughly a 10-year period covering from 2.5 to 12.5 years prior to the survey (from 10-14 years to 0-4 years) ranged from 23 per cent in the Republic of Korea to 38 per cent in Fiji. In absolute terms, Fiji experienced the largest decline, 2.57 children per woman; and the Republic of Korea had the lowest, 1.27 children per woman, over the 10-year period. A close look at the rates of decline indicates that the pace of fertility declines had accelerated in these countries during the early 1970s, compared with the previous quinquennium. An exception to this pattern is the Republic of Korea, which showed a less rapid rate of decline in the most recent period.

The age pattern of the fertility declines varied quite considerably across countries, with a different pace of decline at different ages, thus affecting the current age pattern of fertility. Although decline had taken place in all age groups in all countries over the 10-year period, three countries (Fiji, Malaysia and Sri Lanka) showed the most rapid declines in age group 15-19 (ranging from 48 to 59 per cent). In another three countries (the Philippines, the Republic of Korea and Thailand), the decline also had occurred among women aged 15-19 years, but at a slower pace, with a range from 19 to 26 per cent. Age groups 35-39 and 30-34 also had experienced significant declines in fertility, as high as 55 per cent in Fiji and 50 per cent in the Republic of Korea for age group 35-39. For age group 30-34, the decline ranged from 39 per cent in Fiji to 19 per cent in Malaysia. In all countries, a considerable decline is also noted in the high-fertility group (20-24) over the 10-year period, and the pace of decline had accelerated over the most recent five years in most cases, except in Malaysia and the Republic of Korea. In the latter country, the decline had virtually halted in the most recent five years, while in the former, the decline had slowed down over the recent five years in age group 20-24. In the next high-fertility group—those aged 25-29 years—the pace of decline had accelerated in the most recent five years, as compared with the previous five years, in all countries except the Republic of Korea, where the decline in this age group was almost negligible. In the Republic of Korea, most of the decline had occurred at the extreme ends of the reproductive ages—15-19, and 35-39 and 40-44. The fertility level for the two older age groups already appeared to be low, however, and the rapid decline in these two age groups thus did not have much effect on the total fertility rate. The overall shape of the decline in the region appeared to be U-shaped, with sharp decline for two extreme age groups —those under 20 and those 30 or over—and slower decline for age groups 20-29. An exception to this pattern

TABLE 140. LIVE BIRTH RATES BY AGE GROUP AND TOTAL FERTILITY RATES FOR THE FIVE YEARS PRECEDING THE SURVEY, SELECTED COUNTRIES IN THE ESCAP REGION

Country	\multicolumn{7}{c}{Live birth rates for age group}	Total fertility rate
	15-19	20-24	25-29	30-34	35-39	40-44	45-49	
Bangladesh	0.219	0.304	0.260	0.214	0.142	0.064	0.012	6.08
Fiji	0.061	0.247	0.225	0.165	0.092	0.045	0.009	4.22
Indonesia	0.124	0.249	0.226	0.167	0.112	0.050	0.018	4.73
Malaysia	0.063	0.232	0.252	0.201	0.132	0.041	0.011	4.66
Nepal	0.131	0.283	0.287	0.236	0.159	0.079	0.027	6.01
Pakistan	0.152	0.283	0.312	0.252	0.180	0.064	0.010	6.26
Philippines	0.054	0.214	0.253	0.239	0.179	0.089	0.022	5.25
Republic of Korea	0.012	0.188	0.319	0.196	0.094	0.040	0.006	4.28
Sri Lanka	0.038	0.151	0.207	0.181	0.116	0.045	0.012	3.75
Thailand	0.069	0.213	0.220	0.179	0.154	0.071	0.020	4.63

Source: Chapter I, table 12, in the present volume.

TABLE 141. MARITAL FERTILITY RATES BY AGE GROUP AND TOTAL MARITAL FERTILITY RATES FOR THE FIVE YEARS PRECEDING THE SURVEY, SELECTED COUNTRIES IN THE ESCAP REGION

Country	\multicolumn{7}{c}{Marital fertility rates for age group}	Total marital fertility rate
	15-19	20-24	25-29	30-34	35-39	40-44	45-49	
Bangladesh	0.275	0.315	0.261	0.215	0.142	0.065	0.012	6.43
Fiji	0.344	0.344	0.242	0.172	0.094	0.046	0.009	6.26
Indonesia	0.274	0.293	0.235	0.170	0.114	0.051	0.018	5.78
Malaysia	0.432	0.402	0.296	0.213	0.135	0.041	0.011	7.65
Nepal	0.213	0.310	0.303	0.254	0.180	0.099	0.035	6.97
Pakistan	0.313	0.344	0.331	0.260	0.182	0.064	0.010	7.52
Philippines	0.429	0.432	0.330	0.267	0.194	0.094	0.024	8.85
Republic of Korea	0.364	0.403	0.347	0.198	0.094	0.040	0.006	7.26
Sri Lanka	0.363	0.348	0.284	0.201	0.123	0.047	0.012	6.89
Thailand	0.377	0.348	0.264	0.197	0.162	0.074	0.021	7.22

Source: Chapter I, table 13, in the present volume.

TABLE 142. TRENDS IN LIVE BIRTH RATES BY AGE GROUP AND IN TOTAL FERTILITY RATES IN SELECTED COUNTRIES IN THE ESCAP REGION, PERIODS 0-4, 5-9 AND 10-14 YEARS PRIOR TO THE SURVEY

Country and period prior to survey	\multicolumn{6}{c}{Age group}	Total fertility rate (to 40-44)
	15-19	20-24	25-29	30-34	35-39	40-44	
Fiji							
			Rate				
10-14	0.142	0.324	0.308	0.271	0.205	0.099[a]	6.75
5-9	0.094	0.290	0.260	0.201	0.141	0.099	5.43
0-4	0.061	0.247	0.225	0.165	0.092	0.045	4.18
			Percentage change				
10-14 to 5-9	-33.0	-10.5	-15.6	-25.8	-31.2	..	-19.56
5-9 to 0-4	-35.1	-14.8	-13.5	-17.9	-34.8	-54.6	-23.02
10-14 to 0-4	-57.0	-23.8	-27.0	-39.1	-55.1	..	-38.07
Malaysia							
			Rate				
10-14	0.120	0.298	0.306	0.248	0.181	0.073[a]	6.13
5-9	0.087	0.257	0.291	0.225	0.144	0.073	5.39
0-4	0.063	0.232	0.252	0.201	0.132	0.041	4.61
			Percentage change				
10-14 to 5-9	-27.5	-13.8	-4.9	-9.3	-20.4	..	-12.07
5-9 to 0-4	-27.6	-9.7	-13.4	-10.7	-8.3	-43.8	-14.47
10-14 to 0-4	-47.5	-22.2	-17.7	-19.0	-27.1	..	-24.80
Philippines							
			Rate				
10-14	0.073	0.261	0.328	0.307	0.243	0.125[a]	6.69
5-9	0.073	0.249	0.310	0.287	0.223	0.125	6.34
0-4	0.054	0.214	0.253	0.239	0.179	0.089	5.14
			Percentage change				
10-14 to 5-9	0.0	-4.6	-5.1	-6.5	-8.2	..	-5.23
5-9 to 0-4	-26.0	-14.1	-18.4	-16.7	-19.7	-28.8	-18.93
10-14 to 0-4	-26.0	-18.0	-22.9	-22.1	-26.3	..	-23.17

TABLE 142 (continued)

Country and period prior to survey	Age group						Total fertility rate (to 40-44)
	15-19	20-24	25-29	30-34	35-39	40-44	
Republic of Korea			Rate				
10-14	0.016	0.234	0.331	0.266	0.188	0.069[a]	5.52
5-9	0.015	0.189	0.320	0.217	0.129	0.069	4.70
0-4	0.012	0.188	0.319	0.196	0.094	0.040	4.25
			Percentage change				
10-14 to 5-9	−6.3	−19.2	−3.3	−18.4	−31.4	..	−14.86
5-9 to 0-4	−20.0	−0.5	−0.3	−9.7	−27.1	−42.0	−9.57
10-14 to 0-4	−25.0	−19.7	−3.6	−26.3	−50.0	..	−23.01
Sri Lanka			Rate				
10-14	0.093	0.242	0.282	0.237	0.187	0.063[a]	5.52
5-9	0.064	0.185	0.259	0.223	0.145	0.063	4.70
0-4	0.038	0.151	0.207	0.181	0.116	0.045	3.69
			Percentage change				
10-14 to 5-9	−31.2	−23.6	−8.2	−5.9	−22.5	..	−14.86
5-9 to 0-4	−40.6	−18.4	−20.1	−18.8	−20.0	−28.6	−21.49
10-14 to 0-4	−59.1	−37.6	−26.6	−23.6	−38.0	..	−33.15
Thailand			Rate				
10-14	0.085	0.266	0.310	0.292	0.239	0.122[a]	6.57
5-9	0.080	0.256	0.293	0.239	0.197	0.122	5.94
0-4	0.069	0.213	0.220	0.179	0.154	0.071	4.53
			Percentage change				
10-14 to 5-9	−5.9	−3.8	−5.5	−18.2	−17.6	..	−9.59
5-9 to 0-4	−13.8	−16.8	−24.9	−25.1	−21.8	−41.8	−23.74
10-14 to 0-4	−18.8	−19.9	−29.0	−38.7	−35.6	..	−31.05

Source: United Nations (1983).
[a] Rate not available. Total fertility rate calculated assuming rate from period 5-9 years prior to survey.

was Thailand, where the declines increase at successive higher age groups, except for women aged 35-39, where the percentage decline was slightly less.

Changes in marital fertility rates are of particular interest because they can provide information on the onset of fertility control and the pattern of control occurring with age. Table 143 shows the rates and the percentage changes. For all countries included here, the singulate mean age of marriage is over 20, and the rates at ages 15-19 are therefore based on a small number of cases, which might have affected their representativeness. In any case, there has been some increase in fertility over the 10-year period for this age group in most countries, except Fiji and Sri Lanka. Excluding this group (15-19), it can be seen that the percentage decline over the 10-year period increases with age in most countries, but the rate of decline is nowhere near as fast as it is in the case of age-specific fertility rates, particularly in the younger and peak fertility groups where marital fertility rates are higher. The rates of decline in the older age groups in the two sets of rates (age-specific fertility rates and age-specific marital fertility rates) are very similar, which is largely due to fertility control within marriage. If the two sets of rates given in tables 142 and 143 for the younger age groups (15-19, 20-24 and 25-29) are compared, the significant effect of changing age at marriage on fertility in countries in the ESCAP region can be seen. Another notable feature of the pattern of decline can be seen in the Republic of Korea, where the increase in marital fertility rates in the three most fertile age groups has almost compensated for the very rapid decline in older age groups and thus the total marital fertility rate remained almost unchanged over the 10-year period. However, the increase in marital fertility in the younger, more fertile age groups may be indicative of a new pattern of childbearing by women in the Republic of Korea, whereby the span of childbearing might have been squeezed into the early part of the reproductive ages. This new pattern may represent the future scenario in countries entering the advanced stage of fertility control. The similarity in the pace of declines in the two sets of rates for higher ages only confirms that a considerable part of almost all the declines at higher ages is due to fertility control.

D. DETERMINANTS OF FERTILITY

The level of fertility in a society is directly determined by a set of intermediate variables that either as a matter of individual volition or as a result of socio-economic and cultural practices interfere with or impinge on the biological conditions of birth. Any socio-economic, cultural and environmental change affects fertility through a change in one or more of the biological variables. In order to explain this behavioural and biological influence on fertility, the discussion is divided into two parts. The first deals with the biological variables, in particular, those which have a direct bearing on reproduction in societies where childbearing is restricted to unions, namely, age at marriage and post-partum and lactational infecundability. In the second part, an attempt is made to demonstrate the bivariate relationship between socio-economic variables and fertility. To complete the discussion, the findings from several multivariate analyses are briefly summarized.

TABLE 143. TRENDS IN MARITAL FERTILITY RATES BY AGE GROUP AND IN TOTAL MARITAL FERTILITY RATES IN SELECTED COUNTRIES IN THE ESCAP REGION, PERIODS 0-4, 5-9 AND 10-14 YEARS PRIOR TO THE SURVEY

Country and period prior to survey	15-19	20-24	25-29	30-34	35-39	40-44	Total marital fertility rate (to 40-44)
Fiji			Rate				
10-14	0.381	0.393	0.328	0.276	0.209	0.101[a]	8.44
5-9	0.356	0.364	0.280	0.208	0.144	0.101	7.27
0-4	0.344	0.344	0.242	0.172	0.094	0.046	6.21
			Percentage change				
10-14 to 5-9	−6.6	−7.4	−14.6	−24.6	−31.1	..	−13.92
5-9 to 0-4	−3.4	−5.5	−13.6	−17.3	−34.7	−54.5	−14.52
10-14 to 0-4	−9.7	−12.5	−26.2	−37.7	−55.0	..	−26.42
Malaysia			Rate				
10-14	0.387	0.413	0.337	0.255	0.183	0.077[a]	8.26
5-9	0.404	0.397	0.325	0.236	0.146	0.077	7.93
0-4	0.432	0.402	0.296	0.213	0.135	0.041	7.60
			Percentage change				
10-14 to 5-9	4.4	−3.9	−3.6	−7.5	−20.2	..	−4.06
5-9 to 0-4	6.9	1.3	−8.9	−9.7	−7.5	−46.8	−4.16
10-14 to 0-4	11.6	−2.7	−12.2	−16.5	−26.2	..	−8.05
Philippines			Rate				
10-14	0.389	0.427	0.390	0.336	0.263	0.133[a]	9.69
5-9	0.427	0.440	0.376	0.317	0.237	0.133	9.65
0-4	0.429	0.432	0.330	0.267	0.194	0.094	8.73
			Percentage change				
10-14 to 5-9	9.8	3.0	−3.6	−5.7	−9.9	..	0.41
5-9 to 0-4	0.5	−1.8	−12.2	−15.8	−18.1	−29.3	−9.53
10-14 to 0-4	10.3	1.2	−15.4	−20.5	−26.2	..	−9.91
Republic of Korea			Rate				
10-14	0.233	0.357	0.339	0.268	0.188	0.069[a]	7.27
5-9	0.298	0.373	0.338	0.218	0.129	0.069	7.13
0-4	0.364	0.403	0.347	0.198	0.094	0.040	7.23
			Percentage change				
10-14 to 5-9	27.9	4.5	−0.3	−18.7	−31.4	..	−1.99
5-9 to 0-4	22.1	8.0	2.7	−9.2	−27.1	−42.0	1.47
10-14 to 0-4	56.2	12.9	2.4	−26.1	−50.0	..	−0.55
Sri Lanka			Rate				
10-14	0.364	0.372	0.332	0.250	0.192	0.064[a]	7.87
5-9	0.369	0.350	0.318	0.242	0.149	0.064	7.46
0-4	0.363	0.348	0.284	0.201	0.123	0.047	6.83
			Percentage change				
10-14 to 5-9	1.4	−5.9	−4.2	−3.2	−22.4	..	−5.21
5-9 to 0-4	−1.6	−0.6	−10.7	−16.9	−17.5	−26.6	−8.45
10-14 to 0-4	−0.3	−6.5	−14.5	−19.6	−35.9	..	−13.21
Thailand			Rate				
10-14	0.346	0.378	0.346	0.310	0.251	0.127[a]	8.79
5-9	0.349	0.381	0.340	0.257	0.206	0.127	8.30
0-4	0.377	0.348	0.264	0.197	0.162	0.074	7.11
			Percentage change				
10-14 to 5-9	0.9	0.8	−1.7	−17.1	−17.9	..	−5.57
5-9 to 0-4	8.0	−8.7	−22.4	−23.4	−21.4	−41.7	−14.34
10-14 to 0-4	9.0	−7.9	−23.7	−36.5	−35.5	..	−19.11

Source: United Nations (1983), table 14.

[a] Rate not available. Total marital fertility rate calculated assuming rate from period 5-9 years prior to survey.

Biological determinants

Davis and Blake (1956) and Bongaarts (1978) emphasize the "proximate" determinants by which the observed social and economic differentials in fertility levels are produced between the various subgroups of the population. These factors include pattern of social union (marriage), stability of union, breast-feeding practices, use of contraception, frequency of intercourse and induced abortion. In recent years, with the availability of WFS data, the understanding of these determinants has increased tremendously. However, the data constraints still leave certain portions of the model untested. Very little is known about induced abortion and frequency of intercourse in the countries of the ESCAP region. Even much of the information for other variables is available only for a few of the ESCAP countries, those which participated in the WFS programme. From the foregoing discussion of this paper, it is apparent that fertility has been declining at a rapid rate in the majority of the countries considered here. It is also evident that much of the decline has been caused simultaneously by the rising age at marriage and the dramatic rise in contraceptive use over the 10-year period prior to the surveys. The three main proximate determinants are discussed below.

Marriage

Marriage has long been recognized as one of the principal proximate determinants of fertility, particularly in countries of the ESCAP region, where procreation occurs primarily within unions. In most societies, women spend a substantial proportion of their potential reproductive years out of marriage, either before first marriage or after a marriage has ended due to divorce, separation or death of the husband. In addition, some women never marry (see chapter III).

Marriage is universal in nearly all the countries of the ESCAP region. Historically, marriage fulfilled what was seen as women's primary role, that of reproduction. In nearly all the cultures of the region, a newly married couple is usually subjected to strong pressure for the "family to become three". This situation is changing, but in some cultures social pressure still has a very strong bearing on the course of fertility. The age at which women marry is therefore an important factor which can influence the rate of population growth, particularly in countries where contraceptive prevalence is not very high. In these countries, any delay in age at marriage invariably means a potential loss of reproductive period. However, the relationship between age at marriage and subsequent fertility is much more complex.

The data presented in table 144 show that as the marriage age increases, the number of children ever born decreases. A much clearer picture emerges when age at first marriage is controlled for women who had completed their reproductive life (ages 45-49), as can be seen from table 145. Interestingly, the negative association between age at marriage and fertility is quite strong within each country, particularly for older (18 years and over) age-at-marriage cohorts.

In the countries of the ESCAP region, where most reproduction takes place within marriage, marital status exerts a dominant influence on childbearing. It is interesting to study the completed family size of ever-married women aged 40-49 according to the current status of their first marriages, which is examined in table 146 for 10 countries of the ESCAP region. It is seen that for most countries, the women in stable marriages, that is, those who had continued in their first marriage, had at least one child more than those whose first marriage had been dissolved by the death of the husband (rows 2 and 3) or by divorce (rows 4 and 5). Among these countries, the highest proportion of widowed among the ever-married women aged 40-44 was 19.7, in Bangladesh, and the highest proportion of divorced and separated was 7.5, in Indonesia (Kabir, 1980). Changes in these proportions in the countries of the region, which are likely to occur as a result of modernization and reduction in mortality, can potentially influence completed family size.

Breast-feeding practices

In the absence of contraceptive use, historically, breast-feeding has been an important determinant of fertility differentials. Its effect in inhibiting ovulation increases the length of the birth interval and results in lower completed fertility. In modern countries, the average duration of lactational infecundity is very low because many women do not breast-feed their babies. In the traditional societies of the ESCAP region, where lactation is usually long and often lasts until the next pregnancy, the fertility reduction effect is substantial. It can be seen from table 147 that the proportion of women who breast-fed their last child exceeded 90 per cent in 7 out of 10 countries and was nowhere less than 73 per cent. The mean duration of breast-feeding exceeded 12 months in all countries except Fiji and Malaysia. The longest duration observed, 29 months, was in Bangladesh. This considerable breast-feeding duration has a significant impact on post-partum amenorrhoea. Due to limitations of the data from these countries, it is not possible to establish the specific relationship between duration of breast-feeding and duration of post-partum amenorrhoea. However, the WFS data from outside the region confirmed this relationship (see chapter IV). The mean (or median) duration of amenorrhoea appears to be roughly predictable from the mean duration of breast-feeding (Léridon and Ferry, 1985, figure 7.4). Using one of the functions proposed by Corsini (1979), Bongaarts (1983), and Lesthaeghe and Page (1980), seven months of amenorrhoea are experienced for 12 months of breast-feeding, 12 for 18 months, and perhaps 17 for 24 months. This extends the interval between births substantially and thereby affects the level of fertility.

Contraception

Within marriage, contraceptive practice is primarily responsible for the wide range in the levels of fertility observed across countries. Contraceptive practice is a recent phenomenon in the countries of the ESCAP region. Use levels are low and marital fertility is relatively high. On the other hand, in the more developed of the developing countries as well as in developed countries, where marital fertility is low, well over half the married women of reproductive ages are current users of contraception. Here, the results based on a simple model developed by Bongaarts (1978) are presented. The index of contraception, C_c, is a measure of the fertility-reducing effects of contraception (for definition of the index and more detailed discussion, see chapter VI). The estimates of various indices are shown in table 148. Not surprisingly, the proportion using contraceptives varied substantially between the countries: only 2.4 per cent reported current use in Nepal as against 37 per cent in Fiji (see chapter V and column (2) of table 148). The results indicate that the impact of contraception is negligible in Bangladesh, Nepal and Pakistan (0.95). In Indonesia, Malaysia, the Philippines, the Republic of Korea and Sri Lanka, the fertility-reducing effects of contraception are similar. In Fiji and Thailand, the impact is somewhat greater. The impact of contraception on fertility as reflected by the index of contraception is consistent with the classification of countries according to programme effort (see table 5 in the Introduction to this volume). In Fiji, Indonesia, Malaysia, the Philippines, the Republic of Korea, Sri Lanka and Thailand, each of which had

TABLE 144. MEAN NUMBER OF CHILDREN EVER BORN TO EVER-MARRIED WOMEN, BY AGE AT FIRST UNION, COUNTRIES IN THE ESCAP REGION[a]

Country	Under 15	15-17	18-19	20-21	22-24	25-29	30+	All ages	Number in sample
				(number of children)					
Bangladesh	4.21	3.10	2.62	1.97	2.09	1.91[b]	9.06[b]	3.97	6 515
Fiji	5.78	4.22	3.27	3.18	2.93	2.53	2.10	3.82	4 928
Indonesia	3.92	3.33	3.10	3.00	2.64	2.19	1.39	3.46	9 155
Malaysia	5.46	4.89	4.25	3.36	2.89	2.45	1.61	4.22	6 321
Pakistan	4.70	4.07	3.75	3.10	2.49	2.18	1.93[b]	4.17	4 952
Philippines	6.16	5.44	4.83	4.38	3.79	3.16	2.12	4.58	9 627
Republic of Korea	6.20	5.28	4.01	3.18	2.44	1.97	1.18[b]	3.59	5 430
Sri Lanka	5.75	4.73	3.97	3.44	2.82	2.24	1.62	3.94	6 810
Thailand	4.59	4.38	4.12	3.75	3.28	2.67	1.70	3.93	3 820

Source: Economic and Social Commission for Asia and the Pacific (1982), table 4.

[a] Data for Nepal were not available.
[b] Fewer than 20 cases.

TABLE 145. MEAN NUMBER OF CHILDREN EVER BORN TO EVER-MARRIED WOMEN AGED 45-49, BY AGE AT FIRST MARRIAGE, COUNTRIES IN THE ESCAP REGION

Country	Mean age at first marriage, current age 45-49	Completed fertility[a] (number of children)	15	15-17	18-19	20-21	22-24	25+
					(number of children)			
Bangladesh	11.7	6.7	6.7	7.3	—	6.3	—	—
Fiji	17.6	6.3	7.4	7.0	6.0	5.7	5.4	3.7
Indonesia	15.6	5.2	5.4	5.4	5.1	5.1	4.4	3.2
Malaysia	17.8	6.3	6.0	6.5	6.8	6.1	5.4	4.0
Pakistan	15.7	7.1	7.3	7.4	7.7	6.4	6.3	4.4
Philippines	18.8	7.0	8.8	8.8	7.5	7.3	6.2	4.2
Republic of Korea	18.4	5.8	6.9	6.2	5.2	4.4	4.1	3.5
Sri Lanka	19.0	6.0	7.1	7.0	6.3	5.9	5.2	3.5
Thailand	18.4	6.8	7.0	7.2	7.7	6.1	6.3	4.7

Source: World Fertility Survey standard recode tapes.

[a] Completed fertility is based on responses for women aged 45+ in all countries except Fiji, where it refers to women aged 40+.

[b] Completed fertility is based on responses for women aged 45+ in all countries except Fiji, where it refers to women aged 40+; and Malaysia, Pakistan and Thailand, where it is derived from data on years since first marriage rather than age, as follows: <15, 30+ duration; 15-17, 30+ duration; 18-19, 25+ duration; 20-21, 20+ duration; 25+, 15+ duration.

TABLE 146. MEAN NUMBER OF CHILDREN EVER BORN TO EVER-MARRIED WOMEN AGED 40-49, BY CONTINUITY OF FIRST MARRIAGE AND WHETHER REMARRIED, COUNTRIES IN THE ESCAP REGION

Country	First marriage not dissolved	Widowed Remarried	Widowed Did not remarry	Divorced or separated Remarried	Divorced or separated Did not remarry	Number in sample
			(number of children)			
Bangladesh	7.67	5.58	5.54	5.98	6.61	1 121
Fiji	6.64	5.36	5.78	4.90	3.91	1 056
Indonesia	6.31	4.59	4.75	4.43	2.93	2 214
Malaysia	6.57	5.85	6.02	4.93	3.61	1 757
Nepal	5.88	-----4.75[a]-----		-----3.00[a]----		1 236
Pakistan	7.29	6.45	5.47	5.33	1.97	1 123
Philippines	6.96	6.50	6.42	6.19	4.52	2 610
Republic of Korea	5.76	4.69	4.56	4.00	3.24	1 544
Sri Lanka	6.00	6.18	5.08	4.71	3.31	2 003
Thailand	6.71	6.47	5.59	5.53	3.67	1 040

Source: Economic and Social Commission for Asia and the Pacific (1982a), table 7.

[a] Data on breakdown not available.

an index of contraception below 0.80, programme efforts were classified as strong or moderate, while Bangladesh, Nepal and Pakistan had a weak programme effort and a high index of contraception.

A surprising finding is that in the mid-1970s, contraception apparently affected fertility more in Thailand, where the major diffusion of birth control began only in the early 1970s, than in the Republic of Korea. One

TABLE 147. DURATION OF BREAST-FEEDING AND PERCENTAGE OF CHILDREN EVER BREAST-FED, COUNTRIES IN THE ESCAP REGION

Country	Duration of breast-feeding Median[a] (months)	Duration of breast-feeding Mean[a] (months)	Percentage of children ever breast-fed
Bangladesh	30.7	28.9	98
Fiji	9.2	9.9	86
Indonesia	22.2	23.6	97
Malaysia	2.6	5.8	73
Nepal	23.6	25.2	98
Pakistan	19.4	19.0	95
Philippines	12.7	13.0	86
Republic of Korea	16.6	16.3	93
Sri Lanka	20.8	21.0	95
Thailand	18.9	18.9	92

Source: Ferry and Smith (1983).
[a] Current status estimated for all births in the preceding five years.

TABLE 148. CONTRACEPTION INDEX AND ITS COMPONENTS, COUNTRIES IN THE ESCAP REGION

Country	Index of contraception, C_c (1)	Proportion using contraception, u (2)	Method-effectiveness, e (3)
Bangladesh	0.930	0.078	0.817
Fiji	0.672	0.366	0.889
Indonesia	0.771	0.230	0.874
Malaysia	0.736	0.294	0.817
Nepal	0.976	0.024	0.951
Pakistan	0.960	0.052	0.827
Philippines	0.739	0.300	0.790
Republic of Korea	0.753	0.291	0.849
Sri Lanka	0.771	0.265	0.842
Thailand	0.688	0.296	0.915

Source: Casterline and others (1984), tables 7 and 9.
NOTE: For details of the construction of the index, see Casterline and others (1984), which gives some modifications for combined effects of age-specific construction and correction for overlap between breast-feeding and contraception. However, the combined effect at national level is small on Bongaarts' formula: $C_c = 1 - 1.08ue$.

reason for this may be that levels of use among younger women were higher in Thailand than in the Republic of Korea, and this use was only partially offset by higher contraceptive prevalence among older women in the Republic of Korea. As the model used in this analysis is constructed on an age-specific basis, the greater fertility impact of use at younger ages is taken into account in the contraceptive index. In addition, method-effectiveness is relatively high in Thailand (one of the highest for all 10 countries), reflecting the predominance of the pill and of injectables. It is entirely the high effectiveness of the methods used in that country which sets Thailand apart from Malaysia and the Philippines, where overall contraceptive prevalence is almost the same. Another factor in the low ranking of the Republic of Korea is the exclusion of abortion from the construction of the index.

Socio-economic determinants

When fertility declines, it does not generally decline uniformly in all segments of the population. The decline first appears, in particular, among the more advanced and modernized segments of the population. Therefore, the appearance of differentials in fertility by socio-economic variables is a sensitive indicator of the early phase of fertility decline in the population. Furthermore, the study of fertility differentials can provide useful information for the projection of future fertility as the population passes through the various stages of the development process.

Place of residence

In societies undergoing social and economic transition in the process of development, urban living and life-styles promote the desire for smaller families and a reduction in fertility. This factor is examined in table 149, which shows total fertility rates and age-specific marital fertility rates by current residence. The data in general show that women who were residing in urban areas had lower fertility than those living in rural areas. The differentials emerged uniformly for almost all age groups and became more pronounced at the higher ages. There are two exceptions, however, Indonesia and Pakistan, where urban fertility was slightly higher than rural fertility. In fact, in Pakistan, fertility in other urban areas was higher than rural fertility but major urban areas had lower fertility than rural areas. In Indonesia, possibly owing to more complete urban reporting, as well as greater stability of marriage in urban areas, urban fertility was higher than rural fertility.

Wife's education

The relationship between the wife's education and fertility can be seen in table 150. In general, the total marital fertility rates are inversely related to education in all countries except Indonesia and Sri Lanka. In fact, in Sri Lanka, the fertility of women with no schooling was almost equal to that of women with seven or more years of education and there is not much difference in the fertility levels between the four levels of education; it appears that fertility levels are converging to a common level. In Indonesia, however, the fertility of educated women was considerably higher than that of women with no education. In this case, Singh and Casterline (1985) suggest that in the short run the better-educated group may show higher fertility because fertility regulation efforts do not compensate for the loss of traditional restraints, resulting in a curvilinear, or simple positive, relationship between education and fertility. In the long run, the negative relationship will probably become dominant, as shown by those countries which are past the transitional stage. The inverse relationship between education and fertility is often violated by the groups with from one to three years and from four to six years of education, especially where these groups contain few respondents. When the marital fertility rates are considered, the effect of nuptiality is eliminated and the range of difference between educational categories becomes narrow. The range of differences across educational categories not only expands when the effect of nuptiality is allowed, as in total fertility rate, but a fertility-reducing impact of primary education is sometimes evident where no such impact on marital fertility is apparent. The powerful effect of schooling beyond primary level on reproductive behaviour can be seen by comparing the total fertility rate of those with from four to six years of schooling with that of the group with seven or more years of schooling; the latter group without exception shows the lowest rate, usually two births or more less than the former group. This evidence of a "threshold effect" (fertility declines sharply once a certain level of education

TABLE 149. AGE-SPECIFIC MARITAL FERTILITY RATES, BY CURRENT RESIDENCE, 1975-1980, COUNTRIES IN THE ESCAP REGION

Country and current residence	\multicolumn{7}{c	}{Marital fertility rate for age group}	Total marital fertility rate (20-49)	Total fertility rate
	15-19	20-24	25-29	30-34	35-39	40-44	45-49		
Bangladesh									
Major urban	372	339	260	203	170	86	0	5.29	5.73
Other urban	303	337	303	212	137	66	27	5.41	5.76
Rural	283	324	272	237	166	82	17	5.49	6.11
Fiji									
Major urban	360	327	249	123	57	19	6	3.90	3.30
Other urban	330	352	244	159	72	30	0	4.28	3.79
Rural	351	362	252	191	118	63	13	5.00	4.59
Indonesia									
Major urban	372	379	319	208	132	54	28	5.59	4.61
Other urban	385	368	293	193	109	47	21	5.15	4.32
Rural	288	302	244	182	131	63	23	4.72	4.87
Malaysia									
Major urban	452	401	301	169	113	25	8	5.09	3.47
Other urban	499	452	321	221	154	52	10	6.05	4.48
Rural	433	406	303	235	155	53	16	5.83	5.04
Nepal									
Urban	335	343	269	162	57	65	0	4.48	4.31
Rural	216	311	308	265	189	104	38	6.08	6.22
Pakistan									
Major urban	314	383	377	263	178	32	17	6.25	5.90
Other urban	354	361	360	294	211	98	4	6.64	6.25
Rural	296	340	339	276	204	90	14	6.31	6.32
Philippines									
Major urban	425	417	284	220	116	37	9	5.41	3.53
Other urban	432	434	324	245	154	73	17	6.23	4.03
Rural	431	441	347	290	228	116	31	7.26	5.97
Republic of Korea									
Major urban	368	389	346	150	55	16	0	4.77	3.33
Other urban	332	389	369	198	69	41	9	5.38	4.18
Rural	376	438	344	249	141	64	12	6.23	5.03
Sri Lanka									
Major urban	432	359	279	169	96	22	4	4.64	3.11
Other urban	382	389	308	172	115	31	0	5.07	3.23
Rural	359	349	290	221	141	58	18	5.38	3.89
Thailand									
Major urban	375	381	271	142	85	26	15	4.60	2.53
Other urban	447	345	224	207	133	56	19	4.92	3.63
Rural	383	358	276	213	187	88	25	5.74	4.96

Source: Alam and Casterline (1984), tables A1 and A2.

is attained) in many countries cautions against specifying linear effects of education (Alam and Casterline, 1984).

Women's work status

Because the relationship between women's employment and fertility is of great policy interest, this important topic is discussed here on the basis of the WFS results. There have been numerous studies on the topic, which suggests that the relationship between work and fertility is not a simple inverse one but rather that it is ambiguous: it is generally accepted that the relationship is not unidirectional (Singh and Casterline, 1985). Although employment may affect fertility more often than the reverse, a woman's fertility (either childlessness or past high fertility) may also influence her ability or need to work. The WFS data, however, do not permit examination of these questions. Therefore, the simple relationship between fertility (TMFR for ages 20-49) and employment status in work since marriage (no work, family or self-employed, other non-family employee) is examined in table 151. Rodríguez and Cleland (1981) conducted a large-scale comparative study on this relationship and found a strong relationship between work status and fertility, with non-family workers having the lowest fertility, as expected (given that they are most likely to work away from home and to be paid in cash), and those who had not worked since marriage showing the highest fertility. In this study, no such simple and strong relationship is found. Only in Bangladesh, Fiji, Indonesia and the Philippines did women employed by others have the lowest fertility and women recorded as not working have the highest, with those who worked for the family or were self-employed in-between. Each of the six countries—Malaysia, Nepal, Pakistan, the Republic of Korea, Sri Lanka and Thailand — is different and represents a peculiar situation. Women who worked for the family or were self-employed in Nepal, the Republic of Korea and Thailand had the highest fertility. The "no work" group had the highest fertility only in Malaysia. In Pakistan alone, the group

TABLE 150. AGE-SPECIFIC MARITAL FERTILITY RATES, BY RESPONDENT'S EDUCATION, 1975-1980, COUNTRIES IN THE ESCAP REGION

Country and years of education	\multicolumn{7}{c}{Marital fertility rate for age group}	Total marital fertility rate (20-49)	Total fertility rate
	15-19	20-24	25-29	30-34	35-39	40-44	45-49		
Bangladesh									
Zero	281	321	267	230	164	84	20	5.43	6.07
One to three	256	331	311	255	178	39	0	5.57	6.35
Four to six	311	351	301	274	162	93	5	5.93	6.72
Seven or more	349	321	265	210	221	67	0	5.42	4.98
Fiji									
Zero	311	385	218	132	85	39	12	4.35	..
One to three	347	324	227	150	85	66	10	4.30	..
Four to six	399	334	266	201	122	58	7	4.94	..
Seven or more	333	359	255	182	90	44	7	4.68	..
Indonesia									
Zero	288	311	228	178	125	55	24	4.60	..
One to three	310	287	272	180	178	120	23	5.30	..
Four to six	293	308	274	226	142	77	12	5.20	..
Seven or more	398	396	352	203	82	22	11	5.33	..
Malaysia									
Zero	442	417	297	236	154	56	19	5.89	5.30
One to three	453	424	315	217	145	47	0	5.74	5.26
Four to six	443	406	305	219	140	30	9	5.54	4.81
Seven or more	418	415	305	197	121	6	0	5.22	3.19
Nepal									
Zero	209	311	308	263	186	104	37	6.04	..
One to three	217	308	375	209	275	0	0	5.83	..
Four to six	229	383	308	244	147	136	0	6.08	..
Seven or more	352	302	217	92	0	0	0	3.05	..
Pakistan									
Zero	305	343	345	283	205	88	14	6.39	6.51
One to three	290	308	330	238	284	0	0	5.80	5.41
Four to six	322	400	378	270	158	100	0	6.52	6.12
Seven or more	366	401	334	209	34	0	0	4.89	3.12
Philippines									
Zero	410	383	313	291	186	122	24	6.75	5.45
One to three	418	430	375	300	256	106	41	7.54	6.97
Four to six	438	439	347	285	217	111	21	7.10	6.15
Seven or more	425	440	305	237	143	66	9	5.99	3.84
Republic of Korea									
Zero	308	427	350	248	143	63	12	6.22	5.71
One to three	282	404	332	227	107	66	0	5.68	5.46
Four to six	400	421	353	193	92	32	0	5.45	4.48
Seven or more	292	381	357	179	40	16	20	4.97	3.35
Sri Lanka									
Zero	353	325	296	208	138	64	26	5.28	..
One to three	332	339	274	196	141	61	11	5.11	..
Four to six	366	351	299	219	138	45	7	5.29	..
Seven or more	395	381	292	214	127	38	9	5.30	..
Thailand									
Zero	384	330	282	197	195	86	29	5.59	..
One to three	323	328	314	249	192	67	0	5.75	..
Four to six	400	363	273	210	167	86	26	5.62	..
Seven or more	307	383	228	153	110	20	0	4.47	..

Source: Alam and Casterline (1984), tables A1 and A2.

who worked for others had the highest fertility. It is also important to note, however, that in the Republic of Korea, Sri Lanka and Thailand, where the full inverse relationship was not found, those employed by others still had the lowest fertility. This means that in the majority of the countries (7 out of 10), the women employed by others had the lowest fertility and the differences between the categories "no work" and "work for others" were of considerable magnitude. Because countries in the ESCAP region are at the transitional stage with respect to female employment, the condition depicted here is consistent with prior expectations. In the long run, women's employment will affect fertility as more and more women begin to participate in activities outside the home or farms in the vicinity.

For better understanding of the relationship between work and fertility, it is necessary to control the common antecedent factors, such as education or social status, which determine both work and fertility. Rodríguez and Cleland (1981) analysed the effect of the wife's work

TABLE 151. AGE-SPECIFIC MARITAL FERTILITY RATES, BY RESPONDENT'S WORK STATUS, 1975-1980, COUNTRIES IN THE ESCAP REGION

Country and work status	15-19	20-24	25-29	30-34	35-39	40-44	45-49	Total marital fertility rate (20-49)
Bangladesh								
No work	286	328	282	238	168	84	17	5.59
Family and self	255	316	234	213	145	58	31	4.99
Others	292	302	226	214	150	66	7	4.83
Fiji								
No work	358	364	253	182	102	47	13	4.80
Family and self	137	279	265	148	138	81	0	4.56
Others	313	324	226	169	68	38	0	4.12
Indonesia								
No work	319	347	303	232	179	83	39	5.91
Family and self	249	296	227	158	115	61	24	4.40
Others	299	285	234	190	117	43	6	4.37
Malaysia								
No work	438	431	322	228	141	44	4	5.85
Family and self	431	364	273	232	151	53	22	5.48
Others	457	408	307	205	149	44	14	5.63
Nepal								
No work	244	325	317	267	162	101	26	5.99
Family and self	186	305	308	255	200	108	44	6.10
Others	266	315	264	283	163	84	0	5.55
Pakistan								
No work	306	351	349	276	197	84	11	6.34
Family and self	316	316	335	275	223	98	13	6.30
Others	279	359	337	296	211	86	22	6.55
Philippines								
No work	440	448	358	295	209	100	30	7.20
Family and self	448	418	305	264	195	107	28	6.58
Others	393	428	324	251	192	84	15	6.47
Republic of Korea								
No work	386	422	377	185	84	36	7	5.55
Family and self	365	397	331	220	114	51	10	5.61
Others	282	348	324	181	66	46	0	4.82
Sri Lanka								
No work	392	372	303	219	136	50	18	5.49
Family and self	316	338	283	235	165	66	11	5.49
Others	284	320	273	181	116	49	9	4.73
Thailand								
No work	371	380	220	230	152	63	35	5.40
Family and self	403	359	278	212	177	86	23	5.68
Others	364	349	274	174	170	63	22	5.26

Source: Alam and Casterline (1984), tables A1 and A2.

status on marital fertility after controlling for those factors and found that in nearly all countries the effect remains significant. A fuller discussion of this topic can be found in chapter IX of this volume.

E. SUMMARY AND DISCUSSION

In this review, an attempt has been made to portray the fertility profile of women in countries in the ESCAP region by analysing recent levels and patterns of fertility, as well as fertility changes and their associated causes. The WFS data were drawn from surveys conducted in these countries during the mid-1970s. Most parts of the analysis refer to 10 countries of the region: Bangladesh; Fiji; Indonesia; Malaysia; Nepal; Pakistan; the Philippines; the Republic of Korea; Sri Lanka; and Thailand. This review is based on the reports prepared on designated topics of fertility analysis carried out in implementing the United Nations Minimum Research Programme for Comparative Analysis of World Fertility Survey Data and the other reports published by WFS.

Despite the limitations of the WFS data, several interesting points emerge which have important implications for population policy formulation in the region. These findings, of course, need further confirmation with more recent data.

The evidence presented here tends to indicate that the majority of women in the region who were at the end of their reproductive life in the 1970s had given birth to a large number of children. The high proportion of women with six or more children clearly indicates the climate of high fertility in the ESCAP region. There is very little evidence of child-spacing within the first few years of marriage. Childbearing appears to slow down among different marriage cohorts in different countries; the earliest cohort observed was that for marriage duration of 10-14 years; and by that time, the women had at least three children.

The current fertility levels, indicated by the total fertility rates, are from four to six births per woman. If these countries aspire to achieve replacement level in fertility, it would appear that the current fertility level must be cut by at least 50 per cent. The total marital fertility rates are still very high (from six to eight births per woman), compared with levels in the developed countries. Even countries of the region where marital fertility is known to have been declining over the past decade or so still have total marital fertility rates well over seven births per woman.

Considerable variation exists in the age pattern of childbearing among women in the region. On the one hand, one finds the birth "squeeze" in the most fertile age groups of women in the Republic of Korea; and, on the other hand, childbearing was fairly widespread over the total span of reproductive life in Bangladesh and Pakistan.

The cross-sectional analysis of the fertility changes indicates a modest to moderate amount of change in the fertility levels over the 10-year period from the early 1960s to the early 1970s. With few exceptions, there were declines in fertility levels in all countries and for all age groups. A more rapid decline observed in the total fertility rates suggests the onset of a fertility transition in the region. What is very discouraging, however, is the relatively slower decline in marital fertility and even in some cases a notable increase in marital fertility in the most fertile age groups, which overshadowed the decline in the older age group. However, the increase in marital fertility in the fertile age groups may be only a temporary phenomenon which may have resulted from the change in age at marriage during that period.

Analysis of the determinants of fertility changes tends to show that rising age at marriage, increases in contraceptive prevalence and place of residence have a clear relationship with fertility changes. Other factors, such as education and work status, have been found to be associated with changes, but less clearly, and the relationship is not entirely straightforward.

F. POLICY IMPLICATIONS

The evidence found so far on the fertility situation appears to indicate the following policy implications:

(*a*) The recent decline in fertility in the ESCAP region should not be viewed complacently. Fertility levels are still high and far from the regional goals of achieving replacement level by the year 2000. The high level of fertility warrants more concerted efforts in reducing fertility through structural and programmatic changes;

(*b*) Younger women in general are not spacing their children until they achieve a certain number of children which is well above the replacement level. These young women need to be approached more vigorously for spacing, if not for controlling their fertility at younger ages. Efforts directed towards internalizing the small-family norm at the beginning of their reproductive life would be of great value;

(*c*) Marital fertility rates are still very high; this should indicate to those responsible for family planning programmes that their programmes should increase their contribution to the fertility decline, as the major part of the observed decline in fertility in some countries is due to the postponement of marriage;

(*d*) In the corresponding period of fertility declines, contraceptive practice levels have also risen in the countries of the ESCAP region, with varying magnitudes. At the same time, development efforts have induced changes in socio-economic and demographic conditions, which in turn affect the fertility level. The relative contribution of these factors *vis-à-vis* the family planning programme should be determined to provide a rational basis for allocation of resources.

NOTES

[1] Only in Bangladesh and Pakistan was the mean number of children for age group 45-49 found to be lower than that for age group 40-44 (see table 137).

[2] This period was chosen to minimize the sampling errors of the estimated rates. The ideal period would be the year before the survey but this short period would lead to large sampling errors. It is admitted that the selection of the longer reference period will hide the effect of recent changes in fertility.

[3] Childlessness is measured as the percentage of ever-married women with no children ever born. For alternative definitions of childlessness, see chapter I.

REFERENCES

Alam, Iqbal and J. B. Casterline (1984). *Socio-economic Differentials in Recent Fertility*. World Fertility Survey Comparative Studies, No. 33; Cross-National Summaries. Voorburg, The Netherlands: International Statistical Institute.

Bongaarts, John (1978). A framework for analyzing the proximate determinants of fertility. *Population and Development Review* 4(1): 105-132.

_____ (1983). The proximate determinants of natural marital fertility. In Rodolfo A. Bulatao and Ronald D. Lee, eds., with Paula E. Hollerbach and John Bongaarts, *Determinants of Fertility in Developing Countries*, vol. 1, *Supply and Demand for Children*. Report of the National Research Council Committee on Population and Demography, Panel on Fertility Determinants, New York: Academic Press, 103-138.

Casterline, John B. and others (1984). *The Proximate Determinants of Fertility*. World Fertility Survey Comparative Studies, No. 39. Voorburg, The Netherlands: International Statistical Institute.

Chidambaram, V. C., J. G. Cleland and Vijay Verma (1980). *Some Aspects of WFS Data Quality: A Preliminary Assessment*. World Fertility Survey Comparative Studies, No. 16. Voorburg, The Netherlands: International Statistical Institute.

Cleland, John and John Hobcrafts, eds., in collaboration with Betzy Dinesen. *Reproductive Change in Developing Countries: Insights from the World Fertility Survey*. Oxford: Oxford University Press.

Corsini, C. (1979). Is the fertility-reducing effect of lactation really substantial? In Henri Léridon and Jane Menken, eds., *Natural Fertility*. Proceedings of a seminar organized by the International Union for the Scientific Study of Population. Liège: Ordina Editions, 195-215.

Davis, Kingsley and Judith Blake (1956). Social structure and fertility: an analytic framework. *Economic Development and Cultural Change* 4(4):211-235.

Economic and Social Commission for Asia and the Pacific (1982). Age at first marital union and fertility. Paper submitted to the Fifth Meeting of the United Nations Working Group on Comparative Analysis of World Fertility Survey Data. Geneva, 26-29 January 1982. UN/UNFPA/WFS.V/20, table 4.

_____ (1982a). Marital status composition and fertility. Paper submitted to the Fifth Meeting of the United Nations Working Group on Comparative Analysis of World Fertility Survey Data. Geneva, 26-29 January 1982. UN/UNFPA/WFS.V/13, table 7.

Ferry, Benôit and David P. Smith (1983). *Breast-feeding Differentials*. World Fertility Survey Comparative Studies, No. 23; Cross-National Summaries. Voorburg, The Netherlands: International Statistical Institute.

Hodgson, Maryse and Jane Gibbs (1980). *Children Ever Born*. World Fertility Survey Comparative Studies, No. 12; Cross-National Summaries. Voorburg, The Netherlands: International Statistical Institute.

Kabir, Mohammed (1980). *The Demographic Characteristics of Household Populations*. World Fertility Survey Comparative Studies, No. 6; Cross-National Summaries. Voorburg, The Netherlands: International Statistical Institute.

Léridon, Henri and Benôit Ferry (1985). Biological and traditional restraints on fertility. In John Cleland and John Hobcraft, eds., in collaboration with Betzy Dinesen, *Reproductive Change in Developing Countries: Insights from the World Fertility Survey*. Oxford: Oxford University Press, 139-164.

Lesthaeghe, Ron and H. J. Page (1980). The post-partum non-susceptible period: development and application of model schedules. *Population Studies* 34(1):143-169.

Rodríguez, Germán and John Cleland (1981). Socio-economic determinants of marital fertility in twenty countries: a multivariate analysis. In *World Fertility Survey Conference 1980: Record of Proceedings*. London, 7-11 July 1980. Voorburg, The Netherlands: International Statistical Institute, vol. II, 337-414.

Singh, Susheela and John Casterline (1985). The socio-economic determinants of fertility. In John Cleland and John Hobcraft, eds., in collaboration with Betzy Dinesen, *Reproductive Change in Developing Countries: Insights from the World Fertility Survey*. Oxford: Oxford University Press, 199-222.

Smith, David P. (1980). *Age at First Marriage*. World Fertility Survey Comparative Studies, No. 7; Cross-National Summaries. Voorburg, The Netherlands: International Statistical Institute.

United Nations (1983). Department of International Economic and Social Affairs. Population Division. *Fertility Levels and Trends as Assessed from Twenty World Fertility Surveys*. Non-sales publication ST/ESA/SER.R/50. New York.

_____(forthcoming). *A Comparative Evaluation of Data Quality in Thirty-eight World Fertility Surveys*. Non-sales publication ST/ESA/SER.R/50/Rev.1. New York.

XI. A REVIEW OF THE FERTILITY SITUATION IN COUNTRIES IN THE REGION OF THE ECONOMIC COMMISSION FOR LATIN AMERICA AND THE CARIBBEAN

*Economic Commission for Latin America and the Caribbean**

Abstract

This review of the fertility situation in 13 countries in the region of the Economic Commission for Latin America and the Caribbean (ECLAC) that participated in the World Fertility Survey highlights the major differences and similarities between countries. In most cases, fertility rates estimated from these data apply to the early or mid-1970s and show a moderately high level of five children per woman on average. A general description of recent fertility trends in each country as well as a review of related topics (prevalence of childlessness and infecundity, strength of sex preferences and trends in infant and child mortality) provides a backdrop for the discussion of socio-economic determinants of fertility.

Cross-tabulations of fertility rates with socio-economic characteristics of survey respondents and their husbands show the overall patterns of fertility differentials. In the majority of cases, the usual continuum was observed: fertility of urban and more educated respondents was lower than that of rural and less educated respondents. Fertility was also highest among women with no recorded work and with husbands employed in agriculture. A multivariate analysis measures the impact of each socio-economic variable on cumulative fertility with other fertility determinants controlled. Because of the importance of marital duration in determining achieved fertility, the effect of each socio-economic variable is estimated in relation to this factor, and the strength and even the direction of effects is found to depend upon it. The statistical significance of education as an independent factor affecting fertility is reduced when other factors are controlled.

Some proximate determinants of fertility and their socio-economic correlates are examined next. The Caribbean countries provide an exception to the commonly observed pattern of later marriage among more educated and urban residents. The proportion who had ever used contraception ranges widely, with use of modern methods varying from 32 per cent of all users in Haiti to 49 per cent in Peru. Urban women had the highest levels of use but the gap is widest in countries where the overall use levels were low. In most countries, modern methods were used to roughly the same extent in rural and urban areas, but use was higher among more educated women.

In general, the countries of the ECLAC region fall into several distinct groups. Smaller socio-economic differentials in reproductive behaviour are found in the anglophone Caribbean countries. In certain cases, Costa Rica and Panama, which are relatively advanced economically, fall in this group. Other countries, such as Colombia, Ecuador, Mexico, Peru and Venezuela, display large socio-economic differences. In these countries, it appears that social change has affected primarily the urban, educated and professional groups.

During the latter half of the 1970s, 13 fertility surveys were carried out in the region served by the Economic Commission for Latin America and the Caribbean (ECLAC), as part of the programme of the World Fertility Survey (WFS). This body of new data came at an opportune moment in the demographic history of the region, since during the past 20-25 years, there has been a widespread decline in fertility, in most cases of notable proportions. In fact, the WFS data, along with other empirical evidence, have been instrumental in documenting this profound change. More than establishing current levels and past trends in fertility, however, the WFS data offer a rich source of information for the study of more detailed characteristics of this secular change and for the investigation of the reasons behind it. These twin objectives form the purpose of the present chapter.

---
*Centro Latinoamericano de Demografía.

A. LEVELS AND TRENDS IN FERTILITY

Before examining levels and trends for the 13 countries that participated in WFS, however, the situation that pertains in the region as a whole deserves comment. For the most part, fertility during the latter two decades declined notably. According to ECLAC estimates (1983, 1983a), this is certainly true of Brazil, the most populous country in the region: total fertility is estimated to have declined by more than one third. The same can be stated for many of the smaller Caribbean countries as well. One way of gauging the decline that has occurred in fertility in the past 20 years or so is to note that whereas in the period 1960-1965 the modal total fertility rate (TFR) for the ECLAC region was between six and seven live births per woman and only two countries, Argentina and Uruguay, experienced rates below four, by the period 1980-1985, the modal figure lay between three and four live births and five countries (Barbados, Chile, Cuba, Trinidad and Tobago, and Uruguay) had estimated rates below three.

Decline in fertility, however, did not occur in all ECLAC countries. In the "southern cone" countries of Argentina and Uruguay, for instance, fertility either remained stationary over the period or declined only slightly. In Bolivia and Haiti also, fertility remained high with little or no decline detected. In El Salvador, Honduras, Nicaragua and Suriname, some decline in total fertility apparently occurred, on the order of 10-20 per cent over the 20-year period. Lastly, to place the regional decline in fertility in perspective, the most recent estimates available indicate TFRs greater than five live births per woman in nine countries and TFRs above six live births in three countries. Thus, while fertility declined in most countries, its current level is still from moderately high to high in a considerable portion of Latin America.

For each of the 13 WFS countries in the ECLAC region, this chapter presents a number of fertility estimates (TFR) for the period 1960-1985. From an examination of these estimates, it is obvious that not all merit the same degree of confidence. Older figures, for instance, were arrived at before many important estimation techniques became available. Some data sources are more reliable than others and the type of fertility information collected varies in its adequacy for estimating fertility. Thus, a margin of error should surround the total fertility rates. At least three TFRs are available for each country covering this period. One is the rate estimated from the WFS data set itself. The estimate is based on births that occurred in the five years preceding the date of survey. The central date to which these TFRs refer, therefore, is approximately 2.5 years prior to the date of the survey. In the case of Peru, where only ever-married women were interviewed, proportions ever married by age (from the household survey) were used to deflate age-specific fertility rates. Similar procedures were used in Guyana, Jamaica, and Trinidad and Tobago, where women aged 15-19 who were attending school were not interviewed; and in Mexico, where unmarried women aged 15-19 were not interviewed unless they reported one or more live births. Lastly, since in Costa Rica and Panama women aged 15-19 were not interviewed, registration data for this age group were used for computing TFRs.

As a whole, TFRs derived from WFS data and referring in most cases to the first half of the 1970s display moderately high levels of fertility, the average being about five live births per woman for all 13 countries. Fertility was considerably above replacement level in all countries during this period. In the Dominican Republic, Haiti, Mexico and Peru, on the other hand, the level of fertility recorded by the surveys was even higher. In Mexico, in particular, the WFS data demonstrate that by the early 1970s, fertility had declined only slightly from its historically high level.

A second set of TFRs available for all 13 WFS countries come from ECLAC (1983, 1983a) estimates for 1960-1965 and 1980-1985, which were derived from a variety of sources and methods. For the period 1980-1985, however, some of the figures given are projected rather than estimated because no recent, reliable data are available. At any rate, most countries have conducted the 1980 round of censuses, so recent estimates from census data, though often suffering from reporting biases, were possible. None the less, as can be seen in some countries (e.g., Ecuador and Haiti), estimates for 1980-1985 may be revised in the light of recent survey findings. A final data source comes from the 13 Contraceptive Prevalence Surveys (CPS) carried out in the ECLAC region (three of which were repeat surveys).

Caution is warranted in using fertility estimates calculated from data from these surveys, because some have been found to have sampling biases. Nevertheless, others have been found to yield useful estimates despite having a much simpler questionnaire format (Anderson and Cleland, 1984). With these comments in mind, the fertility situation in each of the 13 WFS countries is described below.

Colombia

Evidence for Colombia indicates that fertility has fallen substantially from the early 1960s (TFR = 6.5-7.0) to 1975, the year before the survey (TFR = 4.5) (Hobcraft, 1980). The 1973 census yields an even lower estimate (4.4) but this is probably an underestimate due to omissions in birth reporting. The first Contraceptive Prevalence Survey (TFR = 3.7, 1977) also may have underestimated period fertility for similar reasons. It is considered by ECLAC (1983) that fertility has continued to decline in Colombia, and in 1985 may have been slightly below four live births per woman. As nuptiality has apparently experienced only minor changes over the same period, the fall in fertility can be attributed almost exclusively to declines in marital fertility (Flórez and Goldman, 1980). Furthermore, the largest drops were found, using WFS data, among women at reproductively "older" ages—e.g., women aged 30-34 at the time of the survey.

Costa Rica

Like Colombia, Costa Rica has experienced a sharp decline in period fertility during the past 20-25 years. Compared with Colombia, however, the decline, beginning at an equally high TFR (7.0-7.5), has been more rapid, falling to about 3.8 live births per woman averaged over the five-year period preceding the WFS programme (1971-1975). More interestingly, recent data reveal that the rapid decline stopped during the mid-1970s and that since then fertility rates have risen slightly (Rosero, 1981). Part of this trend reversal can be explained by birth postponement, from the earlier to the later half of the decade. In addition, it is possible that the difficult legal situation encountered by two contraceptive methods, intra-uterine devices (IUD) and sterilization, after 1975 contributed to this trend (Rosero, 1980). The latter method has apparently become more difficult to obtain since that date despite a favourable judgement in the courts. Another characteristic of the trend reversal in Costa Rican fertility is that fertility rates among older cohorts have continued to fall, but this has been more than compensated for by the tendency of fertility rates of younger cohorts to rise since about 1975 (Rosero, 1981). Thus, the future trend in fertility (rising or falling) will depend in part upon whether women in the earlier part of their childbearing years continue their pattern of behaviour of the past few years or begin to emulate that of their older counterparts.

Dominican Republic

A notable decline in fertility has also been documented in the Dominican Republic. In the early 1960s, high fertility, with TFRs between 7.0 and 7.5, obtained in the Dominican Republic as in other countries in the region (ECLAC, 1983; Conning, 1982). Fertility began falling during the mid-1960s. This change has been linked by some to political changes at that time which led to a liberalization of policies related to family planning (Guzmán, 1980). By the year before the first WFS survey (1974/75), the total fertility rate was estimated to have dropped to about five live births per woman. With little change observed in age at first union, the decline can be attributed mainly to lower marital fertility (Guzmán, 1980). The most recent evidence indicates that the decline has continued into the 1980s and that current total fertility is probably on the order of 4.0-4.5 (Hobcraft and Rodríguez, 1982).

Ecuador

Fewer data on fertility are available for Ecuador than for the countries described above. Nevertheless, a decline in fertility has been documented from the WFS data, although the change has not been large. According to ECLAC (1983) estimates, high fertility prevailed during the early 1960s, with TFR about 7.0. By the period 1975-1979, the rate had dropped to 5.2 (see chapter I), a decline of 24 per cent over a period of about 15 years. Despite this decline, fertility in Ecuador is still moderately high, certainly above the average for the region.

Guyana

Vital registration data for recent periods in Guyana are considered fairly reliable (Balkaran, 1982). Total fertility rates calculated from this source show a steady decline: 6.2 (1960); 5.1 (1970); 3.8 (1974). Similar rates calculated from the 1975 WFS maternity history show an equivalent trend, but with fertility at a consistently higher level. For 1974, for example, the WFS data yield an estimated TFR of 4.3, suggesting a systematic underreporting of births by vital registration statistics. Some of this decline may be due to a rise in age at first union documented in the WFS marriage history data, but the major change appears to have occurred in marital fertility (Balkaran, 1982, p.22).

Haiti

Until recently, data were lacking for estimating fertility levels and trends in Haiti. During the 1970s, however, three sources of data (the 1971 census, a multi-round demographic survey and WFS) became available, confirming moderately high fertility (a TFR of about 5.5 for the mid-1970s). There are indications also that the level of fertility had not differed greatly in the past. These sources provide meagre evidence concerning fertility trends, but a slight decline may have occurred. The pattern of Haitian fertility, unusual for a population with relatively low use of efficient contraception, may partially be explained by relatively late average age at first union and union history patterns that are among the most complex in the entire region (Allman, 1982).

Jamaica

Available evidence points to a rising trend in Jamaican fertility from the post-war period until the early 1960s (Singh, 1982). This rise has been linked to improvements in biomedical and social conditions which would tend to increase the "supply" of children. During the same period, declines in age at first union and proportions of women not in unions generally also acted so as to increase the proportion of women at risk of pregnancy. Since the early 1960s, estimates from the same sources indicate a decline in fertility, with the total fertility rate falling below 5.0 by the mid-1970s. Towards the end of the decade, vital registration, which probably suffers under-reporting of births to an unknown extent, showed the rate dropping below 4.0 live births (Jamaica, 1980). Although reporting errors common to maternity history data may have exaggerated the extent of the decline in the 12 years or so preceding the survey, there appears to be little doubt that by the 1980s total fertility in Jamaica hovered around 3.5. The most recent vital registration data, however, appear to show that the decline in fertility may have been arrested at this level (United Nations, 1982 and 1984).

Mexico

Mexico is the most populous of the ECLAC countries participating in WFS. Its fertility experience is also one of the most dramatic. A number of estimates indicate that high fertility, with TFRs of about 6.5, persisted in Mexico until the early 1970s. Subsequently, however, a notable decline occurred so that by the 1980s, total fertility most probably stood at below 5.0 live births, and its current level may be around 4.5 (Zavala, 1984). Rising age at first union among younger cohorts and lower marital fertility among older cohorts largely account for this change. This abrupt change in the trend in fertility coincides with important population policy changes by the Mexican Government accompanied by a series of organizational changes directed to implementation of new anti-natalist goals (Cabrera, 1984). Despite the apparent success of these public actions, the current level of fertility in Mexico must still be classified as moderately high and above the average of the region taken as a whole.

Panama

Of the countries participating in WFS, Panama appears to have been among the earliest to experience a fertility decline. At the beginning of the 1960s, total fertility appears to have been already below 6.0 live births per woman and data from various sources show an approximately continuous decline since then. By the early 1970s,

WFS data indicate a rate of about 4.5, while the Contraceptive Prevalence Survey data for 1978/79 yield an estimated rate of about 3.5. The most recent provisional vital registration data (Panama, 1983, 1983a, 1984), however, do not follow the declining trend of the 1970s and may imply that in Panama, as in other countries described in this section, fertility may have reached a plateau.

Paraguay

Fertility appears to be declining in Paraguay although not all evidence points in the same direction. For the early 1960s, TFRs higher than 6.5 have been estimated, while two surveys conducted in 1977 and 1979, the latter being in the WFS programme, give evidence that total fertility had fallen to below five births by the mid-1970s (Schoemaker, 1981). Because of the retrospective nature of the data collected in these surveys, however, it is possible that response error has led to an overestimation of past fertility and hence to an overstatement of the fall in fertility in the 15 or so years before the surveys. In fact, other recent data from the Contraceptive Prevalence Survey of 1977 yield a very high TFR of 6.8. Although the methodology employed and small sample size of that survey cast some doubt on the reliability of the fertility estimate, it seems safe to suggest at least that fertility may not have fallen beyond the level recorded in the mid-1970s, that is, about 4.9. In sum, Paraguay appears to have experienced some reduction in fertility during the period 1960-1978.

Peru

Data from a number of sources give a consistent picture of moderately declining fertility in Peru during the period 1960-1980. As in most countries of the region, fertility was quite high in the early 1960s, with TFRs close to seven live births. In a gradual and apparently continuing fashion, estimated TFRs during the 1970s (Peru, 1983) and early 1980s show a decline to 5.2 by 1980, a drop of about 25 per cent over the 20-year period. Current fertility is still too high to speculate whether the observed decline will continue at the same rate or will reach a plateau as seen in several other countries of the region. Until recently, governmental policy concerning fertility was one of non-intervention, so fertility decline must be viewed principally as a consequence of changing attitudes towards contraception among individuals without programmatic support (with nuptiality changes possibly contributing to the decline in a minor way).

Trinidad and Tobago

That fertility change is at a relatively advanced stage in Trinidad and Tobago is reflected by the fact that even for the early 1960s, TFRs of fewer than six have been estimated. By mid-1970, both vital registration and WFS data lead to estimates in the range from 3.1 to 3.4 (Trinidad and Tobago, 1981). The WFS maternity history data, which have been shown to be of high quality (Hunte, 1983), demonstrate also that this decline has affected all age groups, the fertility rates for younger women declining partially in response to rising age at first union (documented from WFS union history data). The most recent vital registration data indicate a continuing decline to levels lower than any other country included here and raise the possibility of Trinidad and Tobago reaching a replacement level of fertility during the current decade.

Venezuela

In the case of Venezuela, fewer data sources are available to assess fertility levels and trends. The two principal sources are WFS and vital registration, but the latter is considered unsuitable because of problems caused by underregistration as well as by the recording of births by date of report rather than date of event. Nevertheless, TFRs apparently had fallen from around 6.5 live births to 4.6 by the mid-1970s. This decline has been attributed both to an increase in age of mother at first birth (and in age at first union) and to a fall in higher order births (Vielma, 1982). Despite this decline, fertility in Venezuela remains at a moderately high level.

Entire region

In sum, evidence in most WFS countries in the ECLAC region, excluding Haiti, point to declining fertility over the period considered. Most countries began the 1960s with high fertility (TFRs of 6.5-7.0). Panama and Trinidad and Tobago, countries with high ratings in socio-economic indices compared with the other WFS countries in the region (see Introduction to this report), are exceptions, because fertility decline apparently began sometime before 1960. By the early 1980s, however, much more diversity in fertility levels was observed. Fertility decline, at least to a level of four or five live births, occurred in most countries, sometimes—as in Mexico—over a very short period. Several countries (Costa Rica, Guyana, Jamaica, Panama, and Trinidad and Tobago) had even lower fertility, between three and four live births per woman, as of the early 1980s. Whether fertility decline will continue at the same rate below the 3.5-4.0 level, however, is open to question. Of the 13 countries, only in Trinidad and Tobago has fertility clearly declined to levels approaching the level generally found in developed countries. Several other countries, namely, Costa Rica, Jamaica, Panama and possibly Paraguay, seem to have experienced a slow-down in fertility decline after a period during which fertility fell at a roughly constant rate. Most of the other WFS countries still have moderately high, but declining, levels of fertility. Whether a fertility plateau will be reached in these countries will be known only in the future. Meanwhile, the reasons for the fertility "slow-down", some of which have been touched on above (e.g., change to a pro-natalist stance on the part of certain sectors of the national authority structure), form an important topic for investigation because they may have a wider significance for the fertility of the region as a whole.

B. LEVELS AND TRENDS IN SOME VARIABLES RELATED TO FERTILITY

The first section of this chapter focused on national fertility estimates and the phenomenon of declining levels of fertility was assessed in general terms. In later sections, factors associated with levels and trends in fertility differentials are considered. To begin, however, some of the variables that impinge upon fertility are described. The first topic—infecundity—merits attention both as an important by-product of WFS data sets and because it constitutes an intermediate factor with an obvious although, in the Latin American context, minor influence on fertility. Secondly, infant and child mortality are described. Although the relationship between these factors and fertility is difficult to analyse for methodological reasons (Economic and Social Commission for Asia and the Pacific, 1984), there are good reasons to believe that high infant mortality is a powerful motive for continued high fertility. Thirdly, sex preference for children, a topic not usually broached in the Latin American and Caribbean context, is discussed to see to what extent such preferences are likely to influence fertility behaviour.

Childlessness and infecundity

Little attention has been paid to the topic of childlessness and infecundity in the demographic literature for the ECLAC region. Yet the WFS data can be used to measure, at least indirectly, both major aspects of infecundity, namely, primary and secondary infertility. A comparative analysis of infecundity is important in itself, even though it is somewhat tangential to the main focus of this chapter, because in many countries of the region population policy is directed not only to assisting couples who wish lower fertility but to aiding those who are unable to achieve the number of children desired.

Columns (1) and (2) of table 152 present measures closely linked to primary infertility: proportions of women in the indicated age groups who have had no live births nor were pregnant at the time of the survey.[1] The sample is restricted to women currently in a marital union who have been in a union for at least five years. By using a minimum period of observation of five years this measure tends to overestimate childlessness, because some women who may first bear children at marital durations longer than five years will thus be included. The degree of overestimation, however, is likely to be quite small for two reasons. First, very early marriages, where adolescent subfecundity may inflate the proportion of nulliparous women with durations of more than five years, are controlled by restricting the samples to women aged 25 or over at survey. Secondly, it has been demonstrated (Hobcraft and McDonald, 1984) that first birth intervals longer than five years occur infrequently, particularly in the Latin American context.

A further problem with the measure of childlessness given in table 152 is that it does not distinguish between biological infecundity and infecundity induced by periods of marital separation due either to a history of dissolution and remarriage or to temporary geographical separation of spouses. Such conditions are more likely to bias these estimates in Caribbean countries, which have more complex union history patterns and in which high rates of migration may also lead to greater frequency of spousal separation.

With all these caveats in mind, it is seen that proportions of childless women vary substantially between countries in the region. For women aged 40-44,[2] childlessness varies from as low as 1.5 per cent in Panama to as high as 7.0 per cent in Guyana. The proportion childless in Guyana is probably upwardly biased by age-misreporting of childless women who may have transferred into the 40-44 age group from surrounding age groups (Vaessen, 1984, p. 9). Nevertheless, the Caribbean countries (the Dominican Republic, Guyana,[3] Haiti, Jamaica, and Trinidad and Tobago) display rates of childlessness that are substantially higher than those in other countries of the region, particularly Costa Rica, Panama, Peru and Venezuela, where less than 2 per cent of women aged 40-44 were childless. As mentioned above, peculiar marriage and migration patterns may partially account for this difference, but differentials related to disease and other biological factors cannot be ruled out.

With regard to women aged 25-49, representing a wider spectrum of experience, a somewhat lower average level of childlessness is found although in several countries the level is higher. The most notable change, in Trinidad and Tobago, results from high levels of childlessness (10-15 per cent) for women aged 15-29, reflecting almost certainly deliberately delayed childbearing among younger married women and paralleling trends noted in other modern societies with high contraceptive use. In fact, in all cases where childlessness is higher among women aged 25-49 than for women aged 40-44 high levels of contraceptive use are also found. The measure used

TABLE 152. MEASURES OF CHILDLESSNESS AND BEHAVIOURAL INFECUNDITY FOR VARIOUS AGE GROUPS, COUNTRIES IN THE ECLAC REGION

Country	Percentage of women with no pregnancies at ages: 40-44 (1)	25-49 (2)	Behavioural infecundity[a] for age group <25 (3)	25-34 (4)	35-44 (5)	45+ (6)	Total (7)
Colombia	3.2	2.3	0.5	4.6	18.7	50.6	11.8
Costa Rica	1.7	2.3	0.6	3.8	16.5	39.3	10.4
Dominican Republic	5.2	3.7	1.1	9.0	27.8	66.4	16.1
Ecuador	1.5	1.7	..	..	..	..	..
Guyana	7.0	4.1	0.7	9.2	37.5	64.5	17.5
Haiti	3.6	3.0	1.3	6.7	20.5	43.0	12.7
Jamaica	4.7	4.9	1.2	7.5	28.2	54.2	14.9
Mexico	2.6	2.3	0.9	4.9	21.4	61.1	13.5
Panama	1.5	1.7	0.6	8.0	24.5	56.0	14.1
Peru	1.7	1.4	0.6	4.3	17.4	52.0	13.1
Paraguay	3.4	3.1	0.7	5.9	19.1	50.7	13.4
Trinidad and Tobago	4.6	6.4	1.7	5.8	21.0	36.4	12.1
Venezuela[b]	1.9	2.1	0.5	4.2	20.5	—	7.0

Source: World Fertility Survey standard recode tapes.

[a] Among currently married non-sterilized women, percentage who were married continuously for 5+ years with open birth interval of 5+ years and no contraceptive use in this interval.
[b] For women aged 15-44 only.

cannot distinguish childlessness caused by deliberate contraception from other causes of childlessness. The lower figures given in column (2) of table 152 suggest a trend towards lower levels of primary infertility in certain countries. This trend may be even greater than the comparison of columns (1) and (2) indicates, because a trend towards delayed childbearing, in some countries, would tend to mask a decline in childlessness.

With WFS data, a number of measures can be devised for secondary infertility, although none is completely satisfactory. One method is to use responses to a direct query on fecundity. Unfortunately, women, especially at older ages, cannot always accurately judge their fecundity status and this is generally reflected in substantial proportions of respondents who answered "don't know". The measure adopted here relies on behavioural indications of infecundity (Vaessen, 1984). Behaviourally infecund women are defined as those continuously married for at least the past five years who reported no use of contraception in the open birth interval and had an open interval of five or more years.[4] One important bias in this measure occurs in situations of high prevalence of contraceptive use. The assumption is that women who use contraception are fecund, but this is not necessarily so, particularly at later ages where women may be uncertain whether they are fecund but use contraception anyway. Comparison of self-reported and behavioural infecundity in fact points to sizeable proportions of such women in high-use countries.

Columns (3)-(7) in table 152 present the proportions behaviourally infecund by age group. Costa Rica, and Trinidad and Tobago are almost certainly cases where infecund women who nevertheless use contraceptives are numerous enough to lead to serious underestimation of infecundity. The low percentages of behaviourally infecund women aged 45-49 (39 and 36 per cent, respectively) must be considered unreliable estimates of the true level of infecundity in these countries. Countries where infecundity appears to be relatively high, as much as double other countries in the region, include the Dominican Republic, Guyana, Jamaica and Panama. Given the fact that contraceptive use is high in Panama, infecundity among older cohorts is probably even higher than shown. It is interesting to note that in these four countries, 8-9 per cent of women in the relatively young group aged 25-34 are infecund, well above the average for the region as a whole (6 per cent).

Levels and trends in infant and child mortality

Despite the fact that empirical studies have proven inconclusive, from a theoretical point of view conditions of high infant and child mortality should induce couples to maintain a high level of fertility (United Nations, 1972; Preston, 1978). At the same time, the reduction of birth intervals caused by infant deaths induces a fertility-increasing effect (Knodel and van de Walle, 1967). This interval effect, however, is important in countries with long breast-feeding durations and low use of contraception, conditions that are found in few WFS countries in the ECLAC region.[5]

Estimates from the WFS data for both infant mortality, $_1q_0$, and mortality under five years of age, $_5q_0$, are presented in table 153. There is a positive relationship between mortality rates and fertility rates,[6] as measured by the correlation coefficient between the total fertility rate and child mortality, confirming, at the aggregate level at least, an association between infant and child mortality and fertility. It is also evident that infant and child mortality rates vary in a similar way so that the same story is told by either measure. In passing, however, it is interesting to observe that as child mortality declines, infant mortality comprises a progressively larger share of it. For instance, in the three countries where infant and child mortality is highest (Haiti, Peru and the Dominican Republic), about 34 per cent of children who die before age 5 are aged 1-4 years at death, but in the three WFS countries where mortality has declined the most (Panama, Trinidad and Tobago and Jamaica), only 22 per cent of child deaths are in this age group. From the point of view of this chapter, however, the importance of table 153 lies in the fact that a wide range of infant and child mortality rates is found. Where such mortality was still high, particularly in the Dominican Republic, Haiti and Peru, one may reasonably expect less enthusiasm about the use of contraception. It has also been shown for Colombia (Baldión, 1981) that educational level is one of the strongest predictors of infant mortality.

Table 153 also gives some idea of the dynamics in infant and child mortality over the period 0-19 prior to survey. For both infant and child mortality, the period 0-4 years prior to the survey is compared with the period 10 years earlier.[7] In almost all countries, significant declines in both mortality measures occurred over this period. Costa Rica and Panama experienced particularly large declines even though mortality was already at a moderate level. On the other hand, in Jamaica, Paraguay, Trinidad and Tobago, and Venezuela, infant mortality remained stationary or showed a slight increase while only modest gains are noted with respect to child mortality. These countries, which had not shown much improvement in health conditions related to childhood mortality during the 10 years preceding the survey, also rank in the group with relatively low levels of infant mortality. In several other countries in the region, both the high level of infant and child mortality and the slower progress in its reduction may be contributing to the moderately high levels of fertility estimated in those countries. In others, however, where much more favourable conditions exist, infant and child mortality probably has a weaker effect on fertility behaviour.

Preference for sex of children

The topic of parental preferences concerning the sex composition of their families and the implications such preferences have for fertility decisions has attracted considerable attention in recent literature for some developing regions (Repetto, 1972; Williamson, 1976). This has not, however, been the case in the ECLAC region, where sex preferences are not thought to be strong. For that reason, it is useful to present the comparative data obtained in the WFS programme.

Most interest in sex preferences has centred on the desire for sons, a well-known phenomenon in many Asian countries. Preferences for certain family compositions, however, may take several forms comprising both sex preferences and size preferences or even balances between the sexes of children. In fact, a variety of sex preferences may coexist in the same population whose effects would go undetected when aggregate measures were used (McClelland, 1979). It has also been questioned whether

TABLE 153. LEVELS AND TRENDS OF INFANT AND CHILD MORTALITY, COUNTRIES IN THE ECLAC REGION

Country	Infant mortality rate, $_1q_0$ (1)	Child mortality rate, $_5q_0$ (2)	(1)/(2) (3)	$_1q_0$ (10-14)/ $_1q_0$ (0-4) (4)	$_5q_0$ (10-14)/ $_5q_0$ (0-4) (5)
Colombia	70	108	0.65	120	130
Costa Rica	53	61	0.87	158	198
Dominican Republic	89	129	0.69	123	134
Ecuador[b]	80	126	0.63	..	..
Guyana	58	77	0.75	108	99
Haiti	123	191	0.64	129	136
Jamaica	43	56	0.77	97	112
Mexico	72	96	0.75	120	141
Panama	33	46	0.72	135	171
Peru	97	149	0.65	121	137
Paraguay	61	85	0.72	98	107
Trinidad and Tobago	43	50	0.86	95	113
Venezuela	53	64	0.83	82	105

Columns 4 and 5 are under "Trends"[a]; columns 1-3 under "Levels for period 1-4 years prior to the survey".

Source: Rutstein (1983), table 3, 5 and 8.
[a] Sample restricted to children whose mothers were aged 20-29 at their births. Expressed as a ratio.
[b] Period 0-9 years prior to the survey.

TABLE 154. PERCENTAGE WHO WERE CURRENTLY USING CONTRACEPTION AMONG WOMEN WITH TWO LIVING CHILDREN, BY SEX COMPOSITION OF LIVING CHILDREN, COUNTRIES IN THE ECLAC REGION

Country	All boys	Balance	All girls
Colombia	53	49	56
Costa Rica	70	81	74
Dominican Republic	44	34	31
Guyana	26	36	31
Haiti	25	26	19
Jamaica	40	51	42
Mexico	38	46	38
Panama	63	65	61
Peru	35	45	39
Paraguay	51	56	43
Trinidad and Tobago	56	62	65
Venezuela	56	64	57

Source: Cleland and others (1983), table A.3.

stronger preferences would have a significant fertility effect since the random nature of the gender of future births means that unfavourable compositions have roughly equal chances of growing worse or becoming less acute.

Keeping in mind these limitations, data on the stated preferences for the sex of the next child of female respondents (Cleland and others, 1983) show that in the majority of Latin American and Caribbean countries, women with two, three or four living children expressed a desire for a balanced composition. Where sons outnumbered daughters among living offspring, women typically preferred the next child to be a girl and vice versa. Where a balance prevailed, preferences were more or less evenly split, while results for two countries (Mexico and Peru) show a moderate tendency towards a son preference in balanced families; and the analogous results for four countries (Colombia, Jamaica, Venezuela, Trinidad and Tobago) display a somewhat milder tendency towards a daughter preference. Even in these countries, however, a balanced composition seems to be an important desire. It is interesting to note that daughter preference, and to a large extent balance preference, is confined to the Latin American and Caribbean region, being rare in Africa and in Asia and Oceania.

Table 154 shows the percentage of women using contraception grouped by family sex composition. Although some variability is noted, more detailed analysis (Cleland and others, 1983, p. 22) shows that statistically significant differences in contraceptive use occur only in the Dominican Republic and Mexico. In the former country, the prevalent preference for sons apparently translates into fertility-related behaviour for families with two, three or four living children. For instance, 44 per cent of women with two sons and no daughters were using contraception but only 31 per cent were users if their family comprised two daughters and no sons, table 154 also shows similar differences in Paraguay.

Interestingly, women with just two living children are more likely to use contraception when sexes are balanced (46 per cent versus 38 per cent). In fact, this pattern is generally found in the entire region, excluding the Dominican Republic, Colombia, and Trinidad and Tobago (in the latter two countries, little difference by family composition is noted in any case). The regularity of these results suggests a greater willingness among younger cohorts to limit families through contraception if they are ideally balanced. This finding, with its implication for future levels of fertility, is probably the most significant result of this comparative sex-preference analysis since, aside from a consistent preference for sons in the Dominican Republic, behaviour as it relates to contraceptive use does not appear to be related to stated sex preferences.

C. SOME SOCIO-ECONOMIC DETERMINANTS OF FERTILITY

As is well-known (Davis and Blake, 1956; Bongaarts, 1978), fertility levels are proximately determined by a set of intermediate socio-biological variables which affect the ability to conceive, exposure to the risk of conception, the probability of a pregnancy resulting in a live birth and the duration of post-partum amenorrhoea. Some of these factors, such as fecundability and post-partum infecundity, in so far as differential infant mortality affects them, were discussed in the previous section. Other proximate determinants are analysed below; still others, such as abortion, are not discussed because of lack of data. In the present section, socio-economic determinants of fertility are investigated, but it should be kept in mind that such factors act on fertility only through intermediate variables affecting exposure and fecundity.

This section is divided into two parts, each based on a different measure of fertility—recent fertility and cumulative fertility. A multi-variable analysis was considered preferable to the choice of just one aspect of fertility because, as shall be seen, each aspect of fertility has its own distinct story to tell. Recent fertility is defined for the five-year period preceding the survey date in each country: rates are the ratios of births in the interval to women-years of exposure for the pertinent subgroup of women. Note that age-specific fertility rates (and therefore total fertility rates) are subject to biases of unknown magnitudes in certain countries where straightforward, all-women samples were not taken. In the case of Peru, for instance, birth histories are available only for ever-married women, so that proportions ever-married by age available from the household survey must be used as multipliers not only for overall rates but for subgroup rates. The extent to which this procedure is defensible in the case of numerically small subsamples has not been carefully examined. Peculiarities in the samples in Guyana, Jamaica, Mexico, and Trinidad and Tobago, already mentioned, mean that to varying degrees certain age-specific fertility rates also are partially based on multipliers from other sources.[8] Another source of error in estimates of recent fertility lies in the biases introduced by age and event misstatement. Evaluation of WFS data shows at least moderate levels of age-heaping. Misdating of events related to the age of the mother, is also a common feature of WFS birth history data. In this regard, evidence of the so-called "Potter effect" (Potter, 1977) has been cited in several country-level data evaluations. The review of the data quality presented in chapter I shows that estimates of recent fertility rates for all Latin American and Caribbean countries are reliable and in only two cases was there evidence that trends estimates might be exaggerated—the Dominican Republic and Panama. From the point of view of the present analysis, the most serious consequence of such misreporting errors is the likelihood that they are not spread evenly through different socio-economic groups. In fact, a standard practice in WFS data evaluation is to use differences by educational level to demonstrate misreporting errors by assuming more accurate reporting among better educated women. This assumption is reasonable but can throw doubt on the source of observed socio-economic differentials in recent fertility where errors are known to be prevalent. In most countries included here, however, this is unlikely to be a significant problem.

Differentials in recent fertility

Table 155, columns (1)-(6), shows differentials in total fertility rates and marital fertility by respondents' current residence. Residence definitions vary considerably between countries (see chapter VII), so some caution must be exercised in making cross-national comparisons. The dominant pattern of TFRs is one of monotonic decline in fertility from rural to other urban to major urban. In several countries, however, little difference between the two urban categories is observed (especially Costa Rica, the Dominican Republic, Panama, and Trinidad and Tobago). In Haiti, major urban fertility is actually somewhat higher than other urban. The fact that these are all geographically small countries, and mostly islands, suggests that there may not be any semi-urban areas where fertility behaviour might display an intermediate level.

Rural TFRs are highest in all countries except Guyana, where women in "other urban" areas experience slightly higher recent fertility than women in rural areas. In Colombia, Paraguay and Venezuela, rural rates are about twice the major urban rates. In the Dominican Republic and Peru, large absolute rural/urban differentials are also observed in TFRs, while in most other countries somewhat smaller but still considerable differentials are found. In Guyana and in Trinidad and Tobago, on the other hand, relatively small absolute differences are noted by residence.

Except for Guyana, TMFRs exhibit the same patterns as TFRs. These marital rates are duration-specific and are calculated on the experience (i.e., fertility for the five years preceding the survey) of women whose first union was 0-24 years before the survey (for details, see Alam and Casterline, 1984). Thus, as expected, differentials in recent marital fertility largely reflect those in overall fertility. In general, differences between the two fertility rates are greater for urban areas than for rural areas. Changes in nuptiality in urban areas, particularly later ages at first union, would account for these differences. These inferred differentials in rural/urban nuptiality also result in smaller rural/urban marital fertility differentials. Excluding Guyana and Trinidad and Tobago, the average rural/urban differential based on TMFR is 2.25 live births, compared with 2.87 for TFR. The cases of Guyana, and Trinidad and Tobago is somewhat distinct from the other countries in the region. First, while rural/urban differences exist, they are quite small and of less significance. Moreover, in these two countries, there does not seem to be a fertility effect of rural/urban differences in nuptiality, as noted above for other countries. One explanation is that the rural/urban dichotomy is fundamentally different in these countries. Another is that Caribbean

TABLE 155. RECENT FERTILITY, BY CURRENT RESIDENCE AND RESPONDENT'S EDUCATION,[a] COUNTRIES IN THE ECLAC REGION

| | Recent fertility by current residence |||||| Recent fertility by respondent's education[a] ||||||||
| | Total fertility rate[b] ||| Total marital fertility rate[c] ||| Total fertility rate[b] |||| Total marital fertility rate[c] ||||
Country	Major urban (1)	Other urban (2)	Rural (3)	Major urban (4)	Other urban (5)	Rural (6)	Zero (7)	One to three (8)	Four to six (9)	Seven or more (10)	Zero (11)	One to three (12)	Four to six (13)	Seven or more (14)
Colombia	2.89	3.86	6.95	3.66	4.45	7.37	7.03	6.04	3.85	2.59	6.78	6.31	4.33	3.20
Costa Rica	2.52	2.73	4.20	3.19	3.43	4.99	4.46	4.07	3.11	2.54	5.06	4.91	3.79	3.22
Dominican Republic	4.23	4.43	7.39	4.93	5.12	7.68	6.99	7.29	5.37	2.98	6.88	7.20	5.86	3.79
Ecuador	3.13	4.88	6.65	3.82	5.70	7.14	7.84	7.25	5.33	2.69	7.43	7.37	5.85	3.32
Guyana	4.05	5.91	5.25	4.26	5.68	5.88	6.55	6.97	5.56	4.84	6.70	7.65	5.81	5.14
Haiti	3.98	3.40	6.19	4.24	3.80	6.24	6.05	4.75	4.06	2.85	5.94	4.92	4.96	3.91
Jamaica	3.86	5.16	5.65	3.67	5.01	5.42	6.19	5.92	5.76	4.83	5.65	4.80	5.07	4.66
Mexico	4.81	5.72	7.63	5.54	6.45	8.15	8.06	7.47	5.75	3.34	7.90	7.73	6.27	4.09
Panama	2.90	2.88	5.10	3.80	3.72	6.21	5.70	5.58	4.12	2.71	6.73	6.66	5.21	3.41
Paraguay	3.15	3.96	6.31	3.60	4.63	6.61	8.23	6.61	4.62	2.94	7.66	6.64	4.98	3.29
Peru	3.88	5.41	7.18	5.02	6.39	7.78	7.32	6.75	5.06	3.27	7.65	7.10	5.64	4.23
Trinidad and Tobago	2.88	3.31	3.67	2.98	3.63	4.24	4.63	3.45	4.13	3.21	6.05	2.24	4.43	3.45
Venezuela	3.29	4.30	7.65	4.10	5.33	8.26	7.02	6.36	4.57	2.64	7.40	6.63	5.11	3.57

Source: Alam and Casterline (1984).
NOTE: For full discussion of residence, see chapter VII.
[a] Years of schooling completed.
[b] Ages 15-49, except for Costa Rica and Panama, ages 20-49; and for Venezuela, ages 15-44.
[c] Marital duration, 0-24 years.

marriage patterns (prevailing also in Guyana) are such that rural or urban environment becomes an irrelevant factor. It is also possible that measurement of "age of first union", particularly difficult in these societies, is so imprecise that such differentials are submerged within the response error.

Table 155, columns (7)-(14), presents total fertility rates for four educational groups. A pattern of smaller total fertility rates with higher respondent education is evident in all countries with a maximum differential (measured as the difference between the extreme groups) of 5.3 live births observed for Paraguay and a differential of from four to five live births in Colombia, the Dominican Republic, Mexico, Peru and Venezuela. In the three anglophone Caribbean countries, on the other hand, differentials by education are much less significant. In the majority of countries, "thresholds" are not very evident, but a predominant pattern is that the largest differential is observed between groups with from one to three or from four to six years of schooling. In Trinidad and Tobago, however, there is no consistent pattern.

Total marital fertility rates follow a similar pattern but, in general, differentials are reduced, indicating that part of the fertility effect of education operates through differential patterns of nuptiality, principally through delayed first union among more educated women. This conclusion is analagous to that described above for rural/urban differences.

Evidently, there is a great deal of correspondence in the observed differentials by rural or urban residence and those by education. In fact, it is well known that the two factors are substantially interrelated so that the effects of one factor are bound to be largely mirrored in those of the other. The present analysis of recent fertility differentials does not allow more detailed breakdowns; and it is not possible to measure, say, the fertility effect of education controlling for rural or urban residence. None the less, it can be assumed that the independent effect of either factor would be weaker. As to the causal ordering of residence and education, technically speaking, respondent's education is prior to current residence. In fact, however, replacing current residence with "long-term" residence as defined in chapter VII by making use of the survey question on childhood residence makes very little difference in most analyses (e.g., Sathar and Chidambaram, 1984). In that case, residence is most probably causally prior to or concurrent with education.

Age-specific and duration-specific fertility rates (upon which TFRs and TMFRs are based) provide further insights into the fertility behaviour of socio-economic groups. For brevity, these rates are analysed only for educational categories, but similar results are observed for other factors. Age-specific fertility falls into two patterns: in Costa Rica, Guyana, Jamaica, and Trinidad and Tobago, different educational groups are not clearly distinguished; in other countries, lower fertility rates are found at all ages as higher levels of education are considered. Figure 76, top panel, illustrates these distinct findings for Paraguay and for Trinidad and Tobago, typical examples of each pattern. The more common pattern, illustrated by Paraguay, demonstrates that reduced fertility occurs at all ages. Differential age-specific marital fertility rates by educational group (figure 76, middle panel) can also be summarized by two typical examples, in this case, Colombia and Peru. While marital fertility rates largely reflect all-women rates, Mexico, Peru, Venezuela and to some extent Costa Rica show a convergence of rates at ages 15-19 regardless of educational level. This suggests that fertility differentials at the earliest reproductive ages are determined more by differences in age at union than by differential contraceptive use in this group of countries. Another group of countries, Colombia, the Dominican Republic, Haiti and Paraguay, displays age-specific differentials beginning at the youngest age group (15-19), thus implying that greater practice of contraception occurs among the more educated women even at the youngest reproductive ages, perhaps for spacing reasons.

Using Guyana and Mexico as the examples, the bottom panel of figure 76 illustrates the two principal patterns of rates according to duration of union. In one pattern (Guyana, Haiti, Jamaica, and Trinidad and Tobago) the proportion of total fertility contributed by women in a union 20 or more years does not vary by education. For example, in Guyana, such women contribute 9.5 per cent (no education) and 10.8 per cent (seven or more years of schooling). The other pattern is found in the remaining countries: a declining contribution with increasing education. In Mexico, for example, the corresponding percentages are 16.8 and 7.5 per cent. In these Hispanic countries, long-married uneducated women continue to reproduce at substantial rates, whereas more educated women have largely stopped bearing children after two decades of marriage.

Recent marital fertility (TMFR) for women of 0-24 years of marital duration is shown by occupation of current husband or partner in table 156, columns (1)-(4). The pattern common to the region, except Venezuela, is for agricultural groups to have the highest rates and professional/clerical groups the lowest. In Venezuela, the "sales and service" category has the highest fertility, while the agricultural category is not greatly differentiated from the other occupational groups. In general, fertility differentials are of the same magnitude as those observed for residential and educational categories. Agricultural occupations are predominantly rural, while professional ones are mainly urban; a similar association between occupation and education obtains (because husband's and wife's education are closely related). Hence, although at this level of analysis it is not possible to consider independent effects, it is clear that they must be much smaller than indicated by simple differences between TMFRs. In fact, to the extent that occupation depends upon residence and education, its independent effect may be quite small.

Table 156 also presents TMFRs for categories of respondents' work status: not working, working for self or within the family enterprise, or working for others (i.e., outside the family). As already discussed in chapter IX, work definitions are far from uniform in these surveys, making cross-national interpretation difficult. Within the fairly homogeneous ECLAC region, however, somewhat more confidence may be placed in work measures. The general pattern, although differentials are much smaller than for the three factors already analysed, is that TMFRs for non-working women are largest while those for women working for others are smallest. Haiti is an exception to this pattern, as family workers have the highest fertility; and in Guyana and Peru, non-workers and family workers have virtually identical rates. In Jamaica and Venezuela, on the other hand, family and non-family workers exhibit approximately the same level of fertility.

Figure 76. Age-specific and duration-specific fertility rates, by educational category, selected countries in the ECLAC region

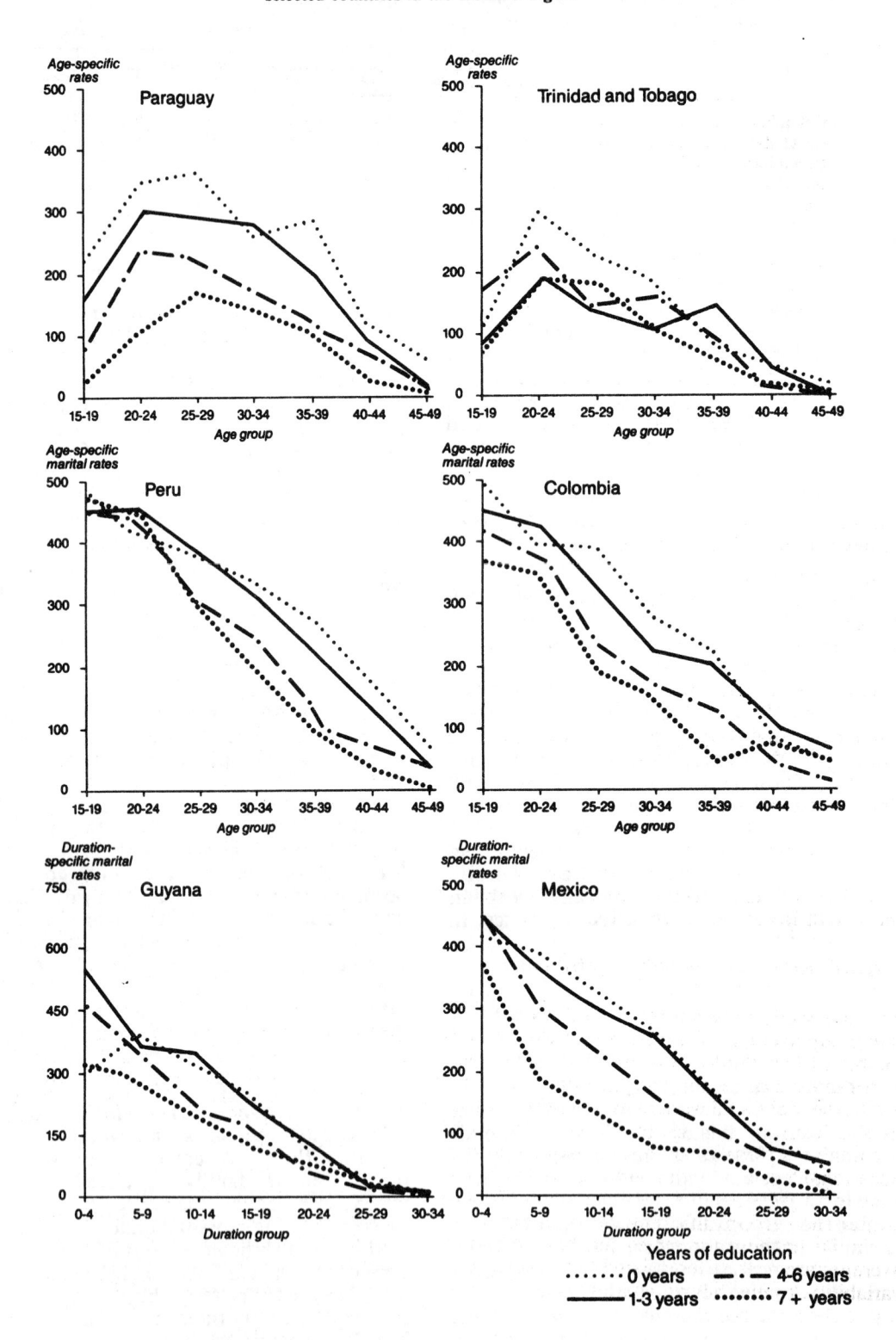

Years of education
- ······· 0 years
- —·— 4-6 years
- ——— 1-3 years
- •••••• 7+ years

Source: Alam and Casterline (1984), tables A1, A2 and A3.

Again, the work-status variable is intimately interrelated with the other socio-economic factors considered. For instance, family work is more common in agricultural, rural households, while "work for others"

TABLE 156. RECENT MARITAL FERTILITY, BY HUSBAND'S OCCUPATION AND RESPONDENT'S WORK STATUS, COUNTRIES IN THE ECLAC REGION

	Total marital fertility rate, by						
	Husband's occupation				Respondent's work status		
Country	Agriculture	Skilled/ unskilled	Sales/ services	Professional/ clerical	No work	Family or self	Other (non-family)
Colombia	7.21	4.48	4.40	3.19	6.03	5.17	4.26
Costa Rica	5.08	3.81	4.03	2.93	4.53	3.76	3.46
Dominican Republic	7.91	5.45	5.30	3.55	6.88	6.15	5.18
Ecuador	7.48	5.91	5.04	3.45	6.60	5.59	4.94
Guyana	6.60	5.59	5.12	3.95	5.44	5.20	4.05
Haiti	6.33	4.95	4.80	3.45	5.40	5.98	4.75
Jamaica	5.93	5.03	3.76	3.43	7.18	5.06	4.79
Mexico	8.09	7.12	6.14	4.60	7.38	6.79	5.35
Panama	6.49	4.45	4.44	3.44	5.69	4.91	3.93
Paraguay	7.00	4.59	3.85	3.53	6.11	5.54	4.06
Peru	7.66	6.57	5.65	4.45	6.82	6.78	5.35
Trinidad and Tobago	4.97	4.04	3.28	2.51	4.34	3.72	3.00
Venezuela	5.70	5.62	8.12	4.00	6.07	5.17	4.26

Source: Alam and Casterline (1984).
NOTE: Marital duration, 0-24 years.

predominates among urban, educated women. Considered by itself, the condition of female work participation is seen to have some influence on fertility.

To summarize the findings of this section, rural or urban residence, educational attainment and occupational status all appear to have influenced recent fertility in the sense that urban, better educated women whose partners have white-collar occupations have substantially lower fertility than rural, uneducated women. In the anglophone Caribbean countries, however, differentials in fertility were of a lesser magnitude, implying less influence of these socio-economic factors on fertility behaviour. The analysis, however, was unable to apportion the relative importance of these three determinants, nor was it able to say anything about the independent effects of any one factor keeping the other two constant. Work status, on the other hand, seems less important, although in most countries women working outside the household environment had lower recent fertility.

Differentials in cumulative fertility

The previous section concentrated on presenting differences in group averages. Cumulative fertility (specifically, number of live children ever born, CEB) is easily available for individual respondents and analysis of this variable with the individual woman as the units of observation is the focus of this section. Figure 77, which presents cumulative fertility by age of woman and by three educational levels for two countries typical of patterns found in all WFS countries (Guyana and Mexico), demonstrates that group differentials in children ever born are similar to those for recent fertility.[9] Although group averages are well differentiated, analysis of individual variability, as the following paragraphs will show, leads to less clear-cut conclusions.

Space does not permit a full explanation of the regression model on which the present analysis is based.[10] The model is log-linear in form with interactions between union duration and other independent variables emphasized. Besides union duration, age at first union and child-death experience are added to the model as demographic variables, while the socio-economic variables considered are respondent's education (number of years of schooling) and rural or urban residence.[11]

Effects of demographic variables on cumulative fertility as portrayed by regression coefficients are shown in table 157. Because of the form of the model, regression coefficients are not interpretable in a straightforward way. Their effect on CEB is shown graphically in figure 78, but first some general patterns may be noted. With regard to age at first union a finding common to most countries is a positive coefficient for the main effect coupled with a stronger negative coefficient for the interactive term (duration times age at marriage). This means that, in general, during the first few years of marriage the age-at-union variable exerts a positive influence but that among women married for longer periods age at first union is negatively associated with CEB. According to the results presented in table 157, the point at which the relationship becomes negative occurs early in the union history of women—after three or four years of union in most cases. A plausible explanation of this pattern is that women who enter unions later are more anxious to begin family-building immediately. Since pre-marital conceptions and births are included in CEB, it is also possible that women who marry at older ages are more likely to have experienced such events. The negative effect which becomes predominant a few years after marriage, on the other hand, is evidence of the fact that women marrying late are older and therefore less fecund at any given marriage duration.

Note that in three countries, Haiti, Panama and Venezuela, statistically significant effects of age at union are found, while in several others the main effect is insignificant. In still other countries, both effects are significant, but the interactive one is much more so than the main effect. One conclusion to be drawn is that it is important to consider age at marriage as affecting CEB together with marital duration.

Experience of the death of one or more children may lead to a desire for more children, as mentioned above in the section on child mortality. The effect of a variable that measures this experience[12] is also shown in table 157. Note first that the variable (main effect) is significant in all countries (and in most cases highly significant), even

Figure 77. **Children ever born to ever-married women, by current age and educational level, Guyana and Mexico**

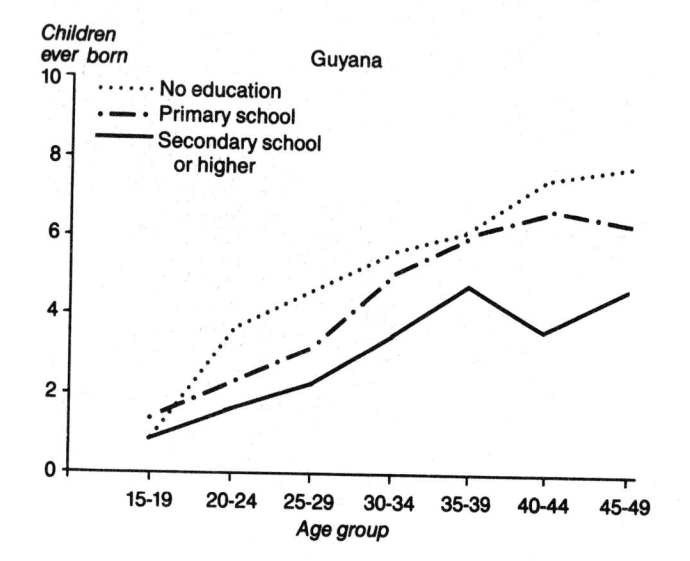

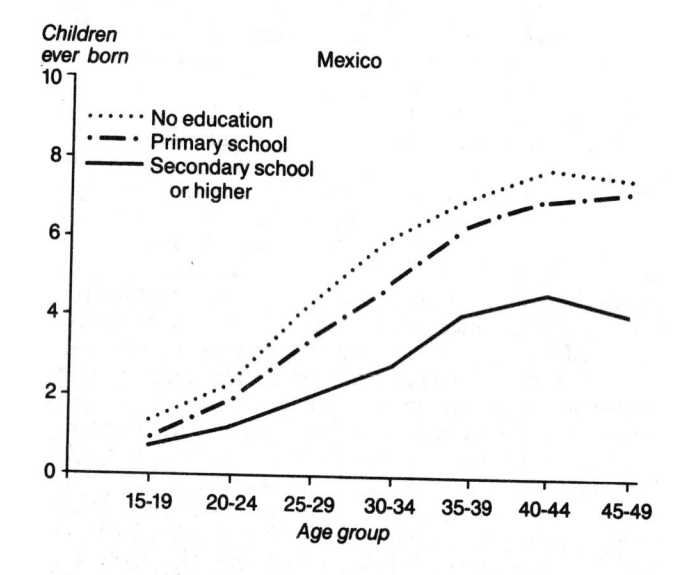

[Graph: Guyana — Children ever born vs Age group (15-19 to 45-49), three lines: No education, Primary school, Secondary school or higher]

[Graph: Mexico — Children ever born vs Age group (15-19 to 45-49), three lines: No education, Primary school, Secondary school or higher]

Source: Hodgson and Gibbs (1980).
NOTE: The definition of primary and secondary schooling varies between countries and was coded at the country level. Reference can be made to table 109 for the number of years included in the primary level for each country.

TABLE 157. REGRESSION COEFFICIENTS FOR LOG-LINEAR MODEL WITH CHILDREN EVER BORN AS DEPENDENT VARIABLE AND UNION DURATION, AGE AT FIRST UNION AND CHILD-DEATH EXPERIENCE AS INDEPENDENT VARIABLES, COUNTRIES IN THE ECLAC REGION

Country	Age at first union Main effect (1)	Age at first union Interactive[a] effect (2)	Child-death experience Main effect (3)	Child-death experience Interactive[a] effect (4)
Colombia	0.01	−0.01[b]	0.29[b]	0.04
Costa Rica	0.02[b]	−0.01[c]	0.54[c]	−0.04
Dominican Republic	0.03[b]	−0.02[b]	0.38[b]	−0.04
Ecuador	0.02[b]	−0.01[c]	0.31[c]	0.04
Guyana	0.02	−0.02[b]	0.79[c]	−0.14[b]
Haiti	0.01	−0.01	0.41[c]	0.04
Jamaica	0.03[b]	−0.02[c]	0.56[b]	−0.03
Mexico	0.00	−0.01[b]	0.27[c]	0.04
Panama	−0.01	−0.01	0.60[c]	−0.10[b]
Paraguay	0.03[c]	−0.02[b]	0.34[b]	0.04
Peru	0.01	−0.01[c]	0.24[c]	0.06[b]
Trinidad and Tobago	0.02[b]	−0.02[c]	0.74[c]	−0.09
Venezuela	−0.01	−0.01	0.41[c]	−0.02

Source: World Fertility Survey standard recode tapes.
[a] Interactive with duration of union.
[b] Statistically significant ($F \geq 5.0$, degrees of freedom: 2+ and infinity. Similar degrees of freedom apply throughout tables.
[c] Statistically significant ($F \geq 20.0$).

with several other independent variables in the regression equation (union duration, age at union). Moreover, the direction of the effect is clearly positive, meaning higher fertility among women who experience child deaths. The interactive effect with duration, however, is in general non-significant and always much smaller in magnitude. In fact, where signs differ between effects, the magnitude of the interactive-effect coefficient is too small to imply that the total effect of child-death experience would cease to be positive during the normal reproductive life span. It should also be emphasized, however, that the relationship between cumulative fertility and child-death experience may merely reflect the increasing probability of a child's death among women with more live births (who have more children at risk of dying as well as children with longer exposure times).

Two clear patterns are evident in the coefficients for child-death experience. Countries where the main effect is large in magnitude (Costa Rica, Guyana, Jamaica, Panama, Trinidad and Tobago, and Venezuela) have interactive effects with negative signs. Although the combined effect is always positive, its magnitude is reduced among women with long marital durations, possibly implying that recently married women can more effectively alter fertility behaviour, compared with older marriage cohorts, in the face of an infant or child death. This is plausible in view of the fact that contraceptive use is relatively elevated in this group of countries. The remaining seven countries display a somewhat different pattern: a positive main effect of a smaller magnitude; and a positive but non-significant interactive effect. In general, these countries have lower levels of contraceptive use and hence presumably less control over fertility in the event of the death of a child.

The combination of main and interactive effects is best described graphically. In figure 78, six countries are selected to demonstrate the range of predicted patterns in CEB resulting from variations in the three demographic variables modelled. For age at first union, the selection of examples was determined by statistical significance: Jamaica has two significant coefficients; Peru one (the interactive effect); and Panama none. Even though similar patterns are shown in all three examples, the probable margin of error would be much wider for Panama than for Jamaica. The crossing-point of the lines for ages at first union of 18 and 23 years indicates the marital duration at which the negative (interactive) effect begins to predominate.

Figure 78. **Number of children ever born according to union duration, by child-death experience and age at first union, countries in the ECLAC region: predicted values from regression models**

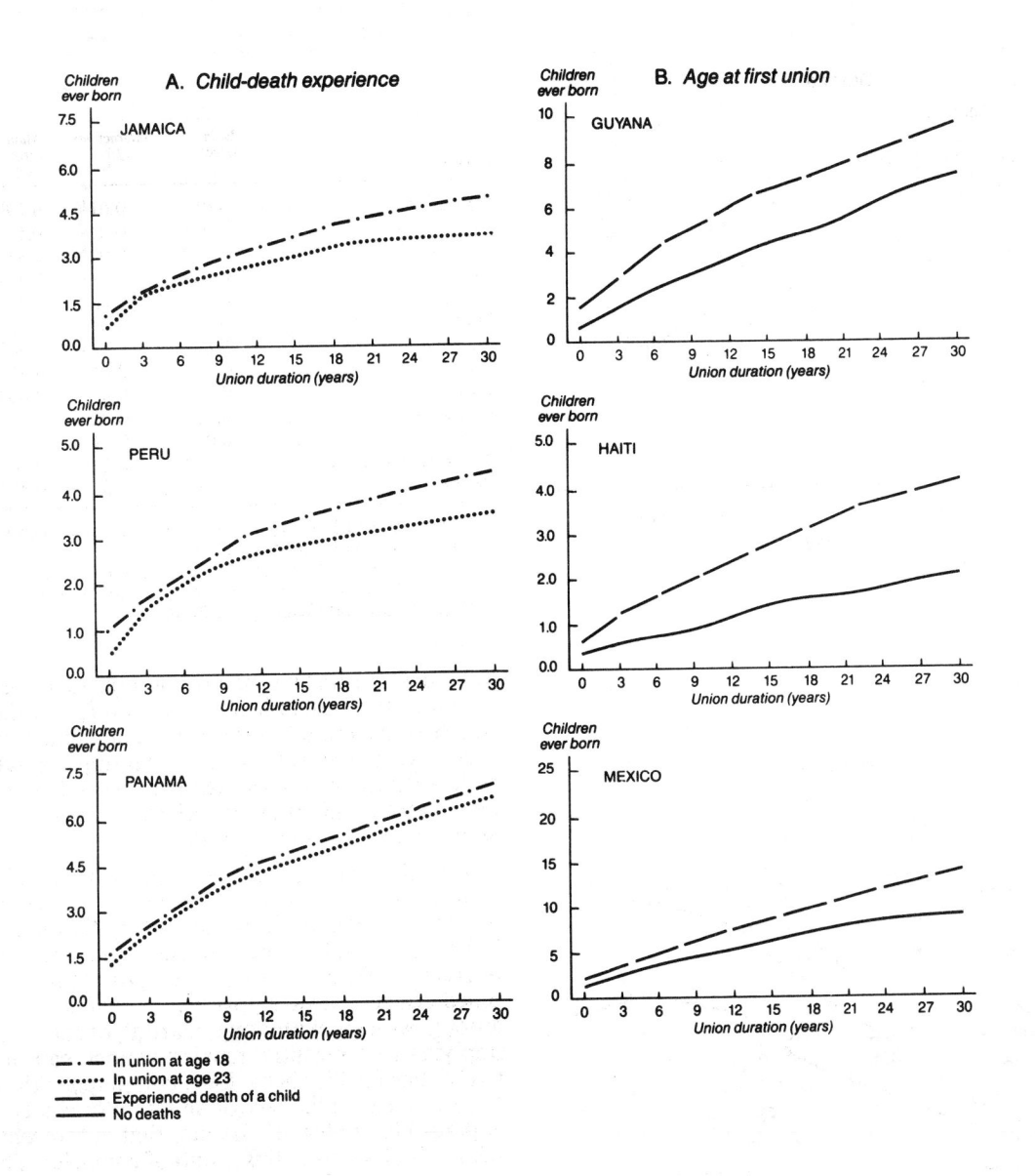

A. *Child-death experience*

JAMAICA

PERU

PANAMA

B. *Age at first union*

GUYANA

HAITI

MEXICO

— · — In union at age 18
········· In union at age 23
— — Experienced death of a child
——— No deaths

Source: World Fertility Survey standard recode tapes.
NOTES: Six years of schooling assumed in Haiti, Mexico and Peru; otherwise, eight years.
In Jamaica, Panama and Peru, average experience of child deaths assumed.
In Guyana, Haiti and Mexico, age at union assumed to be 20 years.

Three countries, Guyana, Haiti and Mexico, which were chosen on the basis of the magnitude of the main effect and the sign of the interactive effect, illustrate the range of results for child-death experience. Guyana has coefficients with the largest absolute values while Mexico is representative of countries with relatively small absolute values and a positive sign for the interactive effect. Haiti lies in between the two extremes.

Residential status influences CEB in a manner similar to the TFR differentials discussed above, as is shown in table 158. In this part of the analysis, residence is measured in three categories based on information on both current and childhood residence: continuous urban; continuous rural; and migrant, where childhood and current residence are different. The predicted differences after 25 years of marriage, however, are less impressive than was the case with recent fertility.[13] In most cases, when education is not considered, the predicted CEBs for urban women are 15-25 per cent below those of rural women, with migrant women occupying a middle position. Peru is an exception in that migrant women have significantly higher fertility than rural women except among the oldest marriage cohorts (25 or more years of union). Also, except for Peru, rural/migrant differences

TABLE 158. PREDICTED CUMULATIVE FERTILITY AT 8 AND 25 YEARS OF MARITAL DURATION, BY RESIDENTIAL STATUS OF RESPONDENTS, COUNTRIES IN THE ECLAC REGION[a]

(Rural fertility = 100)

Country	Marital duration: 8 years			Marital duration: 25 years		
	Long-term rural	Migrant[b]	Long-term urban	Long-term rural	Migrant[b]	Long-term urban
A. Not controlling for education						
Colombia	100	82	80[c]	100	83	81
Costa Rica	100	86	75[c]	100	84	69
Dominican Republic	100	86	78[c]	100	81	71
Ecuador	100	90	84[c]	100	92	81
Guyana	100	..	75[c]	100	..	83
Haiti	100	85	70	100	82	67
Jamaica	100	..	82[c]	100	..	89
Mexico	100	94	92	100	94	90
Panama	100	90	78[c]	100	94	77
Paraguay	100	90	73[c]	100	87	69
Peru	100	105[c]	96	100	100	94
Trinidad and Tobago	100	..	83	100	..	86
Venezuela	100	81	75[c]	100	87	75
B. Controlling for education						
Colombia	100	88	79	100	90	77
Costa Rica	100	89	82	100	88	78
Dominican Republic	100	78	70[c]	100	73	62
Ecuador[d]	100	90	85[c]	100	91	80
Guyana[d]	100	..	84	100	..	86
Haiti	100	99	76[c]	100	93	68
Jamaica	100	..	83	100	..	87
Mexico[d]	100	93	88[c]	100	92	81
Panama	100	94	88	100	96	83
Paraguay[d]	100	98	83	100	95	79
Peru[d]	100	93[c]	87[c]	100	88	85
Trinidad and Tobago[d]	100	..	92	100	..	90
Venezuela	100	81	74	100	88	73

Source: World Fertility Survey standard recode tapes.

[a] Model evaluated with following constants: age at union = 20 years; average child-death experience; six years of schooling (panel B).
[b] Childhood and current residence different.
[c] Statistically significant ($F \geq 5.0$).
[d] Significant interaction between residence and education.

are not significant, in many cases possibly because of the small number of cases in the migrant category. In Haiti and Mexico, women do not have significantly different cumulative fertility when categorized by residence if respondents' residence is considered without their education.

When education is brought into the model (table 158, panel B), several changes occur in the CEB-residence relationship. First, there is a considerable loss of statistical significance in several countries (Colombia, Costa Rica, Guyana, Jamaica, Panama, Trinidad and Tobago, and Venezuela). In these countries, whatever influence residence status has on cumulative fertility appears to operate principally through education or the factors represented by education. In fact, in Guyana and in Trinidad and Tobago, the direction of the relationship, although non-significant, reverses, urban fertility being higher than rural.[14] Secondly, at 25-year duration predicted urban CEB values remain about 20 per cent below rural figures even though the direct influence of residence is reduced. This difference is due to residence-education interactions which, except for the anomalous case of Paraguay, act in the following way: compared with rural women, higher education among urban women has a more negative impact on cumulative fertility. (Interactions are significant in Ecuador, Guyana, Mexico, Paraguay, Peru, and Trinidad and Tobago.) This is illustrated in figure 79 for the typical case of Mexico. Paraguay, where results yield a positive (and significant) interaction, is also shown. These results may say something about the relative influence of rural and urban educational systems over fertility behaviour, the former perhaps being relatively "inefficient" in this regard (in countries where notable interactions were found). Alternatively, these interactions may not be due to differences in the educational system, but rather to rural/urban differences in contraceptive availability and/or strength of the family planning programme effort if education is conceived as enhancing knowledge and use of contraception. Such enhancement could conceivably be affected by differential availability.

In table 159 and figure 80, results of adding educational attainment to the regression model for cumulative fertility are shown. In panel A of table 159, predicted CEB values for women with no education show a significant (except for the Dominican Republic) negative impact of education on fertility when residence is omitted from the model. In many cases, the differentials approach the magnitude of those found above for recent fertility,[15] but in some countries (Mexico and the anglophone Caribbean countries) differences are small or non-existent, particularly among older marriage cohorts. These latter countries

Figure 79. **Predicted number of children ever born, by duration of union for residential-educational groups, Mexico and Paraguay**

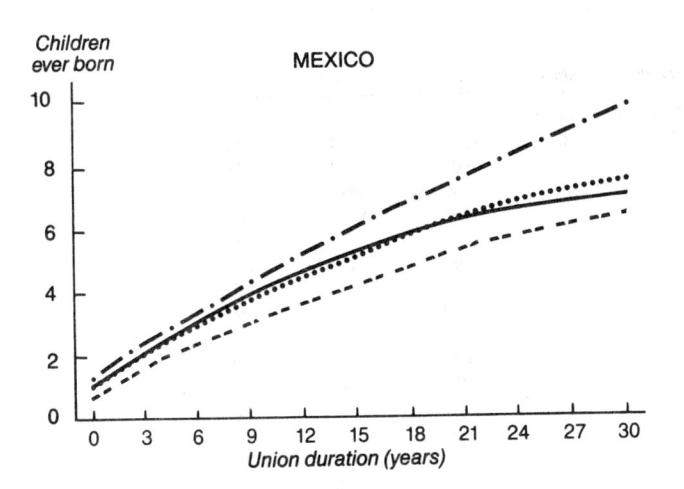

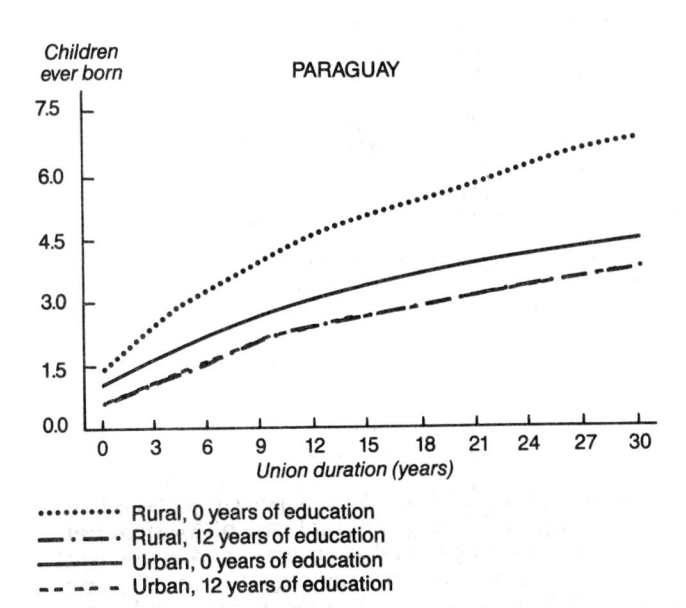

MEXICO

PARAGUAY

········· Rural, 0 years of education
— · — · Rural, 12 years of education
———— Urban, 0 years of education
— — — Urban, 12 years of education

Source: World Fertility Survey standard recode tapes.

display an interesting pattern of non-linearity: at smaller durations, a negative effect of education is apparent, but this disappears at longer durations.

As has already been amply demonstrated, fertility effects of residence, education and other socio-economic measures are interrelated. It is therefore worth while to examine the influence of education independent of residence status (table 159, panel B). The residence measure chosen, which includes "childhood" residence, in most instances can be considered prior to education in the causal sequence, so introducing it as a control variable is not illogical. Statistical significance of the independent effect is considerably reduced; but more interestingly, it changes sign, becoming positive, in several countries: Haiti, Jamaica and Mexico show statistically significant positive effects. In only a few countries (Costa Rica, Panama, Paraguay, Peru and Venezuela) does a fairly strong negative effect remain. Unfortunately, the WFS data do not permit (Arguëllo, 1980) more than speculation as to the reasons underlying this interesting division of countries. Of course, from a policy point of view, the total effect of education, direct and indirect, is of more importance than its independent effect alone. Therefore, these findings should not be misconstrued to suggest that more education would lead to higher fertility for the country as a whole, when in fact, the opposite is clearly true, as can be seen from table 155.

D. DIFFERENTIALS IN PROXIMATE DETERMINANTS OF FERTILITY

The socio-economic differentials in fertility discussed above are obviously not the result of direct relationships, but rather of indirect ones mediated by so-called "intermediate" or "proximate" determinants (Davis and Blake, 1956; Bongaarts, 1978). In this section, differentials in three proximate determinants, age at first marriage, contraceptive use and post-partum infecundity, and their relative contributions to fertility differentials are discussed.

Age at first union

Nuptiality patterns in the ECLAC region have proved to be a rich subject for research both in and of themselves (i.e., the formation and dissolution of sexual unions) and with respect to their impact on fertility (e.g., Roberts and Braithwaite, 1962; Ebanks and others, 1974; Camisa, 1978; Rosero, 1978; United Nations, 1984b). Furthermore, within the region, the anglophone Caribbean countries exhibit unique patterns (e.g., visiting relationships) which distinguish them from the Spanish-speaking countries. It has also been claimed that nuptiality in Haiti is among the most complex of all WFS countries, since migration patterns interact with union stability to a considerable degree in that case (Allman, 1982). While noting this complexity, the present section is limited to describing age-at-union patterns and differentials with respect to residence and education. Table 160 provides the basic comparative results for this analysis.

Age at first union, as measured by the median age for the cohort aged 25-29, varies from about 18 to 22 years.[16] The younger ages are concentrated in the Caribbean countries, including the Dominican Republic. Age at first birth for women aged 40-49, however, has a considerably smaller range (about 20-22 years) implying, perhaps, that estimates of age at first union do not faithfully measure the effective age of commencement of cohabitation both because of the inclusion of early non-permanent relations and because of the omission of pre-marital sexual relations (McDonald, 1984). Disaggregating the samples for Guyana and Trinidad and Tobago into those of Indian ancestry and non-Indian ancestry reveals an important difference in both countries: Indian subgroups appear to begin sexual relations about three years earlier, on average, than their non-Indian counterparts (tabulations not shown). The confounding effect of racial background helps to explain part of the unique Caribbean patterns discussed below.

Table 160, column (2), compares median ages at first union for two cohorts 10 years apart (20-24 and 30-34). These cohorts were chosen to avoid comparing older cohorts for whom an increase in marital age is noted in almost all samples. Because some or all of this increase

TABLE 159. PREDICTED CUMULATIVE FERTILITY AT 8 AND 25 YEARS OF MARITAL DURATION, BY YEARS OF EDUCATION, COUNTRIES IN THE ECLAC REGION[a]

(Zero education = 100)

Country	Marital duration: 8 years			Marital duration: 25 years		
	Zero	6 years	12 years	Zero	6 years	12 years
A. Not controlling for residence						
Colombia[b]	100	87	76	100	88	77
Costa Rica[b]	100	87	65	100	76	58
Dominican Republic	100	100	100	100	100	100
Ecuador[b]	100	81	65	100	76	57
Guyana[c]	100	81	65	100	98	96
Haiti[b]	100	79	61	100	81	65
Jamaica[c]	100	73	53	100	100	99
Mexico[c]	100	94	89	100	102	103
Panama[c]	100	82	67	100	83	68
Paraguay[b]	100	81	65	100	82	67
Peru[b]	100	86	73	100	80	64
Trinidad and Tobago[b]	100	70	48	100	94	87
Venezuela	100	80	63	100	75	56
B. Controlling for residence						
Colombia	100	115	133	100	114	130
Costa Rica[b]	100	87	75	100	81	66
Dominican Republic	100	109	118	100	116	135
Ecuador	100	93	87	100	94	88
Guyana[b]	100	83	69	100	87	93
Haiti[b]	100	101	102	100	109	119
Jamaica[c]	100	79	61	100	107	114
Mexico[b]	100	101	102	100	108	117
Panama	100	87	76	100	88	77
Paraguay[b]	100	81	65	100	82	67
Peru[b]	100	92	85	100	86	74
Trinidad and Tobago[b]	100	74	53	100	92	85
Venezuela	100	92	85	100	86	74

Source: World Fertility Survey standard recode tapes.

[a] Model evaluated with following constants: age at first union = 20 years; child-death experience average; residence status = migrant status in panel B. For migrant status, childhood and current residence different.

[b] Statistically significant (F ≥ 5.01).

[c] Statistically significant (F ≥ 20.01).

may well be due to misreporting of dates or events by older women (moving the date of first union towards survey date or omitting first unions altogether), it is better to avoid using results from such cohorts when analysing trends. A modest increase in median age is noted in all countries except Jamaica, where age at first union seems to have declined slightly over the decade prior to the survey (this decrease is noted in other cohorts as well). In general, increases are smaller in the Caribbean subregion, while in Peru, a large increase of 1.7 years was added to the median age over this period.

The remaining columns of table 160 report singulate mean ages of marriage (SMAM), a summation based on age-specific proportions single (Hajnal, 1953). It should be cautioned that SMAMs are most suited for use in populations not affected by changes in migration and other demographic phenomena, so the comparisons presented here must be treated as liable to a wide margin of error.

Rural/urban[17] and especially educational differences in marital age are substantial in most countries (see also Rosero, 1978). The direction of these differentials (higher age at first union among urban or more educated women) is consistent with the differentials noted in fertility since the long-term effect of later unions is to reduce fertility. As can be seen from the averages given in table 160, basic differences exist between the Caribbean and other countries: differentials by residence are somewhat negative in the former group (i.e., rural ages at union are somewhat higher on average), but positive and in the order of two years in the latter group. Similarly, differentials by education are much less important among Caribbean women. In these countries, possibly, female employment (associated with urban, educated women) is more compatible with marriage or other forms of sexual union so that rural/urban differences are diminished. On the other hand, the percentages given in column (7) show that in most countries with a large age-at-union differential by education (Mexico being a notable exception) the greatest share of the total differential is between respondents with from four to six years or seven or more years of schooling. This seems to imply that unions are delayed by further education in most cases but not in the Caribbean countries.[18]

Lastly, disaggregated SMAMs for five-year periods zero and five years before the survey are compared in columns (4) and (6) of table 160. Given the probable margins of error inherent in this measure, a general conclusion would seem to be that changes in age at union are not occurring at different speeds among the various residence and educational groups. The only exception to this observation is Trinidad and Tobago, where, according to SMAM estimates, women with no schooling entered a union 2.3 years later than women with seven or more years of schooling, so that, by the survey date, SMAM was actually higher for uneducated women.

Figure 80. Predicted number of children ever born according to duration of union, by years of education: Jamaica and Peru

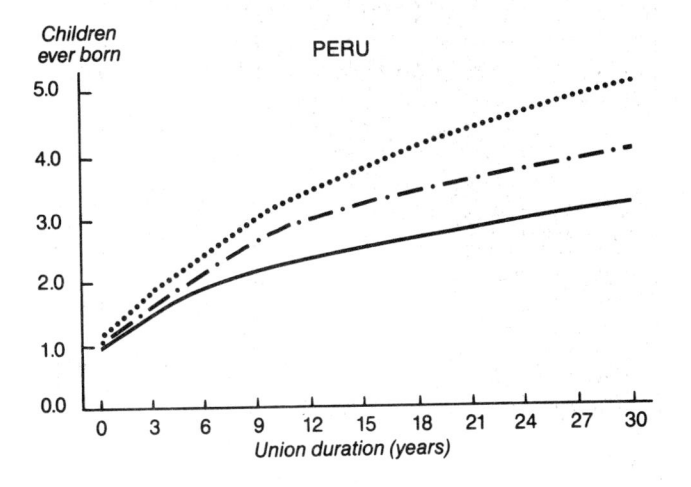

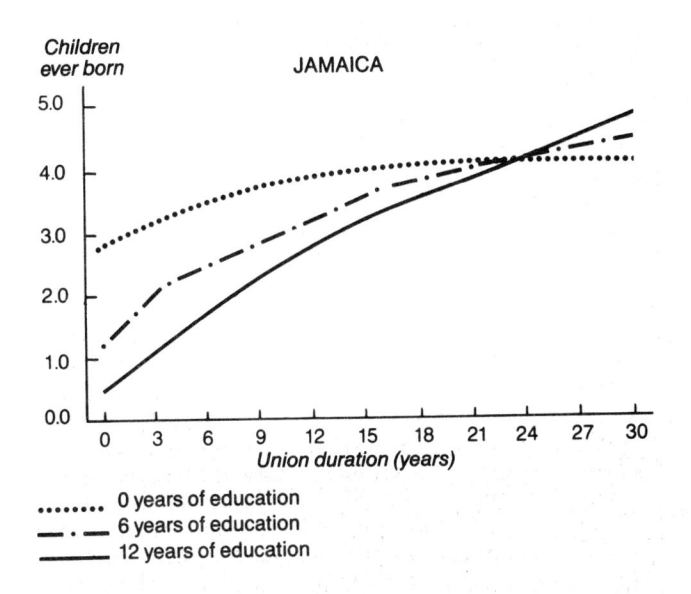

PERU

JAMAICA

······ 0 years of education
─·─·─ 6 years of education
───── 12 years of education

Source: World Fertility Survey standard recode tapes.

Contraceptive use

In most WFS countries of the ECLAC region, the voluntary use of means to prevent conception is widespread and in certain groups of women, the prevalence of contraceptive use reaches levels comparable to that found in Europe or Northern America. The composition of methods used is an important topic, especially for government planners involved in implementing population policies, but such detail is beyond the scope of the present chapter. Here reference is made only to two groups of contraceptive methods usually termed "modern" and "traditional" (for full discussion, see chapter V).[19] The discussion also focuses on ever-use of contraception among currently married women aged 15-49. Current-use rates will always be lower than ever-use rates, but it has been shown that a fairly strong linear relationship exists between the two measures so that they are largely interchangeable in comparative analysis (Sathar and Chidambaram, 1984).

Among all currently married women considered as a whole, ever-use varied from 37 and 48 per cent in Haiti and Mexico, respectively, to 81 and 85 per cent in Trinidad and Tobago and Costa Rica, respectively. On average, about three fifths of all women in the samples had used contraception at some time in the past. Another important feature of contraceptive practice in the region is the high proportions of ever-users (80-90 per cent) who had, at some time, used modern methods, except in Haiti (32 per cent) and Peru (49 per cent). Combining ever-use and percentage of modern use, one finds ever-use of modern methods low compared with the regional average in Haiti (12 per cent), Peru (25 per cent), Mexico (38 per cent) and the Dominican Republic (41 per cent). In Haiti, more than two thirds of the women were currently using rhythm, withdrawal or abstinence (Allman, 1982), while in Peru, these three traditional methods accounted for about half of all current users (United Nations, 1981). At the other extreme, Costa Rica and Trinidad and Tobago, where three quarters of women had used a modern method at some point in their reproductive career, hormonal pills and female sterilization accounted for more than half of users in the former country, while pills and condoms were similarly popular in the latter.

Table 161 presents differentials in ever-use by current residence.[20] Lower use, expected among rural residents, was found in all cases. Women in non-major urban areas had somewhat lower ever-use rates but their contraceptive behaviour on the whole was much more like that of women in major urban areas than like rural women. Interestingly, less significant rural/urban differentials were found in those countries (Costa Rica, Guyana, Jamaica, Panama, and Trinidad and Tobago) where prevalence of use was high and family planning had been well established for several years. This suggests that in the remaining countries family planning knowledge and services had not yet widely diffused beyond urban centres.

In terms of method mix, much smaller rural/urban differences were found. Only in Haiti and Peru, the two WFS countries with low use of modern methods, were large differentials found. The result is an even wider rural/urban gap in percentage of ever-use of modern contraceptive methods: 5 versus 29 per cent in Haiti; and 4 versus 47 per cent in Peru. In other countries, however, the methods used were not appreciably more "traditional" in rural areas, signifying that although fewer rural women used contraception, those who did have recourse to scientific and clinical methods, made use of them roughly to the same degree as urban women.

Rural/urban differences also occur when the foregoing analysis is broken down by age group (not shown). In general, urban distributions are broader and less peaked than rural ones, mainly because of relatively greater use of contraception by young urban women than their rural counterparts. In Venezuela, for instance, over 60 per cent of currently married urban women aged 15-19 had ever used contraception but the corresponding rural figure is only about 25 per cent. In several other countries, more than half of young married urban women were ever-users: Colombia; Ecuador; Peru; Guyana; Jamaica; Trinidad and Tobago.[21] In such urban settings, it appears that contraceptive use is fast becoming or has already become

TABLE 160. MEDIAN AGE AT FIRST UNION AND DIFFERENTIALS IN SINGULATE MEAN AGE AT MARRIAGE, BY RESIDENCE AND YEARS OF EDUCATION, COUNTRIES IN THE ECLAC REGION

			\multicolumn{5}{c	}{Singulate mean age at marriage in years}	
Country	Median age for women, 25-29 (1)	Differential in median age (20-24) − (30-34) (2)	Urban/ rural differential (3)	Urban-rural change, over five years (4)	Education differential (seven years; zero education) (5)	Change in education differential over five years (6)	Percentage of educational differential between highest groups[a] (7)
Colombia	20.7	0.8	2.1	0.3	5.2	0.5	69
Costa Rica	21.7	0.2	2.5	0.4	−1.1	−0.9	..
Dominican Republic	17.9	0.6	1.8	0.4	4.7	0.4	70
Ecuador	20.5	0.9	1.8	0.0	5.0	0.4	70
Guyana	18.4	0.9	−0.1	−0.6	3.7	0.2	22
Haiti	19.8	0.3	0.8	0.6	1.2	−0.8	142
Jamaica	17.8	−0.3	−0.3	−0.4	−0.3[b]	−0.6[b]	..
Mexico	20.1	0.7	2.0	−0.2	4.5	−0.5	4
Panama	19.9	1.0	2.4	0.2	4.3	−0.3	81
Paraguay	20.6	0.3	2.1	0.1	4.9	−0.8	37
Peru	20.6	1.7	1.5	−0.1	4.0	−0.5	85
Trinidad and Tobago	19.2	0.5	−0.9	−0.4	−0.8	−2.3	..
Venezuela	19.9	1.1	2.3	0.3	4.0	0.9	65
Averages:							
Guyana, Haiti, Jamaica, Trinidad and Tobago	18.8	0.35	−0.13	−0.19	0.95	−0.88	..
Other countries	20.2	0.81	2.06	0.16	3.94	−0.09	60

Source: World Fertility Survey standard recode tapes.

[a] $(SMAM(7+) - SMAM(4-6) / (SMAM(7+) - SMAM(0)) \times 100$.

[b] From one to three years of schooling because of lack of observations for women with no schooling.

TABLE 161. PERCENTAGE OF EVER-USERS OF CONTRACEPTION AMONG CURRENTLY MARRIED WOMEN AND PERCENTAGE USING MODERN[a] METHODS, BY CURRENT RESIDENCE, COUNTRIES IN THE ECLAC REGION

	\multicolumn{3}{c	}{Percentage who had ever used}	\multicolumn{3}{c	}{Percentage of users of modern methods among ever-users}
Country	Major urban	Other urban	Rural	Major urban	Other urban	Rural
Colombia	80	72	44	83	85	70
Costa Rica	80	85	81	91	91	88
Dominican Republic	65	60	40	83	85	70
Ecuador	77	68	38	86	81	71
Guyana	70	67	51	84	84	84
Haiti	53	59	30	55	56	17
Jamaica	78	66	62	90	91	86
Mexico	68	60	26	84	80	65
Panama	80	77	61	91	91	79
Paraguay	76	67	47	84	82	68
Peru	77	60	21	61	45	19
Trinidad and Tobago	83	83	77	94	93	93
Venezuela	78	66	42	86	85	79

Source: Sathar and Chidambaram (1984).

[a] Oral pill, intra-uterine device, injectables, condom, female and male sterilization and other female scientific methods.

the normative behaviour for the entire marital span for spacing of children (and perhaps for pre-marital years as well), and use is not solely restricted to "stopping" behaviour. The "stopping" pattern is clearly to be seen in the age-specific ever-use rates, which peak sharply at ages 30-34 among rural women in several countries—Colombia, Ecuador, Guyana, Mexico and Venezuela. In countries where ever-use is generally high (Costa Rica, Panama, Jamaica, and Trinidad and Tobago), however, rural women have broad, flatter distributions implying substantial "spacing" behaviour in rural areas at most ages.

Table 162 displays similar ever-use differentials by the respondent's educational attainment. In general, educated women have made significantly greater use of contraception and also relatively greater use of modern methods. Uneducated women in Ecuador, Mexico and Peru had particularly low rates of ever-use, compared with women with seven or more years of schooling. On the other hand, only in Costa Rica and in Trinidad and Tobago are differentials by education probably not very important, implying a fairly thorough percolation of the contraceptive mode of behaviour through all social classes in these countries. When one focuses on ever-use of efficient methods only, differences by education become more pronounced in several countries.

The percentage of currently married women who had ever used a modern method is given below for those countries:

	\multicolumn{2}{c	}{Years of schooling}
	None	Seven or more
Ecuador	14	70
Haiti	6	34
Mexico	14	70

Panama	37	76
Paraguay	21	68
Peru	4	54

Thus, it is clear that in several countries in the ECLAC region scientific and clinical methods, which often but not always are more efficient contraceptives, are unequally shared by all sectors either because of ignorance (one possible effect of lack of education, but not an insuperable one as demonstrated in other countries e.g., Costa Rica, and Trinidad and Tobago) or because less privileged socio-economic classes are effectively denied access to contraceptive technology.

Age-specific ever-use differentials by education (results not shown) display the same two patterns as found among rural and urban groups. On the one hand, in countries where family planning is relatively new and not as yet widespread (Colombia, Peru, and Ecuador), a high proportion of educated women had used contraception in all age groups for spacing and delaying childbearing, whereas among uneducated women use was concentrated in women aged 30+. Mexico is an extreme example: among married women 15-19, a 22:1 ratio of users was found between the educated (7 or more years) and the uneducated, but at ages 30-34, a ratio of only 3:1 was recorded. On the other hand, in countries where contraception has become normative behaviour, either due to government policy or because of a long diffusion process, both educated and uneducated use contraception widely at all ages and differentials are much less.[22]

Lactational infecundity

The third important proximate determinant of fertility, post-partum infecundity linked to breast-feeding practices, has received little attention in the ECLAC region.[23] This is due in part to the feeling that, compared with other regions where breast-feeding durations are known to be long, average durations in the ECLAC region are relatively short. The inclusion of breast-feeding questions in the WFS core questionnaire,[24] however, provided considerable data on the subject and made the analysis of breast-feeding an important new contribution to the demographic knowledge of the region.

The analysis is based on responses to the question whether the respondent was currently breast-feeding (at the time of survey). Estimating breast-feeding durations from current status data using life-table techniques has been shown to be preferable to other methods (Page and others, 1982), but the question itself suffers from a lack of specificity. Post-partum amenorrhoea (and more particularly anovulation) are more closely related to "full breast-feeding", the period when the baby is being fed only with mother's milk, than to the total breast-feeding period, which may include periods when the baby's diet is being supplemented with other food. In such circumstances, it is quite probable that the fertility-suppressing effect of breast-feeding has been lost (for a full discussion, see chapter IV).

Duration of breast-feeding varies widely in the ECLAC region, as the findings given in table 163 show. In Ecuador, Haiti, Paraguay and Peru, prolonged average durations of one year or more were found, while in Costa Rica and the anglophone Caribbean countries, durations of six months to a year or less are found. Large variations are observed in terms of both residence and education in all countries except the anglophone Caribbean countries, where urban or more educated women had only moderately shorter breast-feeding durations, on average. Rural and uneducated women in Peru and Haiti lactate for periods of more than 1.5 years, suggesting that in these groups breast-feeding may play a role in controlling the spacing between births. In Costa Rica and Panama, on the other hand, it can be easily seen that urban and more highly educated women have to a large extent abandoned the practice of breast-feeding and that its influence in suppressing conception has all but vanished. Other countries fall between these two extremes but in almost all cases the influence of increased education (and to a lesser degree, of urban residence) is clearly evident in drastically reducing the average duration of breast-feeding.

E. CONTRIBUTIONS OF PROXIMATE DETERMINANTS TO FERTILITY REDUCTION

To summarize the analysis of the three proximate determinants considered above, a comparison is made of the relative weight attributable to each factor. The method used is that proposed by Bongaarts (1978, 1982)

TABLE 162. PERCENTAGE OF EVER-USERS OF CONTRACEPTION AMONG CURRENTLY MARRIED WOMEN AND PERCENTAGE USING MODERN METHODS, BY YEARS OF EDUCATION, COUNTRIES IN THE ECLAC REGION

	Percentage who had ever used, by years of eduction				Percentage of users of modern methods among ever-users, by years of education			
Country	Zero	One to three	Four to six	Seven or more	Zero	One to three	Four to six	Seven or more
Colombia	37	54	72	89	73	78	83	84
Costa Rica	73	79	83	91	93	89	88	91
Dominican Republic	30	45	58	76	80	73	83	87
Ecuador	23	37	61	81	61	68	80	86
Guyana	27	39	49	62	96	97	86	84
Haiti	29	51	65	67	21	45	52	51
Jamaica	37	53	60	72	92	98	98	88
Mexico	22	38	59	80	64	76	78	87
Panama	53	55	72	83	70	76	85	92
Paraguay	37	42	62	79	57	69	76	86
Peru	21	41	67	83	20	34	51	65
Trinidad and Tobago	77	63	73	83	95	92	97	93
Venezuela	37	53	70	77	86	85	83	88

Source: Sathar and Chidambaram (1984).

TABLE 163. MEAN DURATION OF BREAST-FEEDING[a] FOR SURVIVING CHILDREN, BY CURRENT RESIDENCE AND YEARS OF EDUCATION, COUNTRIES IN THE ECLAC REGION

(*Months*)

Country	Current residence Rural	Current residence Urban	Years of schooling Zero	Years of schooling One to three	Years of schooling Four to six	Years of schooling Seven or more
Colombia	11.7	8.0	11.9	11.4	8.3	5.3
Costa Rica	6.4	3.7	..	8.1	4.6	3.2
Dominican Republic	11.8	6.6	12.2	10.5	8.6	5.2
Ecuador	15.3	9.9	17.0	14.5	13.0	8.9
Guyana	8.3	5.8	..	9.2	7.7	6.6
Haiti	19.2	11.1	19.0	14.1	..	..
Jamaica	8.9	7.6	..	..	8.9	6.2
Mexico	12.3	7.1	12.9	10.9	8.3	3.8
Panama	10.8	4.2	..	13.0	9.2	2.4
Paraguay	13.6	8.7	15.7	14.6	11.4	6.1
Peru	18.9	11.3	19.3	16.6	12.0	7.0
Trinidad and Tobago	9.4	7.4	..	..	10.0	7.1
Venezuela	11.5	6.5	11.6	10.0	6.7	3.5

Source: Ferry and Smith (1983).

[a] Using current status method explained in chapter IV.

which focuses on only four intermediate variables using the following identity:

$$TFR = C_m \cdot C_c \cdot C_a \cdot C_i \cdot TF$$

where TFR = total fertility rate;
C_m = index of proportion married;
C_c = index of contraception;
C_a = index of induced abortion;
C_i = index of lactational infecundability;
TF = total fecundity rate.

Each index, in so far as it takes a value less than its maximum of 1.00, reduces the potential capacity to bear children, TF. Thus, for example, in a population with no users of contraception, $C_c = 1.00$, and no reduction of potential fertility is attributed to contraceptive practice. The magnitude of the indices may be compared to gauge the contribution of each factor to fertility reduction. In practice, reliable abortion data is scarce and the C_a index must be disregarded—this is the case in the present analysis of WFS data. The identity given above may then be written

$$TFR = C_m \cdot C_c \cdot C_i \cdot \phi$$

where ϕ represents total fecundity to the extent that abortion and other proximate determinants are of negligible importance. There may also be variations in ϕ because of measurement error in the three factors (or because the models used to determine the indices are incorrectly specified) and/or because of real variation in potential fecundity between populations. The necessary omission of abortion is an important drawback of this procedure; and, to the extent that other determinants and total fecundity remain constant, variations in ϕ (calculated from the above-mentioned identity) may be taken to reflect the role of induced abortion in lowering fertility. This, in fact, will be seen to be among the important products of this exercise.

Bongaart's procedure is used in table 164 to examine the contribution of the three proximate determinants to fertility differentials by socio-economic groups. The left side of the table refers to differences in recent fertility (TFR) between respondents in rural areas and those in major urban areas.[25] With one exception, the direction of the contributions is as expected. For instance, in Colombia, 40 per cent of the rural/urban difference in total fertility rates is attributed to the difference in nuptiality patterns in rural and urban areas (urban women married later); 54 per cent to higher use and effectiveness of contraception among urban women; and a negative 10 per cent to smaller durations of breast-feeding among urban women.[26] Different rural and urban nuptial patterns make a substantial contribution in many countries, notably in Costa Rica, Haiti and Panama, where this factor accounts for the largest share of each fertility differential, compared with the other two factors. For example, in Costa Rica, nuptiality differences are about three times more important in accounting for lower urban fertility than differences in contraceptive practice. This confirms that family planning in that country is as effectively practised in rural as in urban areas. In Haiti, on the other hand, the ratio of 40:20 between C_m and C_c suggests that contraceptive use is at an equally low level of effectiveness among rural and urban women. In Trinidad and Tobago, Jamaica and Guyana, C_m is relatively unimportant, probably because the complex marital patterns in these societies have not been well captured by the WFS data at hand. Moreover, the fact that rural/urban fertility differentials in these countries, especially in Trinidad and Tobago, are quite small probably increases the instability in the values of the three indices.

The index of contraceptive use, C_c attains greater values than the other indices in the majority of the Latin American and Caribbean countries. Hence, rural/urban differences in contraceptive practice are, in general, the most important in explaining differential fertility, exceptions having already been noted. The anglophone Caribbean countries, and Mexico, Peru and Venezuela all have $C_c:C_m$ ratios approaching 2:1, indicating that the differentials in contraceptive use existing between rural and urban areas are roughly twice as important in causing lower urban fertility as are rural/urban differences in age at union.

The contribution of breast-feeding to lower rural fertility, C_i, is consistent across all countries and is, in

318

TABLE 164. RELATIVE CONTRIBUTIONS OF THREE PROXIMATE DETERMINANTS TO DIFFERENTIALS IN RECENT FERTILITY BETWEEN RESIDENCE AND EDUCATIONAL GROUPS, COUNTRIES IN THE ECLAC REGION

Country	Rural/urban differential in TFR	Contribution to rural/urban differential[a] of: Index of marriage C_m[c]	Index of contraception C_c[d]	Index of post-partum infecundability C_i[e]	ϕ[f]	Education differential in TFR	Contribution to education differential[b] of: Index of marriage C_m[c]	Index of contraception C_c[d]	Index of post-partum infecundability C_i[e]	ϕ[f]
Colombia	3.52	40	54	−10	16	4.64	47	51	−10	12
Costa Rica	1.77	50	17	−10	43	1.06	44	12	−25	69
Dominican Republic	3.12	36	52	−24	34	4.84	52	40	−11	19
Guyana	1.27	19	34	−19	66	1.46	50	26	−38	62
Haiti	2.20	40	20	−36	76	3.26	44	39	−27	44
Jamaica	1.48	12	46	−10	52	1.71	−3	99	−45	49
Mexico	2.80	46	88	−30	−4	4.49	56	67	−21	−2
Panama	2.36	46	44	−21	31	2.95	56	44	−25	25
Paraguay	2.85	39	43	−21	39	3.89	47	42	−19	30
Peru	2.99	45	67	−36	24	4.22	59	51	−26	16
Trinidad and Tobago	.81	−11	34	−13	90	2.08	22	50	−14	42
Venezuela	4.32	33	59	−17	25	3.97	48	44	−19	27
AVERAGE	2.42	37	49	−22	36	3.10	46	47	−21	28

Source: Singh and others (1985); and for definitions, chapter VI in the present volume.
NOTES: TFR = total fertility rate.
[a] Rural/urban differential: rural or major urban current residence.
[b] Education differential: difference between none and seven or more years of education.
[c] Contribution of later age at first union.
[d] Contribution of increased contraceptive use.
[e] Contribution of reduced breast-feeding duration.
[f] Contribution of omitted factors, inaccurate measurement and/or genuine differences in fecundity.

general, less variable in its effect than the other proximate determinants. Fairly high contributions are noted in Haiti, Mexico and Peru, where the effect of earlier marriage in rural areas (i.e., increased fertility) is approximately cancelled by the effect of longer rural breast-feeding (decreased fertility). Conversely, decreased fertility among urban women due to later marriage is being offset by increased fertility due to reduced breast-feeding. The policy implication of this finding is that in these countries changes in breast-feeding practices, which seemingly will occur inevitably, will tend to diminish the fertility-reducing effects of increased contraceptive use: fertility decline may temporarily slow down even while practice of family planning is growing. In several other countries, as is shown in table 164, differences in the incidence of lactation have ceased to be of major importance in determining differential fertility.

The right half of table 164 presents the same analysis for differentials by education, focusing only on two educational groups (those with no education and those with seven or more years of schooling). Many of the points made above with reference to rural/urban differences are also true here and therefore need not be repeated. One major difference, however, is that marital age supplants contraceptive use as the most important determinant in explaining fertility differences between educational groups. This is not surprising, because marital age and educational attainment are linked in a mechanical way (marriage generally occurring after completing studies), as well as in the more usual socio-economic sense. The contribution of breast-feeding, C_i, is of the same average magnitude here as in the rural/urban case, but the countries where it has an especially strong effect, notably Guyana and Jamaica, change. In these two countries, differential practice of breast-feeding between uneducated and more educated women (but not between rural and urban women) apparently is an important source of variation in fertility. Since the former group is numerically quite small in these countries, however, the practical significance of these findings is probably not large.

As mentioned above, ϕ represents a residual category of contributions to differential fertility. If it is assumed that total fecundity is fairly constant between populations and subpopulations, variation in ϕ can be attributed to poor measurement (a distinct possibility in cases where the fertility differential to be explained is small) or to omitted variables. One obvious measurement problem is how to assign weights in calculating the index of contraceptive use to reflect the presumed average use-effectiveness of the mix of contraceptive methods observed. The most significant of the omitted variables is the incidence of induced abortion. As can be seen, both rural/urban and educational variation in ϕ is large in the majority of countries. The implication, with all the caveats noted above, is that induced abortion is of considerable importance especially in urban areas and, to a somewhat lesser extent, among more educated women (the two subgroups, of course, largely overlap). Deduction based on a complicated procedure and several assumptions is not the preferred approach to estimating the contribution that abortion makes to lowering fertility, but lack of reliable data currently prevents better estimation. Without being able to quantify the contribution of abortion, since so many factors are involved in determining ϕ, the findings given in table 164 nevertheless appear to suggest the possibility of greater abortion incidence among urban, educated women, especially in certain countries.

F. CONCLUSION

In the many topics touched upon in this chapter a recurring finding was that the 13 countries in the ECLAC region that participated in WFS generally fell into two or three groups. One group, in particular, which was quite homogeneous within itself but distinct from other countries comprised the three anglophone countries of the Caribbean: Guyana (see note 3); Jamaica; and Trinidad and Tobago. Within this cluster, results showed that socio-economic groups were not very different either with respect to fertility behaviour or to nuptiality, contraception or lactation. In some analyses, such as age patterns of fertility and contraceptive use, Costa Rica and Panama displayed patterns similar to the Caribbean countries. This enlarged group (plus Venezuela) comprises the most socio-economically advanced countries studied. This suggests that the strength and sometimes even the direction of certain relationships change as countries attain higher levels of development. Several other countries, Colombia, Ecuador, Mexico, Paraguay, Peru and Venezuela, showed large socio-economic differentials by residence, education or occupational status. In terms of fertility behaviour and factors affecting fertility, these societies seem to be subdivided into distinct classes. Possibly rapid social change has so far affected mainly the urban, educated, professional groups in these countries while the diffusion process has left less privileged groups as yet untouched. Other interpretations, of course, are also possible. Lastly, Haiti (and in some respects, the Dominican Republic) does not seem to fit well into any of the above-mentioned groups. Fertility is high in Haiti, but not as high as the low level of contraceptive use would suggest. Breast-feeding is prolonged and union patterns are complex. In such circumstances, it is perhaps not surprising that socio-economic differentials are less notable in Haiti.

Thus, a major finding of this comparative analysis must be that even though many Latin American and Caribbean countries appear to behave in a homogeneous fashion, in important aspects fertility behaviour and fertility-related relationships differ between countries in the region. One cause of this cross-country variation may be the level of socio-economic development; another, as suggested by Caribbean results, may be cultural differences resulting from distinct colonial experiences. Countries in the ECLAC region that did not participate in WFS but that want to take advantage of this rich source of data should therefore maintain this comparative perspective when applying WFS findings to their own situations.

While keeping in mind the variability in estimates and relationships found between countries, several findings are universal enough to merit emphasis here. One such result concerns infant and child mortality experience, which, aside from duration of union, had the strongest and clearest influence on cumulative fertility. Women throughout the region who had experienced one or more child deaths also had more children than other women. This finding, together with the obvious association of infant and child mortality with fertility levels at the national level, highlights the importance that programmes directed to reducing these mortality rates have for subsequent changes in fertility behaviour.

The multivariate analysis of cumulative fertility brought out the importance of considering simultaneously, rather than one by one, factors that may affect fertility. Place of residence (rural or urban) is a less significant determinant once child-death experience has entered the analysis. Then, when the respondent's education is also considered, rural or urban residence has even less independent effect, although the direction remains consistent in all countries (i.e., lower fertility is associated with urban residence). Moreover, residence and education interact in several countries to produce significantly different fertility-residence patterns as education varies (and vice versa). When the education-fertility relationship was investigated, it was similarly found that the independent effect of education is generally small and sometimes not in the expected direction (i.e., lower fertility among women with little or no education). This means that the fairly strong differentials noted in fertility among educational groups are mainly through linkages between education and age at marriage, child-death experience, rural or urban residence and the other intermediate factors discussed in the previous section.

Using methodology proposed by Bongaarts, the contributions of age at first union, contraception and breast-feeding to differences in fertility by socio-economic groups were reviewed. The results are useful to planners in several respects. First, countries where fertility differences between residential or educational groups are to a great extent the result of contraceptive-use differentials are clearly distinguished from countries where rural/urban inequalities in family planning are less important. This knowledge is useful in evaluating the causes of differential fertility: in so far as they are the result, for example, of different nuptiality patterns they may be of less concern; where contraceptive-use differentials loom large, however, policy emphases in family planning programmes may need to be changed.

The presentation of relative contributions of the proximate determinants also gives planners new insights into mechanisms that may affect the future course of fertility change. In Haiti, Mexico and Peru, it was found that breast-feeding practice among the rural and uneducated was prolonged. Therefore, if such women change their lactational practices in the future in imitation of urban, more "modern" models, it may lead to slowing of fertility decline. In other cases, the analysis showed that differential nuptiality contributed most to fertility differentials. Here, too, the future course of fertility change may depend upon the degree that habits among the rural and uneducated change towards later age at first union, as in urban areas.

Lastly, indirect evidence was presented which suggested that in several countries in the ECLAC region induced abortion may contribute to both rural/urban and uneducated/educated differences in fertility. Although conclusions in this regard must remain quite tentative because many unmeasured factors besides abortion may be involved, the potential implications are significant: part of the lower fertility observed among urban, educated groups may be due to a greater incidence of induced abortion and correspondingly less to other variables traditionally associated with these socio-economic groups. These findings also give family planning officials new clues about the extent to which contraceptive prevalence would have to increase, by groups, in order to eradicate abortion practised as a form of fertility control.

Although the comparative analysis of WFS data leads to several advances in knowledge and to related policy implications as just outlined, limitations inherent in the data should also be mentioned. One shortcoming already commented upon is that the WFS socio-economic data are rather superficial. The two major socio-economic variables available are current place of residence and educational attainment. Occupational status was found to be a close approximation to education in its effect on fertility, while women's work experience, an important topic, was operationalized by variables that do not allow a deep analysis of this subject. It should be recalled, however, that comparative analysis requires, for the sake of generality, compromises in measures used and that in certain countries a richer set of socio-economic data is available. Studies of women's work role and fertility in particular countries, for instance, have allowed deeper insights into these relationships (e.g., Gougain, 1983; and Schoemaker, 1981). Also regrettable is the lack of reliable information on the practice of abortion. As has been seen, abortion could be of major importance in explaining fertility levels in certain socio-economic groups, but the evidence for this came indirectly through a complex set of inferences. The first priority in combating the effects of abortion practised as a form of contraception must be to obtain accurate information and in this regard the WFS experience was, unfortunately, a missed opportunity.

Notes

[1] Previous pregnancies that did not result in live births are excluded. For this reason, the measures differ slightly from the usual medical definition of primary infertility.

[2] Because of known reporting errors among women aged 45-49, the younger age group is preferred. For more detail, see Vaessen (1984, p. 8).

[3] Although Guyana is in South America, it is included with the Caribbean countries because the union histories are similar.

[4] Therefore, this measure is not restricted to secondary infertility but includes primary infertile women.

[5] Other research has attempted to demonstrate an opposite causal direction: increased use of contraception diminishing infant mortality by reducing births of high risk, such as high-parity births (Taucher, 1982).

[6] The correlation coefficient between child mortality and total fertility rates for the five years preceding the survey date is 0.65 for the region of the Economic Commission for Latin America and the Caribbean. This is statistically significant but less than the 0.87 found by the Economic and Social Commission for Asia and the Pacific (1984) for that region. A lower correlation in Latin America and the Caribbean fits into the general theoretical perspective, because that region has a lower level of child mortality, on average; therefore, the "replacement" or "insurance" motivations may well be correspondingly weaker.

[7] Therefore, the central years compared are 5 and 15 years prior to the survey.

[8] It should also be recalled that in Costa Rica and Panama, women aged 20-49 were interviewed; and in Venezuela, women aged 15-44. In these cases, normal total fertility rates (ages 15-49) cannot be calculated.

[9] For an analysis of group averages for five World Fertility Survey countries, see Gonzalez and Ramirez (1980).

[10] For a full description, see Hermalin and Mason (1980) and United Nations (1984a).

[11] This variable, which measures long-term residence, is made up of three categories: rural (both in childhood and currently); urban (both in childhood and currently); and migrant (either of the other two possibilities). See chapter VIII.

[12] The variable is dichotomous: 0 = no dead children; 1 = one or more dead children. No attempt was made to restrict deaths to those which occurred before a certain age.

[13] The log-linear model includes union duration, age at union, child-death experience and (optionally) education.

[14] Abstracting from residence-education interaction effects.

[15] However, the category "12 years of schooling" shown in table 159 represents a higher educational attainment than does the category "seven years" used earlier.

[16] A comparison of these median ages, estimated from nuptial life tables, with estimates using the Coale-Trussell model (e.g., Goldman, 1981) shows a consistent difference of about 0.6-0.8 years, the latter being greater in all cases.

[17] Based on current residence.

[18] Since Mexico and the three anglophone Caribbean countries had sampling peculiarities affecting school-age respondents, problems caused by special estimation procedures cannot be ruled out. In Mexico, the differential is shared more between women with less education, e.g., between those with from one to three years and those with from four to six years of schooling, implying a different mechanism because so little education would not generally compete with marriage plans.

[19] "Modern" methods include the oral pill, intra-uterine device, injectables, condom, female and male sterilization; and female scientific methods, such as gel, suppositories, diaphragm, cervical cap and foam. Traditional methods include douche, withdrawal, rhythm, abstinence and folk methods (see chapter V).

[20] Analysis by long-term residence yields essentially the same findings.

[21] Although data on women aged 15-19 were not collected in Costa Rica and Panama, it is certain that they also belong in this list.

[22] Ever-use differentials by work status of respondent (no work, work within household, work for others) are modest and probably not significant. Although surprising, this finding probably reflects the quality of the data more than anything else. Differentials by partner's occupation, on the other hand, are large and to a high degree mirror differences by education as discussed in the text. It is probable that the same dimension is being measured. For these reasons, further discussion of these differentials is not made here (for details, see Sathar and Chidambaram, 1984).

[23] See, however, Delgado and others (1978), Yunes (1975) and Mier y Teran (1978) for studies in Guatemala, Brazil and Mexico.

[24] The module for factors other than contraception affecting fertility (FOTCAF) contains many more questions on breast-feeding and other post-partum variables. Of the countries in the region, however, only Haiti included the module as part of the questionnaire.

[25] Algebraic differences in total fertility rates (TFR) are shown in columns (1) and (6) but the contributions presented in table 164 refer to ratios (e.g., $TFR_i:TFR_u$) rather than to algebraic differences.

[26] Positive five years mean that that factor contributes to lower urban fertility; negative signs mean that the contribution is to higher urban fertility.

References

Alam, Iqbal and J. B. Casterline (1984). *Socio-economic Differentials in Recent Fertility*. World Fertility Survey Comparative Studies, No. 33; Cross-National Summaries. Voorburg, The Netherlands: International Statistical Institute.

Allman, James (1982). Fertility and family planning in Haiti. *Studies in Family Planning* 13(8/9):237-245.

Anderson, John E. and John G. Cleland (1984). The World Fertility Survey and Contraceptive Prevalence Surveys: a comparison of substantive results. *Studies in Family Planning* 15(1):1-13.

Arguëllo, Omar (1980). Variables socio-económicas y fecundidad. *Notas de Población* 8(23):123-148.

Baldión, Edgar (1981). Mortalidad infantil en relación al nivel de fecundidad. Santiago, Chile, Centro Latinoamericano de Demografía (mimeographed).

Balkaran, Sundat (1982). *Evaluation of the Guyana Fertility Survey 1975*. World Fertility Survey Scientific Reports, No. 26. Voorburg, The Netherlands: International Statistical Institute.

Bongaarts, John (1978). A framework for analyzing the proximate determinants of fertility. *Population and Development Review* 4(1): 105-132.

_____ (1982). The fertility-inhibiting effects of the intermediate fertility variable. *Studies in Family Planning* 13(6/7):179-189.

Cabrera, G. (1984). Some aspects of population policy: the Mexican case. Paper presented at a workshop organized by the International Union for the Scientific Study of Population, 22-25 October 1984, Liège (mimeographed).

Camisa, Zulma. (1978). La nupcialidad de las mujeres solteras en la América Latina. *Notas de Población* 6(18):9-75.

Cleland, John, Jane Verrall and Martin Vaessen (1983). *Preferences for the Sex of Children and Their Influence on Reproductive Behaviour*. World Fertility Survey Comparative Studies, No. 27; Cross-National Summaries. Voorburg, The Netherlands: International Statistical Institute.

Conning, Arthur H. (1982). Tendencias de la fecundidad en los países de América Latina, 1950-1975. In Alan B. Simmons, Arthur H. Conning and Miguel Villa, eds., *El contexto social de cambio de la fecundidad en América Latina rural*. Santiago, Chile: Centro Latinoamericano de Demografía and International Development Research Centre.

Davis, Kingsley and Judith Blake (1956). Social structure and fertility: an analytic framework. *Economic Development and Cultural Change* 4(4):211-235.

Delgado, Hernán and others (1978). Nutrition and birth interval components: the Guatemala experiences. In W. Henry Mosley, ed., *Nutrition and Human Reproduction*. New York and London: Plenum Press, 385-399.

Ebanks, G. Edward, P. M. George and Charles E. Nobbe (1974). Fertility and number of partnerships in Barbados. *Population Studies* 28(3): 449-461.

Economic Commission for Latin America and the Caribbean (1983). Situación demográfica de América Latina evaluada en 1983: estimaciones para 1960-1980 y proyecciones para 1980-2025. Paper submitted to the meeting of the Comité de Expertos Gubernamentales de Alto Nivel, Havana, 30 September 1983. E/CEPAL/CEGAN/POB.2/L.2.

_____ (1983a). Some population estimates and projections for the English-speaking Caribbean. Paper submitted to the meeting of the Comité de Expertos Gubernamentales de Alto Nivel, Havana, 30 September 1983. E/CEPAL/CEGAN/POB.2/L.2/Add.1.

Economic and Social Commission for Asia and the Pacific (1984). The influence of infant and child mortality on fertility in the countries of the ESCAP region: an analysis of data from the WFS. Paper submitted to the Sixth Meeting of the United Nations Working Group on Comparative Analysis of World Fertility Survey Data, New York, 22-25 October 1984. UN/UNFPA/WFS.VI/5.

Ferry, Benoît and David P. Smith (1983). *Breast-feeding Differentials*. World Fertility Survey Comparative Studies, No. 23, Cross-National Summaries. Voorburg, The Netherlands: International Statistical Institute.

Flórez, Carmen Elisa and Noreen Goldman (1980). *An Analysis of Nuptiality Data in the Colombia National Fertility Survey*. World Fertility Survey Scientific Reports, No. 11. Voorburg, The Netherlands: International Statistical Institute.

Goldman, Noreen (1981). Dissolution of first unions in Colombia, Panama and Peru. *Demography* 18(4):659-679.

Gonzalez, G. and V. Ramirez (1980). Diferenciales socio-económicas de la fecundidad en América Latina. Santiago, Chile, Centro Latinoamericano de Demografía (mimeographed).

Gougain, L. (1983). Fecundidad y participation laboral femenina en Panama. Santiago, Chile, Centro Latinoamericano de Demografía (mimeographed).

Guzmán, José Miguel (1980). *Evaluation of the Dominican Republic National Fertility Survey 1975*. World Fertility Survey Scientific Reports, No. 14. Voorburg, The Netherlands: International Statistical Institute.

Hajnal, John (1953). Age at marriage and proportions marrying. *Population Studies* 7(2):111-136.

Hermalin, Albert I. and William M. Mason (1980). A strategy for the comparative analysis of WFS data, with illustrative examples. In *The United Nations Programme for Comparative Analysis of World Fertility Survey Data*. New York: United Nations Fund for Population Activities, 90-168.

Hobcraft, John N. (1980). *Illustrative Analysis: Evaluating Fertility Levels and Trends in Colombia*. World Fertility Survey Scientific Reports, No. 15. Voorburg, The Netherlands: International Statistical Institute.

_____ and John McDonald (1984). *Birth Intervals*. World Fertility Survey Comparative Studies, No. 28; Cross-National Summaries. Voorburg, The Netherlands: International Statistical Institute.

_____ and Germán Rodríguez (1982). *The Analysis of Repeat Surveys: Examples from Dominican Republic*. World Fertility Survey Scientific Reports, No. 29. Voorburg, The Netherlands: International Statistical Institute.

Hodgson, Maryse and Gibbs (1980). *Children Ever Born*. World Fertility Survey Comparative Studies, No. 12; Cross-National Summaries. Voorburg, The Netherlands: International Statistical Institute.

Hunte, Desmond (1983). *Evaluation of the Trinidad and Tobago Fertility Survey 1977*. World Fertility Survey Scientific Reports, No. 44. Voorburg, The Netherlands: International Statistical Institute.

Jamaica (1980). Department of Statistics. *Demographic Statistics 1979*. Kingston.

Knodel, John and Etienne van de Walle (1967). Breast feeding, fertility and infant mortality: an analysis of some early German data. *Population Studies* 21(2):109-131.

McClelland, Gary H. (1979). Determining the impact of sex preferences on fertility: a consideration of parity progression ratio, dominance and stopping rule measures. *Demography* 16(3):377-388.

McDonald, Peter (1984). *Nuptiality and Completed Fertility: A Study of Starting, Stopping and Spacing Behaviour*. World Fertility Survey Comparative Studies, No. 35. Voorburg, The Netherlands: International Statistical Institute.

Mier y Teran, M. (1978). El espaciamiento de los nacimientos en zonasrurales de Mexico y algunos factores que lo condicionan. In *Memorias de la I Reunion sobre la Investigación Demográfica en Mexico*. Mexico: Consejo Nacional de Ciencia y Technológia.

Page, Hilary J., R. J. Lesthaeghe and I. H. Shah (1982). *Illustrative Analysis: Breastfeeding in Pakistan*. World Fertility Survey Scientific Reports, No. 37. Voorburg, The Netherlands: International Statistical Institute.

Panama (1983). Dirección de Estadística y Censos. *Situación demográfica: estadísticas vitales, año 1980*.

_____ (1983a). Dirección de Estadística y Censos. *Situación demográfica: estadísticas vitales, año 1981*.

_____ (1984). Dirección de Estadística y Censos. *Situación demográfica: estadísticas vitales, año 1982*.

Peru (1983). Instituto Nacional de Estadísticas. *Aspectos demográficos y prevalencia de anticonceptivos en el Perú*.

Potter, J. E. (1977). Problems in using birth-history analysis to estimate trends in fertility. *Population Studies* 31(2):335-364.

Preston, Samuel, ed. (1978). *The Effects of Infant and Child Mortality on Fertility*. New York: Academic Press.

Repetto, Robert (1972). Son preference and fertility behaviour in developing countries. *Studies in Family Planning* 3(4):70-76.

Roberts, George W. and Lloyd Braithwaite (1962). Mating among East Indian and non-Indian women in Trinidad. *Social and Economic Studies* 11(3):203-240.

Rodriguez, Sepúlveda, Bienvenida (1984). *Evaluación de la Encuesta Nacional de Fecundidad de la República Dominicana de 1980*. World Fertility Survey Scientific Reports, No. 63. Voorburg, The Netherlands: International Statistical Institute.

Rosero Bixby, Luis (1978). Nupcialidad y exposición al riesgo de embarazo en Costa Rica. *Notas de Población* 6(17):33-62.

_____ (1980). La situacion demográfica de Costa Rica. San José, Universidad de Costa Rica (mimeographed).

_____ (1981). *Fecundidad y anticoncepción en Costa Rica, 1981*. San José: Asociación Demográfica Costarricense and Westinghouse Health Systems.

Rutstein, Shea Oscar (1983). *Infant and Child Mortality: Levels, Trends and Demographic Differentials*. World Fertility Survey Comparative Studies, No. 24; Cross-National Summaries. Voorburg, The Netherlands: International Statistical Institute.

Sathar, Zeba A. and V. C. Chidambaram (1984). *Differentials in Contraceptive Use*. World Fertility Survey Comparative Studies, No. 36; Cross-National Summaries. Voorburg, The Netherlands: International Statistical Institute.

Schoemaker, Juan F. (1981). *Participación laboral femenina y fecundidad en Paraguay*. CELADE Series D, No. 98. Santiago, Chile: Centro Latinoamericano de Demografía.

_____ (1984). *Evaluación de la Encuesta Nacional de Fecundidad del Paraguay de 1979*. World Fertility Survey Scientific Reports, No. 62. Voorburg, The Netherlands: International Statistical Institute.

Singh, Susheela (1982). *Evaluation of the Jamaica Fertility Survey 1975-76*. World Fertility Survey Scientific Reports, No. 34. Voorburg, The Netherlands: International Statistical Institute.

_____, J. B. Casterline and J. G. Cleland (1985). The proximate determinants of fertility: sub-national variations. *Population Studies* 39(1):113-135.

Taucher, Erica (1982). Effectos del descenso de la fecundidad sobre los niveles de mortalidad infantil: un estudio basado en datos de cinco países latinoamericanos. Santiago, Chile, Centro Latinoamericano de Demografía (mimeographed).

Trinidad and Tobago (1981). Central Statistical Office. *Population and Vital Statistics 1977 Report*. Port of Spain.

United Nations (1972). Department of Economic and Social Affairs. Population Division. *Measures, Policies and Programmes Affecting Fertility, with Particular Reference to National Family Planning Programmes*. Population Studies, No. 51. New York. Sales No. E.72.XIII.2.

_____(1981). Department of International Economic and Social Affairs. Population Division. *Variations in the Incidence of Knowledge and Use of Contraception: A Comparative Analysis of World Fertility Survey Results for Twenty Developing Countries*. Non-sales publication ST/ESA/SER.R/40. New York.

_____(1982). Department of International Economic and Social Affairs. Statistical Office. *Population and Vital Statistics Report; Data Available as of 1 April 1982*. Series A, 34(2); ST/ESA/STAT/SER.A/140. New York.

_____(1984). *Population and Vital Statistics Report; Data Available as of 1 July 1984*. Series A, 36(3); ST/ESA/STAT/SER.A/150. New York.

_____(1984a). Department of Economic and Social Affairs, Population Division. Education and fertility. Paper prepared for the Sixth Meeting of the United Nations Working Group on Comparative Analysis of World Fertility Survey Data, New York, 22-25 October 1984. UN/UNFPA/WFS/VI/12. New York.

_____(1984b). *Some Relationships between Nuptiality and Fertility in Countries of the West Indies*. Non-sales publication ST/ESA/SER.R/46. New York.

Vaessen, Martin (1984). *Childlessness and Infecundity*. World Fertility Survey Comparative Studies, No. 31; Cross-National Summaries. Voorburg, The Netherlands: International Statistical Institute.

Vielma, Gilberto (1982). *Evaluation of the Venezuela Fertility Survey 1977*. World Fertility Survey Scientific Reports, No. 35. Voorburg, The Netherlands: International Statistical Institute.

Williamson, Nancy E. (1976). *Sons or Daughters: A Cross-Cultural Survey of Parental Preferences*. Beverly Hills, California: Sage Publications.

Yunes, J. (1975). Estudo da lactaçao em muheres do distrito de São Paulo, Brasil. *Saude Publica* 9(2):191-213.

Zavala, E. (1984). *Niveles y tendencias de la fecundidad en México 1960-1980*. Mexico: El Colegio de México, Centro de Estudios Demográficos y de Desarrollo Urbano.

XII. COMPARATIVE ANALYSIS OF WORLD FERTILITY SURVEY DATA: AFRICA, SOUTH OF THE SAHARA

Economic Commission for Africa*

ABSTRACT

This chapter describes the findings of the World Fertility Survey programme in nine countries of sub-Saharan Africa (Benin, Cameroon, Côte d'Ivoire, Ghana, Kenya, Lesotho, Mauritania, Senegal and the Sudan). Marriage and type of marital union, educational attainment and other factors, such as the post-partum non-susceptible period, desired family size and the knowledge and use of contraception, are studied in the context of their implications for fertility; and similarities and variations between these nine countries are highlighted.

Levels of fertility ranged from over eight births in Kenya to slightly less than six in Lesotho and the Sudan. Although the evidence points to an increase in fertility in some countries, the quality of data on trends does not permit any firm conclusions. In most countries, fertility rates have remained more or less constant at high levels. The incidence of sterility among women 45-49 was less than 5 per cent in all countries but Cameroon and the Sudan.

The proportion of ever-married women aged more than 15 years with no education ranged from a high of 80-90 per cent in Senegal, Benin, Côte d'Ivoire and the Sudan to a low of 8 per cent in Lesotho. The nature of the relationship between fertility and education differed among countries, depending upon the proportion of women with seven or more years of education. In Ghana and Lesotho, where more than 20 per cent of women had seven or more years of education, fertility levels were lower at each higher level of educational attainment. In the remaining countries, fertility was higher among women with a few years of education than for those with no education. In most countries, over 40 per cent of ever-married women aged 20-24 were married before age 18. Strong differentials were observed in age at marriage between women in different residence and educational groups. A woman's type of marital union was strongly related to her educational attainment. Women with more education are more likely to remain in a monogamous union and are less susceptible to divorce and remarriage. The incidence of polygamy was found to be high in most countries, from 30 to 47 per cent. Among women who were currently married and married once, those with a monogamous husband had a higher mean number of children than those with a polygamous husband.

The average desired family size among women who responded numerically was between six and nine children. Although there is widespread knowledge of contraception, less than 10 per cent of ever-married women were using in nearly all countries.

The 13 African countries that participated in the World Fertility Survey (WFS) programme were Benin, Cameroon, Côte d'Ivoire,[1] Egypt, Ghana, Kenya, Lesotho, Mauritania, Morocco, Nigeria, Senegal, the Sudan and Tunisia. In the case of the Sudan, the survey was conducted only in the northern part of the country. Although the WFS programme began in 1973 and ended in 1984, African countries joined the programme rather late, with the result that most of the analytical reports were not completed by the end of the programme. This has limited the number of comprehensive studies on the African countries that participated.

This study covers only the nine sub-Saharan countries, namely, Benin, Cameroon, Côte d'Ivoire, Ghana, Kenya, Lesotho, Mauritania, Senegal and the Sudan. Where certain data are not available for some countries, those countries are not reflected in the study. Hence, some of the countries do not appear in tables because the relevant data were not available.

WFS has significantly contributed to the knowledge and information on fertility in the African countries that participated in the programme. In addition, it has provided some information on infant and childhood mortality; this topic, however, is not dealt with in this chapter.

This chapter first provides brief background information on the educational attainment of ever-married women. Marriage and types of marital unions are covered

---
*Population Division.

next, followed by the section on fertility. Section D covers the post-partum non-susceptible period, and section E discusses desired family size, and knowledge and use of contraception. Lastly, a summary of the findings and the policy implications are presented.

A. BACKGROUND

In most African Countries, there has been a slow albeit steady improvement in availability of population data. Many countries have conducted at least one census since independence. Many of the countries, however, did not collect information directly on fertility or mortality. Some countries have had demographic surveys conducted to collect needed data on fertility and related characteristics not collected in censuses. It should be pointed out that some of the demographic surveys carried out earlier were on a small scale and did not provide representative estimates at the national level that could be used for comparative studies.

The participation of African countries in WFS offered the first opportunity to collect considerable information, some of it for the first time, that can be used for comparative studies on fertility, nuptiality and characteristics affecting them. Although the WFS findings do not in all cases agree with results from other sources of information, there appears to be general agreement that the WFS data are of reasonable quality (see Introduction to this report). Errors in data due to misreporting of events or inaccurate dating of events are particularly frequent in surveys like WFS where women in the sample were asked to recall certain information for some years back. Low education, especially among women, contributes to women's inability to report information accurately.

In view of the fact that the educational level of women generally affects fertility and nuptiality, the rest of this background section examines the educational attainment of ever-married women in the nine countries under study.

Table 165 presents data on the distribution of ever-married women aged 15 and over by educational attainment. The countries are ordered from highest to lowest with respect to the proportion of women with no education. For all nine countries combined, as much as 64 per cent of ever-married females aged 15 and over had no education, about 12 per cent had from one to three years of education,[2] 14 per cent had from four to six years and 11 per cent had seven or more years. However, there are wide differences between countries. For example, the proportion of women with no education varied from 80-90 per cent in Senegal, Benin, Côte d'Ivoire and the Sudan to 50-70 per cent in Cameroon, Ghana and Kenya. In Mauritania, about 40 per cent had no education (see note 2) and the proportion was as low as 8 per cent in Lesotho. Lesotho had the highest percentage of ever-married women with from four to six years of education, 54 per cent; Cameroon and Kenya followed with 18 per cent each. The other countries had a range from 2 per cent in Mauritania to 8 per cent in Côte d'Ivoire. In Ghana, 29 per cent of ever-married women had seven or more years of education; in Kenya and Lesotho, the corresponding figures were 17 and 25 per cent, respectively. In the remaining countries, these figures ranged from 2 per cent in Mauritania to 6 per cent in Cameroon.

Next to be considered is the experience of two age groups of women, 20-29 and 30-39. The younger age group was selected because it is most sensitive with respect to a country's current policy towards providing female education, and the older group was chosen to show any differential trend between the countries with regard to the provision of educational opportunities for women.

TABLE 165. PERCENTAGE DISTRIBUTION OF EVER-MARRIED WOMEN AGED 15 OR OVER, BY LEVEL OF EDUCATION, COUNTRIES IN SUB-SAHARAN AFRICA

Country	Zero (1)	One to three (2)	Four to six (3)	Seven or more (4)	Number of women (5)
Senegal	90.2	2.2	4.9	2.7	3 455
Benin	88.1	2.8	6.3	4.5	3 570
Côte d'Ivoire[a]	83.8	3.5	8.2	4.5	4 987
Sudan	81.4	7.1	7.3	4.0	3 113
Cameroon	69.9	6.0	18.2	5.6	7 264
Ghana	59.9	3.3	7.3	29.4	4 931
Kenya	53.6	12.0	17.9	16.5	6 310
Mauritania	40.7	55.6	2.1	1.7	3 502
Lesotho	7.8	12.9	54.3	24.7	3 603
ALL COUNTRIES	63.9	11.7	14.1	10.4	40 735

Source: World Fertility Survey standard recode tapes.
[a] Formerly called the Ivory Coast.

As can be seen from table 166, the nine countries keep roughly the same order when the educational attainment of women aged 20-29 is considered as was observed for women of all ages. In both Benin and Senegal, the proportion of women aged 20-29 with no education was about 85 per cent. These two countries are followed by Côte d'Ivoire and the Sudan, with corresponding proportions of approximately 75 per cent. The proportion with no education drops to about 50 per cent for Cameroon and about 40 per cent for Ghana and Kenya. The case of Mauritania, where women with no education comprised 38 per cent, is not very clear, as explained above (see note 2). Mauritania is the only country where the proportion of women with from one to three years of education was exceptionally high while the proportions with from four to six and with seven or more years were quite low. (The difference in the effect on fertility of from one to three years of education as compared with no education is discussed in a later section of this chapter.) Lesotho also was unique in that no more than 5 per cent of the women had no education. These comments should be borne in mind when considering fertility differentials, in view of the effect educational level exerts on fertility (see chapter VIII).

Equally important is the speed at which education is spreading in a country, which can be seen by comparing educational levels for several cohorts. In this particular case, attention is confined to age groups 20-29 and 30-39. A crude index that measures the educational trend over roughly a 10-year period is the proportion with no education in age group 20-29 as a percentage of the proportion with no education in age group 30-39 (see column (6) of table 166).

The four countries with the highest proportion of women with no education,—Benin, Senegal, Côte d'Ivoire and the Sudan (where illiteracy was over 70 per cent for women aged 20-29)—are the same countries that had the least improvement in educational attainment (column (6) of table 166). Among the remaining five countries, there are two, Lesotho and Mauritania, where the change was small. In the case of Lesotho, the proportion of women

TABLE 166. PERCENTAGE DISTRIBUTION OF EVER-MARRIED WOMEN AGED 20-29 AND 30-39, BY LEVEL OF EDUCATION, COUNTRIES IN SUB-SAHARAN AFRICA

Country and age group	Zero (1)	One to three (2)	Four to six (3)	Seven or more (4)	Number of women (5)	Women aged 20-29 with no education as percentage of women aged 30-39 with no education (6)
Benin						
20-29	86.4	3.7	6.9	3.0	1 586	98
30-39	87.9	2.7	6.3	3.1	1 055	
Senegal						
20-29	84.4	3.3	7.0	5.3	1 288	90
30-39	94.1	1.5	2.9	1.5	988	
Côte d'Ivoire[a]						
20-29	75.6	5.2	12.1	7.1	2 041	81
30-39	92.9	1.4	3.0	2.7	1 316	
Sudan						
20-29	73.9	10.1	9.8	6.2	1 230	86
30-39	86.0	6.2	5.0	2.8	1 089	
Cameroon						
20-29	52.0	8.5	29.5	10.0	2 587	64
30-39	81.0	4.6	11.4	3.0	2 062	
Ghana						
20-29	42.1	3.7	8.6	45.6	2 005	60
30-39	70.7	3.0	7.4	18.9	1 490	
Kenya						
20-29	40.7	10.8	21.0	27.4	2 553	67
30-39	60.7	12.7	16.8	9.8	1 914	
Mauritania						
20-29	37.5	57.2	3.0	2.3	1 368	85
30-39	44.3	54.2	0.8	0.7	980	
Lesotho						
20-29	5.6	9.3	53.7	31.4	1 448	75
30-39	7.5	12.8	59.2	20.5	996	

Source: World Fertility Survey standard recode tapes.
[a] Formerly called the Ivory Coast.

with no education was quite low by most standards and therefore further improvements in educational attainment would necessarily be small. In Mauritania, while these data do not rule out the possibility of more recent changes, no change is evident for these cohorts. In Cameroon, Ghana and Kenya, there is evidence of considerable change (that is, younger cohorts appeared to be obtaining better educational opportunities, as compared with the older cohorts).

So far the discussion has been concentrated on the proportion of women with no education and the changes in this proportion between cohorts. It is equally important to consider the remaining educational categories because of the close association between number of years of education, on the one hand, and type of marital union and fertility, on the other.

Little needs to be said about the proportion of women aged 20-29 with from one to three years of education, except that it was highest in Mauritania (57 per cent) followed by Kenya, the Sudan, Lesotho and Cameroon, where the proportion was about 10 per cent. Comparison of the proportions of ever-married women aged 20-29 with those aged 30-39 with from four to six years of education indicates a marked increase in the trend in education among young women in Senegal, Côte d'Ivoire, the Sudan, Cameroon and Kenya. Changes were also occurring in the highest educational category (seven years or more). Ghana, Kenya and Lesotho stand out particularly because of increases of 10 percentage points or more in the proportion of women at this level.

Within this group of nine countries, very different levels and trends in the educational attainment of women are apparent. Ghana, Kenya and Lesotho differed sharply from the other countries with respect to the percentage of women with seven or more years of schooling. These countries had higher levels of educational attainment and had shown relatively rapid progress over the decade between the years when the cohorts aged 20-29 and 30-39 were of school age. On the other hand, women with schooling were very much in the minority in Benin, Senegal, Côte d'Ivoire and the Sudan. A minimum of a few years of schooling was becoming more common in Cameroon.

B. MARRIAGE AND TYPES OF MARITAL UNIONS

In sub-Saharan Africa, where the use of modern methods of contraception is limited to a very small percentage of the population (as shown later), other factors become more dominant in determining fertility. One of these factors is marriage and types of marital unions (Henin, 1969).

In the WFS programme, a wide definition of marriage was used to obtain all types of reproductive unions. The results given here therefore describe the age at first exposure within a socially recognized union. For convenience, the term "marriage" in this chapter should be understood to include all types of reproductive unions. This section examines the proportions of women married between the ages of 15-19 and 45-49 at the time of the survey. The singulate mean age at first marriage (SMAM) is used to measure the average age at first marriage (for definition, see chapter III).

Proportions marrying and age at marriage

It should be noted that age at first marriage and chances thereof are of particular interest in explaining fertility levels as well as trends since, in general, childbearing begins when marriage takes place, although some childbearing also occurs to women before they enter into union (chapter III). The proportion of women entering into a union for the first time at a given age provides information on the proportion of women exposed to the risk of childbearing in the absence of effective country use. Based on this reasoning, larger proportions of women entering into a first union at an early age would be associated with higher fertility risks and larger proportions of women entering into first union at later ages would be associated with lower fertility risks.

It can be seen from table 167 that Cameroon, Côte d'Ivoire and Senegal all had over 50 per cent ever married among females aged 15-19, while Benin had 44 per cent. At ages 25-29, over 95 per cent of the females in Benin (99 per cent), Cameroon (96 per cent), Ghana (97 per cent); Côte d'Ivoire, Kenya and Senegal (96 per cent) were ever married. In Lesotho, the proportion married in this age group was about 93 per cent; in Mauritania, 92 per cent; and only 89 per cent in the Sudan.

The female singulate mean age at marriage shows noticeable variation between the countries under consideration. It was highest in the Sudan (21.3 years), followed by Kenya (19.9 years), Lesotho (19.6 years) and Mauritania (19.2 years), and lowest in Cameroon (17.5 years). In between are Senegal, where SMAM was 17.7 years, and Côte d'Ivoire with 17.8 years.

Trends in proportions marrying

Table 168 shows the proportions of women who are married by ages 18, 20 and 24 for five age cohorts. The youngest (15-19) and the oldest (45-59) cohorts are omitted from the analysis, the former because of incomplete exposure and the latter because of possible errors resulting from recall lapse. There is evidence from the proportions married by age 18, 20 and 24 that the age at first marriage may have risen in four countries: Kenya; Mauritania; Senegal; the Sudan. Côte d'Ivoire, Ghana and Lesotho appear to have experienced a decline in the age at first marriage. While there appears to have been a decline in young marriages in Benin and Cameroon, proportions married at slightly older ages were higher among the youngest cohorts. It must be added, however, that any conclusions reached about long-term trends must be treated with caution in view of the unreliability of date reporting in the marriage history data (see chapter I).

Differentials in age at marriage for ever-married women by place of residence and education

Age at first marriage for women does vary according to place of residence: for example, there are generally differentials between rural and urban areas. Similarly, there are usually differentials in age at first marriage by levels of education of a woman. This section examines these differentials.

Place of residence

Senegal had the highest proportion married among the 15-19 cohort of rural women, about 76 per cent (table 169). In Benin, Cameroon and Côte d'Ivoire, more than 50 per cent of the rural women aged 15-19 were ever married. Comparing rural and urban residence for ever-married women in age group 15-19, for the eight countries for which data were available, there were higher proportions of married women in rural areas than in urban areas except in Kenya, where the reverse was true. In most cases, leaving out the extremes, rural/urban differences were between 10 and 20 per cent.

Except for Mauritania, table 169 shows that in the remaining countries, the proportions of married women in the age groups from 20-24 to 45-49 were, in most cases, higher in rural areas than in urban areas. In Mauritania, the data show an opposite pattern, for which there is no apparent explanation.

The singulate mean age at first marriage was higher for urban women than for rural women in all countries except Mauritania. A difference of roughly two years or more was found in Benin, Cameroon, Senegal and the Sudan. Much smaller differences were observed in Côte d'Ivoire, Ghana and Kenya. The observed higher mean age at marriage in urban areas than in rural areas must be related to better educational opportunities for women in the urban areas than their counterparts have in rural areas. The duration of education has a delaying effect on age at first marriage.

TABLE 167. PROPORTION OF WOMEN EVER MARRIED, BY AGE GROUP, AND SINGULATE MEAN AGE AT MARRIAGE, COUNTRIES IN SUB-SAHARAN AFRICA

Country	\multicolumn{7}{c	}{Percentage of ever-married women in age group}	Singulate mean age at marriage (years)
	15-19	20-24	25-29	30-34 (percentage)	35-39	40-44	45-49	
Benin	43.8	90.2	98.8	99.7	99.8	99.7	99.6	18.2
Cameroon	53.1	89.6	96.3	98.3	99.1	98.9	98.2	17.5
Côte d'Ivoire[a]	56.0	89.6	95.5	98.1	99.3	99.8	99.7	17.8
Ghana	30.9	84.6	97.0	99.1	99.1	99.5	99.8	19.3
Kenya	27.4	79.2	95.5	98.7	99.2	99.2	99.7	19.9
Lesotho	31.5	85.5	92.8	94.9	96.9	98.0	97.3	19.6
Mauritania	37.1	75.9	91.6	95.3	98.0	98.0	98.4	19.2
Senegal	59.3	85.9	95.8	99.6	100.0	99.7	99.6	17.7
Sudan[b]	21.8	63.7	89.0	95.6	98.0	98.6	99.2	21.3

Source: Ebanks and Singh (1984), p. 23, table 1.
[a] Formerly called the Ivory Coast.
[b] Northern part only.

TABLE 168. PROPORTION OF WOMEN MARRIED BY SPECIFIED AGES FOR SELECTED COHORTS, COUNTRIES IN SUB-SAHARAN AFRICA
(Percentage)

Country and age at first marriage	20-24 (1)	25-29 (2)	30-34 (3)	35-39 (4)	40-44 (5)
Benin					
18	42.4	49.0	50.3	49.6	41.6
20	73.5	71.2	71.3	71.0	63.6
24	96.6	92.5	89.3	89.9	86.9
Cameroon					
18	61.3	62.5	65.7	57.2	60.1
20	81.0	77.9	79.5	72.2	72.5
24	92.9	92.8	92.4	88.5	84.5
Côte d'Ivoire[a]					
18	60.2	58.0	62.2	57.4	53.8
20	79.3	77.1	77.6	77.0	72.0
24	92.2	91.7	92.9	92.0	88.8
Ghana					
18	61.5	59.0	62.2	63.7	58.5
20	72.4	69.3	71.2	72.1	68.2
24	93.5	91.7	91.4	89.2	86.9
Kenya					
18	45.1	49.4	59.9	55.3	53.3
20	65.0	73.3	76.0	75.6	73.5
24	87.4	90.5	94.5	92.6	90.9
Lesotho					
18	39.4	37.1	41.3	36.7	40.8
20	69.9	66.5	69.4	66.1	67.5
24	89.8	89.4	88.0	87.2	87.4
Mauritania					
18	61.7	69.8	74.7	76.5	73.3
20	71.5	79.5	82.4	83.4	82.7
24	79.0	89.1	90.1	92.9	91.2
Senegal					
18	61.6	66.1	80.0	80.8	77.1
20	76.7	79.3	90.4	90.3	88.0
24	90.8	92.2	96.4	97.0	97.5
Sudan					
18	46.7	58.9	69.2	65.1	66.9
20	56.9	74.5	79.8	77.4	76.4
24	71.2	85.9	91.6	89.1	90.9

Source: Ebanks and Singh (1984), appendix table 1.
[a] Formerly called the Ivory Coast.

Education

One of the most important determinants of the age at marriage (and fertility) in the context of sub-Saharan Africa is education (Anker and Knowles, 1982; Henin, 1973). In the following paragraphs, an analysis is made concerning the proportions married and the singulate mean age at first marriage by level of education. One of the problems in this type of analysis in the case of sub-Saharan Africa is that of small sample size for higher levels of education.

Table 170 shows the proportions married among women aged 15-29 in four educational categories: none; from one to three years; from four to six years; seven years or more. Among the youngest age cohort (15-19), it can be seen that, in general, the proportions ever married decrease with increases in the level of education. This pattern is maintained except in Benin, where the proportion ever married rises from 24.1 for the group with from one to three years of education to 32.5 for those with from four to six years. For age group 20-24, the proportions married decline similarly with an increase in education in Benin, Cameroon, Côte d'Ivoire, Ghana and Kenya. Senegal and the Sudan are exceptions to this observation: in both countries, the proportions of women with no education were slightly lower than of those with from one to three years; thereafter, the usual decline pattern is maintained. Although there are some fluctuations in the data for age group 25-29 for Benin, Côte d'Ivoire, Ghana and Kenya, the data for Cameroon, Senegal and the Sudan conform to the inverse relationship. For the oldest age groups, there are no differences in the proportions married by educational levels since nearly all women were married in all educational categories (not shown).

It is seen that the difference in the proportions ever married is relatively large if women aged 15-29 and 20-24 with no education are compared with those with seven or more years. These are the cohorts where the effects of current educational policy can be most directly observed. Only in Benin and the Sudan do any sizeable differentials appear among women older than 25. Differences of 40 per cent or more in proportion ever married are apparent in every country among women aged 15-19, but this can be partially explained by the fact that women still enrolled in school are less likely to marry. Women aged 20-24 are likely to have completed their education. Among women in this age group, it can be seen that the proportion married does not begin to show a notable decline until from four to six years of education has been achieved. In all countries, the larger difference in proportions married is between the group with from four to six years and that with seven or more.

Column (4) of table 170 gives the singulate mean age at first marriage by educational category. Almost without exception, SMAM rises with the increase in the number of years of education. The difference in SMAM between women with no education and those with seven or more years ranges from seven years in Benin to three years in Ghana.

Types of unions

In the foregoing section, attention was given to age at marriage, the proportions marrying, and the trends and differentials for these two marital variables. In this section, other aspects of marriage, which relate more particularly to Africa in that they play a significant role in determining fertility, are discussed. These factors are polygamy and marital instability (Henin, 1969).

Table 171 gives an overall view of differences in current marital status among the eight countries under consideration. The first distinction of interest is the differential incidence of monogamous versus polygamous unions in these countries. The incidence of polygamy (women who reported themselves to be in current unions with co-wives) ranged from 7.5 per cent of ever-married women in Lesotho to 46.6 per cent in Senegal. A high incidence of polygamy also was found in Côte d'Ivoire (38.5 per cent), Benin (36.5 per cent), Cameroon (37.2 per cent), Ghana (30.8 per cent) and Kenya (27.1 per cent). If younger women and older women are compared (panels B and C of table 171), the predominant pattern is a larger proportion of women in polygamous unions towards the end of the reproductive ages. The exceptions to this pattern can be found in Lesotho; Mauritania, where the incidence of polygamy was relatively low and did not show much difference; and Benin and Cameroon, where a relatively high incidence of polygamy (35.9 and 36.5 per

TABLE 169. AGE-SPECIFIC PROPORTIONS OF WOMEN EVER MARRIED AND SINGULATE MEAN AGE AT MARRIAGE, BY PLACE OF RESIDENCE, EIGHT COUNTRIES[a] IN SUB-SAHARAN AFRICA
(*Percentage*)

Country and place of residence	\multicolumn{7}{c	}{Ever-married women in age group}	Singulate mean age at marriage (8)
	15-19 (1)	20-24 (2)	25-29 (3)	30-34 (4)	35-39 (5)	40-44 (6)	45-49 (7)	
Benin								
Urban	21.1	75.6	96.5	98.9	99.3	100.0	98.5	20.0
Rural	63.1	97.1	99.8	100.0	100.0	99.6	100.0	16.8
Cameroon								
Urban	34.9	75.4	93.0	95.8	97.2	96.7	96.9	19.5
Rural	58.8	94.2	97.2	98.9	99.5	99.4	98.4	16.9
Côte d'Ivoire[b]								
Urban	52.2	88.7	94.7	97.5	98.9	100.0	98.6	17.9
Rural	59.5	91.3	96.2	98.5	99.5	99.7	100.0	17.6
Ghana								
Urban	24.8	76.1	95.3	99.3	99.1	99.4	99.0	20.0
Rural	34.2	89.4	98.1	99.1	99.1	99.5	100.0	18.9
Kenya								
Urban	34.3	71.3	92.5	94.7	97.2	96.0	100.0	20.6
Rural	26.4	81.0	96.0	99.2	99.3	99.4	99.6	19.8
Mauritania								
Urban	37.4	78.1	91.2	95.9	98.0	98.3	98.9	19.1
Rural	39.9	74.2	90.6	95.0	98.0	97.7	98.2	19.1
Senegal								
Urban	31.3	72.4	91.4	100.0	100.0	100.0	98.7	19.9
Rural	76.2	94.6	98.4	99.4	100.0	99.7	100.0	16.2
Sudan[c]								
Urban	14.6	50.9	83.5	92.9	96.8	97.6	98.2	22.8
Rural	25.4	69.6	91.1	96.7	98.5	99.2	99.7	20.9

Source: Ebanks and Singh (1984), table 7.
[a] Data for Lesotho not available.
[b] Formerly called the Ivory Coast.
[c] Northern part only.

cent, respectively) showed little or no difference at the older ages.

Since it concerns current marital status, it would be useful to apportion women classified as "divorced or separated" or "widowed" according to type of previous union. These groups of women are in fact a relatively large proportion among women aged 40 or more years in Cameroon, Lesotho and Mauritania. The incidence of polygamy even among younger women was over 20 per cent in all countries but Lesotho and Mauritania. The highest rates were found in Benin, Cameroon, Côte d'Ivoire and Senegal (over 35 per cent). Higher proportions in polygamous unions were found among older women in Côte d'Ivoire (44.7 per cent) and Senegal (61.7 per cent).

Women currently in polygamous unions can be divided into those in their first union and those in higher order unions. In the latter case, it is not known whether earlier unions were monogamous or polygamous, as type of union was determined only for current situations. The proportion of ever-married women currently in polygamous unions who had had a previous union ranges from 1 per cent in Lesotho to 15 per cent in Senegal (column (5) of table 171). In all countries, the proportion of ever-married women currently in a polygamous union who had had a previous union rises with age; Benin, Côte d'Ivoire and Senegal had differences of 10 per cent or more. This comparison refers to age groups 20-29 and 40 or over. The pattern with respect to the proportion of women currently in a first polygamous union was not so consistent. In three countries (Ghana, Kenya and Senegal), the increase in proportion suggests the possibility that some women who enter monogamous unions at a younger age may find themselves acquiring co-wives in the course of the marriage at a later stage of the life cycle.

The proportion currently divorced or separated varied widely across the countries, from 2.2 per cent in Benin to 13.9 per cent in Mauritania. The high proportion in Mauritania could be explained by the social status of such women, particularly among the Maure ethnic group, who consitute the majority. Traditionally, high social status is accorded Maure women who experience several marriages. Among women aged 20-29, the proportion was uniformly low (below 8 per cent) but at the older ages (40 or over) it varied from 2.8 per cent in Senegal to 18 per cent in Mauritania. The incidence of widowhood was also very low at younger ages. Among older women, proportions ranged from 1.8 per cent (Senegal) to 18.9 per cent (Lesotho), a range that cannot be explained solely by differential mortality patterns or age differences between spouses. In Senegal, it is notable that only 4.6 per cent of older ever-married women (sum of columns (7) and (8)) were not currently married.

While Senegal had the highest proportion of women in higher order marriages (23.7 per cent, sum of columns (2) and (5)), four other countries had proportions exceeding 15 per cent: Benin, 16.3; Côte d'Ivoire, 19.8; Ghana, 17.4; Mauritania, 19.5.

The proportion of ever-married women who were currently in polygamous unions is shown for four educational groups (table 172). Because of known relationships between age and education as well as between age and the incidence of polygamy, both age and marital duration have been controlled. In all countries, more educated women are less likely to be in polygamous unions. Differences of 10 per cent or more between

TABLE 170. PROPORTION OF WOMEN EVER MARRIED IN SELECTED AGE GROUPS AND SINGULATE MEAN AGE AT MARRIAGE, BY LEVEL OF EDUCATION, SEVEN COUNTRIES[a] IN SUB-SAHARAN AFRICA

Country and years of education	Ever-married women in age group 15-19 (percentage) (1)	20-24 (2)	25-29 (3)	Singulate mean age at marriage (4)
Benin				
Zero	60.5	96.9	99.7	16.9
One to three	24.1	96.6	96.9	18.9
Four to six	32.5	83.8	100.0	19.5
Seven or more	13.7	31.5	78.1	24.1
Cameroon				
Zero	82.1	98.0	98.5	15.4
One to three	59.7	95.1	96.9	17.6
Four to six	45.7	88.0	94.3	17.2
Seven or more	22.8	66.0	88.2	22.1
Côte d'Ivoire[b]				
Zero	66.4	92.8	96.3	17.1
One to three	58.6	90.8	100.0	17.7
Four to six	47.5	86.0	92.2	18.5
Seven or more	20.3	73.2	88.7	21.8
Ghana				
Zero	56.4	93.6	98.7	17.4
One to three	45.7	93.0	100.0	18.2
Four to six	32.1	89.7	97.4	19.2
Seven or more	19.3	77.6	95.1	20.5
Kenya				
Zero	61.4	91.6	97.2	17.2
One to three	36.8	90.0	99.4	18.7
Four to six	21.0	83.3	96.2	19.5
Seven or more	15.8	64.1	90.5	21.8
Senegal				
Zero	71.9	92.1	97.4	16.7
One to three	53.8	95.7	95.5	17.6
Four to six	33.9	70.0	87.2	20.4
Seven or more	10.1	52.8	82.1	22.8
Sudan[c]				
Zero	42.9	62.5	92.9	21.2
One to three	25.7	66.3	85.8	21.1
Four to six	13.3	53.6	83.3	22.8
Seven or more	4.0	22.6	63.2	24.7

Source: Ebanks and Singh (1984), table 8.
[a] Data for Lesotho and Mauritania not available.
[b] Formerly called the Ivory Coast.
[c] Northern part only.

extreme educational groups were found in all countries but Ghana and Lesotho. Differences do not progress systematically across the age groups, however; in some countries, the proportions do not begin to drop sharply until women have from four to six years of schooling (Benin, Cameroon and Senegal) and in others not until seven or more years of education have been reached (Côte d'Ivoire and Mauritania). Other countries show fluctuating patterns (Ghana, Kenya and Lesotho). Despite the tendency for women with higher levels of education to have a lower incidence of polygamy, prevalence levels among women with seven or more years of schooling were above 20 per cent in Benin, Côte d'Ivoire, Ghana, Kenya and Senegal.

Time spent in union

Exposure to the risk of conception is difficult to measure for Africa south of the Sahara, given the available data on marital status. While it is often assumed that women in polygamous unions experience less exposure than women in monagamous unions, this is likely to vary over the course of the life cycle and the marriage and may relate also to a woman's position in relation to her co-wives. Data are not available on changes in the type of union a woman might have experienced over her life cycle but only on the current status of her union as monagamous. Thus, variation in exposure among these countries is best calculated by using a measure of time spent in various marital statuses computed from the marital status distributions at the time of the survey (see chapter III and table 173).

The countries are ranked in descending order of the proportion of time spent in marriage. The proportion of time spent in marriage, column (3), is dependent upon the proportion of time spent single, on the one hand, and time spent divorced and widowed, on the other hand. The highest proportion of time spent single is found in Lesotho, Mauritania and the Sudan, where these proportions ranged between 15 and 19 per cent, followed by Ghana and Kenya, with 13 and 14 per cent, respectively. In the remaining four countries—Benin, Cameroon, Côte d'Ivoire and Senegal—the proportions were between 9 and 10 per cent.

With regard to time spent in divorce and widowhood, their share was relatively high in Mauritania and Lesotho (17 and 12 per cent, respectively), two countries that also led in the proportion of the woman's reproductive life spent in a "single" state. In the remaining seven countries, the share of "divorce and widowhood" was less than 10 per cent (no more than 4 per cent in Benin and Senegal). This share is surprisingly low, given the incidence of marital disruption in these countries (see table 171) and indicates the prevalence of remarriage among widowed and divorced women in many of these countries.

C. FERTILITY

This section examines levels in crude birth rates (CBR) and total fertility rates (TFR), incidence of sterility, fertility patterns, fertility trends, fertility and nuptiality, and fertility differentials by residence and education.

Fertility levels

Fertility levels in Africa in general are the highest in the world, as is reflected in the crude brith rates and total fertility rates of the countries reviewed here (see table 174). For the five years preceding the survey, the crude birth rates ranged from 54.0 in Benin to 40.2 in Lesotho. Côte d'Ivoire and Senegal also recorded extremely high crude birth rates, over 50 per 1,000. The estimated total fertility rate per woman was highest in Kenya, with 8.3 births per woman. Only Lesotho and the Sudan had total fertility rates below six births. These high fertility levels are a reflection of a number of factors, such as socio-economic circumstances, cultural attitudes, age at marriage and limited or lacking deliberate control on family size.

Incidence of sterility

The problem of sterility is of great concern in parts of some African countries. Sterility is the inability of a woman to produce a live birth, although the problem also relates to men. Sterility in women can be primary or secondary. Primary sterility arises when a woman is

TABLE 171. DISTRIBUTION OF EVER-MARRIED WOMEN BY CURRENT MARITAL STATUS, SELECTED AGE GROUPS, COUNTRIES IN SUB-SAHARAN AFRICA
(*Percentage*)

Country	Monogamous unions - First (1)	Monogamous unions - Second or more (2)	Monogamous unions - Total (3)	Polygamous unions - First (4)	Polygamous unions - Second or more (5)	Polygamous unions - Total (6)	Divorced or separated (7)	Widowed (8)
A. Age group 15-49									
Benin	52.8	7.0	59.8	27.2	9.3	36.5	2.2	1.3
Cameroon[a]	46.8	6.6	53.4	30.9	6.3	37.2	4.1	5.2
Côte d'Ivoire[b]	44.7	9.8	54.5	28.5	10.0	38.5	5.3	1.7
Ghana	44.8	9.8	54.6	23.2	7.6	30.8	8.4	1.9
Kenya	60.3	4.3	64.6	23.8	3.3	27.1	5.1	3.7
Lesotho	78.5	1.3	79.8	6.3	1.2	7.5	5.2	7.4
Mauritania[a]	51.5	15.8	67.3	11.1	3.7	14.8	13.9	3.8
Senegal	40.1	8.8	48.9	31.7	14.9	46.6	3.7	1.3
B. Age group 20-29									
Benin	57.4	4.8	62.2	30.2	5.7	35.9	1.1	0.6
Cameroon[a]	55.0	4.5	59.5	31.3	5.2	36.5	2.7	1.2
Ghana	55.6	8.7	64.3	21.8	5.2	27.0	7.9	0.5
Côte d'Ivoire[b]	49.9	9.0	58.9	27.4	8.0	35.4	5.3	0.4
Kenya	65.5	4.0	69.5	20.7	2.3	23.0	6.1	1.2
Lesotho	84.0	1.0	85.0	6.6	1.0	7.6	4.9	2.5
Mauritania[a]	56.2	15.0	71.2	11.6	3.0	14.6	0.9	0.9
Senegal	48.1	7.5	55.6	29.4	9.4	38.8	4.6	0.8
C. Age group 40+									
Benin	45.2	10.6	55.8	20.2	15.7	35.9	4.5	3.6
Cameroon[a]	33.2	9.7	42.9	27.6	9.5	37.1	6.1	14.1
Côte d'Ivoire[b]	28.5	14.2	42.7	26.9	17.8	44.7	6.9	5.7
Ghana	37.1	12.0	49.1	23.2	12.4	35.6	9.7	5.5
Kenya	47.3	5.1	52.4	29.7	4.4	34.1	3.5	9.8
Lesotho	65.7	1.1	66.8	6.6	1.3	7.9	6.4	18.9
Mauritania[a]	35.1	21.2	56.3	8.8	5.0	13.8	18.0	11.7
Senegal	21.1	12.5	33.6	36.4	25.3	61.7	2.8	1.8

Source: World Fertility Survey standard recode tapes.
[a] Current marriages not classified by type of union are distributed in proportion to the distribution of unions by type in each category.
[b] Formerly called the Ivory Coast.

TABLE 172. PROPORTION OF EVER-MARRIED WOMEN IN POLYGAMOUS UNIONS, BY LEVEL OF EDUCATION,[a] COUNTRIES IN SUB-SAHARAN AFRICA
(*Percentage*)

Country	Zero (1)	One to three (2)	Four to six (3)	Seven or more (4)	Difference (1) − (4)
Benin	38.7	38.2	32.8	24.0	14.7
Cameroon	44.8	41.3	32.3	18.8	26.0
Côte d'Ivoire[b]	42.3	41.4	39.4	28.5	13.8
Ghana	37.6	26.9	31.0	30.0	7.6
Kenya	34.0	23.9	27.4	22.0	12.0
Lesotho	10.6	14.1	8.1	6.4	4.2
Mauritania	21.0	15.7	23.3	11.0	10.0
Senegal	49.3	50.5	41.4	33.6	15.7
AVERAGE	34.8	31.5	29.5	21.8	—

Source: World Fertility Survey standard recode tapes.
[a] Age and marital duration are controlled using multiple classification analysis.
[b] Formerly called the Ivory Coast.

unable to bear a live child throughout her reproductive life, while secondary sterility arises after a woman has had at least one child born.

No attempt is made here to present a detailed comparative analysis of primary and secondary sterility. With regard to primary sterility, the proportion of ever-married women aged 45-49 who reported that they had never had a child provides an index of infertility or sterility. The percentages of ever-married women aged 45-49 who reported that they had no child were: Benin, 4.0; Cameroon, 13.7; Côte d'Ivoire, 5.0; Ghana, 2.1; Kenya, 4.6; Lesotho, 4.1; Mauritania, 3.7; Senegal, 3.5; and the Sudan, 8.6 (Economic Commission for Africa, 1986, annex, table 3A). Thus, the problem of infertility is more pronounced in Cameroon, followed by the Sudan. Owing to reporting errors and misinterpretation of the question in collecting data on childlessness, these figures should be considered rough indications. Concerning secondary sterility, it would appear to affect a growing number of women in some countries covered in this study, particularly Cameroon (Economic Commission for Africa, 1986, para. 23). Some of the main causes of sterility in Africa, documented in the literature, include venereal diseases, in particular, syphilis and gonorrohoea.

Fertility patterns

Table 175 shows that the average age-specific fertility rates for African countries are higher in all age groups than those for Latin America and the Caribbean and for Asia and Oceania, especially in age groups 25-29 and 30-34, where the differences between the average for Africa and that for Latin America and the Caribbean were 65 and 63 births per 1,000 women, respectively. The age patterns of fertility for Asia and Oceania and for Africa are similar in that peak fertility occurred at ages 25-29 but the former region had lower rates than the latter in all age groups.

TABLE 173. PROPORTION OF WOMEN'S REPRODUCTIVE YEARS EXPECTED TO BE SPENT IN VARIOUS MARITAL STATES, COUNTRIES IN SUB-SAHARAN AFRICA
(*Percentage*)

Country	Total (1)	Single (2)	Married Total (3)	First union (4)	Later union (5)	Divorced (6)	Widowed (7)
Senegal	100	9	87	62	25	3	1
Benin	100	10	86	69	17	2	2
Côte d'Ivoire[a]	100	9	84	63	21	5	2
Cameroon	100	10	81	69	12	4	5
Ghana	100	13	78	61	17	7	2
Kenya	100	14	77	71	7	4	4
Sudan	100	19	73	64	9	4	4
Lesotho	100	15	72	70	2	4	8
Mauritania	100	15	68	50	19	13	4

Source: Chapter III, table 46, in the present volume.
[a] Formerly called the Ivory Coast.

TABLE 174. CRUDE BIRTH RATES AND TOTAL FERTILITY RATES FOR THE FIVE YEARS PRECEDING THE SURVEY DATE, COUNTRIES IN SUB-SAHARAN AFRICA, AND AVERAGES COMPARED WITH OTHER REGIONS

Country and region	Crude birth rate (per 1,000)	Total fertility rate, ages 15-49
Sub-Saharan Africa		
Kenya	48.4	8.3
Côte d'Ivoire[a]	52.6	7.4
Senegal	51.9	7.2
Benin	54.0	7.1
Ghana	43.5	6.5
Cameroon	45.5	6.4
Mauritania	45.5	6.2
Sudan	40.6	5.9
Lesotho	40.2	5.8
AVERAGE	46.9	6.8
Latin America and the Caribbean		
AVERAGE[b]	35.0	4.9
Asia and Oceania		
AVERAGE[b]	39.1	5.7

Source: Chapter I, table 10, in the present volume.
[a] Formerly called the Ivory Coast.
[b] Thirteen countries in the region participated in the World Fertility Survey.

As is shown in table 176, childbearing in African countries generally begins at an early age. The contribution to total fertility among all women by those under 20 years of age accounted for 9 per cent in Lesotho and the Sudan, 11 per cent in Benin and Kenya, 13 per cent in Mauritania and Senegal, 14 per cent in Côte d'Ivoire and 15 per cent in Cameroon. However, women aged 20-29 and 30-39 contributed more or less similar proportions to total fertility—over 40 per cent. In general, the data indicate that the countries under study have a broad peak pattern extending over ages 20-29 years (chapter I, table 12).

Fertility trends

It is difficult to study fertility trends in African countries because reliable time-series on fertility levels at different periods are not available for the most part. Fertility trends estimated from WFS birth histories have the usual problems associated with misdating and omission of distant births. This section draws on results of a paper prepared for the Economic Commission for Africa (ECA) by the International Statistical Institute (ISI) in January 1986 (ECA/ISI, 1986, p. 8). The data given in table 177, covering cumulated fertility up to age group 30-34 during the 20 years before the survey date, is the basis for analysis of fertility trends. It has been noted that fertility increased in the 1960s in Kenya, Mauritania and the Sudan (North). The poor quality of data, however, was seen to have contributed to some of the increase (Henin, Korten and Werner, 1982; Rizgalla, 1985). The data for Cameroon indicate with reasonable reliability a rising level in fertility, in response to a decline in pathological sterility (Santow and Bioumla, 1984). In the case of Senegal, it has been found that there is no reason to doubt the persistently high levels of fertility since the early 1960s (Gueye, 1984). There is slight evidence of decline in fertility in Ghana. As for Benin and Lesotho, fertility levels had remained more or less constant during the 20 years preceding the survey date.

Fertility and nuptiality

The relationship between fertility and the different types of marital unions is not easy to untangle. There may be an element of selectivity in that women who are childless or at low parities may be more likely to have husbands who take on another wife. Achieved fertility may affect the timing and stability of marital unions. The timing of the first marriage may be determined by the occurrence of a pregnancy, if sexual activity begins before marriage, as is the case among some ethnic groups in some African countries. Also, involuntary childlessness may lead to divorce.

The effect of polygamy on fertility is controversial. It is claimed that low fertility in polygamous unions may be the result of favouritism, in that some wives may be favoured by the husband over others, or may be due to lower coital frequency (Lorimer, 1954, p. 98; Musham, 1956; Romaniuk, 1968, p. 214).

Table 178 presents the mean number of children ever born to women aged 40 years or over, according to current marital status. Fertility was highest among women who were currently married, married once and with no co-wives. Women who had married more than once had lower fertility than those who married once (columns (2) and (4)), irrespective of whether they were in monogamous or polygamous unions. Women who were either divorced or separated had the lowest fertility in most cases. The exceptions are Cameroon and Lesotho, where

TABLE 175. AVERAGE AGE-SPECIFIC FERTILITY RATES FOR EVER-MARRIED WOMEN DURING THE FIVE YEARS PRECEDING THE SURVEY, SUB-SAHARAN AFRICA, LATIN AMERICA AND THE CARIBBEAN, AND ASIA AND OCEANIA

Region	15-19	20-24	25-29	30-34	35-39	40-44	45-49	Total fertility rate
A. Rate
Sub-Saharan Africa[a]	158	291	300	254	186	114	047	6.75
Latin America and the Caribbean	103	239	235	191	136	065	018	4.93
Asia and Oceania	104	258	278	231	160	079	022	5.66
B. Percentage
Sub-Saharan Africa[a]	11.7	21.6	22.2	18.8	13.8	8.4	3.5	100
Latin America and the Caribbean	10.4	24.2	23.8	19.4	13.8	6.6	1.8	100
Asia and Oceania	9.2	22.8	24.6	20.4	14.0	7.0	1.9	100

Source: Chapter I, table 12, in the present volume.
[a] Including nine countries covered in this report.

TABLE 176. PERCENTAGE CONTRIBUTION TO TOTAL FERTILITY RATES OF ALL WOMEN AGED UNDER 20, 20-29 AND 30-49 YEARS, COUNTRIES IN SUB-SAHARAN AFRICA

Country	Under 20	20-29	30-34
Benin	11	45	44
Cameroon	15	45	40
Côte d'Ivoire[a]	14	41	45
Ghana	10	42	48
Kenya	11	42	47
Lesotho	9	45	46
Mauritania	13	44	43
Senegal	13	44	43
Sudan	9	46	45

Source: Economic Commission for Africa (1986).
[a] Formerly called the Ivory Coast.

TABLE 177. TRENDS IN FERTILITY LEVELS IN THE RECENT PAST, COUNTRIES IN SUB-SAHARAN AFRICA

Country	0-4 years	5-9 years	10-14 years	15-19 years
Benin	4.7	4.5	4.5	4.5
Cameroon	4.3	4.2	3.9	3.6
Côte d'Ivoire[a]	4.9	5.0	4.8	4.6
Ghana	3.9	4.1	4.2	4.2
Kenya	5.2	5.5	5.7	5.1
Lesotho	3.7	3.6	3.6	3.5
Mauritania	4.2	4.9	4.6	4.2
Senegal	4.9	4.8	4.9	4.9
Sudan	3.9	4.9	4.7	4.3

Source: Economic Commission for Africa/International Statistical Institute (1986).
[a] Formerly called the Ivory Coast.

the lowest fertility was found among women in higher order marriages.

While the magnitude of the difference in fertility between older women currently in monogamous unions and those in polygamous unions is not sizeable in most cases, differences of 1.2 children per woman were found in Côte d'Ivoire and Kenya for women still in their first unions. Among women in higher order unions, achieved fertility was almost identical for monogamous and polygamous wives except in Mauritania, where polygamous wives had 1.1 children fewer.

As a rough estimation of the loss in fertility due to differences in the proportions of women in different types of marital union in the eight countries being considered, the overall mean number of live births among ever-married women aged 40 and over is related to the average for women who were currently married, married once and with no co-wives, taking the latter as 100 (table 179). Differences are not extremely large, but proportions of less than 90 per cent were found in Cameroon, Côte d'Ivoire, Mauritania and Senegal.

Factors behind the prevalence of childlessness in the countries under study were referred to earlier. The proportion of childless women among women aged 40 and over in each type of marital union is given in table 180. Differences in the incidence of childlessness may explain some of the differences in the mean number of live births shown above. The proportion of childless women was lowest for women in monogamous unions who had married once and highest among those who had married more than once as well as those who were divorced or separated.

Very high proportions of childless women are noticeable for women who had married more than once, particularly in Cameroon and Lesotho, where these proportions reached from 33 to 28 per cent among women in polygamous unions. These high percentages of childless women could be due in part to sterility in the case of Cameroon and to migration of males to South Africa in the case of Lesotho. Childlessness appears to be particularly high among the divorced and separated for almost all countries. More than 20 per cent of divorced or separated women in Cameroon and Senegal were childless and between 10 and 17 per cent in Kenya, Côte d'Ivoire, Benin, Mauritania and Lesotho were childless, (column (5) of table 180).

Fertility differentials by type of place of current residence and education

Type of place and residence

The definition of rural and urban localities differs widely between countries. Some countries distinguish localities on the basis of population size, the most common criterion for an urban locality being 5,000 or more inhabitants. This figure is quite arbitrary, for in many sub-Saharan African countries, localities with such a population may be no more than large-sized villages. Bearing this in mind, it can be seen from table 181 that

TABLE 178. MEAN NUMBER OF CHILDREN EVER BORN TO WOMEN AGED 40 OR OVER, BY CURRENT MARITAL STATUS, COUNTRIES IN SUB-SAHARAN AFRICA

Country	Monogamous union First (1)	Monogamous union Second or more (2)	Polygamous union First (3)	Polygamous union Second or more (4)	Divorced or separated (5)	Widowed (6)	Never married (7)
Benin	6.5	5.9	6.2	6.0	4.6	5.3	0.0[a]
Cameroon	5.7	3.3	5.6	3.4	3.5	5.5	2.2
Côte d'Ivoire[b]	8.0	6.2	6.8	6.2	5.2	6.0	4.5[a]
Ghana	6.7	6.4	6.3	6.3	6.0	6.3	1.0[a]
Kenya	8.6	6.3	7.4	6.4	6.0	6.8	7.0[a]
Lesotho	5.5	3.6[a]	5.1	3.5[a]	4.1	4.9	..
Mauritania	6.8	6.6	6.9	5.4	4.3	6.3	..
Senegal	8.0	6.0	7.6	5.9	4.2[a]	6.4[a]	4.5[a]

Source: World Fertility Survey standard recode tapes.
[a] Fewer than 20 cases.
[b] Formerly called the Ivory Coast.

TABLE 179. MEAN NUMBER OF LIVE BIRTHS TO EVER-MARRIED WOMEN AS A PROPORTION OF MEAN NUMBER OF LIVE BIRTHS TO WOMEN MARRIED AND WITH NO CO-WIVES, WOMEN AGED 40 OR OVER, COUNTRIES IN SUB-SAHARAN AFRICA

Country	Women married once and no co-wives (1)	Overall mean number of live births (2)	Index (1) = 100 (3)
Kenya	8.6	7.7	90
Côte d'Ivoire[a]	8.0	6.8	85
Senegal	8.0	6.9	86
Benin	6.5	6.2	95
Ghana	6.7	6.4	96
Cameroon	5.7	5.0	88
Mauritania	6.8	6.0	88
Lesotho	5.5	5.2	95

Source: World Fertility Survey standard recode tapes.
[a] Formerly called the Ivory Coast.

the rural fertility rates were higher than the "major urban" rates. This pattern is repeated when comparing rural areas with "other" urban, except in the case of Cameroon, where the total fertility rate was slightly higher for "other" urban than for rural areas.

Education

A close examination of table 182 shows that the countries included in this study can be divided into two groups. In one group, the pattern is such that higher fertility is observed among women with from one to three years of education, as compared with women with no education and those with additional years of education. This is the case with Benin, Cameroon, Côte d'Ivoire, Kenya and Senegal. Taking Senegal as an example, the total fertility rate among women with no education was 7.3, compared with 9.4 for women with from one to three years; then it declines to 6.3 with from four to six years and to 4.5 with seven or more years of education.

In the case of Cameroon and Kenya, fertility does not fall below the level for uneducated women until women have at least seven years of schooling. At the early stages of educational development, women with some education may be more appreciative of the value of pre-natal care and generally more aware of the importance of hygiene than women with no education. This factor, in the absence of changes in ideals as to family size, may contribute to the higher number of live births for this category (Henin, 1973). Beyond three or four years of education, the total fertility rate tends to decline.

With regard to the second group of countries, which includes Ghana, Lesotho and the Sudan, fertility among women with some education was lower than that for women with no education. An explanation can be advanced for Ghana and Lesotho in that these two countries enjoy the highest educational levels, as can be seen from tables 165 and 166. It is not immediately clear why the Sudan follows the second pattern despite the relatively low level of educational attainment.

D. POST-PARTUM NON-SUSCEPTIBLE PERIOD

The post-partum non-susceptible period is discussed under three headings: post-partum amenorrhoea; abstinence; and breast-feeding. The averages presented in this section are calculated using the current status method (chapter IV), which uses information on the current status of post-partum women at the time of the survey. The mean duration of various post-partum states is estimated using information on the proportion of all women who had given birth X months before the survey and who were in a particular post-partum state at the time of the survey. Further details on the method can be found in chapter IV. It should be added that in sub-Saharan Africa, where modern methods of contraception are either unknown or little used, factors that contribute to the length of the non-susceptible period are very important because of their inhibiting effect on fertility (Bongaarts, 1980; Bongaarts, 1981; Bongaarts, Frank and Lesthaeghe, 1984).

Post-partum amenorrhoea

Post-partum amenorrhoea is a biological variable which is determined to a large extent by the mother's breast-feeding of the infant. All women have a period of amenorrhoea after birth but those who do not breast-feed have a short one of about 1.5-2.0 months, whereas if breast-feeding is prolonged, amenorrhoea may last up to 15-24 months.

Table 183 (column (6)) shows that the mean duration of post-partum amenorrhoea was longest in Ghana (12.4 months) and shortest in Mauritania (8.8 months). It can also be seen (columns (3)-(5)) that for all eight countries included in the table, there is a common pattern of a decline in the mean with age, from the older to the younger ages. The mean duration of amenorrhoea decreased with modernization from rural to urban women and from less educated to more educated women (not shown) (Singh and Ferry, 1984, pp. 26-27). In other

TABLE 180. PROPORTION OF ALL EVER-MARRIED WOMEN AGED 40 OR OVER WHO WERE CHILDLESS, BY TYPE OF MARITAL UNION, COUNTRIES IN SUB-SAHARAN AFRICA

(*Percentage*)

Country	Monogamous union First (1)	Monogamous union Second or more (2)	Polygamous union First (3)	Polygamous union Second or more (4)	Divorced or separated (5)	Widowed (6)
Benin	1.7	2.9	2.2	3.9	16.7	8.3
Cameroon	8.8	33.2	11.0	33.3	23.4	9.4
Côte d'Ivoire[a]	2.8	4.8	2.5	5.1	11.5	3.9
Ghana	1.3	2.5	2.1	5.6	3.1	1.8
Kenya	0.9	9.6	4.5	2.5	14.9	2.6
Lesotho	4.6	34.2	7.7	28.2	11.4	1.3
Mauritania	0.0	0.0	0.0	5.4	9.5	4.5
Senegal	0.0	6.2	1.7	6.1	22.2	0.0

Source: World Fertility Survey standard recode tapes.
[a] Formerly called the Ivory Coast.

TABLE 181. TOTAL FERTILITY RATE, BY TYPE OF PLACE OF CURRENT RESIDENCE, COUNTRIES IN SUB-SAHARAN AFRICA

Country	Total fertility rate Major urban	Total fertility rate Other urban	Total fertility rate Rural
Benin	5.75	6.70	7.40
Cameroon	5.30	6.70	6.51
Côte d'Ivoire[a]	6.42	6.86	7.72
Ghana	5.41	6.26	6.79
Kenya	5.90	6.08	8.48
Lesotho	–	4.79	6.23
Senegal	6.76	6.32	7.47

Source: Ashurst and Casterline (n.d.), table 2.
[a] Formerly called the Ivory Coast.

TABLE 182. TOTAL FERTILITY RATE FOR AGES 15-49, BY RESPONDENT'S EDUCATION, EIGHT COUNTRIES[a] IN SUB-SAHARAN AFRICA

Country	Years of schooling Zero (1)	One to three (2)	Four to six (3)	Seven or more (4)
Benin	7.35	8.50	5.79	4.26
Cameroon	6.38	6.98	6.77	5.18
Côte d'Ivoire[b]	7.45	8.02	6.36	5.83
Ghana	6.84	6.67	6.69	5.49
Kenya	8.28	9.21	8.43	7.34
Lesotho	6.24	5.63	5.97	4.76
Senegal	7.32	9.44	6.31	4.47
Sudan	6.47	5.56	4.98	3.37

Source: Ashurst and Casterline (n.d.), table 3.
[a] Data for Mauritania not available.
[b] Formerly called the Ivory Coast.

words, with increased modernization, the birth interval will shorten in the absence of the use of contraception.

Post-partum abstinence

Post-partum abstinence was found among women in all nine countries studied here. The Sudan and Kenya had the shortest period of abstinence, averages of about 2.6 and 2.9 months, respectively, while Benin had the longest, 15.5 months. Most of the remaining countries had a period ranging from 10 to 13 months (column (10)). Furthermore, it can be seen that there is a decrease in the duration from older to younger women in all countries (columns (7)-(9)).

The period of non-susceptibility, which is defined as the period during which a woman is either amenorrhoeic or obtaining, is therefore substantially lengthened beyond the duration of amenorrhoea because of the prolonged abstinence: in Lesotho, from 9.6 to 16.5 months; in Benin, from 12 to 17 months; and in Cameroon, from 12 to 16 months.

The decline in the duration of abstinence will have a more immediate effect on the non-susceptible period, and on the birth interval where abstinence is longer than the period of amenorrhoea. The effect of decline in breast-feeding and amenorrhoea will be more important for countries where abstinence is short (Lesthaeghe and others, 1981).

Breast-feeding

Full breast-feeding differs from one country to another. The longest duration, 8.0 months, was reported in Mauritania; and the shortest, 2.2 months, in Kenya (column (2) of table 183). There was little difference by age in the duration of full breast-feeding (not shown), except in few cases where duration declined with age (in Cameroon and the Sudan); this may well be due to physical changes in the quantity of milk produced with age. Differences among residential groups show the expected pattern of longer breast-feeding in rural than in urban areas. In some areas, the difference was as much as two months. Similar differentials were observed from the group with no education to those with seven or more years of schooling groups (not shown) (Singh and Ferry, 1984, p. 29).

The average duration of breast-feeding (column (1)) is longer than the average duration of amenorrhoea (column (6)); the latter is still longer than the average duration of abstinence (column (10)). This was generally the case for all countries except Kenya and the Sudan, which had short periods of abstinence.

In Benin, over 80 per cent of breast-feeding women abstained during the first six months and about 70 per cent continued to do so to the end of the breast-feeding period if they were no longer amenorrhoeic (not shown). In the case of Kenya and the Sudan, about 80 per cent of breast-feeding women were amenorrhoeic for up to six months and resumed sexual relations after the third month from birth. On the other hand, Benin, Cameroon and Lesotho had long periods of abstinence—as was shown earlier—while Côte d'Ivoire, Ghana, and Mauritania had a middle position (Singh and Ferry, 1984, p. 22).

TABLE 183. MEAN DURATION OF BREAST-FEEDING, POST-PARTUM AMENORRHOEA, ABSTINENCE AND NON-SUSCEPTIBILITY,[a] SELECTED AGE GROUPS AND ALL AGES, EIGHT COUNTRIES IN SUB-SAHARAN AFRICA
(Months)

Country	Full breast-feeding, all ages (1)	Breast-feeding, all ages (2)	Amenorrhoea 15-24 (3)	Amenorrhoea 25-34 (4)	Amenorrhoea 35+ (5)	Amenorrhoea All ages (6)	Abstinence 15-24 (7)	Abstinence 25-34 (8)	Abstinence 35+ (9)	Abstinence All ages (10)	Susceptibility, all ages (11)
Benin	2.6	19.2	10.9	12.0	13.7	11.9	15.6	15.1	16.2	15.5	17.2
Cameroon	5.1	17.5	10.4	12.2	13.8	11.8	12.8	13.7	16.5	13.9	15.9
Côte d'Ivoire[b]	5.0	17.5	8.5	11.7	13.0	10.4	11.4	14.0	16.0	13.1	14.7
Ghana	4.5	17.9	11.8	12.2	14.1	12.4	9.4	9.6	11.7	10.0	14.6
Kenya	2.2	16.9	7.8	10.7	11.9	9.9	2.3	2.9	3.8	2.9	10.3
Lesotho	2.5	19.1	8.0	9.8	12.0	9.6	15.6	16.0	15.4	15.0	16.5
Mauritania	7.9	15.6	8.5	9.0	9.0	8.8	..	..	..	..	..
Sudan	5.6	15.8	9.5	11.6	10.3	10.8	2.5	2.6	2.8	2.6	11.2

Source: Singh and Ferry (1984), tables 5-8.
[a] Defined as the period during which a woman is either amenorrhoeic or abstaining.
[b] Formerly called the Ivory Coast.

E. DESIRED FAMILY SIZE AND KNOWLEDGE AND USE OF CONTRACEPTION

In this section, a brief treatment of desired family size and of knowledge and use of contraception is presented. Information on these topics would be most useful for planners and policy-makers in countries where intervention on fertility is of policy concern, and it also helps to explain prevailing levels of fertility. Furthermore, such information would be valuable in preparing assumptions for projections of fertility component of population projections.

Desired family size

Table 184 contains data on desired family size and mean wanted family size. A considerable number of women in the countries covered in the study did not give a numerical reply to the question on desired family size: from 33 per cent in Mauritania to 2.3 per cent in Lesotho (column (4)), table 184. Only Ghana and Lesotho show small proportions (2.3 and 10.9 per cent, respectively). This is a further reflection of higher proportions of educated women in these two countries, as seen earlier.

Many women were also unable to indicate a numerical response on additional number of children wanted. The proportion of such women was highest in Senegal with 85 per cent, followed by Cameroon with 75.8 per cent, and lowest in the Sudan and Lesotho (column (5)). For all women who indicated the desired family size, these were very high indeed. In Mauritania, Côte d'Ivoire, Senegal and Cameroon the desired family size was eight and above, while in Ghana and Lesotho six children was the desired family size. The mean wanted family size based on ever-married women who were fecund at the time of the survey was more or less of similar magnitude or slightly less than the desired family size which was asked to all women.

What emerges from these results is that African women in general do not feel at ease in talking about desired family size. Among those who gave a numerical reply to the question on desired family size, the results show that large families were desired. Consequently, it would not be easy for more women to consider reducing their family size until their attitudes on family size change.

Knowledge and use of contraception

With respect to knowledge and use of contraception, the WFS data for some countries indicate that there is widespread knowledge about contraception but only small proportions of women were using a contraceptive method at the time of the survey. The following examples illustrate this: (*a*) in Kenya, 91 per cent of women who were married and fecund at the time of the survey knew of a contraceptive method, but only 9 per cent were using a method at that time; (*b*) in the Sudan, 50 per cent knew of a method and only 6 per cent were using a method; (*c*) in Ghana, women who were using contraception at the time of the survey constituted 9.5 per cent of the married women or 8.6 per cent of ever-married women (United Nations, 1986, p.118; World Fertility Survey, 1983, p.13). As for Senegal, the WFS results indicate that 60 per cent of ever-married women had heard of at least one contraceptive method. However, the proportion of married using a contraceptive method at the time of the survey was as low as 4 per cent. For literate women, the percentage was 13.4 (World Fertility Survey, 1981, pp. 12-13). In Lesotho, only 5 per cent of married women under 50 years were using contraception at the time of the survey (World Fertility Survey, 1981a, p.10). Although no figures are provided on differentials in knowledge and use of contraception, the information available indicates that better educated women are more knowledgeable about contraceptive methods and have higher proportions using a contraceptive method than their less educated counterparts (chapter V).

F. SUMMARY AND POLICY IMPLICATIONS

It has been shown that age at marriage is generally low and marriage is almost universal for African women by age 20. Trends in age at marriage show that some of the countries are experiencing a rise in the age at marriage and a decline in the proportion marrying. This is particularly true of more educated, urban women.

Another aspect of marriage, the type of marital union, was also considered; and it was found that the incidence of polygamy is high—from 30 to 47 per cent in five of the countries. Remarriages are also very common. Further, it was found that there is a relationship between the type of marital union and education in that women with

TABLE 184. DESIRED FAMILY SIZE, COUNTRIES IN SUB-SAHARAN AFRICA

Country	Desired family size[a] (1)	Percentage of women who wanted no more children[b] (2)	Mean wanted family size[c] (3)	Percentage of women without numerical preferences as to Children desired[d] (4)	Children wanted in addition[e] (5)
Benin	7.6	8	f	32.3	43.4
Cameroon	8.0	3	f	28.5	75.8
Côte d'Ivoire[g]	8.4	4	7.6	26.6	19.8
Ghana	6.0	12	5.5	10.9	19.5
Kenya	7.2	17	7.0	19.3	26.5
Lesotho	6.0	15	5.2	2.3	6.2
Mauritania	8.8	11	f	33.0	46.1
Senegal	8.3	8	6.8	27.2	85.0
Sudan[h]	6.4	17	6.4	18.4	12.9

Source: United Nations (1986), table 3.

[a] Mean number of children that women said they would like to have in their whole life if they could choose it. Data refer to all women interviewed.

[b] Based on the question: "Do you want to have another child sometime?" Data refer only to currently married fecund women (but in Senegal only to pregnant women).

[c] Number of living children and the number of additional children wanted ("Wants no more children" responses were coded as zero additional child). Data refer to currently married fecund women (but in Senegal only to pregnant women).

[d] Percentage of women who gave a non-numerical answer to the question concerning desired family size (see note [a]).

[e] Percentage of non-numerical responses as to the number of children additionally wanted, including those who were "undecided" or whose responses were "not stated".

[f] Although information was collected, no data were available at the time this table was finalized.

[g] Formerly called the Ivory Coast.

[h] Northern part only.

more years of education are more likely to remain in a monogamous union and are less susceptible to the incidence of divorce and remarriage.

The average total fertility rate was higher for the nine sub-Saharan African countries than the average for Asia and Oceania (a difference of about one birth) and for Latin America and the Caribbean (a difference of two births). Of the nine countries, one country, Kenya, had a total fertility rate of over eight. Kenya is followed by Côte d'Ivoire, Senegal and Benin, with a total fertility rate slightly over seven; Ghana, Cameroon and Mauritania, slightly over six; the Sudan and Lesotho, slightly less than six. There is a difference of little over two births between the highest, Kenya, and the lowest, Lesotho. Discussion of the incidence of sterility showed that in seven of the countries, from 2.1 to 5 per cent of women aged 45-49 were reported to be childless. In Cameroon, however, the figure was about 14 per cent; and in the Sudan, it was 9 per cent.

There is some evidence that in the 20 years preceding the survey date, fertility had risen in Cameroon, Ghana, Kenya, Mauritania and the Sudan. However, the quality of date reporting in the birth histories accounts for part of the increase in fertility in some of these countries.

In the other countries, the rates have remained more or less constant at high levels. Women who were currently married, married once and to a monogamous husband were found to have the highest fertility, followed by currently married women, married once and to a polygamous husband. The two categories of women with lowest fertility were those who were married more than once, followed by those divorced and separated.

The study of fertility differentials by respondent's years of education showed some interesting results. In some countries, the relation between the mean number of live births and the number of years of education was not linear. Fertility appears to be higher for women with few years of education than for women with no education. Fertility then tends to decline with more years of education. This was not true, however, in the case of Ghana and Lesotho, two countries with high proportions of women with from four to six or seven or more years of education. It was argued that for the expected inverse linear relationship between number of years of education and fertility to prevail, a community must wait until most of its women get at least five or more years of education. Of course, other changes need to accompany the attainment of that minimum level of education. Fertility of women in rural areas was found to be higher than fertility of women in urban areas.

The discussion of desired family size and of knowledge and use of contraception showed that among those who provided a numerical response on desired family size, the figures were quite high, ranging from six to nine children. Many women do not find it easy to talk freely about desired family size or the additional children they want to have. This is a reflection of cultural attitudes about childbearing in most African countries. Although there was widespread knowledge of contraception, the proportions actually using contraceptives were quite small, in nearly all cases less than 10 per cent of the ever-married women. Among those using contraception, most were in urban areas and were among the better educated. The results on desired family size and knowledge and use of contraception provide some explanation of the very high fertility levels in African countries.

There are many policy issues that Governments of African countries need to consider if they want to reduce the high levels of fertility, in view of their overall socio-economic developments, as portrayed in the Kilimanjaro Programme of Action on Population adopted by African Governments in 1984. That programme addresses the high fertility levels in Africa, among other population issues. These high levels accompanied by declining mortality contribute to high population growth rates in Africa —the highest among the regions of the world. These population growth rates in turn pose serious problems for African Governments in providing adequate social service related to education, health, employment, housing, recreation, food etc. These problems are pronounced at this stage when African countries are experiencing serious economic difficulties. With continued population growth, it is likely to be more difficult to achieve the desired objectives of programmes intended to improve the economic situation.

In order to reduce the high levels of fertility, some specific measures that Governments may want to consider, as integral components of socio-economic development strategies, should include:

(a) The need to review age at marriage and pass legislation to increase that age where it is considered to be low. If this is done, it will in the long run have an effect in lowering fertility levels;

(b) Women's education should be improved. They should be given more opportunities to continue with education for many years. This will lessen entry into marriage at an early age, as is the case at present. In addition, adequate education among women would act as a catalyst in changing their attitudes which currently favour large family sizes. Furthermore, adequate education will prepare women to engage in gainful employment outside the home;

(c) Strong educational campaigns should be mounted to educate and persuade the population to accept the benefits of small family size. Means for achieving small family size should be made available;

(d) Mother and child health and family planning should be integrated, wherever possible, in other sectoral areas within the framework of rural and urban development programmes. Special attention should be given to birth-spacing and to a significant reduction of infant and child mortality, which are important determinants of fertility;

(e) Existing programmes to reduce fertility need to be strengthened and improved to achieve their desired objectives. However, attention should also be given to reduce problems of infertility where it exists;

(f) Where there are no clear programmes and policy to reduce fertility, formulation of relevant policies should be given some consideration;

(g) Women's social status should be improved to enable them to participate at all levels in the socio-economic development activities of a country.

Action on the above-listed measures would be of great help in improving the life of the people of African countries. Many African leaders have recently begun to change their perception on population. They no longer want to treat population programmes in isolation but as part of the other programmes and policies on health, housing, food production, education, employment, environment and use of resources. This emphasizes the recent approach of development which has to take into account population, environment and resources. The African Governments have a considerable challenge. The recommendations in the Kilimanjaro Programme of Action on Population provide a framework for meeting the challenge, especially in dealing with problems related to high fertility levels.

NOTES

[1] Formerly called the Ivory Coast.

[2] The distorting effect of 56 per cent for Mauritania should be borne in mind, because the educational system uses both modern and traditional educational methods, which presented difficulties in interpretation of years of education.

REFERENCES

Anker, Richard and James C. Knowles (1982). *Fertility Determinants in Developing Countries: A Case Study of Kenya*. Liége: Ordina Editions for International Labour Office.

Ashurst, H. and J. B. Casterline (n.d.). Socio-economic differentials in current fertility; additional tables. Data for World Fertility Survey Comparative Studies. Voorburg, The Netherlands, Statistical Institute (unpublished).

Benin (1983). Ministère du plan, de la statistique et de l'analyse économique. Institut national de la statistique et de l'analyse économique; Bureau central de recensement. *Enquête sur la fécondité au Bénin: rapport préliminaire*. Cotonou.

Bongaarts, John (1978). A framework for analyzing the proximate determinants of fertility. *Population and Development Review* 4(1):105-132.

_____ (1980). The fertility-inhibiting effects of the intermediate fertility variables. Paper submitted to the International Union for the Scientific Study of Population and World Fertility Survey Seminar on the Analysis of Maternity Histories, London, April 1980.

_____ (1981). The impact on fertility of traditional and changing child-spacing practices in tropical Africa. In Hilary J. Page and Ron Lesthaeghe, eds., *Child-Spacing in Tropical Africa: Traditions and Change* London and New York: Academic Press, 111-129.

_____, Odile Frank and Ron Lesthaeghe (1984). The proximate determinants of fertility in sub-Saharan Africa. *Population and Development Review* 10(3):511-537.

Caldwell, John C., with Nelson O. Addo and others, eds. (1975). *Population Growth and Socioeconomic Change in West Africa*. New York: Columbia University Press for The Population Council.

Cameroon (1983). Ministère de l'économie et du plan. Direction de la statistique et de la comfabilité nationale. *Enquête national sur la fécondité du Cameroon: rapport principal*. Yaoundé.

Côte d'Ivoire (1984). Ministère de l'économie et des finances. Direction de la statistique. *Enquête nationale ivoirienne sur la fécondité, 1980-81: rapport principal*. Abidjan.

Ebanks, G. Edward and Susheela Singh (1984). Socio-economic differentials in age at marriage; preliminary tables. Data for World Fertility Survey Cross-National Summaries. Voorburg, The Netherlands, International Statistical Institute (unpublished).

Economic Commission for Africa (1981). Population Division. Fertility differentials in Africa. In *Population Dynamics: Fertility and Mortality in Africa*. Proceedings of the Expert Group Meeting on Fertility and Mortality Levels and Trends in Africa and their Policy Implications, Monrovia, Liberia, 26 November-1 December, 1979. Addis Ababa.

_____ (1986). Population dynamics in Africa. Addis Ababa, 21 February 1986. E/ECA/PSD.4/29.

_____ and International Statistical Institute. Contribution of World Fertility Survey programme to knowledge about population dynamics in Africa. Addis Ababa, 20 January 1986. E/ECA/PSD.4/30.

Frank, Odile (1983). Infertility in sub-Saharan Africa: estimates and implications. *Population and Development Review* 9(1):137-144.

_____ (1984). Child fostering in sub-Saharan Africa. Paper submitted to the Annual Meeting of the Population Association of America, Minneapolis, Minnesota, 3-5 May 1984.

_____ (1985). *The Demand for Fertility Control in Sub-Saharan Africa*. Center for Policy Studies Working Papers, No. 117. New York: The Population Council.

Ghana (1983). Central Bureau of Statistics. *Ghana Fertility Survey, 1979-80: First Report*. Accra.

Gueye, Lamine (1984). *Enquête sénégalaise sur la fécondité: rapport d'évaluation*. World Fertility Survey Scientific Reports, No. 49. Voorburg, The Netherlands: International Statistical Institute.

Henin, Roushdi A. (1968). Fertility differentials in the Sudan. *Population Studies* 22(1):147-164.

_____ (1969). The patterns and causes of fertility differentials in the Sudan (with reference to nomadic and settled populations). *Population Studies* 23(2):171-198.

_____ (1977). The demography of Tanzania: an analysis of the 1973 National Demographic Survey of Tanzania. In Roushdi A. Henin, Douglas Ewbank and Howard Hogan, eds., *1973 National Demographic Survey of Tanzania*, vol. VI, *An Analysis of the 1973 National Demographic Survey of Tanzania*. Dar es Salaam: Bureau of Statistics of the Ministry of Finance and Planning and University of Dar es Salaam.

_____, Alisa Korten and Linda H. Werner (1982). *Evaluation of Birth Histories: A Case Study of Kenya*. World Fertility Survey Scientific Reports, No. 36. Voorburg, The Netherlands: International Statistical Institute.

Hill, Althea (1981). *The Demographic Situation in Sub-Saharan Africa: A Background Paper*. Washington, D.C.: The World Bank.

Hogan, Howard R. (1977). Childlessness and subfecundity. In Roushdi A. Henin, Douglas Ewbank and Howard Hogan, eds., *1973 National Demographic Survey of Tanzania*, vol. VI, *An Analysis of the 1973 National Demographic Survey of Tanzania*. Dar es Salaam: Bureau of Statistics of the Ministry of Finance and Planning and University of Dar es Salaam, appendix 5.4.

Kenya (1980/81). Ministry of Economic Planning and Development. Central Bureau of Statistics. *Kenya Fertility Survey 1977-78: First Report*. Nairobi.

Lesthaeghe, Ron and others (1981). Child-spacing and fertility in sub-Saharan Africa: an overview of issues. In Hilary J. Page and Ron Lesthaeghe, eds., *Child-Spacing in Tropical Africa: Traditions and Change*. London and New York: Academic Press, 3-23.

Lesotho (1981). Ministry of Planning and Statistics. Central Bureau of Statistics. *Lesotho Fertility Survey, 1977: First Report*. Maseru.

Lorimer, Frank and others, eds. (1954). *Culture and Human Fertility: A Study of the Relation of Cultural Conditions to Fertility in Non-Industrial and Transitional Societies*. Population and Culture Series, No. 1. Paris: International Union for the Scientific Study of Population and United Nations Educational, Scientific and Cultural Organization.

Muhsam, H. V. (1956). The fertility of polygamous marriages. *Population Studies* 10(1):3-16.

Nag, Moni (1984). *Constraints on the Use of Fertility Regulating Methods*. Center for Policy Studies Working Papers, No. 107. New York: The Population Council.

Rizgalla, M. K. (1985). *Evaluation of the Sudan Fertility Survey 1979*. World Fertility Survey Scientific Reports, No. 72. Voorburg, The Netherlands: International Statistical Institute.

Romaniuk, Anatole (1968). Infertility in tropical Africa. In John C. Caldwell and Chukuka Okonjo, eds., *The Population of Tropical Africa*. London, Longmans, Green for the Population Council, 214-224.

Santow, G. and A. Bioumla (1983). An evaluation of the Cameroon Fertility Survey, 1976. World Fertility Survey Technical Papers, Tech. 2173. Voorburg, The Netherlands, International Statistical Institute.

Senegal (1981). Ministère de l'économie et des finances. Direction de la statistique; Division des enquête et de la démographie. *Enquête sénégalaise sur la fécondité 1978: rapport national d'analyse*. Dakar.

Singh, Susheela and Benoît Ferry (1984). *Biological and Traditional Factors that Influence Fertility: Results from WFS Surveys*. World Fertility Survey Comparative Studies, No. 40; Cross-National Summaries. Voorburg, The Netherlands: International Statistical Institute.

Sudan (1982). Ministry of National Planning and Department of Statistics. *The Sudan Fertility Survey, 1979—Principal Report*. 2 v. Khartoum.

United Nations (1986). Department of International Economic and Social Affairs. Population Division. *Policy Relevance of Findings of the World Fertility Survey for Developing Countries*. Non-sales publication ST/ESA/SER.R/59. New York.

Ware, Helen (1976). Motivations for the use of birth control: evidence from West Africa. Demography 13(4):479-493.

World Fertility Survey (1981). *The Senegal Fertility Survey 1978: A Summary of Findings*. WFS Summaries of Findings, No. 30. Voorburg, The Netherlands: International Statistical Institute.

_____ (1981a). *The Lesotho Fertility Survey 1977: A Summary of Findings*. WFS Summaries of Findings, No. 34. Voorburg, The Netherlands: International Statistical Institute.

_____ (1983). *The Ghana Fertility Survey, 1979-1980: A Summary of Findings*. WFS Summaries of Findings, No. 39. Voorburg, The Netherlands: International Statistical Institute.

XIII. A REVIEW OF THE FERTILITY SITUATION IN THE ARAB COUNTRIES OF WESTERN ASIA AND NORTHERN AFRICA

Samir Farid*

ABSTRACT

In this chapter, significant features of the fertility situation in six countries of Western Asia and Northern Africa (Egypt, Jordan, Morocco, the Syrian Arab Republic, Tunisia and Yemen) are reviewed. Within an overall climate of high fertility, diversity was still found with respect to various aspects of reproductive behaviour. The total fertility rate around the survey date was fewer than six children in Egypt, Morocco and Tunisia; between seven and eight in Jordan and the Syrian Arab Republic and more than eight in Yemen. Adolescent fertility was high and there was an average of one live birth to every three or four women aged 20-39. While fertility had not apparently declined in the Syrian Arab Republic and Yemen, data from the Northern African countries, Egypt, Morocco and Tunisia, showed definite declines of from 1.5 to 1.8 children per woman during the decade from the mid-1960s to mid-1970s.

Significant differences in fertility between women residing in urban and in rural areas were found in all countries but Yemen, where most women live in rural areas. Fertility had declined most steeply among urban women and, at all ages, they bore children at a lower rate than women in rural areas. In all six countries, women with successively higher levels of educational attainment had lower completed family size, due not only to fertility control within marriage but to later age at marriage. Nevertheless, fertility among women in the same residential and educational categories differed widely between countries. Socio-economic differentials in fertility preferences followed similar patterns to those observed for fertility.

The demographic significance of age at first marriage is clearly demonstrated in these countries, where childbearing is almost exclusively confined within marriage. Extremes in marriage patterns were found between Yemen, with 60 per cent of women aged 15-19 ever married, and Tunisia, with roughly only 5 per cent. All countries had experienced a trend towards later marriage ages. In Yemen, the shift had been from the early to the late teens, and in Tunisia, from the late teens to the early twenties.

While roughly one third of currently married women were using contraception in Tunisia, the practice was essentially non-existent in Yemen. In most countries, contraceptive use was largely confined to urban areas and increased dramatically as a woman's educational attainment rose.

Current trends in these countries suggest that higher educational levels and continuing urbanization will be forces leading to further increases in marriage age, a moderation of family size ideals and an increase in contraceptive use.

In the Arab countries of Western Asia and Northern Africa, the family is undergoing rapid, important changes. The fact is clearly documented by much evidence from the past two decades, including the data from the World Fertility Survey (WFS) programme in those countries. Virtually all socio-economic indicators are moving in a direction that could only be considered development: the expansion of educational opportunities, and the resulting increase in levels of literacy, enrolment and educational attainment; the improvement of health services and public sanitation, and the resulting declines in mortality; the transformation of the economy from an almost exclusively agricultural base towards a mix of industry and agriculture; the spread of urbanization; the electrification of many rural areas; the expansion of transport networks; and the rapid increase in the proportion of the population reached by the mass media.

Such substantial social and economic changes can only be expected to affect family life. As in most developing countries, however, development efforts have been spread unevenly among the different segments of the population. The WFS results in the region and many other pieces of evidence convey a picture of a striking contrast between the rural and the urban family formation patterns, and

---
*Free-lance statistical consultant.

of the women living in these two different contexts. Not only is urban residence distinguished from rural residence, but within the urban sector, the prime cities are distinctive; and, largely within the major urban areas, women's education is rapidly becoming associated with the emergence of a new pattern of reproductive preference and practice.

For the Arab countries of Western Asia and Northern Africa, the overall crude birth rate averages about 44-45 per 1,000. These rates are well above the average of 29 per 1,000 estimated for the world in 1975-1980, and the 34 per 1,000 estimated for the less developed regions (United Nations, 1985). The crude death rate is roughly 14-15 per 1,000 for the two subregions and the population growth is estimated at roughly 2.9 per cent for the period 1975-1980 in Northern Africa and 3.5 per cent for the Arab countries of Western Asia because of the additional factor of immigration (United Nations, 1985).

Only three Arab countries (Egypt, Morocco and Tunisia) maintain that the current rate of population growth is so high that it impedes development; all three have national family planning programmes. At the other extreme, the Arab countries in the Gulf and the Libyan Arab Jamahiriya have strong pro-natalist sentiments. The remaining countries in these regions adopt non-intervention policies, but family planning services are available through maternal and child health programmes and/or private clinics.

The objective of this chapter is to identify the salient features of the diversity in the reproductive patterns of the countries and of the underlying processes also. The presentation draws upon the WFS results in six countries: Egypt; Jordan; Morocco; the Syrian Arab Republic; Tunisia; Yemen.[1] These countries are at different stages of development and modernization. There are differences between them in the levels of urbanization and industrialization; in the spread of education, particularly among females; in the provision of health services; and in the possibilities generated by the development process for upward social and economic mobility. As can be seen from table 185, the Arab countries of Northern Africa are a more homogeneous group with respect to indicators such as life expectancy and urbanization. Among the Arab countries of Western Asia, Jordan and the Syrian Arab Republic are very different from Yemen with respect to both demographic and socio-economic indicators. With regard to education, however, it is striking that Egypt, Morocco and Yemen compare very poorly with Jordan, the Syrian Arab Republic and Tunisia with respect to women's literacy and, in particular, school enrolment.

In reviewing reproductive behaviour in the Arab countries of Western Asia and Northern Africa, particular emphasis is given to differences in behaviour by residence and education. Not only is fertility discussed but some of its major determinants, including nuptiality, breast-feeding, fertility preferences and family planning, are considered.

A. FERTILITY

As in most developing countries, fertility in most of the Arab countries is the most important determinant of changes in the rates of population growth. While information on fertility patterns and levels in the region has been sparse until recently, the general impression has been one of pro-natalist societies in which the average number of births per woman has been and remains high. The WFS data show high levels of fertility for a majority of women of all ages in almost all the six countries included. The data also reveal large differences in fertility according to residence. Not only is urban residence distinguished from rural residence but within the urban sector, the capital city is distinctive. A major factor in such diversity is the degree of differentiation with respect to the social and economic structure of the urban and rural sectors.

Fertility levels and trends

For all six countries included here, the number of children ever born reported in the WFS data was found to be as high or higher than parity reported in other sources, suggesting that enumeration of births was at least

TABLE 185. SELECTED DEMOGRAPHIC INDICATORS FOR SIX ARAB COUNTRIES IN WESTERN ASIA AND NORTHERN AFRICA

Country	Date of World Fertility Survey	Population, 1980 (millions)	Crude birth rate, 1975-1980 (per 1,000)	Crude death rate, 1975-1980 (per 1,000)	Annual population growth rate (percentage)	Life expectancy, 1975-1980	Percentage of population living in urban areas 1950	1980
Egypt	1980	41.3	41	14	2.6	55	35	45
Jordan	1976	2.9	47	11	2.3	60	35	60
Morocco	1980	20.1	45	14	3.0	55	26	41
Syrian Arab Republic	1978	8.8	46	9	3.4	64	31	47
Tunisia	1978	6.4	36	11	2.6	58	31	52
Yemen	1979	5.8	49	24	1.9	41	2	15

	Percentage of persons aged 15 and over who can read and write				Number enrolled in primary school as percentage of age group			
	Male 1970	Male 1980	Female 1970	Female 1980	Male 1960	Male 1980-1982	Female 1960	Female 1980-1982
Egypt	50	58	20	28	80	90	52	63
Jordan	50	82	20	58	94	105	59	100
Morocco	33	41	11	18	67	97	27	60
Syrian Arab Republic	59	72	21	35	89	112	39	89
Tunisia	44	61	17	34	88	119	43	92
Yemen	9	24	1	2	14	82	—	12

Source: For data in upper panel, United Nations (1985); for data on literacy and school enrolment, United Nations Children's Fund (1985).

as complete or more complete for WFS than for previous censuses and surveys in these countries (see chapter I). The reported completed fertility of all ever-married women aged 45-49 ranged from about seven children in Egypt, Morocco and Tunisia to about eight in the Syrian Arab Republic and almost nine in Jordan (table 186). The data on achieved fertility by current age also shows that among ever-married women aged 25-29, the mean number of births was in excess of three children in all but one country. The mean was also about two children for women aged 20-24 in three of the six countries included.

The level and age pattern of current fertility may be compared across the six countries, using the total fertility rate (TFR). Age-specific fertility rates and total fertility rates, averaged over the five years preceding each survey, are shown in table 187. The region shows quite a wide range in current fertility. The total fertility rate is fewer than six children in three countries, Egypt, Morocco and Tunisia; between seven and eight in Jordan and the Syrian Arab Republic and more than eight children in Yemen.

All six countries had high fertility rates over a broad peak extending over ages from 20 to 34, with maximum fertility occurring at ages 25-29 and with fertility rates in age group 20-24 ranking second to those in the peak group.[2] Fertility rates were also high among adolescents (women aged 15-19), being well above 100 births per 1,000 women in three of six countries. There is, however, considerable variation in the age pattern of fertility of these six countries, with the largest variation in the youngest and the oldest age groups. This is to be expected, as it is at these ages that most fertility reduction takes place during the early stages of fertility transition. Variation in rates at the ages of peak fertility also is substantial. In age group 20-24, there was reportedly one birth per three women per annum in Jordan, the Syrian Arab Republic and Yemen, but one birth per four women in Egypt, Morocco and Tunisia. In age group 30-34, there was a little over one birth for every five years of exposure in Egypt and Morocco, about one birth for every four women in Tunisia and about one birth for every three women in the remaining countries.

The fertility schedule for each of the six countries thus represents a high level of reproductive activity, especially for ages 20-39 years, where, on average, there was one live birth to every three to four women each year. Fertility remains high throughout the childbearing years, with from 11 to 13 per cent of all births that occurred among women in their forties in Morocco, the Syrian Arab Republic and Tunisia.

Trends in fertility can be inferred by comparing the completed fertility of women aged 45-49 at the time of the survey with the level of current fertility as measured by the total fertility rate. Alternatively, by combining data from the birth histories of the women interviewed and basic information obtained in the household interview, age-specific fertility rates and total fertility rates can be derived for intervals of time prior to the survey date in five-year periods. As is common to other surveys, these data are subject to errors of various forms. Three types of error can distort estimates of levels and trends in fertility: misreporting of the age of the respondent; omissions of live births; and displacement of dates of birth. The assessment of the quality of WFS data presented in chapter I contains evidence of the occurrence of these types of errors in the surveys in the countries reviewed here. In particular, date reporting in Yemen was found to be sufficiently weak as to reduce significantly the confidence that can be placed in the recent fertility levels estimated from that survey. The exact trends implied by the birth histories may be problematical also in the cases of Egypt and Jordan because of evidence of possible irregularities and date-reporting biases.

TABLE 186. MEAN NUMBER OF CHILDREN EVER BORN TO EVER-MARRIED WOMEN, BY CURRENT AGE,[a] SIX ARAB COUNTRIES IN WESTERN ASIA AND NORTHERN AFRICA

Country	<20	20-24	25-29	30-34	35-39	40-44	45-49	All ages
Egypt	0.63	1.81	3.07	4.61	5.79	6.46	6.87	4.23
Jordan	0.92	2.45	4.23	5.90	7.34	8.57	8.80	5.43
Morocco	0.27	1.92	3.25	4.91	6.13	7.11	7.08	4.55
Syrian Arab Republic	0.88	2.16	3.70	5.21	6.62	7.50	7.83	4.74
Tunisia	0.63	1.52	2.88	4.53	5.81	6.60	7.04	4.50
Yemen	0.60	1.81	3.36	5.05	6.09	6.59	7.10	3.74

Sources: Egypt (1983); Jordan (1976); Morocco (1984); Syrian Arab Republic (1982); Tunisia (1982); Yemen (1983).
[a] As of the survey date.

TABLE 187. AGE-SPECIFIC FERTILITY RATES AND TOTAL FERTILITY RATES FOR THE PERIOD 0-4 YEARS PRIOR TO THE SURVEY, SIX ARAB COUNTRIES IN WESTERN ASIA AND NORTHERN AFRICA

Country	Overall quality	<20	20-24	25-29	30-34	35-39	40-44	45-49	Total fertility rate
Egypt	B	99	256	286	217	130	48	16	5.26
Jordan	B	124	343	365	332	240	103	19	7.63
Morocco	B	93	265	296	222	178	98	29	5.90
Syrian Arab Republic	A	123	297	339	312	245	136	44	7.48
Tunisia	A	34	225	304	260	199	112	36	5.85
Yemen	C	175	346	346	334	229	197	75	8.51

Sources: Chapter I, table 62 in the present volume; and World Fertility Survey standard recode tapes.

NOTE: Rates assessed as: A = good quality; B = acceptable quality; C = less reliable.

In an elaborate evaluation of the WFS fertility and nuptiality data from Egypt, Coale (1985) shows that the proportion ever-married at the younger ages as reported in the survey and in the 1960 and 1976 censuses was substantially understated because of the overstatement of age among younger women. One of the implications of this overstatement of current age is that "age-specific marital fertility rates are also understated in recent years at ages in the teens" (Coale, 1985). Coale then applied a series of complex and multiple adjustments to allow for the overreporting of age among younger women. The final consequence for estimates of fertility in 1980 is that the estimated total fertility rate for the most recent period was increased to about 5.5. Coale's analysis of Egyptian data, however, confirmed the occurrence of a substantial decline in fertility between the mid-1960s and the mid-1970s. The decline was caused by an increase in age at marriage, a decline in the marriage rate and a decline in marital fertility at higher ages and longer durations of marriage.

An evaluation of the WFS data for Jordan indicates the possibility of omission of female births, and underestimates and overestimates of fertility in the periods 20-24 and 10-19 years prior to the survey, respectively (Abdel-Aziz, 1983). These errors may be largely the result of either forward displacement of dates of birth or selective age misstatement for the highly fertile women, among respondents with reported ages of 40-44. Abdel-Aziz (1983), however, concludes that the reported level of fertility for the five-year period preceding the survey was correct and that the estimated total fertility rate of 7.7 appears to be almost one child lower than that of earlier periods.

In the Syrian Arab Republic, a similar pattern of omission of female births in earliest periods and overestimates of fertility for the period 10-14 years before the survey was also observed (Ali, 1984). In Yemen, an evaluation study attributes an apparent increase in fertility in recent years to changes in marital exposure following the civil war in the 1960s and early 1970s and/or the effects of omission, misplacement of dates of vital events and age misreporting (Al-Tohamy and Kalule-Sabiti, 1985).

Considering recent trends in fertility, as implied by the retrospective birth histories, and keeping in mind the data quality problems already discussed, it may be seen from table 188 that, according to reported data, little if any change in fertility had taken place in two of the six countries: the Syrian Arab Republic and Yemen. In the remaining countries, a decline in total fertility of about one child per woman was implied by the retrospective birth histories in Jordan, and larger declines on the order of from 1.5 to 1.8 children per woman were implied by the data in Egypt, Morocco and Tunisia. The steepest decline was estimated for Egypt: from about 7.0 to 5.3 live births, between 1960 and 1980. The major part of this decline occurred prior to 1975; since then, the decline in Egyptian fertility has been very modest.

The fertility rates considered so far have referred to women regardless of age at marriage. It was noted earlier that a commonly observed feature of fertility decline is an increase in the age at first marriage, and hence in the age at birth of the first-born. Similarly, subnational variations, as is shown below, may in part reflect differences in age at marriage rather than a genuine difference in the tempo of fertility among married women. Trends in cumulative fertility up to marital duration 15-19 years, according to age at first marriage, are shown in table 189 for the four most recent five-year periods prior to the survey. A notable feature of this table is that the expected inverse relationship between cumulative fertility and age at marriage is shown for only two countries—Egypt and Tunisia—where the effect of increasing age at marriage on achieved fertility becomes evident only for those who are married after reaching age 22 years. The remaining four countries show a somewhat curvilinear relationship, reflecting the effect of adolescent infecundity on achieved fertility for women with very young ages at marriage.

Fertility differentials

The First Country Reports for the six countries included here all show, to varying degrees, evidence of the existence of certain socio-economic differentials in fertility. The most significant factors are place of residence and women's educational status. Other social and economic factors are also associated with differentials in marital fertility, although none is as powerful as residence and education. The remainder of this section therefore documents, in a comparative context, the socio-economic differentials in current fertility levels, for groups classified by type of place of current residence and respondent's years of schooling, for these six Arab countries.

Three types of rates are examined: total fertility rates (TFR), total marital fertility rates by age (age-TMFR), and total marital fertility rates by duration (duration-TMFR). The age-specific total marital rate is obtained by the cumulation of the age-specific marital fertility rates by five-year age groups over ages 20-49 years. It may be interpreted as the mean number of births to a woman if she were to remain within a union during ages 20-49 and were to experience the observed within-union fertility schedule. The duration-specific total marital fertility rate is obtained by the cumulation of duration-specific marital rates to duration 25 years.[3]

TABLE 188. ESTIMATED TOTAL FERTILITY RATES FOR FIVE-YEAR PERIODS PRIOR TO THE SURVEY, CALCULATED FROM BIRTH HISTORY DATA, SIX ARAB COUNTRIES IN WESTERN ASIA AND NORTHERN AFRICA

Country	Overall quality trends	Year of survey	0-4	5-9	10-14	15-19
Egypt	C	1980	5.27	5.53	6.53	7.09
Jordan	C	1976	7.70	8.54	8.94	8.78
Morocco	B	1980	5.91	6.89	7.10	7.32
Syrian Arab Republic	B	1978	7.51	7.84	8.46	8.05
Tunisia	A	1978	5.86	6.13	7.21	7.33
Yemen	C	1979	8.51	8.69	8.07	8.52

Sources: Overall quality derived from chapter I in the present volume; total fertility rates derived from Farid (1984).

NOTE: Rates assessed as: A = good quality; B = acceptable quality; C = less reliable.

TABLE 189. CUMULATIVE FERTILITY TO MARITAL DURATION 15-19 YEARS, BY AGE AT MARRIAGE, SIX ARAB COUNTRIES IN WESTERN ASIA AND NORTHERN AFRICA

Country and age at marriage	0-4	5-9	10-14	15-19
Egypt				
16	5.75	5.62	6.17	6.30
16-17	5.45	5.27	5.65	6.52
18-21	5.20	4.93	5.45	5.94
22+	3.88	4.01	5.15	a
All ages	5.31	5.22	5.83	6.31
Jordan				
16	7.39	7.28	7.44	6.99
16-17	7.34	7.40	7.62	6.56
18-20	7.14	7.58	7.22	6.55
21+	5.91	6.33	a	a
All ages	7.11	7.28	7.43	7.08
Morocco				
15	5.47	5.47	5.43	5.14
15-17	5.81	6.11	6.12	6.01
18-20	5.55	5.98	5.53	5.43
21+	5.11	6.02	5.46	a
All ages	5.62	5.88	5.76	5.60
Syrian Arab Republic				
16	7.17	6.67	6.71	6.22
16-18	6.74	6.81	7.36	6.76
19-22	6.52	6.43	7.24	a
23+	5.55	5.82	a	a
All ages	6.64	6.54	7.06	6.66
Tunisia				
18	6.10	6.06	6.29	6.09
18-19	6.04	5.84	6.08	6.55
20-22	5.80	5.50	6.18	a
23+	4.81	4.80	a	a
All ages	5.76	5.69	6.22	6.31
Yemen				
14	5.68	5.15	4.55	4.94
14-15	6.10	5.91	5.01	5.28
16-18	5.77	6.08	5.30	4.68
19+	6.13	6.20	5.72	a
All ages	6.01	5.73	4.98	5.12

Source: Singh (1984), table 8.

[a] These cells have incomplete exposure because of the combination of high ages at marriage with samples restricted to ages under 50.

Rural or urban residence

Urban residence is consistently related to both the tempo and the level of fertility in the countries considered, perhaps excluding Yemen. The age-specific fertility schedules by current residence (table 190) are all broadly similar in shape, with a flatter peak, or later tapering-off, among rural women; and the sharpest peak and greatest concentration of childbearing at young ages among women living in major urban areas. In Tunisia, for example, about 22 per cent of all urban births were to women aged 35-49 years, compared with 31 per cent of births to rural women.

The figures given in table 190 also show that not only is urban residence distinguished from rural residence, but whithin the urban sector, the capital city is distinctive.[4] In the Syrian Arab Republic, for example, 20 per cent of all births at Damascus (major urban) were among women aged 35-49, compared with 27 per cent of births to women in "other urban" areas and 30 per cent of births to rural women.

Aside from the difference in the proportionate distributions of births, the urban/rural differentials in the age-specific fertility rates follow the expected pattern: the rates were lowest in major urban areas, followed by other urban areas, and highest among rural women. Even in the peak years of childbearing, 25-29 years, there was a sizeable difference in annual fertility rates between residence groups, ranging from 30 per cent in Jordan to 56 per cent in the Syrian Arab Republic.[5] This pattern indicates earlier completion of childbearing to be a major factor in formation of the smaller urban family.

The size of the differentials in total fertility rates according to residence groups, however, varies between the six countries—from one child in Yemen to more than two in Egypt and Tunisia, more than three in Jordan and Morocco, and more than four in the Syrian Arab Republic (table 191). These recorded differences in total fertility are achieved through a markedly lower level of reproductive activity among urban women at all ages, and particularly—in both relative and absolute terms—at the older ages.

This pattern of differentials in total fertility rates is largely repeated by both the age and duration marital fertility rates, but the size of the absolute differences is reduced by between 30 and 40 per cent for four of six countries. It is also of interest to note that the duration total marital fertility rates exceeded the corresponding TFRs among all three residential groups for all the countries except Yemen. The differences were largest for major urban areas and smallest for rural areas. As Alam and Casterline (1984) suggest, this indicates that in these populations the equivalent of 25 years of exposure after marriage at the observed duration-specific rates is not achieved at the current age-specific rates, and that this situation is largely due to postponement of marriage. Further, the duration-specific fertility rates according to residence (not shown here) show a notable urban/rural divergence of fertility rates with marriage duration. This finding indicates that in urban areas—particularly in the capital cities—in most of the countries included, later marriage rather than a longer first birth interval accounts for any delay in the onset of childbearing, and lower fertility is produced through a lower tempo of fertility after the first few years of marriage and an earlier completion of childbearing.

Data on fertility trends according to residence from the retrospective birth histories (not shown) imply a decline in "major urban" fertility in five countries (Egypt, Jordan, Morocco, the Syrian Arab Republic and Tunisia), dating from at least the mid-1960s; a slightly later and smaller decline among "other urban" women in four countries (Egypt, Morocco, the Syrian Arab Republic and Tunisia); and a much smaller decline in rural fertility in two countries (Egypt and Tunisia). The size of the reduction in fertility implied for these countries was a decline in the total fertility rate of two to three live births per woman in major urban areas, between one and two live births per woman in other urban areas and about one live birth per woman in rural areas.

A major factor in the urban fertility decline has been the reduction in marital fertility, which was most extensive and consistent among women aged 20 years or more at first marriage. In major urban centres, fertility rates had fallen in all age groups and in all but the shortest marriage durations, though again it was within the older age groups and longer marriage durations that it was most distinct. The reduction in marital fertility among women residing in other urban areas was smaller in each age

TABLE 190. AGE-SPECIFIC FERTILITY RATES AND TOTAL FERTILITY RATES, BY CURRENT RESIDENCE, SIX ARAB COUNTRIES IN WESTERN ASIA AND NORTHERN AFRICA

Country and area of residence[a]	15-19	20-24	25-29	30-34	35-39	40-44	45-49	Total fertility rate
Egypt								
Major urban	59	179	234	167	95	28	7	3.84
Other urban	82	242	279	211	114	32	14	4.86
Rural	126	302	315	244	153	64	20	6.12
Jordan								
Major urban	100	303	319	268	193	66	12	6.30
Other urban	103	335	380	337	256	105	24	7.70
Rural	181	403	415	410	284	167	30	9.45
Morocco								
Major urban	32	168	223	167	109	53	17	3.85
Other urban	67	229	260	175	132	74	26	4.81
Rural	123	308	338	258	219	124	34	7.02
Syrian Arab Republic								
Major urban	91	204	251	213	121	54	11	4.72
Other urban	119	281	312	284	225	122	31	6.87
Rural	140	343	392	378	315	175	64	9.04
Tunisia								
Urban	24	196	255	214	116	70	24	4.75
Rural	43	254	354	304	233	154	49	6.95
Yemen								
Major urban								
Other urban	152	384	333	317	170	172	34	7.81
Rural	178	340	348	337	240	199	78	8.60

Sources: Alam and Casterline (1984); and additional tables prepared by the World Fertility Survey.
[a] For definition of residence groups, see chapter VII in the present volume.
[b] As of the survey date.

TABLE 191. CURRENT LEVELS OF FERTILITY ACCORDING TO CURRENT RESIDENCE, SIX ARAB COUNTRIES IN WESTERN ASIA AND NORTHERN AFRICA

Country	Total fertility rate, ages 15-49 All	Major urban	Other urban	Rural	Total marital fertility rate, ages 20-49 Major urban	Other urban	Rural	Total marital fertility rate, durations 0-24 Major urban	Other urban	Rural
Egypt	5.27	3.84	4.86	6.12	5.02	5.73	6.39	5.19	6.10	6.75
Jordan	7.70	6.30	7.70	9.45	7.27	8.49	9.37	7.83	9.03	10.09
Morocco	5.91	3.85	4.81	7.02	5.26	5.78	7.27	5.34	6.09	7.53
Syrian Arab Republic	7.51	4.72	6.87	9.04	5.83	7.72	9.64	6.10	7.86	9.27
Tunisia	5.86	— 4.75 —		6.95	5.65	6.72	8.15	5.35	6.40	7.95
Yemen	8.51	— 7.81 —		8.60	— 7.82 —		8.44	— 7.73 —		7.86

Source: Ashurst, Balkaran and Casterline (1984).

group and commenced at a later marriage duration. Some evidence of a very recent reduction in rural fertility at longer durations may herald a rural decline as well.

Education differentials

A uniformly inverse relationship between current levels of fertility and women's educational status is shown for the six countries included, although the size of the differential is greater where substantial decline in urban fertility has occurred (table 192). The total fertility rate by educational attainment, available for four of six countries, decreases from the lowest educational category to the highest, the difference between extreme educational groups ranging from 4.7 births in the Syrian Arab Republic to 2.2 in Morocco.

The total marital rates by age show a similar pattern, although the differentials across education groups are generally reduced because a large part of the effect of education arises from its effect on the timing of first marriage. The fertility rates by duration, however, show a mixed pattern: uniformly inverse in Egypt, Jordan and the Syrian Arab Republic; curvilinear in Yemen; and irregular in Morocco and Tunisia. These education differentials in fertility appear to be even larger than those shown for Latin America and the Caribbean, where the differentials in marital fertility are at least twice what they are in sub-saharan African countries.

When the data on current marital fertility by women's education were classified according to place of residence (not shown), a different pattern emerged for Egypt, the Syrian Arab Republic and Yemen; the inverse relationship was found only in urban areas while an inverted U-shaped relationship was shown for rural areas (Hallouda and Cochrane, 1983; and Ali and Callum, 1985). In these cases, women with some years of schooling had higher fertility than those with no education, the differences amounting, on average, to about 5 per cent. This curvilinear pattern has also been noted in several African and a few Asian countries. The reasons for this pattern have

TABLE 192. CURRENT LEVELS OF FERTILITY, BY WIFE'S LEVEL OF EDUCATION,[a]
SIX ARAB COUNTRIES IN WESTERN ASIA AND NORTHERN AFRICA

Country	Total fertility rate, ages 15-49				Total marital fertility rate, ages 20-49				Total marital fertility rate, duration 0-24			
	Zero (1)	One to three (2)	Four to six (3)	Seven or more (4)	Zero (5)	One to three (6)	Four to six (7)	Seven or more (8)	Zero (9)	One to three (10)	Four to six (11)	Seven or more (12)
Egypt	..	..	..	..	6.13	5.90	5.63	4.96	6.53	6.35	6.15	3.78
Jordan	9.34	8.63	6.98	4.91	9.04	7.97	6.96	6.26	9.73	9.27	7.70	6.19
Morocco	6.36	5.15	4.39	4.15	6.70	5.86	5.86	6.17	7.03	5.53	5.82	4.63
Syrian Arab Republic	8.81	6.71	5.59	4.08	9.08	7.29	6.14	6.04	8.97	7.20	6.53	5.42
Tunisia	..	..	..	..	7.53	6.42	6.06	4.67	7.32	5.92	6.01	3.88
Yemen	8.55	— 5.38 —			8.36	— 6.13 —			7.83	— 8.50 —		

Source: Ashurst, Balkaran and Casterline (1984).   [a] Years of schooling completed.

been explained by the fact that while education of women tends to increase the age at marriage and in many environments to reduce the proportion of women who ultimately marry, education may have positive effects on the natural fertility of those who are married because more educated women tend to be healthier and are also likely to breast-feed for shorter periods (Cochrane, 1979).

The extent to which residence variations in fertility were a function of urban residence *per se*, or could equally well be explained by other socio-economic factors, notably mother's education, was investigated in a number of studies. In Egypt and the Syrian Arab Republic, mother's education exhibited a similar range of total fertility as residence. An inverse or curvilinear relationship between educational level and fertility persisted within residence; similarly, the effect of residence was observed irrespective of mother's education. An analysis that controlled for age and marriage duration confirmed the significance of both residence and mother's education, there remaining an effect, though muted, of one after controlling for the other (Hallouda and Cochrane, 1983; and Ali and Callum, 1985). A similar pattern seems also to hold for Jordan and Tunisia.

Thus, the data provide support for the importance of both residence and education (or environment and individual location within it) in relation to current fertility levels in most of the countries considered. Although residence and education explain a large part of the fertility differences found within each country, little of the difference in fertility between countries is explained by these two socio-economic characteristics. Among the three Northern African countries with the lowest fertility in this group (Egypt, Morocco and Tunisia), only in Tunisia was female enrolment at a relatively high level and the proportion urban over 50 per cent (see table 185). Significant and important differences remain between these countries in the level of fertility when comparing residence and educational groups, particularly rural fertility. This may largely be due to the extent of differentiation with respect to the social and economic development of the urban and rural sectors in these countries.

B. NUPTIALITY

In all six countries, virtually everyone ultimately marries, but there are wide variations in the timing of marriage between and within these countries. There are substantial differences according to type of place of residence and across levels of educational achievement. The change from early to later ages at marriage is generally seen as a response to the modernization process in a society, and socio-economic differentials in the age at first marriage are known to constitute one of the intermediate variables accounting for fertility differentials. In fact, a noteworthy finding of the analysis presented in chapter VI of this volume is the importance of nuptiality in most of the Arab countries of Northern Africa and Western Asia, particularly Tunisia, in determining fertility levels and differentials. In the Arab world, therefore, where marriage and fertility are viewed as interrelated, both as social and demographic processes and as sequential phases in the life cycles of women, shifts in the age pattern of first marriage assume special demographic significance.

Proportions ever married

Data on the proportions ever married by five-year age groups, together with estimates of the singulate mean age at marriage (SMAM),[6] are shown in table 193. The proportions ever married among men and women aged 45-49 show that marriage is almost universal in all six countries.

The youngest nuptiality pattern among these six countries for both men and women is found in Yemen and the oldest in Tunisia. The very high level of teen-age marriages in Yemen (60 per cent ever married among women aged 15-19), together with extremely low contraceptive use, are the two most important factors in that country's high fertility level. Women in the remaining countries, Egypt, Jordan, Morocco and the Syrian Arab Republic, had almost identical proportions ever married at ages 15-19 (about 22 per cent) and ages 20-24 (about 63 per cent). The singulate mean age at marriage for females ranged from 17 years in Yemen to 24 years in Tunisia. The remaining four countries had a range of SMAM from 21 to 22 years.

Men show a much older age pattern of marriage than women. The age for males, however, varied within a narrower range than for women, from 26 to 28 years for the countries covered, except Yemen, which had SMAM for males of only 22 years. In all six countries, the mean age at marriage for men exceeded that for women by at least five years.

Transitions in cohort nuptiality

While marriage has remained almost universal in the Arab countries, significant changes have taken place in the tempo of nuptiality in the recent past. An examination of the age patterns of cumulative proportions married for successive age cohorts (not shown here) revealed the prevalence of a very early marriage pattern in Yemen and a relatively late marriage pattern in Tunisia, while the remaining four countries were quite close to each other in the pattern and level of their distributions (Farid, 1984).

TABLE 193. PROPORTIONS EVER MARRIED, BY AGE GROUP AND SEX, AND SINGULATE MEAN AGE AT MARRIAGE, SIX ARAB COUNTRIES IN WESTERN ASIA AND NORTHERN AFRICA

Country	15-19	20-24	25-29	30-34	35-39	40-44	45-49	Singulate mean age at marriage
A. Females								
Egypt	22.5	64.9	86.3	96.4	97.9	97.8	98.5	21.3
Jordan	19.5	64.1	87.0	94.9	97.3	97.9	98.2	21.6
Morocco	22.1	63.7	87.8	97.3	99.2	99.5	99.6	21.3
Syrian Arab Republic	22.7	60.2	82.6	92.5	94.5	97.0	98.2	22.1
Tunisia	5.2	42.6	80.0	93.9	98.1	98.3	98.8	23.9
Yemen	60.5	92.1	96.7	98.1	98.9	97.9	98.2	16.9
B. Males								
Egypt	2.3	20.8	56.9	85.1	94.0	97.6	99.1	26.5
Jordan	1.0	22.3	62.4	89.4	97.2	98.4	99.3	26.3
Morocco	2.3	27.7	63.3	88.7	95.4	98.1	98.7	26.0
Syrian Arab Republic	2.5	21.4	62.6	87.4	95.6	98.0	98.9	26.4
Tunisia	0.1	8.6	48.6	85.6	95.8	97.1	98.6	28.0
Yemen	15.3	62.4	87.5	95.1	98.0	98.4	98.9	21.8

Sources: Ebanks and Singh (1984); and additional tables prepared by the World Fertility Survey.

The data also show substantial decreases over time in the proportions of young marriages, reflecting a clear trend towards later marriage. The change appears to have been in the direction of delaying first marriage from the early teens to the middle teen-ages in Yemen; from the middle teen-ages to the late in Egypt, Jordan, Morocco and the Syrian Arab Republic; and from the late teen-ages to the early twenties in Tunisia, a country that seems to have had the oldest marriage pattern even among the oldest cohorts. There is also evidence that the mean age difference between spouses has been narrowing. This is partially due to the fact that the change in nuptiality was sharper among women than among men.

This important transformation in the tempo of female nuptiality in the Arab countries reflects, of course, an upward trend in age at first marriage. This may be illustrated by an examination of trends in the median age at first marriage, i.e., the age by which 50 per cent of the women of any given cohort had entered into a first marriage. Table 194 shows that the median age at first marriage in all six countries, except for recent cohorts in Tunisia, had always been achieved before age 20. Little, if any, change is shown for Yemen, while increases of about one year for the Syrian Arab Republic and larger increases of from 2.5 to 3 years for the remaining four countries are shown in table 194.[7] It is also of interest to note that, in all the countries studied, except Yemen, women currently aged 15-19 years had not attained the level of 50 per cent ever married.

The substantial decreases in the proportions of very young marriages, and the accompanying rise in age at marriage observed in most of the countries covered in this analysis, suggest that the two dimensions of the tempo of nuptiality, namely, the early/late dimension (i.e., the median age of first marriage) and the rapid/slow dimension (i.e., the speed with which the median age of first marriage is approached from the beginning of the nuptial span), have worked—with only few exceptions—in such a way as to reinforce each other.

Marital stability

In the Arab countries, marriage provides the social setting within which almost all childbearing occurs; and marital dissolution—either by death of a spouse or by divorce or separation—directly diminishes the likelihood of childbearing. A comparison of levels of marital dissolution reveals that Jordan, the Syrian Arab Republic and Tunisia had the lowest proportion of ever-married women widowed within 20 years of marriage (about 5 per cent) and also the lowest proportion divorced within 20 years (4-6 per cent). In Egypt, Morocco and Yemen, there were higher percentages widowed (8-10 per cent); and the proportions divorced ranged from 11 per cent in Egypt to 20 per cent in Morocco (Smith, Cerrasco and McDonald, 1984; Balkaran and Smith, 1984). This wide range of divorce levels indicates that divorce is not readily linked with religion. All the countries covered in this chapter are predominantly Muslim.

Overall rates of dissolution and levels of remarriage, however, are such that an average woman, once married, spends 93-98 per cent of her subsequent reproductive life in a marital union. The percentage of lost reproductive time after first marriage for women younger than age 35 slightly exceeded 5 per cent only in Morocco. Therefore, marital dissolution is likely to have only a minor depressing effect on the overall level of marital fertility in these countries.

Socio-economic differentials

Urban women marry later than rural women; the difference, on average, is about three years in Egypt and Morocco, about two years in Jordan and Yemen and about one year in the Syrian Arab Republic and Tunisia (see column (8), table 195). Further, larger proportions of rural women than urban women were married in the crucial age groups, 15-19 and 20-24. Among rural women aged 15-19, Yemen had the highest proportion ever married (64 per cent), followed by Egypt, Jordan and Morocco (about 29 per cent). For four of six countries, the difference in the proportions ever married between the rural women aged 15-19 and their urban counterparts was from 12 to 20 per cent. In the Syrian Arab Republic, this difference was negligible. At older ages, the rural women in all six countries continue to achieve a given proportion ever married before the urban women.

The First Country Reports for the six countries in the analysis show a persistent relationship between education and age at marriage, with a clear tendency for the mean age at marriage for women marrying before reaching age 25 to vary inversely with the educational level of women in nearly all cases.

TABLE 194. MEDIAN AGE AT FIRST MARRIAGE FOR COHORTS OF WOMEN AGED 15-49,
SIX ARAB COUNTRIES IN WESTERN ASIA AND NORTHERN AFRICA

Country	\multicolumn{7}{c}{Age of cohort[a]}
	15-19	20-24	25-29	30-34 (years)	35-39	40-44	45-49
Egypt	..	19.5	18.8	17.5	16.9	16.9	16.6
Jordan	..	19.4	18.3	17.5	17.5	17.2	16.7
Morocco	..	19.6	18.4	16.9	15.9	16.2	15.7
Syrian Arab Republic	..	20.0	19.3	18.4	19.0	19.2	18.7
Tunisia	..	23.3	20.8	19.2	18.8	19.1	19.4
Yemen	16.0	16.2	16.1	15.2	15.8	15.4	16.0

Source: Farid (1984).
[a] As of the survey date.

TABLE 195. AGE-SPECIFIC PERCENTAGES OF EVER-MARRIED WOMEN AND SINGULATE MEAN AGE AT MARRIAGE,
BY TYPE OF RESIDENCE, SIX ARAB COUNTRIES IN WESTERN ASIA AND NORTHERN AFRICA

Country and area of residence	\multicolumn{7}{c}{Age group}	Singulate mean age at marriage (8)
	15-19 (1)	20-24 (2)	25-29 (3)	30-34 (4)	35-39 (5)	40-44 (6)	45-49 (7)	
Egypt								
Urban	14.3	49.7	80.5	96.0	97.3	97.0	98.8	23.0
Rural	29.4	78.3	92.3	96.0	98.4	98.5	98.3	19.8
Jordan								
Urban	16.1	58.5	84.5	94.4	96.4	97.7	98.1	22.1
Rural	28.7	77.8	94.1	97.4	99.6	98.6	99.1	19.8
Morocco								
Urban	11.5	46.2	83.1	97.0	98.9	99.6	99.0	23.0
Rural	30.4	76.9	91.3	97.5	99.5	99.4	99.9	20.1
Syrian Arab Republic								
Urban	21.8	56.2	79.0	91.0	91.7	95.6	97.1	22.6
Rural	23.7	64.5	86.6	94.3	97.8	98.5	99.2	21.5
Tunisia								
Urban	3.1	37.3	75.5	92.3	97.3	98.1	98.3	24.6
Rural	7.5	48.0	85.1	95.6	97.9	98.4	99.3	23.2
Yemen								
Urban	42.1	81.6	92.9	96.2	99.1	94.2	97.6	17.5
Rural	63.5	93.2	97.1	98.3	98.9	98.4	98.9	15.5

Sources: Ebanks and Singh (1984); and additional tables prepared by the World Fertility Survey.

Information on marital status by age and educational level is available only for Jordan, Morocco and the Syrian Arab Republic. The remaining three countries did not collect information on educational level in the household schedule. For Jordan and the Syrian Arab Republic, the proportions ever married show a curvilinear relationship with education; women with no schooling marry somewhat later than those who have some schooling, while women with seven or more years of schooling marry latest of all (table 196). In interpreting the curvilinear relationship, it should be kept in mind that most of the illiterate women were married to men with the same educational status, while educated women tended to be married to men with at least the same level of education (Kandis, 1977). Thus, illiterate males may delay marriage because of difficulties in securing the necessary resources to marry. On the other end of the scale, better-educated males may have the desire to delay marriage in order to accumulate skills and resources. This explanation, of course, assumes the absence of educational differentials in the age difference between spouses.

Further analysis of data for Egypt, Jordan and the Syrian Arab Republic revealed an inverse relationship between age at marriage and level of education in urban areas. For rural areas in these three countries, a substantial differential only emerges once women complete primary schooling (Sokona and Casterline, 1985; Ali and Callum, 1985; Kandis, 1977). It appears, therefore, that residence and education are important factors in explaining the female age at marriage. Comparing urban and rural residents, the effect of education appears to be of more relevance for urban women. This may be due to the greater variation in educational attainment among urban women, as compared with rural women. It is also possible that in urban areas, decisions about the timing of marriage are less constrained by traditional norms and customs, thus leaving more room for the action of social and economic factors (Sokona and Casterline, 1985).

C. BREAST-FEEDING

In the traditional fertility context, featuring the absence of widespread use of modern methods of contraception, birth-spacing is largely a function of the norms governing behaviour after childbirth. Most important of these, as shown in chapter IV, is the non-susceptible period associated with lactation. Among the majority of women in the six countries considered who did not practise any form of contraception, breast-feeding was one of the most important volitional factors affecting birth-spacing and hence ultimate family size. Breast-feeding also represents one of the mechanisms through which infant mortality

TABLE 196. AGE-SPECIFIC PERCENTAGES OF EVER-MARRIED WOMEN AND SINGULATE MEAN AGE AT MARRIAGE, BY LEVEL OF EDUCATION, JORDAN, MOROCCO AND SYRIAN ARAB REPUBLIC

Country and years of education	15-19	20-24	25-29	30-34	35-39	40-44	45-49	Singulate mean age at marriage
Jordan								
Zero	39.7	80.2	94.1	96.7	98.7	97.9	98.7	19.2
One to three	40.7	76.1	94.7	96.2	99.0	100.0	98.5	18.7
Four to six	35.5	78.0	91.7	95.2	94.0	98.1	96.4	19.3
Seven or more	11.5	50.3	76.5	91.6	93.9	97.5	96.7	23.2
Morocco								
Zero	30.2	73.9	90.9	97.7	99.7	99.4	99.8	20.3
One to three	11.1	44.4	81.7	94.1	95.7	99.9	99.9	23.6
Four to six	9.2	27.5	71.4	96.6	93.3	99.9	99.9	25.1
Seven or more	..	20.0	62.5	99.9	..	..	..	25.9
Syrian Arab Republic								
Zero	32.3	70.2	88.1	95.3	96.3	97.9	98.9	20.5
One to three	28.3	72.4	80.7	89.4	93.8	96.0	92.3	19.6
Four to six	29.6	67.0	85.0	90.8	92.7	95.1	97.4	21.2
Seven or more	10.3	38.7	63.8	83.2	84.1	85.5	86.7	22.8

Source: Ebanks and Singh (1984).

may influence fertility, since the effect of an infant death before it is weaned may be a reduction in the period of non-susceptibility to conception.

Most infants in these six countries are breast-fed. In three countries, 92 per cent of the children born in the 10 months preceding the survey were breast-fed; and in the remaining three countries, 96 per cent. These percentages decrease steadily as children age, particularly for Jordan, the Syrian Arab Republic and Yemen, where under 50 per cent of the children are breast-fed at the time of their first birthday. On average, the duration of breast-feeding was about 12-13 months in Jordan, the Syrian Arab Republic and Yemen; 15-16 months in Morocco and Tunisia, and 19 months in Egypt (see chapter IV).

There are strong differences in breast-feeding behaviour for women in urban and rural areas. For each country, a slightly higher percentage of children were ever breast-fed in rural than in urban areas. The distribution of children who were breast-fed by duration of breast-feeding shows a gap between the proportion of children breast-fed in urban and that in rural areas. This gap widens dramatically for all six countries by the third month of the child's life (Akin and others, 1984; Alwani and Santow, 1985). In addition to residence, mother's education also was strongly related to differences in duration of breast-feeding. In all six countries, women with more education tended to breast-feed for shorter durations.

A multivariate analysis of the determinants of breast-feeding in Egypt, Jordan, Tunisia and Yemen (Akin and others, 1984) indicates that urban residence was the variable most associated with breast-feeding; it lowered the probabilities of ever breast-feeding, of continuing from a short to a moderate duration and of continuing from a moderate to a long duration. The same study also reveals that urban residence apparently had more influence on breast-feeding behaviour than mother's education.

These variations in lactation suggest that modernization is associated with a significant decline in the proportion of infants who are breast-fed for prolonged periods. The traditional pattern of universal and prolonged lactation, and some dependence upon its contraceptive properties, appears to persist only in rural areas, while the modern sector is marked by a diminishing role of lactation in relation to fertility. In general, lactational infecundity appears to have the most impact in the rural areas and the least in urban areas. Counterbalancing and usually dominating this trend, as is shown below, are the differences in the impact of contraception: protection was higher in the urban areas and quite low in the rural areas.

D. FERTILITY PREFERENCES

A preference of a sizeable proportion of women in all six countries for moderate to large family size is shown by responses concerning the preferred number of children. Thus, the mean number of children desired by all currently married women, standardized by the number of living children, was about four in Egypt and Tunisia, five in Morocco and six in the remaining three countries. This pattern of a moderate level of fertility preference in the three countries with significant fertility declines, and high preferences in the remaining three countries, was evident not only among older women who may rationalize their fertility performance by stating the number of children they have as their preference but among younger cohorts. Thus, for women with from five to nine years of marital duration, the mean desired family size is about four children in three countries (Egypt, Morocco and Tunisia), and it exceeded five children in the remaining countries. Further, the proportion of women whose desired family size (standardized by number of living children) was greater than actual family size was 50-60 per cent in the three countries with the lowest desired family size, while it exceeded 70 per cent for the remaining three countries (Lightbourne, 1984). These comparisons lend credence to respondents' stated fertility desires as an actual reflection of preferences.[8]

A second source of information on fertility preferences comes from data on desire for additional children. The proportion of women who wanted no more children, standardized by number of living children, was lowest in Yemen (24 per cent), highest in Egypt (54 per cent) and between 30 and 45 per cent in the remaining four countries. Detailed tabulations also show that the effective family size at which at least 50 per cent of women wished to cease childbearing was three children in Egypt; four in Tunisia; five in Morocco and the Syrian Arab Republic, six in Jordan and seven in Yemen (Lightbourne, 1984).

In all six countries, there are considerable variations in family size preferences, especially by residence and education, just as was observed in the case of actual fertility. Thus, both desired and actual family sizes reached their highest levels among women who were living in rural areas and those with no education, while the smallest families tended to be desired and achieved by urban women who were at least literate, particularly in capital cities. None the less, in at least three of six countries, residential differentials in desired family size appear to converge among the most educated. This suggests that education is a force for both reduction and convergence of family size desires.

The strongest socio-economic differentials in fertility preferences are found in Egypt and the Syrian Arab Republic. Several studies undertaken recently on the Egyptian survey data reveal that four variables were significantly and independently related to fertility desires. Level of education had a significant negative relation with total desired family size. The level of education desired for daughters, reflecting childbearing tastes and preferences, was also significantly related in a negative direction to fertility desires. Previous childbearing experience, represented by the number of living sons and the number of living daughters, was positively associated with fertility desires, and in particular desires for living sons, suggesting that son preference may have some influence on fertility desires in Egypt, especially in rural areas. Variables used as indicators of the extent to which parents expect to rely upon children as a source of support and of the availability of alternative support were not, however, consistently related to fertility desires. Although the women who expected to receive help of some kind from their children were, in general, likely to desire more children, the availability of neither savings nor pensions nor social security was consistently and significantly related to fertility desires (Boraie, McCarthy and Oruch, 1985; Cochrane, Khan and Taha, 1985; Easterlin, Crimmins and Taha, 1985; Taha and Cochrane, 1985). In addition, in a comparison of Egyptian data for husbands and wives, Cochrane, Khan and Taha (1985) indicate that the major factors determining husbands' and wives' desire to continue childbearing appear to be fairly similar.[9]

In the Syrian Arab Republic, a study by Alloush and others (1985) indicates that fertility preferences were influenced by residence and by individual characteristics, particularly education; and the level of living derived from household income also proved important with respect to urban but not rural fertility preferences. Among urban residents, mother's education had a stronger total negative impact on desired family size than her husband's education, while the reverse applied among rural residents.

An analysis of reproductive behaviour in rural areas in Egypt reveals that fertility aspirations are powerfully associated with village characteristics. In larger, less isolated villages, where a larger proportion of the workforce is employed outside of agriculture, where agriculture is more mechanized and monetized, where the social structure is less traditional, where infant mortality is lower, where schooling opportunities are greater and where health care is more readily accessible, women desired smaller families (Casterline and Eid, 1985). The effects of village characteristics on fertility aspirations were found to be much more substantial than the effects on contraceptive use and, in particular, on actual fertility. These results are consistent with other research in Egypt demonstrating the impact of macro social and economic changes on reproductive behaviour (Loza, 1982; Sayed, 1983). Judging from the absence of similar findings in most of WFS data from other countries (Casterline and Eid, 1985), the existence of such macro effects may be a distinctive feature of Egyptian society.

In all six countries, a majority of women considered it important to have at least one child of each sex; beyond that, there was a preference for sons. Nevertheless, a relatively high proportion of women with a balanced sex composition or with more boys than girls were indifferent about the sex of their next child; and it seems that these women had a pure preference for number only and that they would be relatively satisfied with either sex at the next higher parity. This pattern lends credence to the possibility suggested by Cleland, Verrall and Vaessen (1983) that the pro-son sentiments of Arab wives, while apparently real, do not appear to exert any appreciable influence on reproductive behaviour.

E. FAMILY PLANNING

The preceding analysis indicates that the fertility transition in the six countries is strongly influenced by social and economic development, which, through a variety of mechanisms, reduces the family size that couples desire. Individual choices about family size are, however, made effective through fertility regulation. The remainder of this chapter, therefore, focuses on an investigation of the extent to which family planning has contributed to the current pattern of variation in fertility in the six countries being reviewed.

Contraceptive awareness

In five of the six countries, at least 75 per cent of ever-married women had heard of one or more contraceptive methods; and in Egypt, Jordan and Tunisia, 90 per cent or more. Contraceptive awareness was very much lower in Yemen (25 per cent). Detailed results show that the pill was by far the most widely recognized method, followed by the intra-uterine device (IUD). Few women reported knowledge of traditional methods. Contraceptive awareness shows little variation by age or socio-economic characteristics (see chapter V).

Contraceptive use

The percentage of currently married women who had used contraception at some time ranged from 3 per cent in Yemen to 47 per cent in Jordan and Tunisia (table 197). In contrast to knowledge, ever-use of contraceptives varied substantially between socio-economic groups. Urban residence and higher levels of education are the characteristics most associated with ever-use.

Current contraceptive use among currently married women was highest in Tunisia—32 per cent. It drops to only 1 per cent in Yemen and was between 19 and 25 per cent in the remaining four countries. This picture, however, changes when the levels of current use of only modern methods are examined. More than 95 per cent of all current users in Egypt were using modern methods, but the proportion falls to 68 per cent in Jordan. This pattern suggests that the inter-country variation in current

TABLE 197. LEVELS OF EVER-USE AND CURRENT USE OF CONTRACEPTION AMONG CURRENTLY MARRIED WOMEN, SIX ARAB COUNTRIES IN WESTERN ASIA AND NORTHERN AFRICA

(*Percentage*)

	All methods		Modern methods	
Country	Observed	Standardized for age	Observed	Standardized for age
A. *Ever-use*				
Egypt	42	43	41	42
Jordan	47	49	40	41
Morocco	31	32	28	29
Syrian Arab Republic	34	35	30	31
Tunisia	47	46	41	40
Yemen	3	3	3	3
B. *Current use*				
Egypt	24	25	23	24
Jordan	25	26	17	18
Morocco	19	20	16	17
Syrian Arab Republic	20	21	15	16
Tunisia	32	31	25	24
Yemen	1	1	1	1

Sources: Sathar and Chidambaram (1984); and additional tables prepared by the World Fertility Survey.

fertility can be partially accounted for by variations in use of modern methods. In Tunisia, for example, a greater percentage of currently married women were currently using contraception than in Egypt—32 per cent compared with 24 per cent. But the differences between the two countries in the current use of modern methods is much lower—25 per cent in Tunisia compared with 23 per cent in Egypt. Jordan provides an even more striking example. Current use of contraceptives by women in Jordan was one percentage point higher than in Egypt, but the current fertility level in Jordan was higher than that of Egypt by as much as 38 per cent. One reason for this is that use of modern methods was 26 per cent lower in Jordan than in Egypt.

Detailed tabulations show that among current users of modern methods, the pill is by far the most widely employed, followed by IUDs. The only exception is Tunisia, where IUDs and the pill were used by more or less equal proportions of women.

The results also show that women are unlikely to use contraceptives unless they have at least one son. The absence of a daughter in the family is also a deterrent to contraceptive practice, although to a lesser degree. Use becomes more frequent among women with families of balanced sex composition or with more sons than daughters (Farid, 1984).

The practice of contraception was still primarily an urban phenomenon in the six countries. In five of these countries, current use, among currently married women, ranged from 37 to 46 per cent in major urban areas, but only between 6 and 20 per cent in rural areas (table 198). The figures given in table 199 also show that education, measured by years of schooling, was closely associated with contraceptive use. Thus, contraceptive use increases dramatically as women's education rises. There were, however, only small differences in current use between women with from one to three years of schooling and those with from four to six years in Egypt and Jordan, while in the Syrian Arab Republic and Tunisia, current use in the former educational group was slightly higher than in the latter group.

The use of modern methods is generally expected to be more prevalent among more educated women. In the Syrian Arab Republic and Tunisia, however, the figures given in table 199 show no significant variation in relative use of modern methods above the group with from one to three years of education. In Morocco and Tunisia, traditional methods accounted for a higher proportion of the overall use among educated women than among those with no schooling. For example, in Tunisia, use of actual methods accounted for as much as 50 per cent of the overall use among the most educated women, compared with 15 per cent among women with no education.

Further analysis of survey data from Egypt, the Syrian Arab Republic and Tunisia (El-Deeb and Casterline, 1985; Alloush and others, 1985) shows that for women of higher educational attainment and women residing in major urban areas, contraception now appears to be a means of birth-spacing as well as family limitation. In the Syrian Arab Republic, it has been noted that urban women were likely to extend birth intervals through the use of contraception (Alwani and Santow, 1985).

TABLE 198. LEVELS OF EVER-USE AND CURRENT USE OF CONTRACEPTION AMONG CURRENTLY MARRIED WOMEN, BY TYPE OF PLACE OF RESIDENCE, SIX ARAB COUNTRIES IN WESTERN ASIA AND NORTHERN AFRICA

(*Percentage*)

	All methods			Modern methods		
Country	Major urban	Other urban	Rural	Major urban	Other urban	Rural
A. *Ever-use*						
Egypt	69	58	25	68	57	24
Jordan	62	54	22	55	45	16
Morocco	61	54	17	57	48	15
Syrian Arab Republic	73	46	12	67	41	9
Tunisia	67	61	31	59	52	28
Yemen	— 15 —		1	— 14 —		1
B. *Current use*						
Egypt	43	36	12	40	34	12
Jordan	37	28	9	26	19	6
Morocco	39	35	9	33	29	8
Syrian Arab Republic	46	28	6	35	22	4
Tunisia	45	43	20	33	31	18
Yemen	— 6 —		0	— 6 —		0

Sources: See table 197.

TABLE 199. LEVELS OF EVER-USE AND CURRENT USE OF CONTRACEPTION AMONG CURRENTLY MARRIED WOMEN, BY EDUCATIONAL LEVEL,[a] SIX ARAB COUNTRIES IN WESTERN ASIA AND NORTHERN AFRICA

(Percentage)

Country	All methods, by education[a] Zero	One to three	Four to six	Seven or more	Modern methods, by education[a] Zero	One to three	Four to six	Seven or more
A. Ever-use
Egypt	31	48	55	74	30	46	54	72
Jordan	34	41	53	69	28	45	45	59
Morocco	25	—— 68 ——		81	23	—— 61 ——		72
Syrian Arab Republic	20	59	59	65	17	53	54	56
Tunisia	41	58	59	81	37	47	50	62
Yemen	3	—— 16 ——			3	—— 16 ——		
B. Current use
Egypt	17	25	31	54	16	24	30	48
Jordan	15	28	32	42	10	17	22	30
Morocco	15	—— 47 ——		56	13	—— 40 ——		41
Syrian Arab Republic	10	37	34	43	8	30	25	32
Tunisia	27	42	41	56	23	30	30	28
Yemen	1	—— 10 ——			1	—— 10 ——		

Sources: See table 197.   [a] Years of schooling completed.

TABLE 200. PERCENTAGE DISTRIBUTION OF CURRENTLY MARRIED FECUND WOMEN ACCORDING TO INTENTIONS CONCERNING FERTILITY AND CONTRACEPTIVE USE, SIX ARAB COUNTRIES IN WESTERN ASIA AND NORTHERN AFRICA

Country	Ever used	Never used — Intended to use — Wanted more children	Wanted no more children	Subtotal	Never used — Did not intend to use — Wanted more children	Wanted no more children	Subtotal	Total
Egypt	43	15	10	25	23	9	32	100
Jordan	49	13	6	19	25	7	32	100
Morocco	36	9	6	15	38	11	49	100
Syrian Arab Republic	35	7	6	13	43	9	52	100
Tunisia	48	8	6	14	28	10	38	100
Yemen	3	3	2	5	76	16	92	100

Source: Farid (1984).

Potential contraceptive demand

Data on intended use of contraceptives provide evidence of interest in fertility regulation and of potential contraceptive demand. The needs for family planning services in the six Arab countries discussed here are indicated by the figures in table 200, which gives the distribution of currently married fecund women by contraceptive-use status and fertility intentions. The table indicates that family planning has far to go in these countries if a significant reduction in fertility is to occur. The proportion of currently married women who had never used contraception ranged from 51 per cent in Jordan to 97 per cent in Yemen. If those who did not intend to adopt family planning in the future are used as a gauge, resistance to family planning was extremely high in Yemen (where 92 per cent of women did not intend ever to practise contraception), fairly high in Morocco and the Syrian Arab Republic (49 and 52 per cent) and relatively low in Egypt, Jordan and Tunisia (32-38 per cent).

Detailed tabulations for Egypt, Jordan and Tunisia show that current use of contraception by urban women who wanted no more children was very high and showed few substantial variations. Among rural women, while family size preferences notably exceeded urban ones and correspondingly fewer women wanted no more children, among those who wanted no more children contraceptive use was lower than for urban women.

F. CONCLUSION

A reproductive climate in the Arab countries of Western Asia and Northern Africa featuring moderate to high fertility has been described. The generally pro-natalist attitude derives from a social and family organization in which children represent an important continuity in family tradition and in which childbearing and child-rearing, as well as nurturing of the entire family, is still the major recognized role of women. Despite the overall context of high fertility, a distinctive feature of family formation in these countries is a notable diversity in preference and practice. Such diversity is only to be expected in a period of transition where reproductive behaviour will reflect the effects of both traditional and non-traditional factors.

Urban residence, and particularly residence in the capital city, and, largely within urban residence, women's education, are associated with substantially lower desired and actual family size. Lower urban fertility is effected primarily through later age at marriage, an earlier completion of childbearing and, in the case of most educated women, also through longer intervals between births. The primary vehicle of change in urban fertility is use of modern methods of contraception, most importantly, the contraceptive pill. In rural areas, traditional forces are expressed in the form of earlier age at marriage, high desired family size and low contraceptive use.

This rural/urban contrast indicates that in urban areas of these Arab countries, traditional forces are less dominant and less constraining, and that other social and economic factors carry more weight. Throughout these countries, the trend has been towards a greater proportion of the population residing in urban areas, more schooling for women and increased employment in non-agricultural occupations. This trend is expected to continue in the future. Were the education and residence differentials in reproductive preference and practice to persist, a continued rise in the age of marriage, a moderation of family size ideals and an increase in contraceptive use could be anticipated as a consequence of the shifting composition of the population towards higher proportions living in urban areas and greater proportions with more education.

It is edifying that relatively small national sample surveys would have imparted such a sense of the breadth of experience in these countries and of the underlying demographic processes as well. The dynamic demographic scene and the rapid social and economic development, together with the absence of a complete vital registration system in several of the countries, would commend the WFS type of inquiry as an invaluable method of data collection.

NOTES

[1] The six countries conducted national fertility surveys from 1976 to 1980. The Egyptian survey utilized, in addition to the questionnaire for ever-married women, a household economic questionnaire and an individual questionnaire for husbands.

[2] Excluding Yemen, which has identical rates for age groups 20-24 and 25-29; and Tunisia, which has a higher fertility rate in age group 30-34 than that in age group 20-24.

[3] Further detail on methodological considerations is given in Alam and Casterline (1984).

[4] For a full discussion of the differences between major urban and other urban, see chapter VII.

[5] The only exception to this pattern is Yemen.

[6] For definition of singulate mean age at marriage, see chapter III.

[7] In chapter I, the marriage history data for both Jordan and Yemen were considered to be of less reliable quality because of a combination of low proportions of marriage dates reported with month and year, substantial fluctuations in annual rates and distortion in proportion married for certain cohorts. The validity of these estimates for Egypt is questioned by Coale (1985), who proposes that the rise in age at first marriage during the decade or so preceding the survey had been much more modest than the survey data suggest. There are sound reasons to dispute the amount of recent change shown by the Egyptian survey, but the general picture of delayed first marriage, for men and especially women, is unavoidable when all pertinent data sources are assessed.

[8] For a full discussion of fertility presence, see chapter II.

[9] There were two exceptions to this statement. First, educational aspirations for daughters tended to be a significant factor for all husbands except in rural Upper Egypt, but for wives only in urban areas. Secondly, infant and child mortality—as measured by the proportion of births that had died—was significantly positively related to the desire for additional children among husbands only in rural Egypt but among wives in both urban and rural areas.

REFERENCES

Abdel-Aziz, Abdallah (1983). *Evaluation of the Jordan Fertility Survey 1976*. World Fertility Survey Scientific Report, No. 42. Voorburg, The Netherlands: International Statistical Institute.

Akin, John and others (1984). *Breast-feeding Patterns and Determinants in the Near East: A Comparative Summary Analysis for Four Countries*. Carolina Population Center. Chapel Hill: University of North Carolina.

Alam, Iqbal and J. B. Casterline (1984). *Socio-Economic Differentials in Recent Fertility*. World Fertility Survey Comparative Studies, No. 33; Cross-National Summaries. Voorburg, The Netherlands: International Statistical Institute.

Ali, Ibrahim (1984). *Evaluation of the Syria Fertility Survey 1978*. Damascus: Central Bureau of Statistics.

_____ and C. Callum (1986). Socio-economic correlates of fertility. In S. M. Farid and K. Alloush, eds., *Determinants of Fertility in Syria*. Voorburg, The Netherlands: International Statistical Institute.

Alloush, K. and others (1986). Fertility Preferences and Contraceptive Use. In S. M. Farid and K. Alloush, eds., *Determinants of Fertility in Syria*. Voorburg, The Netherlands: International Statistical Institute.

Al-Tohamy, A. and I. Kalule-Sabiti (1985). *Evaluation of the Yemen Arab Republic Fertility Survey 1979*. World Fertility Survey Scientific Reports, No. 76. Voorburg, The Netherlands: International Statistical Institute.

Alwani, M. and Gigi Santow (1986). The proximate determinants of fertility. In S. M. Farid and K. Alloush, eds., *Determinants of Fertility in Syria*. Voorburg, The Netherlands: International Statistical Institute.

Ashurst, Hazel, Sundat Balkaran and J. B. Casterline (1984). *Socio-Economic Differentials in Recent Fertility*. World Fertility Survey Comparative Studies, No. 42; Cross-National Summaries. Rev. ed. Voorburg, The Netherlands: International Statistical Institute.

Balkaran, Sundat and David P. Smith (1984). Marriage dissolution and remarriage; additional tables. Data for World Fertility Survey Comparative Studies. Voorburg, The Netherlands, International Statistical Institute (unpublished).

Boraie, S., J. McCarthy and Morna R. Oruch (forthcoming). Achieved fertility, family size desires and contraceptive use. In A. M. Hallouda and S. M. Farid, eds., *Egypt: Demographic Responses to Modernization*. Cairo: Central Agency for Public Mobilisation and Statistics.

Casterline, J. B. and Ismail Eid (forthcoming). Village characteristics and reproductive behaviour. In A. M. Hallouda and S. M. Farid, eds., *Egypt: Demographic Responses to Modernization*. Cairo: Central Agency for Public Mobilisation and Statistics.

Cleland, John, Jane Verrall and Martin Vaessen (1983). *Preferences for the Sex of Children and Their Influence on Reproductive Behaviour*. World Fertility Survey Comparative Studies, No. 27: Cross-National Summaries. Voorburg, The Netherlands: International Statistical Institute.

Coale, Ansley J. (forthcoming). A reassessment of fertility trends, taking account of the Egyptian Fertility Survey. In A. M. Hallouda and S. M. Farid, eds., *Egypt: Demographic Responses to Modernization*. Cairo: Central Agency for Public Mobilisation and Statistics.

Cochrane, Susan H. (1979). *Fertility and Education: What Do We Really Know?* Baltimore, Maryland: The Johns Hopkins University Press.

_____, M. A. Khan and Ibrahim K. Taha (forthcoming). The determinants of the demand for children among husbands and wives. In A. M. Hallouda and S. M. Farid, eds., *Egypt: Demographic Responses to Modernization*. Cairo: Central Agency for Public Mobilisation and Statistics.

Easterlin, Richard A., Eileen M. Crimmins and Ibrahim K. Taha (forthcoming). Determinants of fertility control. In A. M. Hallouda and S. M. Farid, eds., *Egypt: Demographic Responses to Modernization*. Cairo: Central Agency for Public Mobilisation and Statistics.

Ebanks, G. Edward and Susheela Singh (1984). Socio-economic differentials in age at first marriage; additional tables. Data for World Fertility Survey Comparative Studies, Cross-National Summaries. Voorburg, The Netherlands: International Statistical Institute (unpublished).

Egypt (1983). Central Agency for Public Mobilization and Statistics. *The Egyptian Fertility Survey, 1980*. Cairo.

El-Deeb, Bothaina and J. B. Casterline (forthcoming). Determinants of contraceptive use. In A. M. Hallouda and S. M. Farid, eds., *Egypt: Demographic Responses to Modernization*. Cairo: Central Agency for Public Mobilisation and Statistics.

Farid, Samir (1984). Fertility patterns in the Arab region. Paper submitted to the World Fertility Survey Symposium, London, 24-27 April 1984.

Hallouda, A. M. and Susan H. Cochrane (1983). Effects of education and urbanization on fertility and desired family size in Egypt. Paper submitted to the International Union for the Scientific Study of Population Seminar on Population Policy in Egypt, Cairo, April 1984.

_____ and S. M. Farid (1983). Regional demographic contrasts in Egypt. Paper submitted to the International Union for the Scientific Study of Population Seminar on Population Policy in Egypt, Cairo, April 1984.

Jordan (1976). Department of Statistics. *National Fertility Survey in Jordan, 1972*. Amman.

Kandis, Afaf D. (1977). Female education and fertility decline in a developing country: the case of Jordan. In *Population Bulletin of the United Nations Economic Commission for Western Asia, No. 13*. Beirut: Economic Commission for Western Asia, 17-31.

Lightbourne, Robert E. (1984). Quality of the WFS fertility preference data. Paper submitted to the World Fertility Survey Symposium, London, 24-27 April 1984.

Loza, Sarah F. (1982). *Social Science Research for Population Policy Design: Case Study of Egypt*. Ed. by Carmen Miró. International Union for the Scientific Study of Population Papers, No. 22. Liège.

Morocco (1984). Ministère de la santé publique. *Enquête nationale sur la fécondité et la planification familiale au Maroc 1979-80: rapport national*. Rabat.

Sathar, Zeba A. and V. C. Chidambaram (1984). *Differentials in Contraceptive Use*. World Fertility Survey Comparative Studies, No. 36; Cross-National Summaries. Voorburg, The Netherlands: International Statistical Institute.

Sayed, Hussein A. (1983). *Community and Family Planning: The Case of Egypt*. Cairo: Population and Family Planning Board.

Singh, Susheela (1985). Birth histories: levels and trends in fertility in 41 WFS countries; draft and additional tables. Data for World Fertility Survey Comparative Studies; Cross-National Summaries. Voorburg, The Netherlands: International Statistical Institute (unpublished).

Smith, David P., Enrique Carrasco and Peter McDonald (1984). *Marriage Dissolution and Remarriage*. World Fertility Survey Comparative Studies, No. 34; Cross-National Summaries. Voorburg, The Netherlands: International Statistical Institute.

Sokona, O. and J. B. Casterline (forthcoming). Socio-economic differentials in age at marriage. In A. M. Hallouda and S. M. Farid, eds., *Egypt: Demographic Responses to Modernization*. Cairo: Central Agency for Public Mobilisation and Statistics.

Syrian Arab Republic (1982). Central Bureau of Statistics. *Syrian Fertility Survey 1978: Principal Report*. Damascus, vol. 1.

Taha, Ibrahim K. and Susan H. Cochrane (forthcoming). The determinants of desired family size: a causal analysis for policy. In A. M. Hallouda and S. M. Farid, eds., *Egypt: Demographic Responses to Modernization*. Cairo: Central Agency for Public Mobilisation and Statistics.

Tunisia (1982). Office national du planning familial et de la population. *Enquête tunisienne sur la fécondité 1978: rapport principal*. Tunis.

United Nations (1985). Department of International Economic and Social Affairs. Population Division. *World Population Prospects: Estimates and Projections as Assessed in 1982*. Population Studies, No. 86. New York: United Nations. Sales No. E.83.XIII.5.

United Nations Children's Fund (1985). *The State of the World's Children*. New York.

Yemen (1983). Central Planning Organization. Department of Statistics. *Yemen Arab Republic Fertility Survey, 1979*. Sana'a. Published in English and Arabic.

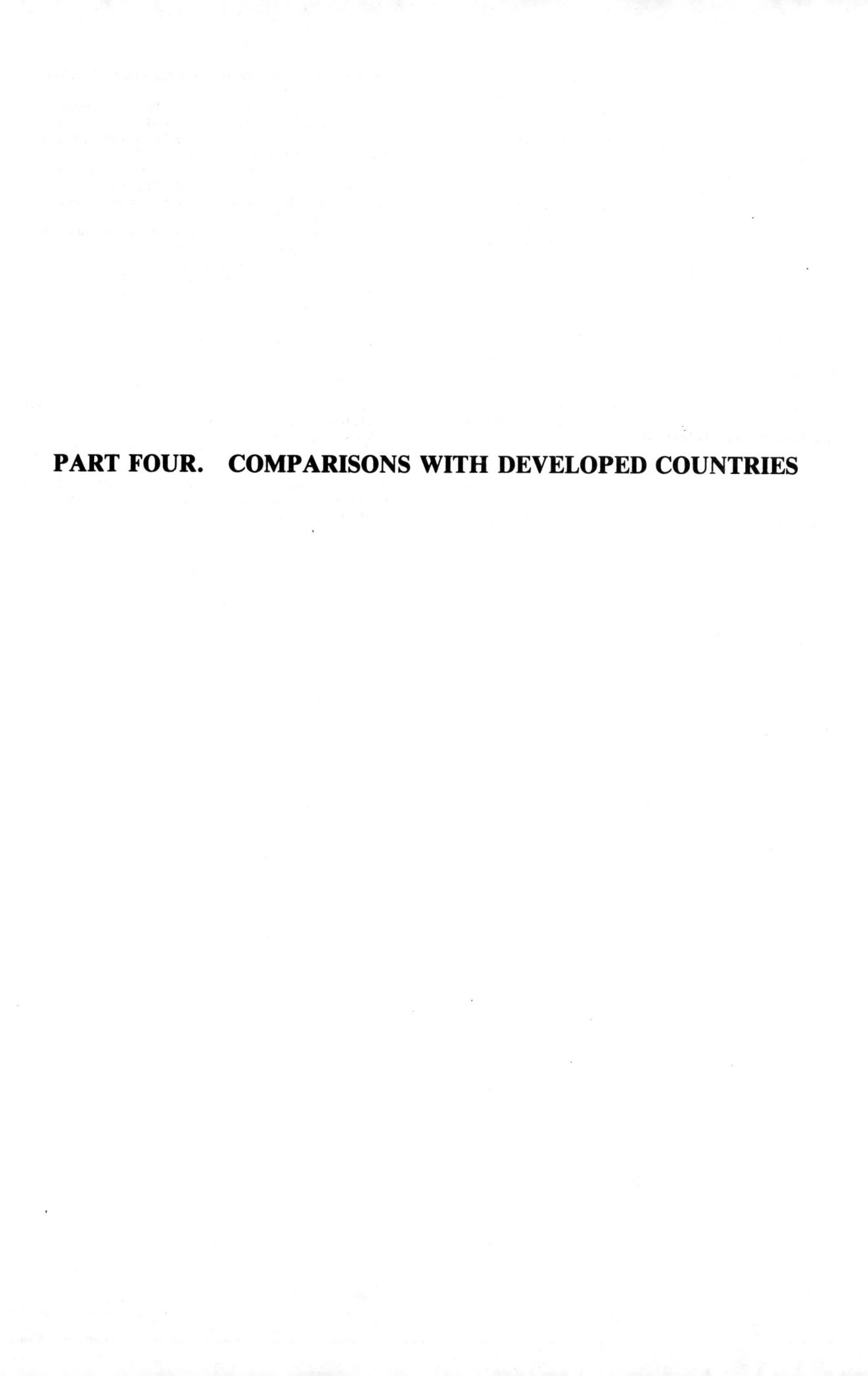

PART FOUR. COMPARISONS WITH DEVELOPED COUNTRIES

XIV. FERTILITY AND FAMILY PLANNING IN THE DEVELOPED COUNTRIES

*Economic Commission for Europe**

ABSTRACT

The findings summarized in this chapter are derived from 15 fertility surveys undertaken between 1975 and 1978 in Europe and a fertility survey carried out in the United States of America in 1974. As of the dates of these surveys, marital fertility had fallen to about 2.0 children or fewer in all countries but Spain and Yugoslavia. This evolution of fertility in the developed countries is the result of a continuous decline during the post-war period. As early as the 1956-1960 marriage cohort, the average expected ultimate family size was above 2.1 children per woman in all countries but Hungary and above 3.0 in Spain and the United States of America. For the 1971 and later cohorts this expected number exceeded 2.1 children in only nine countries, even though ideal family size was shown to be closer to 2.5, on average. Family size desires appeared thus to be above actual fertility. The low fertility levels can readily be linked to the high use of contraception and the incidence of induced abortions in a number of countries. In Romania, Spain and Yugoslavia the proportion of currently married women using contraception remains below 60 per cent; in the other countries, it is 70 per cent or more, reaching 94 per cent in Czechoslovakia.

The effect of contraception on fertility depends not only upon its prevalence but upon its efficiency and use-effectiveness. Thus, fertility can be further reduced when unwanted pregnancies due to contraceptive failure or to non-use are interrupted by abortions. For selected countries with available data, it appears that up to 90 per cent of unwanted pregnancies have sometimes been terminated through that means.

As concerns the socio-economic context that has favoured the observed fertility levels, three major variables were more closely scrutinized. From this standpoint, the traditional hypotheses about fertility differentials were once more brought to the fore. The negative association between contraceptive use and childbearing, on the one hand, and employment experience, on the other hand, stands out clearly in the analysis. Likewise, achieved fertility was consistently higher, and level of use of modern contraceptive methods lower, for women living in rural areas than for their urban counterparts. Lastly, education was negatively associated with number of children ever born, but the differentials were larger for wife's than for husband's education.

The World Fertility Survey (WFS), in accordance with its main purpose of assisting particularly the developing countries in carrying out fertility surveys, was mainly concerned with the participation of countries of the developing world in the programme. Nevertheless, in the developed countries considerable interest existed in the WFS programme; and a large number of them carried out fertility surveys in the second half of the decade, which in broad lines, albeit not in detail, followed WFS recommendations. Compared with the 43 developing countries that participated in the WFS programme, between the mid-1970s and the end of 1980, fertility surveys were conducted in 21 developed countries.

The Economic Commission for Europe (ECE), together with the United Nations Social Development Programme at Geneva and the World Fertility Survey, collaborated in the promotion and implementation of these national surveys and their subsequent comparative analysis. An important contribution in the preparatory stages of the project was made by the Conference of European Statisticians, which, as a subsidiary body of ECE, organized two meetings on fertility surveys under its auspices and in collaboration with the International Statistical Institute. These meetings discussed and endorsed the standard questionnaires proposed by WFS for use in low-fertility countries and formulated recommendations on the scope, format and nature of national reports.

The main responsibility for the comparative analysis of the WFS type of survey in the developed countries was entrusted to the secretariat of the ECE, in part because of the experience acquired from an earlier comparative fertility study (United Nations, 1976). In this context, the United Nations Working Group on Social Demography

---
*Population Activities Unit of the General Economic Analysis Division.

held several meetings of experts involved in the national fertility surveys in order to assist the ECE secretariat in the preparation of the comparative analysis. Members of the working group also played a crucial role in securing the supply of national data for the comparative project.

A working outline for the comparative study was developed by the ECE secretariat in co-operation with the Working Group on Social Demography. Within the overall framework, five general topics were designated for analysis: (*a*) achieved or cumulative fertility; (*b*) tempo of the family-building process; (*c*) family planning and unwanted fertility; (*d*) family size preferences and expectations; and (*e*) reproductive motivations.

The comparative study (Economic Commission for Europe, forthcoming) focuses on 16 countries in the ECE region: Belgium (1975-1976); Bulgaria (1976); Czechoslovakia (1977); Denmark (1975); Finland (1977); France (1977-1978); Hungary (1977); Italy (1979); the Netherlands (1975); Norway (1977-1978); Poland (1977); Romania (1978); Spain (1977); United Kingdom (England, Scotland and Wales) (1976); United States of America (1976); and Yugoslavia (1976).

The comparative study did not attempt a comprehensive presentation of the results of the 16 surveys, but was rather directed to exploring, through the topics listed, two issues of central concern to the countries in the region and to developed societies in general. These issues are, first, the factors associated with low fertility; and secondly, likely trends in childbearing for the near future. The analysis was designed to yield a multi-faceted description of marital fertility and, in so far as possible, to explain these phenomena in terms of their social, economic and cultural determinants. The approach is based primarily on the characteristics and behaviour of individuals, examining the nature and strength of the associations between fertility and these determinants. The background factors are seen as directly determining family size preferences and motivations, which in turn operate through family planning behaviour to influence childbearing, the latter being considered in terms of both the number and the timing of births.

The present chapter summarizes some of the major characteristics of the surveys, the data and methodologies used in this comparative analysis and some of its main findings (Economic Commission for Europe, forthcoming). It draws heavily on published and unpublished papers based on the comparative study (see references). Although, for illustrative purposes, some of the selected results are presented in tables 202-211, many of the findings are discussed without presenting the actual results. It should be noted that, in the tables, the standardized averages are based on a standard distribution of marriage duration which approximately resembled that of the 16 countries combined. The results concerning child-spacing include the median number of months at which the cumulative probability of a birth event reached 0.50. These statistics, derived from the life-table analysis of birth histories, were restricted to intervals beginning from 12 years prior to each survey date.

A. BASIC CHARACTERISTICS OF THE SURVEYS

Although the organizations responsible for the surveys differed between countries, in most, the national statistical offices assumed the major responsibility, with regard both to the initiation of the survey and to its implementation. In some countries, however, the sponsors were universities, university-related institutions or population research institutes collaborating with universities. Statistical offices in almost all countries played the most important role in the execution of the surveys, being involved in the selection of the sample and the respondents as well as in the data collection stage.

As concerns timing, the surveys in the different countries took place over a period of about five years between 1975 and 1980, but most of the 16 surveys considered here were carried out between 1976 and 1978 (see also table 201):

Year of survey	Number of countries
1975	2
1976	5
1977	5
1978	3
1979	1

On the whole, therefore, the comparative study had a reasonably sharp delimitation in time. It may also be noted from table 201 (column (1)) that the time taken to complete the field-work varied considerably, from less than a month in some countries to about a year in one.

One difference between the WFS recommendations for developing countries and the proposals for the surveys in developed countries was the target population. Whereas WFS recommended the inclusion of all ever-married women under age 50, the recommendations for the developed countries suggested samples of women currently in their first marriage under age 45, mainly to assure, at least in this respect, comparability with the 1970 ECE study. Actually, the criteria for selection varied considerably (see columns (2) and (3) of table 201). Only three countries followed the recommendations with respect both to age and to marital status.

As far as marital status was concerned, most countries included all ever-married women (i.e., widowed and divorced women in addition to all currently married women). In another, smaller group of countries, the surveys covered all women, including single women, while in one case, both single women who had children living with them and all ever-married women formed the sample. For the comparative analysis, however, it was possible to select currently once-married women for all countries except two. In the cases of Denmark and Poland, the individual data from the tapes did not include information on the number of times the respondent had been married. The resulting bias was negligible in Poland, but probably more important in Denmark.

In most countries, the upper age-limit for inclusion in the survey was 44 years, although in a few cases it was set at 49 years. In Hungary, however, the upper limit was at 40 years; and the sample for the Netherlands included all women married during the period 1963-1973 irrespective of age, resulting in an underrepresentation of women aged 35 years or over. There were only relatively small differences in the lower age-limit. The exception was France, where the sample excluded women under age 20, thus affecting inter-country comparability for the younger ages (table 201, column (3)).

Considerable differences existed as far as the size of the sample was concerned. Table 201 presents in columns (4) and (5), respectively, the number of women interviewed in the original samples and in the subsamples used for the comparative analysis. The latter varied from a low of about 2,000 to as high as 10,000. These differences

TABLE 201. SOME CHARACTERISTICS OF SURVEYS OF 16 DEVELOPED COUNTRIES

Country	Interview period (1)	Original sample universe definition: marital status (2)	Age limits (3)	Number of women interviewed (4)	Number of women included in ECE sample (5)
Belgium	July 1975-May 1976	All (including single)	16-44	4 863	4 010
Bulgaria	November-December 1976	Ever married	15-44	6 911	6 352
Czechoslovakia	July-September 1977	Currently married, married once	18-44	3 041	2 932
Denmark	April 1975	All (including single)	18-49	5 240	3 129
Finland	March-June 1977	Currently married	18-44	5 449	5 349
France	December 1977-December 1978	All (including single)	20-44	3 018	2 290
Hungary	May-June 1977	Currently married	Under 40	4 009	3 658
Italy	May-December 1979	Ever married	18-44	5 499	5 359
Netherlands	March-May 1975	Currently married	[a]	4 522	4 335[a]
Norway	October 1977-February 1978	All (including single)	18-44	4 137	2 824
Poland	October 1977	Currently married	Under 45	9 799	9 799
Romania	June-July 1978	Currently married	15-49	10 141	8 771
Spain	November-December 1977	Ever married	15-49	6 290	4 618
United Kingdom[b]	May-June 1976	All (including single)	16-49	6 589	3 682
United States of America	January-September 1976	Ever married[c]	15-44	8 611	5 545
Yugoslavia	October 1976	Currently married	15-49	8 115	6 806

Source: Economic Commission for Europe (forthcoming).
[a] All women married between 1963 and 1973, irrespective of age.
[b] Not including Northern Ireland.
[c] Including single women also if they had offspring living in the household.

would seem to be large enough to affect the relative accuracy of the results in terms of statistical significance, particularly in the case of cross-tabulations of two or more variables.

It is much more difficult to assess the various aspects of the field-work, which may affect the results. For the surveys considered here, the interviewing technique was basically the same in all: answers to the questionnaire were provided by the respondent in the course of a personal interview. The interviewers were all female, but the field staff differed to the extent that in a number of countries interviewers were recruited from among public health workers, while in others professional field staff were used. In a few countries, however, social workers and students were trained as interviewers.

The length of the interview and the number of interviewers also varied considerably between countries. In most, the interviews were reported to have lasted, on average, an hour. In some, however, they took only half that time; and, at the other extreme, some countries reported an average duration of one and a half hours. The range in the number of interviewers employed was also very broad and not always related to the number of respondents. There were fewer than 100 interviewers in some countries, but as many as 1,300 in Finland. The number of interviews per interviewer went from a low of 4 in Finland to a high of 180 in Romania (Economic Commission for Europe, forthcoming).

One possible source of distortion in the results is the interval between the selection and the interviews of respondents. If the actual interviews, for example, would only take place one year after the selection, women married for a period of less than one year would be excluded from the investigation. In virtually all countries concerned, the actual time lag between selection and interview did not exceed a few months. In England and Wales, the time-lag was from seven to eight months, but this delay had been foreseen and taken into account when the sample was selected. In the case of Spain, however, the delay between selection and the interview was as much as two years, thus affecting to some extent the comparability of the data.

The sampling design and procedures varied considerably between countries, mainly due to national requirements and past experience. Moreover, the World Fertility Survey did not attempt to standardize sample design. A review of the sample design and procedures in the countries considered here therefore shows considerable divergencies. In all cases, however, the samples were based on carefully considered random designs guided by the aims of precision and economy of cost. Thus, all but two countries used some stratification in the sampling. A two-stage sample was used in about three fifths of the countries; two countries used one-stage sampling, while in the case of the United States of America, a five-stage selection procedure was applied. In the large majority of countries, the designs implied equal probabilities of selection of eligible women and the sample was self-weighting in 11 countries. In the remaining five cases, disproportionate sampling was used, but weights were introduced to correct for the differences in sampling rates. In about one third of the countries, provision was made for the replacement of selected respondents who could not be contacted. In several countries, including Belgium, Italy, the Netherlands and Spain, the proportion of substitutes was very high, amounting to between 25 and 35 per cent of the original selection (Berent, Jones and Siddiqui, 1982, chapter 3).

For various reasons, the questionnaires used in the developed countries, contrary to the situation in the developing countries, were not uniform. Although WFS developed a model questionnaire for national surveys with two variants, one for high-fertility and one for low-fertility countries, the latter was intended rather to indicate the essential minimum of topics to be covered and to serve as a guideline on how to approach them. In addition, the ECE secretariat, in consultation with the International Union for the Scientific Study of Population Committee on Comparative Analysis of Fertility, prepared a special set of questions entitled "A Module on Family Size Preferences and Motivations in Low-Fertility Countries". The low-fertility variant of the WFS questionnaire together with the module constituted the WFS/ECE recommendations for the survey questionnaire.

The questionnaires in only three countries followed closely the WFS/ECE recommendations. In the others, a number of additional topics generally were covered, including in some cases very detailed questions on pregnancies, fecundity and contraceptive practices; on contraceptive methods and the fertility decision-making process; and on the formation of the relationship between couples and so forth. The questionnaires of other countries contained special sections on household composition, women's employment and their employment history.

Nevertheless, in most countries, the questionnaires covered the topics recommended for purposes of the comparative analysis. As concerns the respondent's background, all countries asked for information on age and educational level. Four countries, however, did not include questions on family income; two omitted place of residence; and in one country, the information on husband's education and occupation was not available. Pregnancy histories, including the number of live births, their dates, the survival status of each child and the current pregnancy status, were investigated everywhere. Nevertheless, in one country the total number of pregnancies was not reported. Of the 16 countries, 11 included one or more questions on induced abortions. With respect to fertility regulation, all countries investigated current use of contraceptive methods, but three countries did not include past use. With regard to methods, it may be noted that some countries did not consider sterilization a method of birth control. The recommendations concerning fertility expectations and preferences included questions on family size ideals, which were covered by at least one question in all but two surveys, and on the number of additional children the respondent expected to have, data for which were obtained in some form in all countries. The phrasing of questions on the latter topic, however, differed considerably: reference was made to "wanted", "planned" or "intended", rather than expected number of children, in a number of countries. Lastly, all countries collected information on women's work history, including whether the respondent was currently working, whether she had worked since first married and her occupation. Additional questions on full-time and part-time work and whether working at home or away from home were also included in many of the investigations.

Although in many aspects the survey characteristics were such as to suggest that valid international comparisons of the national results could be made, the preceding summary also reveals differences in organization and execution of national surveys. The impact of such differences on the cross-country comparability of the results cannot be exactly measured. In general, for all countries except two, the survey sample could be reduced to a comparable subsample for marital status and age. Although the differences in questionnaires between countries as far as detail and specific questions are concerned were substantial, all of them focused on the main subject categories selected for the comparative study: achieved fertility; birth-spacing; family size preferences; and family planning. The countries for which data were available are also generally representative for the ECE region. Therefore, on the whole, and subject to some qualifications, the information available lent itself to valid international comparisons.

B. Data and methodology of the comparative analysis

The data utilized by the comparative fertility study were based, as noted, on 16 different fertility surveys conducted between 1975 and 1979. These surveys were designed to be nationally representative, except in the case of Belgium, where the survey referred only to the Flemish part of the country. For analytical purposes and for reasons of maintaining cross-country comparability, the sample studied was restricted to once-married, currently married women under age 45. For the majority of the countries, it was possible to obtain such a subsample. The exceptions, as already noted in the preceding section, were the Netherlands, Hungary and Denmark and Poland. The Netherlands sample referred to women married between 1963 and 1973, the Hungarian survey excluded women over age 40, while for the Danish sample it was not possible to exclude women married more than once. This was also true for Poland but the resulting bias was, unlike the case of Denmark, insignificant.

The 16 surveys were designed and conducted essentially independently of one another; and although an ECE/WFS model questionnaire was developed, the differences between countries in the form and content of the material collected were substantial. These differences necessitated a lengthy and painstaking process of reclassifying variables into comparable standard forms. The annex provides a shortened version of the list of variables selected for the comparative analysis. This list obviously is rather limited, considering the wealth of information available in the individual surveys. Moreover, data on the variables listed were not available for all the countries and the cross-country comparability of many of these variables was a constant concern in the study. Nevertheless, the material utilized in the comparative study has much to offer for valid international comparisons.

As far as analytical methods are concerned, the comparative analyses generally consisted of multi-way cross-classification of the data. In addition, more complex methods, including direct standardization, analysis of variance, multiple classification analysis and life-table analysis, were also utilized. The specific details about data and methodology will appear in the final report of the comparative fertility study (Economic Commission for Europe, forthcoming).

C. Summary of findings

Levels and trends

Table 202 presents some of the indicators describing levels of fertility and the practice of family planning in Europe and the United States. Selected data on trends are presented in tables 203-205. In table 203, the results of 11 countries from the ECE/WFS comparative study (around 1975) are compared with results for the same countries from the previous ECE comparative study (around 1970) (United Nations, 1976). Efforts were made to achieve maximum comparability between the two surveys by adjusting the subsample of either survey to match the other in terms of age, marital status, geographical coverage etc. Tables 204 and 205 are restricted to results from the present comparative study, providing comparisons by marriage cohort.

Fertility

Reflecting the very low levels of fertility reached in Europe and the United States of America, the average number of children ever born to the married women included in the survey varied around two children. The actual values ranged from 1.64 in Hungary to 2.36 in Spain (table 202). Many of the women in these surveys were still in the process of completing their families. Completed family size for the group of cohorts as a whole is likely to be well above replacement levels in most countries. This is supported by data on average ultimate expected number of children, which ranged from 2.08 (Hungary) to 3.3 (Spain) for the 1956-1960 marriage cohort, but not by those on the 1971 and later marriage cohorts. For the latter, the average ultimate expected number exceeds 2.1 children in only nine countries (table 204). Between 80 and 90 per cent of the respondents in all countries expected up to three children, but the mode everywhere was two children. The results also indicate that in each country the average number of children born during the first five years of marriage represent about three fifths of the ultimate expected number of children. The average ideal family size appears to cover the range from 2.21 children in Bulgaria and Italy to 2.76 children in Spain (table 203). The data reveal that the ideal family size concentrates on two or three children and there were virtually no women in Europe (and the United States) who considered a childless family to be ideal.

Changes in achieved and expected fertility between the earlier (around 1970) and the later (around 1975) rounds of surveys provide some insights into trends over time (table 203). The comparisons indicate that the standardized average number of births declined in three countries by about 10 per cent (Belgium, Poland, United States of America) but stayed about the same or changed only slightly in the others. The comparison of data on the average ultimate expected family size suggests a similar pattern, with Belgium and the United States manifesting the largest declines, followed by Poland and Denmark. The data, however, also indicate a slight but noticeable rise in ultimate expected family size in England and Wales. In almost all of the countries for which comparisons were possible, there had been an increase over time in the proportion of women who expected to have a two-child family. In contrast, the proportion of those who expected three or more children declined in many of the countries (table 203). The declining trend in ultimate expected family size is even more pronounced in the data by marriage cohort (table 204). In nine of the 16 countries examined, the average ultimate expected family size declined steadily by marriage cohort, and in only one country (Hungary) did the average expected family size remain virtually constant across marriage cohorts (table 204).

The incidence of pre-marital (or pre-union) births varied across countries, with the highest levels in Finland, Poland and Norway, where from 6 to 9 per cent of the women reported having births before first marriage (Ford, 1984, table A1). Once married, most couples had their first child within five years of marriage. The median interval between marriage and a first birth, however, varied considerably. It was less than one year in Poland and Spain and over two years in the United Kingdom (not including Northern Ireland) and in the United States. The second birth usually came from 33 to 50 months after the birth of the first child. Third births were much less common in the participating countries and the point at which the cumulative probability of a third birth reached 0.25 came from three to four years after the second birth in most countries.

Data on the median number of months between marriage and first birth indicate that in the Netherlands, the United Kingdom (England, Scotland and Wales) and the United States, cohorts married during the early 1970s significantly postponed first births, compared with those who married during the second half of the 1960s (table 204). On the other hand, a trend towards earlier first and second births was noticeable in Eastern Europe and in Yugoslavia. An examination of the data showed significant shifts towards the postponement of second births in France, Norway and the United States.

Family planning

Contraceptive knowledge and use are evidently very high in Europe and the United States. The level of knowledge of individual methods, however, although high, varied notably across countries (table 202). The evidence suggests that many women were not familiar with contraceptives other than those widely used in their own countries. For instance, knowledge of the intra-uterine device (IUD) in Bulgaria, Poland and Spain, where this method was comparatively little used, was below that in some of the other countries where IUD use was more widespread. In Spain, for example, only 33 per cent of women said that they knew of IUDs, as compared with the 91 per cent who stated they had knowledge of the pill.

The level of current contraceptive use among currently once-married women, in the 11 countries for which data are available, varied from 55 per cent in Yugoslavia to 94 per cent in Czechoslovakia (table 202). This proportion, however, does not necessarily portray the complete picture because a number of reasons contribute to the non-use of contraception. A somewhat better indication is provided by the percentage of non-users among women who were exposed to the risk of pregnancy and did not want additional children. Measured with this standard, the incidence of non-use falls below 10 per cent in many European countries and high levels were observed only for Spain (38 per cent) and Yugoslavia (23 per cent).

In spite of uniformly low levels of fertility, the countries of Europe show a very mixed picture of current contraceptive use by method and several distinct patterns seem to exist (see table 205). One pattern is that of the Netherlands, the Nordic countries, the United Kingdom (England, Scotland and Wales) and the United States of America, where couples rely upon modern contraceptives, such as IUDs, the pill and sterilization, and very little upon such conventional methods as rhythm and withdrawal. In the United Kingdom (as in the United States), however, sterilization was more prevalent than IUD use, in comparison with the other countries in this group. In France and Hungary, although the majority of the couples rely upon modern contraceptives, a high proportion also depend upon conventional methods. In Belgium

TABLE 202. LEVELS OF FERTILITY AND FAMILY PLANNING, 16 DEVELOPED COUNTRIES: SELECTED INDICATORS

Indicators	Belgium	Bulgaria	Czechoslovakia	Denmark	Finland	France	Hungary	Italy	Netherlands	Norway	Poland	Romania	Spain	United Kingdom[a]	United States of America	Yugoslavia
Number of respondents	4 010	6 352	2 932	3 129	5 349	2 290	3 658	5 359	4 335	2 824	9 799	8 771	4 618	3 682	5 545	6 806
1. Number of live births																
(a) Average	1.78	1.85	2.00	1.98	1.84	2.02	1.64	1.96	1.51	2.00	2.00	2.03	2.36	1.89	1.99	2.19
(b) Average standardized for marriage duration	1.79	1.78	1.96	2.00	1.86	2.01	..	1.95	..	2.05	2.07	2.00	2.41	1.85	2.08	2.17
(c) Average born before fifth year of marriage	1.43	..	1.41	..	1.46	1.55	1.32	1.50	1.51	1.62	1.56	..	1.71	1.40	1.59	..
2. Family planning																
(a) Percentage who knew at least one contraceptive method	99	92	96	..	100	100	98	100	100	..	95	..	95	..	99	..
(b) Percentage who knew pill	93	68	83	..	100	99	94	98	100	..	69	..	91	..	97	..
(c) Percentage who knew intra-uterine device	66	53	85	..	100	74	70	82	98	..	42	..	33	..	82	..
(d) Current use of contraception (percentage):																
All women	85	75	94	63	80	77	74	78	75	72	75	58	56	77	69	55
Exposed women (including sterilized)	92	80	95	..	84	88	82	85	82	88	83	64	56	81	82	68
(e) Percentage of women who reported having had an induced abortion	0.5	27	26	..	..	..	32	7	..	10	7	48	..	3	3	32
(f) Number of abortions per 100 pregnancies	..	66	14	..	..	..	20	..	..	5	5	35	..	..	..	24
3. Unwanted fertility																
(a) Percentage distribution of pregnancies																
All pregnancies	100	..	100	..	..	100	100	..	100	..	100	100	100	..	100	..
Wanted	71	..	70	..	..	61	65	..	80	..	86	62	92	..	69	..
Unplanned	21	..	13	..	..	23	21	..	18	..	14	38	6	..	21	..
Unwanted	8	..	17	..	..	16	14	..	2	..	..	..	2	..	10	..
(b) Percentage distribution of births:																
All births	100	..	..	100	100	100	100	..	100	..	..	..	100	100	100	..
Wanted	71	..	..	77	66	64	82	..	81	..	..	..	92	73	66	..
Unplanned	21	..	..	15	25	25	14	..	18	..	..	..	6	27	24	..
Unwanted	8	..	..	8	10	11	4	..	2	..	..	..	2	..	9	..
4. Average ideal number of children	2.62	2.21	2.49	2.40	2.68	..	2.46	2.21	..	2.58	2.69	2.49	2.76	2.47	2.33	2.54

Source: Economic Commission for Europe (forthcoming).
NOTE: The symbol .. indicates not available, not pertinent or not applicable.

[a] Not including Northern Ireland.

TABLE 203. SELECTED INDICATORS OF FERTILITY AND FAMILY PLANNING FOR 11 DEVELOPED COUNTRIES, AROUND 1970 AND AROUND 1975

Indicators	Belgium 1966	Belgium 1975	Czechoslovakia 1970	Czechoslovakia 1977	Denmark 1970	Denmark 1975	Finland 1971	Finland 1977	France 1971	France 1977	Hungary 1966	Hungary 1977	Netherlands 1969	Netherlands 1975	Poland 1972	Poland 1977	United Kingdom[a] 1967	United Kingdom[a] 1976	United States of America 1970	United States of America 1976	Yugoslavia 1970	Yugoslavia 1976
1. Average number of live births	2.04	1.78	1.87	2.00	2.02	1.98	1.91	1.84	2.16	2.02	1.68	1.64	..	1.51	2.32	2.00	1.93	1.87	2.31	1.99	2.22	2.19
2. Average number of live births standardized for marriage duration	2.10	1.79	1.96	1.96	2.04	2.00	2.04	1.86	2.12	2.01	..	..	..	..	2.21	2.07	1.81	1.83	2.32	2.08	2.13	2.17
3. Average ultimate expected number of children	2.50	2.25	2.37	2.40	2.55	2.36	2.55	2.46	2.55	2.54	2.14	2.08	..	..	2.71	2.50	2.21	2.31	2.95	2.60	..	..
4. Percentage distribution of ultimate expected number of children																						
All	100	100	100	100	100	100	100	100	100	100	100	100	..	..	100	100	100	100	100	100	..	..
Zero	4	4	1	1	3	3	3	3	3	3	2	2	..	..	1	1	8	4	4	4	..	..
One	20	19	9	8	8	9	10	10	14	13	20	15	..	..	9	10	19	12	7	10	..	..
Two	33	43	58	55	43	50	47	45	40	41	53	64	..	..	43	50	41	50	35	43	..	..
Three	21	21	23	27	31	26	23	28	25	28	16	15	..	..	27	26	18	21	26	25	..	..
Four	13	9	5	6	11	8	10	10	11	8	5	3	..	..	11	8	8	9	16	10	..	..
Five or more	8	4	4	3	4	3	5	4	7	7	3	1	..	..	8	5	5	4	13	8	..	..
5. Average interval length (months):																						
(a) Marriage to first birth	..	19	..	19	16	..	..	16	17	19	..	19	..	20	16	15	26	25[b]	19	21	17	16
(b) First to second birth	..	31	37	38	37	36	..	35	34	32	..	40	..	30	37	35	35	32[b]	31	30	35	34
(c) Second to third birth	..	35	40	40	44	42	..	38	37	34	..	39	..	32	40	37	40	..	34	34	36	32
6. Mean age at first birth	23.4	23.4	22.5	22.4	22.4	23.0	..	23.2	22.6	23.0	..	21.9	..	24.3	23.0	22.6	23.0	23.5[b]	21.3	22.0	..	21.7
7. Percentage of users using:																						
(a) Intra-uterine device	..	4	14	19	4	14	4	35	2	13	—	13	1	6	1	2	2	10	9	9	2	3
(b) Pill	..	38	4	15	37	35	26	14	17	34	—	49	45	66	4	10	19	35	41	34	9	9
(c) Condom	..	8	19	14	30	39	40	40	12	8	18	5	23	14	17	19	41	23	17	11	6	4
(d) Withdrawal	..	27	52	31	7	2	21	21	52	27	64	23	9	3	38	25	25	6	3	3	73	65
(e) Rhythm	..	15	3	7	2	1	1	1	14	9	4	5	19	4	33	41	5	1	8	5	3	8
(f) Sterilization	..	6	..	3	..	..	—	—	—	5	..	2	..	6	..	..	..	20	16	25	..	..

Source: Economic Commission for Europe (forthcoming).
NOTE: The symbol .. indicates not available, not pertinent or not applicable.

[a] Data for England and Wales only, except as noted.
[b] Including data for Scotland.

TABLE 204. AVERAGE ULTIMATE EXPECTED FERTILITY AND MEDIAN NUMBER OF MONTHS BETWEEN MARRIAGE AND FIRST BIRTH, BY MARRIAGE COHORT, SELECTED DEVELOPED COUNTRIES

Country	Average ultimate expected family size by year of marriage				Median number of months between marriage and first birth, by year of marriage	
	1956-1960	1961-1965	1966-1970	1971 or later	1966-1970	1971 or later
Belgium	2.45	2.22	2.06	2.10	17.8	16.9
Bulgaria	2.18	2.13	2.07	1.92	..	..
Czechoslovakia	2.44	2.39	2.38	2.34	15.5	15.1
Finland	2.63	2.35	2.33	2.36	14.5	17.3
France	2.77	2.67	2.44	2.28	14.9	17.5
Hungary	2.08	2.06	2.08	2.09	15.4	14.0
Italy	2.84	2.56	2.40	2.14	14.0	14.4
Netherlands	..	2.35	2.17	2.19	19.7	28.7
Norway	2.85	2.67	2.29	2.30	10.5	13.7
Poland	2.81	2.65	2.42	2.21	12.4	10.6
Romania[a]	2.33	2.37	2.23	2.05	..	..
Spain	3.31	3.03	2.74	2.32	12.5	12.5
United Kingdom[b]	2.60	2.34	2.12	2.03	25.0	34.7
United States of America	3.10	2.61	2.23	2.16	22.9	31.0
Yugoslavia	..	..	..	..	14.1	12.7

Source: Economic Commission for Europe (forthcoming).
NOTE: The symbol .. indicates not available, not pertinent or not applicable.
[a] Marriage cohorts are: 1956-1960 = 1953-1957; 1961-1965 = 1958-1962; 1966-1970 = 1963-1967; 1971 or later = 1968 or later.
[b] Not including Northern Ireland.

TABLE 205. CURRENT USE OF MODERN AND TRADITIONAL METHODS, BY MARRIAGE COHORT, SELECTED DEVELOPED COUNTRIES
(Percentage of all current users)

Country	Modern methods[a]				Traditional methods[b]			
	1956-1960	1961-1965	1966-1970	1971 or later	1956-1960	1961-1965	1966-1970	1971 or later
Belgium	38	45	52	64	54	45	37	28
Bulgaria	5	5	7	6	85	86	81	80
Czechoslovakia	30	35	46	39	43	37	35	38
Finland	51	57	60	53	5	4	2	1
France	37	51	61	58	52	37	30	33
Hungary	42	56	68	76	42	33	25	18
Italy	10	18	25	26	73	60	55	52
Netherlands	..	72	80	80	..	11	6	4
Norway	53	63	72	69	15	12	6	6
Poland	8	12	15	14	69	68	62	64
Romania[c]	—	1	1	2	84	84	85	82
Spain	14	18	25	40	69	67	58	42
United Kingdom[d]	58	65	71	76	11	7	4	5
United States of America	63	71	71	69	12	7	8	7
Yugoslavia	10	11	15	15	78	73	68	68

Source: Economic Commission for Europe (forthcoming).
NOTE: The symbol .. indicates not available, not pertinent or not applicable.
[a] Sterilization, pill, intra-uterine device.
[b] Rhythm, withdrawal.
[c] See note a in table 204.
[d] Not including Northern Ireland.

and Czechoslovakia, conventional methods are almost as much used as the modern methods. In Southern Europe and Poland, the conventional methods outweighed modern methods. Bulgaria and Romania turned out to be extreme cases, where not more than 5 per cent of the couples were utilizing modern contraceptives.

The analysis of the incidence of induced abortion through survey data is admittedly a difficult task. The results are influenced by the designs of the questionnaires and the legal status and history of abortion as well as a number of less tangible factors which affect the reliability of the information provided. In Belgium, Italy, the United Kingdom and the United States of America, for instance, 0.5 to 7 per cent of women reported having had at least one abortion. In these four countries, restrictions on abortions were either in force at the time of the survey or had been only recently relaxed. On the other hand, in Bulgaria, Czechoslovakia, Hungary, Norway, Poland, Romania and Yugoslavia, abortion had been legal and widely available for many years. Except for Poland, where only 7 per cent of the women reported having had an abortion, these countries reported higher levels of abortion than the other countries: from 10 per cent in Norway to 48 per cent in Romania (table 202).

Unwanted and unplanned fertility

In the definitions used in the surveys, a pregnancy that came sooner than it was wanted was called "unplanned", while a pregnancy that came after the couple had already decided to stop childbearing was considered "unwanted". The data for some countries also made it possible to classify not only pregnancies but births in the same manner. The incidence of unplanned pregnancies was found to be quite high in Europe. It is estimated that in at least six countries, one in five pregnancies was unplanned. The percentage of unwanted births varied from 2 to 11 per cent in the nine surveys for which the relevant data were available (table 202). One analysis suggested that a considerable, and in some cases a very high, proportion (from 33 to 92 per cent) of unplanned pregnancies were terminated by induced abortion in Czechoslovakia, Hungary, Poland and Romania (Berent, 1982, table 18). Given the still very high use of traditional contraceptive methods in Eastern European countries, there is no doubt that abortion plays a crucial role in reducing their fertility levels.

The extraordinary variety of contraceptive practices in Europe is evident in both the 1970 and 1975 surveys. Comparisons of the two rounds of surveys clearly indicate that the traditional contraceptives (rhythm and withdrawal) are being progressively replaced by modern methods. Use of IUDs has increased over time in the 11 countries for which two comparable surveys were available. The pill, however, while increasingly used in some countries, has also suffered some setbacks (table 203). Comparison of the marriage cohorts of 1956-1960, 1961-1965 and 1966-1970 also provides further confirmation that there has been a trend towards increased use of modern methods and reduced utilization of rhythm and withdrawal. The shift from traditional towards modern methods was most pronounced in Belgium and France. Bulgaria, Poland and Romania are exceptional cases where the proportion of couples utilizing rhythm and withdrawal has scarcely changed over time (table 203).

Socio-economic differentials

The analysis of differentials in fertility and family planning was a major component of the ECE Comparative Fertility Study. For the purposes of this analysis, a number of demographic and socio-economic characteristics were employed. (The majority of the independent variables used are listed in the annex.) Tables 206-211 provide some of the results for three selected independent variables, i.e., wife's education, residence and work history. These three variables were chosen in part because of their importance as correlates of fertility and family planning and in part because of the wider availability of pertinent data. The discussions in this section, however, are based on analyses not only of these variables but of other socio-economic variables included in the study, but for which data are not presented in this chapter (Economic Commission for Europe, forthcoming).

Achieved fertility

Despite the low fertility in the countries included in the comparative study, it is interesting to note that considerable socio-economic differentials still persist, at least in relative terms. The extreme case was Bulgaria, where the average number of births for the sampled women was 1.8, and yet differences between subgroups were very marked and frequently exceeded 0.5 child in absolute terms. In general, the differences by residence, education, social status and level of living—measured by income, number of rooms in the living-quarters etc.—were found to be more pronounced in Eastern Europe (Czechoslovakia was a frequent exception), Finland and Yugoslavia. This was less true, on the whole, of the characteristics related to women's work, perhaps because the employment of married women is more taken for granted in most of these countries than in other parts of Europe. On the other hand, there appeared to be remarkably little contrast in fertility levels within Belgium, Italy and Spain. For Belgium, this was more or less to be expected from the results of other studies. For Italy and Spain, however, this finding is more surprising, particularly because these countries had experienced fertility decline relatively recently. Problems of measurement may be responsible in the case of certain specific variables, but the situation warrants examination in greater detail. What differentials did appear were most pronounced with respect to the women's work experience, which was particularly important in Belgium (Jones, 1982).

The strongest differentials found in most countries were those by current residence, wife's level of education and wife's work history (table 206). Achieved fertility was consistently higher for women living in rural areas than for their urban counterparts. Education was negatively associated with number of children ever born, but the differentials were larger for wife's than husband's education. Also, in the case of wife's education, the relationship showed a tendency to be stronger at the lower than at the upper educational levels. On the other hand, achieved fertility tends to be positively related to husband's education at the upper end of the educational scale, particularly among urban residents and wives whose husbands were white-collar workers. This pattern emerged in Belgium, Finland and Spain, and to a lesser extent in France, Norway and the United Kingdom (England, Scotland and Wales).

The negative association between childbearing and employment experience stands out clearly in the analyses. However, wife's employment experience often showed a greater effect within the low-status categories (measured by education, husband's occupation and income). This may very well be due to the fact that women who are less well off may need longer hours at jobs that are less flexible and may not have as easy access to alternative forms of child care. This pattern was quite widespread, but it was particularly striking in Belgium, France and the United States of America (Jones, 1982, table 11).

Ultimate expected fertility

The variable "ultimate expected number of children" is the number of live births reported by the respondent at the time of the interview plus the number of children she expects to have in the future (Berent, 1983, p. 7). However, the definition of "expected" number of children varied considerably across countries.

According to the results of this analysis, the differentials in ultimate expected number of children are relatively smaller and less systematic than those observed for achieved fertility. Nevertheless, for those socio-economic variables which showed some bearing on total expected family size, the patterns of differentials were more or less

TABLE 206. AVERAGE NUMBER OF LIVE BIRTHS STANDARDIZED BY MARRIAGE DURATION, BY WIFE'S EDUCATION, RESIDENCE AND WORK HISTORY, SELECTED DEVELOPED COUNTRIES

Country	Wife's education — Primary not completed	Primary completed	Lower secondary	Higher secondary	Post-secondary	Residence — Rural	Urban	Wife's work history — Currently working	Not working, worked since marriage	Worked only before marriage or never
Belgium	— 1.77 —		1.83	1.72	1.90	1.85	1.78	1.54	2.03	2.11
Bulgaria	2.41	1.74	1.55	1.50	1.37	1.97	1.64	1.75	2.11	2.19
Czechoslovakia	— 2.35 —		2.08	1.80	1.62	2.16	1.89	1.88	2.35	3.01
Denmark	— 2.20 —		1.87	1.86	1.85	2.16	1.94	1.86	2.25	2.10
Finland	— 2.01 —		1.80	1.74	1.64	2.09	1.71	1.78	2.07	2.30
France	2.51	2.03	1.86	1.79	1.66	2.19	1.93	1.64	2.24	2.56
Hungary[a]	— 2.59 —		1.67	1.38	1.38	1.79	1.50	1.48	1.83	2.17
Italy	2.45	1.96	1.74	1.68	1.48	1.98	1.89	1.74	1.96	2.15
Norway	— 2.40 —		2.11	1.95	1.86	2.18	1.91	1.90	2.23	2.40
Poland	2.70	2.32	1.95	1.71	1.55	2.47	1.82	2.01	2.18	2.36
Romania	— 2.25 —		1.68	1.52	1.39	2.25	1.74	1.96	— 2.25 —	
Spain	2.63	2.28	2.42	2.27	2.41	2.45	2.40	2.11	2.32	2.56
United Kingdom[b]	— 2.15 —		1.90	1.73	1.72	..	..	1.60	2.11	2.27
United States of America	— 2.76 —		2.34	2.07	1.82	..	..	1.81	2.22	2.58
Yugoslavia	2.43	1.81	— 1.59 —		1.40	2.45	1.96	1.78	1.93	2.50

Source: Economic Commission for Europe (forthcoming).
NOTE: The symbol .. indicates not available, not pertinent or not applicable.
[a] Averages not standardized.
[b] Not including Northern Ireland.

TABLE 207. AVERAGE ULTIMATE EXPECTED NUMBER OF CHILDREN, STANDARDIZED BY MARRIAGE DURATION, BY WIFE'S EDUCATION, RESIDENCE AND WORK HISTORY, SELECTED DEVELOPED COUNTRIES

Country	Wife's education — Primary not completed	Primary completed	Lower secondary	Higher secondary	Post-secondary	Residence — Rural	Urban	Wife's work history — Currently working	Not working, worked since marriage	Worked only before marriage or never
Belgium	— 2.17 —		2.29	2.20	2.36	2.35	2.23	2.02	2.38	2.50
Bulgaria	2.84	2.06	1.88	1.84	1.72	2.33	1.98	..	..	..
Czechoslovakia	3.82	2.71	2.47	2.26	2.13	2.63	2.21	2.35	2.60	3.17
Denmark	— 2.46 —		2.29	2.26	2.39	2.57	2.33	..	..	..
Finland	— 2.51 —		2.43	2.41	2.32	2.72	2.34	2.42	2.62	2.91
France	3.01	2.46	2.38	2.35	2.35	2.67	2.48	2.24	2.67	3.03
Hungary[a]	3.43	2.53	2.06	1.91	1.93	2.22	1.95	1.94	2.32	2.61
Italy	3.13	2.42	2.18	2.12	..	2.46	2.32	2.24	2.26	2.63
Norway	— 2.84 —		2.51	2.45	2.42	2.64	2.39	2.42	2.63	2.88
Poland	3.09	2.77	2.40	2.17	2.00	2.97	2.24	2.48	2.53	2.80
Romania	2.41	2.32	2.13	2.03	1.99	2.30	2.14	..	..	..
Spain	3.05	2.70	2.78	2.72	3.03	2.92	2.83	2.59	2.76	2.99
United Kingdom[b]	— 2.55 —		2.32	2.24	2.32	..	..	2.25	2.50	2.69
United States of America	4.03	3.12	2.86	2.60	2.38	..	..	2.39	2.79	3.09

Source: Economic Commission for Europe (forthcoming).
NOTE: The symbol .. indicates not available, not pertinent or not applicable.
[a] Standardized by the country distribution of marriage duration.
[b] Not including Northern Ireland.

similar to those for achieved fertility. Wife's education showed a significant negative association with ultimate expected family size in Eastern Europe, France, Italy and the United States. As in the case of achieved fertility, this relationship was stronger at the low educational levels but became weaker or disappeared at higher levels. In the case of husband's education, the relationship was somewhat weaker than wife's education. As could be anticipated, rural residents expected more children than urban residents. This differential was more important in Eastern Europe (and Finland) than in the Western European countries. Working women everywhere expected fewer children than non-working women, and the strength of this association varied positively with the length of employment since marriage as related to marriage duration (table 207).

Child-spacing

The nature and strength of the relationship between the length of birth intervals and various socio-economic variables varied across countries and within countries across birth intervals. Higher educational levels of wives were found to be associated with a lower level of pre-marital conception and a longer interval between marriage and first birth. Exceptions to this pattern, however, were found in Belgium, Czechoslovakia and Yugoslavia. The positive relationship between the length of first interval and wife's education was much more pronounced in Finland, Norway and the United States than in the other countries included in the analysis (tables 208 and 209). In the case of husband's education, a similar positive relationship was observed for all countries except

Yugoslavia. As concerns the higher-order intervals, frequent and important exceptions to the relationship observed for the first birth interval were found to exist.

In most countries, women whose husbands were employed in white-collar occupations had the longest median number of months from marriage to first birth. The probability of a pre-marital conception was the highest among blue-collar workers in most of the countries. In general, rural women had shorter birth intervals than women living in urban areas. These differences hold in more countries for the second and third intervals than the first interval. The largest difference in the length of first interval by residence was found in Finland. The analytical results clearly suggest that rapid childbearing is associated with low female labour force participation. Women who were working at the time of the survey had their children at longer intervals and had a lower probability of pre-marital conception than other women (table 208).

TABLE 208. MEDIAN NUMBER OF MONTHS BETWEEN MARRIAGE AND FIRST BIRTH, BY WIFE'S EDUCATION, RESIDENCE AND WORK HISTORY, SELECTED DEVELOPED COUNTRIES

Country	Primary not completed	Primary completed	Lower secondary	Higher secondary	Post-secondary	Rural	Urban	Currently working	Not working, worked since marriage	Worked only before marriage or never
Belgium	— 15.8 —		10.5	16.9	..	16.5	16.5	20.4	14.4	10.8
Czechoslovakia	— 16.3 —		14.0	16.0	..	15.3	15.5	15.7	15.9	12.8
Finland	— 10.3 —		12.1	17.6	25.2	11.7	17.2	16.7	14.2	8.2
France	14.8	14.0	16.6	17.0	24.0	15.9	16.7	20.2	13.9	12.5
Hungary	— 10.2 —		13.6	17.4	..	13.4	16.6	17.3	13.3	9.1
Italy	12.6	13.7	15.2	15.1	..	..	..	15.2	16.4	12.4
Netherlands	..	5.6	20.7	26.0	..	18.7	21.8	37.2	22.5	13.5
Norway	..	..	7.4	11.3	23.6	10.1	13.8	14.2	12.0	6.4
Poland	..	10.5	10.6	11.8	15.4	10.6	11.9	11.9	10.5	9.2
Spain	11.8	12.1	12.4	15.1	..	12.3	12.6	14.7	14.5	11.6
United Kingdom[a]	..	..	21.7	31.2	38.9	..	..	36.7	26.1	12.1
United States of America	..	..	14.2	20.9	37.8	..	..	34.6	24.1	1˜5
Yugoslavia	15.1	12.3	— 11.0 —		15.7	..	..	12.6	12.7	14.5

Source: Economic Commission for Europe (forthcoming).
NOTE: The symbol .. indicates not available, not pertinent or not applicable.

[a] Not including Northern Ireland.

TABLE 209. CUMULATIVE PROBABILITY OF A FIRST BIRTH SEVEN MONTHS AFTER FIRST MARRIAGE, BY WIFE'S EDUCATION AND WORK HISTORY, SELECTED DEVELOPED COUNTRIES

Country	Primary not completed	Primary completed	Lower secondary	Higher secondary	Post-secondary	Currently working	Not working, worked since marriage	Worked only before marriage or never
Belgium	— 0.24 —		0.24	0.15	..	0.19	0.23	0.28
Czechoslovakia	— 0.17 —		0.21	0.15	..	0.16	0.20	0.23
Finland	— 0.36 —		0.33	0.25	0.14	0.27	0.28	0.45
France	0.21	0.26	0.21	0.21	0.10	0.17	0.27	0.26
Hungary	— 0.29 —		0.16	0.11	..	0.11	0.15	0.40
Italy	0.12	0.13	0.16	0.12	..	0.12	0.11	0.15
Netherlands	..	0.20	0.15	0.07	..	0.11	0.11	0.21
Norway	..	..	0.49	0.35	0.12	0.32	0.36	0.57
Poland	..	0.30	0.29	0.24	0.18	0.24	0.30	0.37
Spain	0.10	0.11	0.10	0.07	..	0.08	0.12	0.11
United Kingdom[a]	..	..	0.17	0.12	0.03	0.13	0.13	0.24
United States of America	..	..	0.28	0.14	0.07	0.10	0.12	0.18
Yugoslavia	0.14	0.22	— 0.25 —		0.15	0.21	0.25	0.15

Source: Economic Commission for Europe (forthcoming).
NOTE: The symbol .. indicates not available, not pertinent or not applicable.

[a] Not including Northern Ireland.

Contraceptive knowledge and use

European populations appear to be rather homogeneous within countries as far as the knowledge of contraception is concerned. The knowledge of contraceptives that were widely used in the country varied little across socio-economic groups, but there appeared some differences as to the knowledge of uncommon methods. Knowledge of little-used methods was invariably higher among better-educated women and urban residents. In Eastern Europe and Spain, these differences were wider than in other countries. The data indicate that in Eastern Europe and Spain, diffusion of the knowledge of modern contraceptives had not taken place evenly throughout all segments of the society (Economic Commission for Europe, forthcoming, chapter VI).

Moderate but nevertheless significant levels of socio-economic differentials in the incidence of contraceptive use were observed only for some Eastern and Southern European countries (see table 210). Women with low education and women whose husbands worked in agriculture had lower likelihood of using contraception in these countries. There was some evidence that while poorly educated women had lower levels of contraceptive use, they were also more likely to resort to abortion than their counterparts at higher educational levels. There appeared virtually no difference by type of residence in the current use of contraception, except in Spain and Yugoslavia. In Romania, however, rural women had higher levels of contraceptive use than their urban counterparts (Economic Commission for Europe, forthcoming, chapter VI).

The strength of associations between socio-economic characteristics and propensity to utilize modern or traditional methods varied across countries. In Spain, among women practising contraception, the percentage utilizing modern methods was significantly higher for urban than for rural residents. This was also true, to a lesser extent, in Belgium, Bulgaria, Czechoslovakia and Poland. Similarly, large differences by education in the use of modern

TABLE 210. CURRENT USE OF MODERN METHODS OF CONTRACEPTION,[a] BY WIFE'S EDUCATION, RESIDENCE AND WORK HISTORY, SELECTED DEVELOPED COUNTRIES
(*Percentage of all current users*)

Country	Primary or less	Lower secondary	Higher secondary	Post-secondary	Rural	Urban	Currently working	Not working, worked since marriage	Worked only before marriage or never
Belgium	42	49	56	65	33	51	49	51	42
Bulgaria	4	7	6	8	3	6	..	..	..
Czechoslovakia	28	35	40	42	29	40	37	36	39
Denmark	45	53	50	44	44	50	..	..	..
Finland	53	56	59	56	50	59	56	61	46
France	47	52	60	61	48	54	51	55	51
Hungary	56	63	69	61	60	68	55	71	59
Italy	16	27	32	41	21	24	25	27	18
Netherlands	77	78	79	74	74	79	80	79	76
Norway	61	68	67	60	63	70	66	67	65
Poland	8	13	15	20	9	14	12	11	11
Romania	—	1	1	3	1	1	..	..	..
Spain	22	34	47	73	11	31	32	35	23
United Kingdom[b]	55	67	69	61	..	..	65	67	71
United States of America	71	78	68	64	..	..	70	65	72
Yugoslavia	11	—— 17 ——		13	10	13	14	14	10

Source: Economic Commission for Europe (forthcoming).
NOTE: The symbol .. indicates not available, not pertinent or not applicable.
[a] Sterilization, pill, intra-uterine device.
[b] Not including Northern Ireland.

TABLE 211. CURRENT USE OF TRADITIONAL METHODS OF CONTRACEPTION,[a] BY WIFE'S EDUCATION, RESIDENCE AND WORK HISTORY, SELECTED DEVELOPED COUNTRIES
(*Percentage of all current users*)

Country	Primary or less	Lower secondary	Higher secondary	Post-secondary	Rural	Urban	Currently working	Not working, worked since marriage	Worked only before marriage or never
Belgium	51	43	32	22	60	40	41	43	47
Bulgaria	80	79	80	71	90	79	..	..	..
Czechoslovakia	43	41	37	33	46	36	39	38	37
Denmark	4	3	3	2	3	3	..	..	..
Finland	5	3	2	2	5	2	4	3	4
France	43	39	30	24	44	35	38	35	39
Hungary	36	29	22	24	32	23	30	22	32
Italy	68	47	41	30	59	53	54	52	62
Netherlands	10	7	5	6	11	6	4	7	10
Norway	14	10	8	6	10	8	9	9	8
Poland	71	66	62	55	72	62	65	68	66
Romania	87	81	78	79	88	79	..	..	..
Spain	62	44	35	16	75	51	51	51	60
United Kingdom[b]	16	9	5	4	..	..	8	6	6
United States of America	9	8	9	8	..	..	8	9	10
Yugoslavia	77	—— 59 ——		54	9	70	69	72	76

Source: Economic Commission for Europe (forthcoming).
NOTE: The symbol .. indicates not available, not pertinent or not applicable.
[a] Rhythm, withdrawal.
[b] Not including Northern Ireland.

contraceptives were observed only for Spain, Italy and Poland, while Belgium and Czechoslovakia showed moderate differences (table 210). There were no large differences between urban and rural residents as to the use of traditional methods, except in Spain. However, there was a negative association between the use of traditional methods and education in most of the countries, the strongest being in Spain. In Bulgaria and Romania, where women predominantly utilized traditional methods, this relationship was virtually absent (table 211).

Ideal family size

As was pointed out earlier, the average ideal family size in the countries included in the study varied over a very narrow range, which no doubt also reduced the range of variation by socio-economic variables. No strong associations between ideal family size and socio-economic variables were found; the differences in the average number of children for extreme categories rarely exceeded from 0.2 to 0.3. There were indications in some cases that ideal family size was negatively associated with education, size of place of residence and income. Average ideal number of children was generally higher for women whose husbands worked in agriculture than for wives of white-collar workers (Economic Commission for Europe, forthcoming, chapter VII).

D. CONCLUDING REMARKS

It may be argued that although the surveys on which the ECE comparative survey was based were conducted, for the most part, from five to eight years ago, the findings are not likely to be seriously outdated, because no dramatic changes in fertility have since occurred in the countries concerned. It must be recognized, however, that the findings pertain to marital fertility only. In addition, they were based on analytical approaches that emphasized individual characteristics only. In addition, there were problems of inter-country comparability, although these were reduced to manageable limits through efforts at the data-processing stage and, more importantly, because of the emphasis placed on broad associations and differentials. Subject to these qualifications, some generalizations that emerge from the findings are:

(*a*) Low fertility in Europe and the United States of America is characterized by an increasing trend towards the two-child family and a decline in families with four or more children. Low fertility norms are reaching different socio-economic groups within countries: the small differences in expected family size and virtually non-existent differences in ideal family size across social and economic classes testify to this;

(*b*) In these countries, the strategies of family formation and family planning take a variety of shapes but the end result is low fertility;

(*c*) While traditional methods of contraception coexist with modern methods in many parts of Europe, reliance upon modern contraceptives seems to be on the rise. Unplanned and unwanted births are still experienced by many couples in these countries, but the ability to avoid unwanted births has improved over time;

(*d*) Despite the diffusion of low fertility norms and their narrow range, it is not uncommon to observe some differences in fertility and family planning behaviour by social class and level of living. The relationship between education and fertility is a good example: rural residence and low education were often associated with traditional family planning and high fertility, more so in Eastern than in Western Europe. Women's labour force participation among the countries studied was generally found to be incompatible with high fertility. Nevertheless, exceptions to commonly hypothesized relationships are not infrequent. Further research is, however, required to understand the exact mechanisms through which this factor influences fertility, or vice versa;

(*e*) The nature of information on expected fertility involves attitudinal aspects for which validity is not certain. One can speculate, however, that the recent marriage cohorts are going to have smaller average ultimate family size than their predecessors. It may be that this observation has some value because it not only has consistently emerged in these surveys but is consistent with the previous ECE study (United Nations, 1976). The types of changes that are taking place with respect to the status of women in the developed countries also tend to support this speculation. It is clear from the previous discussion that increased urbanization, rising educational standards and increased labour force participation of women are likely to continue to depress fertility in the developed countries;

(*f*) There are a number of socio-economic and policy implications that may be derived from the foregoing discussion:

(i) Given that marital fertility in Europe and the United States is generally just above replacement levels, general fertility is probably destined to be below replacement, which has long-term consequences for the age structure. The societal costs of the aging of the population are just beginning to be realized. The changing structure of the population will be an unprecedented challenge for policy-makers for years to come;

(ii) With rising aspirations, educational opportunities and the decline in time spent in childbearing, the role of women is changing. The family as a social unit still persists, but it is going through major changes in many countries. The conflict between women's roles as workers and as mothers has wide-ranging consequences for the family and the society. Research is needed to understand these effects and policies are required to moderate the potentially adverse influences. Various measures have been enacted in some developed countries to ease this conflict, e.g., through the improvement of child-care facilities and provision of paid leave to care for sick children, but the contribution of such policies is not yet well known. Furthermore, although these policies may be viewed as family-welfare programmes, they are usually geared towards pro-natalist goals. Relatively little attention has been paid to the improvement of the mother's status as a worker;

(iii) If the continued reliance upon traditional methods of contraception in some countries is due to the inaccessibility of alternative methods, then perhaps the provision of a broader range of contraceptives may be considered one of the policy alternatives. With such a provision, the psychosocial costs of contraceptive practice for the couples would be reduced, the occurrences of unwanted and unplanned pregnancies would decline and, perhaps, there would be less reliance upon abortion. On the other hand, the inaccessibility of modern contraceptives would scarcely influence motivations for childbearing, as the evidence is clear that, in developed societies, couples do resort to traditional methods if deprived of access to modern methods.

REFERENCES

Berent, Jerzy (1982). *Family Planning in Europe and USA in the 1970s*. World Fertility Survey Comparative Studies, No. 20; ECE Analyses of WFS Surveys in Europe and USA. Voorburg, The Netherlands: International Statistical Institute.

_____ (1983). *Family Size Preferences in Europe and USA: Ultimate Expected Number of Children*. World Fertility Survey Comparative Studies, No. 26; ECE Analyses of WFS Surveys in Europe and USA. Voorburg, The Netherlands: International Statistical Institute.

_____, Elise F. Jones and M. Khalid Siddiqui (1982). *Basic Characteristics, Sample Design and Questionnaires*. World Fertility Survey Comparative Studies, No. 18; ECE Analyses of WFS Surveys in Europe and USA. Voorburg, The Netherlands: International Statistical Institute.

Economic Commission for Europe (1984). Socio-economic determinants of achieved fertility in some developed countries: a multivariate analysis based on World Fertility Survey data. In *Fertility and Family: Proceedings of the Expert Group on Fertility and Family, New Delhi, 5-11 January 1983*. New York: United Nations, 201-224.
Sales No. E.84.XIII.7.

_____ (forthcoming). *Fertility and Family Planning in the ECE Region: A Comparative Analysis of WFS Surveys*.

Ford, Kathleen (1984). *Timing and Spacing of Births*. World Fertility Survey Comparative Studies, No. 38; ECE Analyses of WFS Surveys in Europe and USA. Voorburg, The Netherlands: International Statistical Institute.

Jones, Elise F. (1982). *Socio-Economic Differentials in Achieved Fertility*. World Fertility Survey Comparative Studies, No. 21; ECE Analyses of WFS Surveys in Europe and USA. Voorburg, The Netherlands: International Statistical Institute.

United Nations (1976). Department of Economic and Social Affairs. Population Division. *Fertility and Family Planning in Europe Around 1970: A Comparative Study of Twelve National Surveys*. Population Studies, No. 58. New York.
Sales No. E.76.XIII.2.

Annex

VARIABLES SELECTED FOR THE ECONOMIC COMMISSION FOR EUROPE COMPARATIVE ANALYSIS

DEPENDENT VARIABLES

A. Achieved fertility
  1. Total number of children ever born
  2. A set of five variables representing the number of live births occurring during successive spans of marriage durations (0-4, 5-9, 10-14, 0-9, 0-14 years)
B. Tempo of family-building process: measures obtained from life-table analysis concerning first three birth intervals were used.
  1. Cumulative probabilities of a birth in the interval by months elapsed since last event (six monthly intervals)
  2. Median number of months until n^{th} birth
  3. First quartile of number of months until n^{th} birth
C. Family planning and unwanted fertility
  1. Knowledge of contraceptive methods
  2. Ever-use of contraceptive methods
  3. Current use of contraceptive methods
  4. Attitudes towards abortion
  5. Incidence of induced abortion
  6. Number of unplanned pregnancies/births
  7. Number of unwanted pregnancies/births
D. Family size preferences and expectations
  1. Ultimate expected number of children
  2. Ideal number of children for a similar couple
  3. Ideal number of children in the country
  4. Preferred/desired number of children (first and second preference)
  5. Number of children wanted at marriage
E. Reproductive motivations
  1. Reasons for not wanting more children
  2. Willingness to change attitude of not wanting more children
  3. Reasons for changing attitude of not wanting more children
  4. Reasons for wanting a large family

INDEPENDENT VARIABLES

A. Demographic variables
  1. Wife's age
  2. Marriage duration
  3. Wife's age at marriage
  4. Marriage cohort
B. Socio-economic characteristics
  1. Type of current residence
  2. Size of current residence
  3. Type of childhood residence
  4. Size of childhood residence
  5. Wife's level of education
  6. Husband's level of education
  7. Husband's socio-occupational status
  8. Wife's religious affiliation
  9. Wife's intensity of religious feeling
  10. Total family income
  11. Husband's income
  12. Wife's income
  13. Number of rooms in dwelling
  14. Wife's work history
  15. Proportion of time wife worked since marriage
  16. Wife's employment status
  17. Wife's occupation
  18. Wife's place of work

XV. A GLOBAL PERSPECTIVE

Abstract

This chapter compares the findings for developed and developing countries with respect to fertility and its determinants, and discusses the contribution of the World Fertility Survey (WFS) data to understanding of the demographic transition. There is a very substantial gap between the average total fertility rate of the most advanced developing countries participating in WFS (4.6) and the developed countries (2.0). Differences in fertility rates between the developed and developing countries become progressively larger with age. Unwanted fertility occurs in both groups but rates are much lower in the developed group. Unwanted fertility appears to be a by-product of the overall process of fertility decline, arising when reproductive experiences lag behind aspirations for fertility control.

Increases in age of marriage have played an important role in fertility decline in the developing countries, in contrast to the historical experience in Europe. Data on breast-feeding, not collected for the developed countries, demonstrate the demographic significance of this practice in the developing countries, particularly in Africa and in Asia and Oceania. While overall levels of contraceptive use are substantially lower in the developing than the developed countries, modern clinic methods are more prominent among the methods used.

Observed differentials in fertility and contraceptive use by residence and education support the diffusion explanation of the demographic transition in which differentials widen in the course of development and then narrow as the small family norm is broadly accepted. The widest differentials were found in the middle range of developing countries. Fertility also appears to be declining more rapidly among the more educated and urbanized groups. Evidence from both developed and developing countries concerning women's employment shows that reduced fertility is primarily associated with work in the modern sector, probably due not only to the effect of work experience on family size desires but to that of women's childbearing experience on the likelihood of working.

Lastly, certain broad conclusions are drawn. First, the importance of development for the fertility transition is strongly confirmed. Secondly, differences in fertility preferences between developing countries at similar levels of development attest to the importance of other societal fertility determinants, such as differences in household organization and institutional arrangements. Thirdly, evidence that population policy has an independent effect was seen not only in the significant role of modern contraceptive methods in many developing countries but in the high levels of contraceptive use achieved by some poor countries with strong family planning programmes. Thus, while WFS data confirm the inevitability of a demographic transition by documenting common patterns and changes occurring across similar socio-economic groups in various settings, they also illustrate that the process has the potential for many variants.

The World Fertility Survey (WFS) was a product of the concern about population growth and the interest in its interrelations with socio-economic development that gathered momentum in the late 1960s and early 1970s. The World Population Conference at Bucharest in 1974 had similar origins. It was anticipated that the provision of survey data for a very wide range of countries, including some for which no type of demographic information had previously been available, would not only greatly enlarge existing knowledge of fertility levels and trends but would lead from this to better understanding of the process of change, its determinants and how they might be manipulated. Expectations with respect to the expansion of descriptive resources were amply realized, extending even to some topics, such as infant mortality, that had not been given much attention. At the level of analysis, however, while significant progress has been made, many of the central questions remain unresolved. The main contribution of WFS in this area has perhaps been to reformulate the issues and to provoke new areas of inquiry.

The theory of the demographic transition as originally laid out by Notestein and others after the Second World War represented a fresh insight into demographic phenomena, the significance of which can scarcely be overestimated. However, it was essentially a descriptive statement that did not specify the mechanisms linking modernization and changes in the vital rates, and it was thus predictive only at the most general level. Much of the effort of demographic analysis during the past 40 years has gone into the attempt to fill this gap, particularly with respect to the determinants of fertility change, the area where the range of feasible policy options appears to be greatest.

At first, research was necessarily concentrated largely on developed countries for which extensive data resources existed, reaching back in some cases well into the past. Census data of reasonable quality were not available for many developing countries, and vital registration statistics were typically even less reliable if there were any at all. A number of important studies were nevertheless carried out, especially dealing with Asia and Latin America. Moreover, the gradual development of sophisticated techniques for the analysis of deficient data made possible a considerable extension of what was known both about the demographic history of developed countries during the pre-transitional and early transitional periods and about current conditions in less developed parts of the world.

Theories about fertility decline, partial theories and new frameworks for analysis emerged. Prominent among these were the threshold hypothesis (United Nations, 1965), the notion of diffusion as a vehicle of change, the identification of intermediate variables through which the effects of social and economic factors on fertility operate (Davis and Blake, 1956) and the household economics model of fertility decisions (Easterlin, 1975, 1978). Much discussion revolved around the relative importance of the means as opposed to the motivation for fertility control. The level of generalization that could be achieved remained limited, however, because some of the world's major populations had not been systematically studied, and the analytical approaches that had been used were extremely varied.

The surge of information emanating from the World Fertility Survey greatly stimulated further development and testing of explanations for fertility change. The project ultimately achieved remarkable geographical scope,[1] and the data were not only generally of good quality but for the most part, highly comparable from country to country (for further discussion, see the Introduction to this report). The types of problems that could be addressed, however, were necessarily defined by the data that were collected. The model questionnaire, including both the high-fertility and the low-fertility variants of the core and the several modules for use at the discretion of individual countries, focused mainly on fertility events themselves and on specific areas of behaviour directly related to childbearing. The inquiry on socio-economic themes representing potential explanatory factors was of a more exploratory nature. Individual characteristics were selected in part on the basis of previously demonstrated association with one or more aspects of fertility and in part for practical reasons, such as the ease of obtaining reliable responses, but probably to a lesser extent because of theoretical considerations. This applied also to the experimental efforts made in some countries to collect background data at the community level. Some of the individual-level surveys in the developed countries went much further in their investigation of potential determinants, but there is very little possibility of comparing the resulting data across countries.

Hence, it is not surprising that, as far as understanding of the fertility process goes, the overall thrust of the WFS findings appears to have reached in two different directions. The first of these is improved understanding of the role of the intermediate variables. Bongaarts (1978, 1982) took advantage of WFS data in developing his model, which permits quantitative evaluation of the relative importance of the principal intermediate variables (proximate determinants). His and other applications of these concepts, carried out partially at WFS, demonstrated that the effects of a given proximate determinant vary greatly in different settings. Recently, the model has begun to be applied to the study of socio-economic differentials in fertility (Casterline and others, 1984). Some intermediate variables, however, notably abortion, were covered less completely or less successfully than others.

While greater appreciation of the "mechanics" underlying the reproductive process is certainly a step forward, progress with respect to the understanding of fertility—the second major theme in the WFS findings—is less evident, at least in terms of the immediate returns realized. The inability to draw from individual-level data more definitive conclusions concerning the social and economic determinants of reproductive behaviour and the causal antecedents of change has proved frustrating. This is to some extent due to the cross-sectional character of the surveys and the limited scope of the questionnaire, but it should not by any means be viewed as a black-and-white situation. The very volume of the data collected in WFS has permitted constructive review of many underlying theoretical issues (Cleland, 1985).

Nevertheless, the shortcomings of WFS appear to have formed part of the impetus for a growing drive to move beyond the individual and the couple to the broader, institutional context within which individuals function. The need was felt within the WFS organization itself, leading to increasing efforts to collect and exploit community-level information in conjunction with the individual-level surveys and, ultimately, to a special seminar on the methodological and theoretical issues associated with such activities (Casterline, 1985). Proceeding in this direction, researchers at the University of Michigan have pioneered a two-stage approach that combines analyses at the macro and micro levels (Hermalin and Mason, 1980; Entwisle and Hermalin, 1984). Other leaders in the field have spoken out insistently concerning the need to focus attention on forces that affect social entities as a whole (e.g., Caldwell, 1982; McNicoll, 1982; Ryder, 1983; Casterline, 1985).

The decision to include not only developing countries but as many developed countries as possible in the WFS programme was a significant one. Coverage of a cross-section of the world's populations, ranging from some of the least advanced to the most advanced countries, provides maximum scope for generalization of the results. The principal purpose of this chapter is to integrate the two sets of findings.

In cross-sectional samples of individuals, differences across the age dimension are often interpreted as representing the experience of a hypothetical cohort over time. But this is misleading if the current status of actual cohorts has been shaped by events that occurred at specific times in the past which successive cohorts experienced at different stages of their lives. A similar situation holds at the macro level, within the WFS sample of countries, with respect to the development dimension. On the one hand, conditions in countries observed at progressively higher levels of development may be indicative of the course of change to come in countries that are currently less advanced. This point of view is implicit in much of the discussion in this chapter. On the other hand, it is important to recognize that contemporary conditions differ in fundamental ways from those prevailing when the currently developed countries were going through the twin processes of modernization and demographic transition. In particular, the technological advances that have occurred at an ever-increasing pace in the developed countries are an integral part of the environment of change in the rest of the world; this will inevitably have some impact on the outcome. In the demographic area, imported public health and medical techniques have brought about far more rapid declines in death rates, and hence higher rates of population growth, in the developing countries, than were ever experienced in the now developed countries. It also seems likely that modern techniques of fertility control are capable of hastening, at least to some extent, the realignment of fertility with mortality.

The discussion in this chapter is based on the comparative studies that were conducted by the United Nations separately for the high-fertility (developing) and the low-fertility (developed) countries. The results of the former study, which was carried out by the Population Division at United Nations Headquarters, are presented in chapters I-IX of this volume. The latter study was the responsibility of the Population Activities Unit of the Economic Commission for Europe (ECE) at Geneva. The final report, which is in the process of publication (Economic Commission for Europe, forthcoming), is briefly summarized here in chapter XIV.

Each of these studies constituted a major undertaking with its own work programme and goals. Because relatively little was known about the developing countries prior to the WFS programme, a very broad analysis was called for. In contrast, the ECE comparative study was designed to address certain specific issues. Fertility and nuptiality are well documented in the regularly published statistics of virtually all of these countries. The main advantages of fertility surveys, with which several countries had already had some considerable experience, are the information they yield on fertility preferences and contraceptive use and the possibility of relating many aspects of fertility behaviour at the individual level to a far wider range of background characteristics than is typically available for other types of data. Hence, participation in WFS and ultimately in the ECE comparative study was looked upon as an opportunity to gain collective insight into the reasons for the prevailing exceptionally low level of fertility as well as likely trends in childbearing for the near future. In order to focus the inquiry as precisely as possible and also for practical reasons, the comparative analysis was restricted to currently married women in their first marriage.

Thus, bringing together the findings of the two studies is not an entirely straightforward matter. The substantive areas of overlap are limited. In some instances, external sources are called upon to supplement the WFS data for the developed countries. The presentation follows the general sequence of the early chapters in this volume, taking up first fertility levels and preferences, then the proximate determinants and lastly socio-economic differentials. The emphasis throughout is on the themes of socio-economic development and family planning programme effort. It is assumed that for each of these purposes the low-fertility countries represent an extension along the continua according to which the developing countries were grouped. While this assumption seems valid for level of development, there is no real counterpart in the more advanced countries of family planning programme effort. In view of the current low level of fertility, none of these Governments favours the further reduction of fertility and some have policies explicitly designed to encourage childbearing. In general, however, contraceptives are widely available and are often subsidized through the regular system of health care, although specific methods may be difficult to obtain, or even illegal, in a given country.

A. Fertility

Levels

When rapid population growth in many parts of the world first became a major focus of attention, it was quickly recognized that the level of fertility provided one of the most reliable means of distinguishing the developed from the developing countries (United Nations, 1963). Since the advent of substantial declines in a number of developing countries, the distribution of countries by level of fertility is no longer as prominently bimodal as was formerly the case. Even so, there is no question that average reproductive performance is much lower in the developed countries participating in WFS than in their counterparts among the developing countries. Among the countries represented in the ECE comparative study, total fertility rates in the year of the surveys ranged from 1.7 in six countries (Belgium, Finland, Italy, Netherlands, United Kingdom, United States of America) to 2.7 in Spain (United Nations, 1985, table 14). For Europe as a whole, the total fertility rate was 2.0 during the period 1975-1980 (United Nations, 1985, table 11), compared with averages based on the WFS data and representing the five-year period preceding the surveys of 6.5 for Africa, 4.9 for Latin America and the Caribbean and 5.7 for Asia and Oceania (see chapter I, table 10). Thus, in the developed countries, each generation was falling slightly short of reproducing itself, while in other parts of the world, the size of succeeding generations was likely to be at least double that of the current generation of parents.

Viewed in the perspective of the country groupings utilized in this report, the developed countries do indeed extend the negative association found for the developing countries between the level of fertility and both level of development and strength of family planning programme effort (taking the overall availability of services as the equivalent of the latter in the developed countries). There is, however, a very substantial gap in the continuum between the average total fertility rate of even the most advanced group of developing countries (4.6) or those with the most active family planning programmes (4.6) (see chapter I, table 11) and that of the developed countries participating in WFS (2.0) (United Nations, 1985, table 14). It is worth noting that the variation within the ECE region is also in line with these relationships; the average total fertility rates in the survey years for WFS countries in Northern and Western Europe, which are more industrialized on the whole and tend to provide greater support for family planning, are lower (1.8 for both subregions) than the corresponding rates for WFS countries in Eastern and Southern Europe (2.3 and 2.2, respectively) (United Nations, 1985, table 14).

Total expected family size is the measure most similar to a total fertility rate that was calculated directly from the survey data for the countries participating in the ECE comparative study. Hungarian women expected the smallest number of children, fewer than 2.1 on average, while Spanish women expected the largest number, an average of 2.8 per woman (Berent, 1983). There are three main reasons that these figures differ from, and usually exceed, the total fertility rates for the survey years: first, they include a substantial component of future childbearing; secondly, they are based only on currently married women in their first marriage, whose fertility is usually higher than that not only of women who never marry but of women who experience marital disruption; and thirdly, they cover births that had taken place over an extended period in the past during which many of these countries underwent rather sharp fertility declines.

Trends

All of the developing countries where the WFS data are considered to be of sufficiently high quality to provide satisfactory measures of trends in fertility display substantial declines over a 10-year period running from about 12.5 years to 2.5 years before the survey (see chapter I, table 16).[2] Among 19 such countries, the total fertility rate dropped by from 1.7 to 4.9 children. In general, the total fertility rate was decreasing in the developed countries also from the late 1960s to the late 1970s (United Nations, 1985a). However, some Eastern European countries where fertility was at a particularly low level around the period 1965-1970 experienced moderate rises in the total fertility rate during the ensuing decade. In contrast, the declines were particularly sharp in Northern and Western European countries. The survey data on total number of children expected by marriage cohort suggest, moreover, that even the upturn in period rates in Eastern Europe is unlikely to be reflected in rises in completed family size (Berent, 1983, table 17).

Age pattern

Shifts in the age pattern of fertility for developing countries at successively higher levels of development were identified in chapter I (figure 3). In moving from the lower to the upper half of the development range represented, absolute declines in the age-specific fertility rates are greatest at the younger ages, where delay in age at marriage is the principal factor. In moving within the upper half of the range, from the middle-high to the high development group, declines at ages 30 and over predominate, reflecting mainly contraceptive use. A somewhat different progression emerged when the countries were grouped by strength of family planning programme effort. Again, rising age at marriage is important in moving from the lower to the upper half of the overall programme effort range. But marked declines for older women are observed between each category and the next higher one, showing the continually increasing impact of contraceptive practice.

The age-specific rates for the developed countries are far lower throughout the reproductive span. The averages for the 16 countries included in the ECE comparative study (as of the respective year of survey) are as follows (United Nations, 1984, table 3):

Age	Rate per 1,000 women
<20	39.7
20-24	141.3
25-29	126.5
30-34	63.9
35-39	24.4
40-44	6.1
45+	0.5

Whether grouped by level of development or strength of family planning programme effort, all categories of the developing countries display the maximum rates throughout the twenties or a peak at ages 25-29. In contrast, the curve for the developed countries peaks at ages 20-24, forming a pattern similar to that of the developing countries characterized by low age at marriage and moderately high contraceptive use. The early peak for the developed countries is mainly due to the influence of the Eastern European countries, where marriage occurs relatively early. In most of the rest of the developed countries reviewed, the curve is quite flat across the twenties, but particularly in Southern Europe, there may be a late peak at ages 25-29. The relative difference between the developing and the developed countries as a whole becomes much larger as age increases, and throughout the greater part of the age span the primary factor depressing the rates in the developed countries is undoubtedly contraception. In advanced societies, contraception is regularly used to postpone the first birth and to space later births, as well as to limit ultimate family size. These points are elaborated upon further in section B of this chapter, in the discussion of proximate determinants of fertility, including nuptiality and contraception.

Childlessness

The proportion of married women who reach the end of their childbearing years without ever having a live birth can be taken as an indicator of the prevalence of childlessness. Roughly comparable WFS information on this topic exists from the surveys in the developing and developed countries. In the developing countries, the proportion of currently married women aged 30-44 and married for at least a total of five years who were reported as never having had a fertile pregnancy ranged from below 2 per cent (Bangladesh, Ecuador, Malaysia, Mexico, Panama, Peru, the Philippines, the Republic of Korea and Thailand) to 10 per cent (Cameroon) (see chapter I, table 22). Among the developed countries, the range in the proportion of currently married women aged 40-44 and still in their first marriage who had not had a live birth is somewhat narrower, from 3 per cent (Poland) to 7 per cent (Belgium) (Economic Commission for Europe, forthcoming, chapter IV). Although the measure used for the developed countries implies more continuous exposure to the risk of childbearing than that used for the developing countries, the mode in the developed countries is 6 per cent, while in almost three quarters of the developing countries, the proportion lies between 2 and 4 per cent.[3] The very low figures for many of the developing countries probably reflect data problems, e.g., age-misreporting and the tendency of older women to fail to report some births, especially those of children who may have died very young (Vaessen, 1984). In general, childlessness in developing countries is taken to represent primary infecundity, and it tends to be highest in Western Africa and the Caribbean.

Among the countries participating in the ECE comparative study, the proportion childless in Poland may approximate the level of primary infecundity in a country with modern health services. The proportions observed in such countries as Belgium, Denmark, France, the United Kingdom (England, Scotland and Wales) and the United States of America, which are about twice as high as that of Poland, thus probably contain an almost equal component of voluntary childlessness. Given the extent to which fertility is controlled in developed societies, it seems remarkable that relatively few women choose to forgo childbearing altogether. Both for the developed and for the developing countries, these data of course represent the reproductive performance of a generation ago, and the results may be different when women who were in their prime childbearing years at the time of the surveys reach the end of their reproductive life.

Unwanted births

The issue of unwanted fertility is particularly important in policy questions. In principle, the practice of family planning brings down fertility by enabling couples to avoid childbearing beyond the number of children they actually want. Thus, as control over reproduction is established, not only should there be fewer births but the proportion of all births reported as unwanted should diminish. The level of unwanted fertility was found to vary widely among the developing countries that participated in the WFS programme. For Africa, Latin America and the Caribbean, and Asia and Oceania, the total unwanted fertility rates were 0.5, 1.0 and 0.9, respectively; the respective proportions of the total fertility rate were 8, 21 and 16 per cent (see chapter II, table 41).[4] Contrary to expectation, the unwanted total fertility rate was higher both in the more developed of these countries and in those with relatively strong family planning programme effort (chapter II, table 42). Moreover, as development and programme effort increase, the wanted component of the total fertility rate drops sufficiently to bring down the total fertility rate itself, and hence the proportion of total fertility that is unwanted rises. Other research in this area has resulted in similar findings (Westoff, 1978; Retherford and Palmore, 1983).

The data collected in developed countries indicate that unwanted births have by no means disappeared, even in the context of very low overall fertility. Among eight countries, the proportion of children ever born that were reported as unwanted ranged from 2 to 11 per cent (chapter XIV, table 202). These proportions are much lower than those based on the total fertility rates for developing countries given above but they are not comparable because they reflect, on average, the mid-point of the childbearing years; and births considered unwanted are more likely to occur later. The period measure of unwanted fertility used for the developing countries represents experience over the full range of reproductive ages. It nevertheless remains true that the unwanted birth rates per woman would be very much lower in the developed than the developing countries because the overall level of fertility is so much lower.

The implications of these findings are of some interest. Longer exposure to the risk of unwanted childbearing is an inevitable concomitant of reduction in the numbers of births that are wanted. More importantly, however, the persistence of a significant element of unwanted fertility when reproduction has reached replacement level, along with higher proportions of births that are unwanted among the more advanced than among the less advanced developing countries, and also among those where there is more rather than less family planning activity, indicate that unwanted fertility may be a by-product of the overall process of fertility decline itself. To the extent that actual reproductive experience lags behind aspirations for fertility control generated by modernization and the available means of family planning, unwanted births can apparently result at any stage in this process.

B. PROXIMATE DETERMINANTS

Nuptiality

Marriage has traditionally been taken as an indicator of the initiation of exposure to intercourse, which is, of course, the reason that its study is important in relation to fertility. In the Western countries that were for a long time the almost exclusive source of data for demographic analysis, childbearing before marriage was sufficiently small that it could safely be ignored for most purposes. This is no longer the case in Western countries and certainly does not apply on a world-wide basis. In so far as possible, the ECE comparative study utilized a definition of marriage that included regular cohabitation on an informal basis as well as legal union. Similarly, for the participating developing countries, a flexible approach was adopted with the aim of including all unions of a stable character. In the present discussion, marriage can be taken as having this broad and somewhat imprecise meaning.

In many of the currently developed countries, changes in marriage patterns, and consequently the effect of nuptiality on fertility, were quite different during the period of demographic transition from the changes associated with fertility decline in some currently developing countries. Deliberate control of reproduction first became established in north-western Europe, typically during the latter part of the nineteenth century. There, childbearing was already restrained to a considerable degree by customs of late marriage and high proportions of women remaining single throughout their reproductive years (Hajnal, 1965). Along with the decline in marital fertility due to the adoption of birth control practices, the proportions of women who were married generally rose. This exerted upward pressure on the birth rates, although it was by no means sufficient to counterbalance the effect of control of fertility within marriage. Only recently has the average age at first marriage again moved upward; meanwhile, rates of separation and divorce have also tended to rise sharply, lowering the proportions of women living in a sexual union at older ages. The impact of these latter trends on fertility is reduced, however, by the increasing likelihood of sexual exposure among unmarried women.

Around the time of the 16 surveys taken in developed countries, a little less than half of the women aged 20-24 were married, about 7 per cent remained single at ages 45-54, and the singulate mean age at marriage was just over 22 (table 212) (United Nations, forthcoming). These averages hide substantial differences among the subregions of Europe. For instance, two thirds of women aged 20-24 were married in Eastern Europe but less than half were in both Northern and Southern Europe.

TABLE 212. SELECTED MARRIAGE INDICATORS FOR EUROPE: SUBREGIONAL AVERAGES

Subregion	Percentage of women single at ages 20-24	Percentage of women single at ages 45-54	Female singulate mean age at marriage[a]
Europe	46.1	6.8	22.2
Eastern Europe	34.8	3.9	21.4
Northern Europe	55.9	7.6	23.1
Southern Europe	51.5	10.1	22.3
Western Europe	44.8	7.8	22.0

Source: Economic Commission for Europe (forthcoming).
[a] As defined in chapter III of the present volume.

As pointed out in chapter III, women in developing countries tend to marry relatively early and marriage is nearly universal (see table 43). Current experience is nevertheless quite varied, on a regional as well as a country-by-country basis. Especially in Asia and Oceania, age at marriage is sometimes as high as or higher than that prevailing in Europe.

Both the trend towards later age at marriage in developing countries (tables 44 and 45) and the cross-sectional negative association of nuptiality with level of development and strength of family planning programme effort in these countries (table 43) indicate that, in contrast to the historical experience of north-western Europe, falling proportions married are now playing an important role in fertility decline. Analysis of the effects of the principal proximate determinants on fertility likewise shows that nuptiality imposes a greater restraint on fertility at higher than at lower levels of development; it thus reinforces the restraint of contraception which shifts in the same direction, although the change in its fertility impact across the four levels of development is roughly one half that of contraception (chapter VI, table 86).

Because of variation in the length of exposure to the risk of childbearing, a negative relationship would be expected between age at marriage and ultimate family size, everything else being equal. In societies where fertility is highly controlled, however, the effects of differences in exposure should be minimal, since even women who marry relatively late are likely to have sufficient time to equal the low reproductive performance of those who marry earlier. Age at marriage is nevertheless associated with a number of social and economic factors that also influence fertility. In the ECE study, evidence of both preferences for fewer children among women who marry late and selection into very early marriage of women who are predisposed towards higher fertility was found (Economic Commission for Europe, forthcoming, chapter IV). On the other hand, in the developing countries it was observed that although the total marital fertility rate was indeed greater for women who married before age 20 than for women who married later, the latter group actually made up in part for its late start by higher rates of childbearing after marriage (chapter III, table 52). Thus, in developing countries, women who experienced early marriage may be more likely than others to control fertility later. A similar pattern has been noted for some European populations in the pre-transitional period (Blake, 1985).

Breast-feeding and post-partum abstinence

As discussed in the introduction to this chapter, full appreciation of the role of breast-feeding and other forms of behaviour tending, in the absence of contraception, to delay the next conception following a birth has awaited the advent of WFS data. This factor has proved to be particularly important in Africa, a region for which few demographic data had been available. In Africa as a whole, and also in countries falling into the low or middle-low development groups, as well as in countries where family planning programme effort is weak or non-existent, the restraint on fertility imposed by post-partum infecundability associated with breast-feeding is greater than that imposed either by marriage or contraception (chapter VI, table 86). The realization that fertility might actually rise during the early stages of modernization if declines in breast-feeding induced by urbanization and changes in women's activity patterns were not balanced by increases in contraceptive use or reductions in marital exposure represents a major new insight in the field. The WFS data available on these topics are nevertheless very limited; relatively few of the surveys included questions on amenorrhoea, post-partum sexual abstinence or full and partial breast-feeding.

Apart from the paucity of data, one reason that the potential impact of breast-feeding may have not been fully appreciated heretofore is that in pre-transitional Europe it appears to have had less dampening effect than nuptiality on fertility and also less than in many developing countries today (Bongaarts, 1982). Although breast-feeding is reported to have increased during the 1970s in several developed countries (McCann and others, 1981), both the proportion of infants breast-fed at first and the duration of breast-feeding apparently are currently very much lower than in the vast majority of developing countries (McCann and others, 1981). No questions on breast-feeding were included in the recommended WFS questionnaire for use in low-fertility countries.

Contraception

Fertility decline may be assisted by changes in marriage patterns or by maintenance of customs of lengthy breast-feeding, but to achieve and sustain low levels of reproduction, efficient practice of birth control is essential. Both in the developed and in the developing countries, a central purpose of WFS was to document knowledge and use of contraception. Since the WFS staff were actively involved in the questionnaire design phase of the surveys in developing countries, it was possible to achieve a high degree of conformity with the recommended model and hence good comparability of the results. This holds less well for the countries participating in the ECE study, where the execution of the surveys was entirely the responsibility of the countries themselves, and there are some significant differences both in underlying concepts and definitions and in the ways the data were treated during the initial processing stages. These differences relate even to such important topics as current use of a method, contraceptive sterilization and exposure to the risk of conception.

Since fertility control has been well established throughout Europe for a considerable period of time, it is not surprising that knowledge of at least one method of contraception is virtually universal (chapter XIV, table 202). Knowledge of any method is currently as high, or almost as high in many developing countries, particularly those in Latin America and the Caribbean and some in Asia and Oceania, but simple lack of awareness of any method still presents a major obstacle to use in most African and a few Asian countries (chapter V, table 74).

Confining attention to those surveys in developed countries for which the data on current use of contraception appear to be reasonably comparable (Belgium (Flemish population only), Bulgaria, Finland, France, Hungary, Norway, Poland, Romania, Spain, the United Kingdom (England and Wales) and the United States of America), the proportion of married women who were using a method varies from a little over half (Romania, Spain) to four fifths or more (Belgium, Finland) (chapter XIV, table 202; United Nations, 1984a, table 3).[5] Although there are three developing countries where prevalence overlaps the lower end of this range (Costa Rica, Panama, Trinidad and Tobago), by and large there is a substantial gap between the developed and the developing countries (chapter V, table 74). Even in countries that fall into the high development group (I) and in those where the family planning programme effort is strong, scarcely more than two fifths of currently married women reported use of a method at the time of the survey.

It was pointed out in chapter V that the distribution of methods used differs substantially among the developing countries. Thus, there is little to be gained from discussing average levels of use or individual methods or typical distribution patterns. This is also true in the developed countries, and again, availability as well as various dimensions of acceptability, including perceived effectiveness, safety, convenience and ethics, can be assumed to play some part in determining the choice of specific methods. Moreover, in those developed countries where contraception was widely practised before the advent of clinic methods (male and female sterilization, pill, intra-uterine device (IUD)), certain of the older conventional methods (condom, withdrawal) are still relied upon by many couples, and their use follows a distinct regional pattern.

In Northern and Western Europe, from approximately half to two thirds of all contraceptive users were employing one of the modern clinic methods (Berent, 1982; United Nations, 1984a). The proportion tends to be much lower in Southern and Eastern Europe, where the availability of one or more of these methods is often restricted. Among the supply methods, diaphragm, foam etc. were not being used by many women except in the United States, but the condom remained a popular method employed by from about one quarter to two fifths of all couples in Northern Europe and in the Netherlands; thus, when the WFS classification of modern methods is used (clinic and supply methods combined), these particular countries rank very high. Interestingly, however, in the remaining countries, i.e., Eastern Europe, Southern Europe, France and Belgium, where more reliance was traditionally placed upon withdrawal than upon the condom, withdrawal continued to play a significant role. Among the developed countries as a group, the rhythm method is of minor importance except in Poland and to a lesser extent, in Belgium. Few of these countries included abstinence in their roster of methods, and it is highly unlikely that its use would assume any significance as compared, for instance, with parts of Africa.

Modern clinic methods are currently more prominent in the distributions of methods used in most developing countries than they are in many developed countries (United Nations, 1984a). In this respect, the developing countries might be thought of as being in the more advanced position. This reflects the fact that fertility control practices are becoming established in the developing countries at a time when contraceptive technology has progressed significantly; more choices are available and among them the clinic methods are likely to be not only the most effective but the easiest to use. Hence, particular family planning programmes have often stressed one or more of them. There may, nevertheless, be real differences between the two groups of countries in the efficacy with which any given method is used. Even so, the emphasis on these methods no doubt contributes to the rapid rise in the impact of contraception on fertility, from a proportional reduction of nearly zero in the least developed countries and those with minimal family planning activity to around 35 per cent in the more advanced developing countries and those with a strong family planning programme (chapter VI, table 86).

The pattern of current contraceptive use according to family size appears to vary according to the overall level of contraceptive use in the country. Instances of lower levels of use for larger than for moderate family sizes are more common where the general level of contraceptive use is fairly high. In developed countries, the level of current contraceptive use is typically greatest for women with a moderate number of children, usually two children. This is also the case in Latin America and the Caribbean, where the level of use is usually at or near its maximum for women with two children, whereas in Asia and Oceania, it is more common for use levels to peak at three or four children. In countries where use levels are low (including most of Africa), the proportion using contraceptive increases steadily through the larger family sizes. The average pattern for 10 developed countries around 1970 is compared in figure 81, with patterns for several developing countries which illustrate the range of patterns described above. The curve for Costa Rica is quite similar in level and shape to that for the developed countries except that childless women in the developed countries show a higher level of use.

Lower levels of contraceptive use at the higher parities may result partially, and perhaps entirely, from the effects of contraceptive use on the distribution of women by parity. To the extent that contraception is effective, users tend to remain at low or moderate parities, while women who do not adopt contraception—whether out of a desire for a large family or because of ignorance about, aversion to or lack of access to family planning services—progress to higher parities. Especially in societies where a large proportion of women use contraception effectively, the women who are found at the higher parities are quite an atypical group, selected for their failure or unwillingness to control fertility.

Abortion

Voluntary abortion was not covered in the comparative analysis of the proximate determinants of fertility in developing countries mainly because relatively few of the surveys included direct questions on abortion. Moreover, abortion data from other sources are deficient or entirely lacking for most of the developing countries. Careful review of the information that does exist suggests that abortion, whether legal or illegal, is practised virtually everywhere; and in many countries, it is probably sufficiently common to have an appreciable effect on fertility (Tietze, 1983; David, 1983). As pointed out in chapter VI, omission of abortion from the analysis of the proximate determinants means that the estimates of the total fecundity rate are biased downward in varying degrees.

Figure 81. Percentage of currently married women currently using contraception, by number of living children: selected developing and developed countries

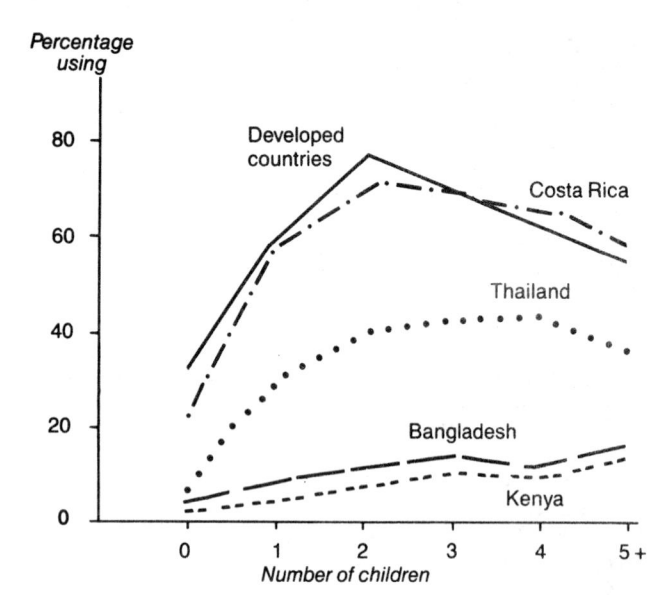

Sources: United Nations (1976) and World Fertility Survey standard recode tapes.

NOTE: Average for 10 developed countries around 1970: Belgium; Czechoslovakia; Denmark; Finland; France; Hungary; Poland; United Kingdom (England and Wales); United States of America; Yugoslavia.

More than half of the surveys covered in the ECE comparative study, including all of those in Eastern European countries, called for the reporting of abortions as a part of the pregnancy history. Even in Eastern Europe, however, where abortion had been legal and, typically, widely available for many years, the results appear for the most part to provide serious underestimates (Economic Commission for Europe, forthcoming). Elsewhere, the completeness of reporting was even worse. Thus, for reasons that are not entirely obvious, the survey instrument appears so far to be unsuccessful as a means of collecting abortion data. On the other hand, published abortion statistics based on medical records are available for quite a few low-fertility countries where abortion is legal. The reported abortion ratios in Europe and the United States in the late 1970s range from below 10 per 100 known pregnancies in the Netherlands to nearly 50 in Bulgaria and Romania (Tietze, 1983, table 2). The relatively high abortion rates and ratios found generally in Eastern Europe are almost certainly a function not only of greater acceptance of abortion as a means of fertility control but of far less reliance upon the modern clinical methods of contraception.

Bongaart's schematic presentation of changes in the relative importance of the major proximate determinants during the course of the fertility transition shows abortion coming into play relatively late in the process and growing in significance (Bongaarts, 1982). However, this may reflect mainly the availability of data. A rather different view is offered by David (1983), who suggests that as contraceptive practice improves, resort to abortion can be expected to decline but not disappear.

C. SOCIO-ECONOMIC DIFFERENTIALS

The diffusion explanation of the process of adoption of fertility control practices suggests that socio-economic differentials in reproductive behaviour within a society, which might well be minimal at first, will emerge and widen for a certain time but subsequently begin to narrow, dwindling to little importance as the small family norm is universally accepted. The characteristics of individuals and couples according to which the greatest contrast would be expected during the transitional period are those indicative of opportunity for direct participation in the modernization process. The results of the WFS data can be interpreted to conform, at least in a very general way, to this pattern. In both the developed and the developing countries, an identical cluster of socio-economic characteristics (residence, education and women's employment) attracted the most attention. Each of these characteristics represents a spectrum not only with respect to participation in the development process but with respect to exposure to new ideas and behaviour patterns.

The approaches to the analysis of differentials that were used in the two sets of countries differed considerably. In principle, the effects of any socio-economic factor on fertility must operate through one or more of the proximate determinants. Since contraception, however, is the only one of these variables that was explicitly covered in both studies, the discussion here is confined to differentials in fertility itself and in contraceptive use. In addition, the dependent variables were not the same and the use of demographic controls differed. The independent variables were also classified differently, although every effort was made to be consistent within each of the two sets of countries. Both comparative studies incorporated some multivariate analysis, but they were quite dissimilar in their overall strategy and procedures. For these and other reasons, only very superficial comparisons of the results are possible.

The methodology used in the comparative study of socio-economic differentials in fertility and contraceptive use for the developing countries is discussed in detail in chapters VII-IX of this report. A brief description of the approach to these topics that was used in the ECE comparative study covering the developed countries is included here as background for the comparisons made in this section because it is not included in chapter IV of this report. Complete details are given in chapters IV and VI of the final report of the ECE study (Economic Commission for Europe, forthcoming). As previously mentioned, the entire study was limited to once-married women in their first marriage. The principal measure of fertility is the number of children ever born (achieved fertility). Averages standardized by duration of marriage are presented for categories of an extensive range of independent variables; and in some cases, cross-tabulations by two or more variables are included. Multiple classification analysis was used for the multivariate analysis of fertility. Marriage duration and age at marriage were introduced as controls (both in the form of categorical variables). The main focus is on three independent variables: wife's level of education; type of place of current residence; and wife's work history. Husband's level of education and socio-occupational status are also considered. The level of contraceptive use is variously measured, based on all respondents; respondents exposed to the risk of pregnancy, excluding contraceptively sterilized women; or exposed respondents, including those contraceptively sterilized. The relative importance of individual methods and classes of methods is evaluated in relation to all users, including the contraceptively sterilized. No multivariate analysis of contraceptive use was carried out.

Residence

Fertility was found to be higher in rural than in urban areas in all regions and also at all levels of development and of family planning programme effort (chapter VII, table 96; chapter XIV, table 206). This relationship between size of place of residence and fertility is usually monotonically negative when the rural-urban continuum is further broken down for the developed countries (Economic Commission for Europe, forthcoming). More detailed data are not available for the developing countries. Within the group of developing countries, it can be seen that the widening of fertility differentials at successively higher levels of development for the first three development groups is due to the declining level of fertility in urban areas. Differentials for the high development group (I) are somewhat smaller mainly because of lower levels of rural fertility. Moreover, residence differentials in fertility for current period rates are larger than differentials observed in the achieved parity of older women (40-49) primarily because of declines over time in urban fertility. The residence differential in fertility is small in most of the countries participating in the ECE study, and comparison with earlier surveys in some of these countries suggests that it has remained stable or declined (Economic Commission for Europe, forthcoming). Control for wife's education in a multivariate framework reduces the effect of residence in both developed and developing countries, as would be expected due to the association of residence and education, although it usually does not eliminate it entirely (Economic Commission for Europe, forthcoming, chapter IV; and chapter VII, table 106, in the present report).

One reason for the differential in fertility in the developing countries is certainly the greater propensity to use contraception in urban areas (chapter VII, table 97). It is interesting to note that when countries are grouped according to the strength of family planning programme effort within levels of development, the results show that, within development groups, countries with stronger family planning programmes tend to have higher proportions using contraception than countries with weaker programmes. In addition, while relatively small rural/urban differentials in use levels are found in countries with weaker programmes at low levels of development and in countries with stronger programmes at high levels of development, larger differentials are found in countries that fall between these two extremes. In contrast, no real difference by residence was found in the proportions of exposed women using some method of contraception in the developed countries[6] (Berent, 1982). Urban contraceptors in these countries were, nevertheless, somewhat more likely to be using modern, clinic methods than rural women (chapter XIV, table 210).

Education

It has frequently been pointed out that the effect of education on fertility has numerous potential meanings. Education *per se* may affect childbearing through the substantive knowledge imparted. More likely, the communication skills acquired, in particular the ability to read, may significantly alter the individual's conceptual frame of reference. Education may also convey the influence of residence, income or socio-economic status or be jointly determined with variables of this type. In addition, women's education is often taken as an indicator of the opportunity costs of childbearing. It is no doubt in part because of these multiple possible links that education emerges so consistently as an important variable in the analysis of fertility-related behaviour. However, it has practical advantages for analytical purposes as well in that it is usually fixed for any given individual before childbearing begins and remains stable throughout adult life, while most other socio-economic indicators are subject to change during the course of the childbearing years.

The observed patterns of association are, nevertheless, quite varied. The presentation in chapter VIII argues that, among developing countries, the shape of the relationship changes systematically with modernization (figure 54). The association is, in general, negative; but the educational range where this effect becomes pronounced tends to shift from the upper towards the lower end of the distribution as development progresses, and in the least developed countries, women with just a few years of education often bear more children than those with no education. This concurs with the conclusions of other analyses of the socio-economic determinants of fertility based on WFS data (Rodríguez and Cleland, 1980) and indeed with more general reviews of findings concerning this relationship (Cochrane, 1983). The circumstances in which the anomalous positive association is found suggest a situation where upward pressure on fertility due to reduced breast-feeding, and perhaps to change in other unmeasured intermediate variables, outweighs the effect of possible initial efforts to use contraception.

According to the formulation given in chapter VIII, the shape of the relationship between fertility and education that would be expected in the most developed countries calls for a moderate decline in fertility from the lower to the middle or upper middle levels of education and then a flattening out or an upturn at the highest levels of education. Here, the emergence of a positive association between education and fertility would be accounted for by the link between education and wealth; everything else being equal, couples for whom the financial restraints are least should be most free to have children. It must be emphasized that the range of educational achievement represented in developed populations overlaps that of the developing countries to a very limited extent; the only categories that can be considered approximately equivalent are the lower end of the distribution for developed countries (primary school not completed and primary school completed) and the top category of the distributions for developing countries (seven or more years of education). In terms of the schematic presentation in figure 54, the line representing the relationship between education and fertility for the most advanced of these countries not only should fall considerably below the next line above it but should be shifted well to the right (United Nations, 1983).

The results shown in chapter VIII generally support the hypothesized relationships for the developing countries, with fertility differentials by education tending to be small and non-monotonic in the least developed countries and larger and monotonic in the more developed. In many of the poorer countries, fertility of women with some education is higher than women with no education. A comparison of current period rates with achieved parity of older women by educational group suggests that differentials have been widening over time in the least developed countries because of declines in fertility among relatively more educated women (with seven or more years of education). No declines are apparent among women with less education in these countries. In the more developed countries, fertility appears to have declined more evenly across the educational groups. Thus, for most countries, the fertility differentials tend to be larger for recent fertility than for cumulative fertility. However, it should be pointed out that while certain patterns can be observed across countries in fertility differentials, levels of fertility vary widely across countries for women with similar levels of education. Uneducated women in some countries have lower fertility than highly educated women in others.

The results of the ECE comparative study are very much in line with this expectation (chapter XIV, table 206). A negative association between the level of education of the respondent and children ever born is evident in all but one of the 15 countries examined. The differences are more pronounced at the lower than at the upper end of the education scale (which includes secondary school and college), and they are larger overall in countries where there are still many women who had not completed secondary school (Economic Commission for Europe, forthcoming, chapter III). The picture is very similar for husband's education, with the additional twist that at the upper end of the education scale, fertility shows a clear tendency to rise with education among urban residents and especially among men whose wives were also well educated (Economic Commission for Europe, forthcoming, chapter IV).

In all cases, the impact of wife's education on fertility diminishes when other socio-economic factors are controlled. In the developing countries, fertility differentials between extreme educational groups become smaller and fewer countries show statistically significant differences by respondent's education when residence, husband's occupation and education are controlled. The impact of other variables has the greatest effect in reducing differentials in the most developed countries, indicating that the fertility effects of education are more strongly interlinked with woman's work and husband's education. The effects of education usually remain important in the multivariate analysis for the developed countries, in terms both of statistical significance and of size of differentials; but in the ECE analysis husbands' education was not controlled and, given the high intercorrelation between husbands' and wives' education, these results are not comparable with those for the developing countries.

The proportion of women in developing countries that use some method of contraception appears to increase monotonically with number of years of education in all regions, at all levels of development and for all degrees of family planning programme effort (chapter VIII, table 122). Within each educational level, contraceptive use increases steadily with level of development. While the slope of the relationship is less steep in Asia and Africa than in Latin America and the Caribbean and in the lower compared with the upper levels of development, the lines are roughly parallel for all strengths of family planning programme effort, suggesting that, as was found for rural women, the presence of such programmes may raise the level of use among women with little or no education above what it might otherwise have been. The evidence also supports the conclusion that the relatively high fertility of women with from one to three years of education in countries just starting along the path to development is not due to lower levels of contraceptive use but must be attributed to some of the other proximate determinants discussed above. In the developed countries, the proportions of non-sterilized, exposed women using a reversible method of contraception tends to be positively associated with education as well, although the differences are usually small and are often limited to the lower portion of the education scale (Economic Commission for Europe, forthcoming). Among contraceptors, reliance upon modern clinic methods rises sharply with education mainly in countries where there is a strong influence of Roman Catholicism (Belgium, Czechoslovakia, France, Italy, Poland and Spain) (chapter XIV, table 210).

Women's employment

The situation with respect to women's employment is considerably more complex than either residence or education, as concerns both measurement of the phenomenon of interest and the nature of the link(s) with fertility that might be expected. The problems connected with the WFS data on women's economic activity obtained from the surveys in developing countries are reviewed in chapter IX. Many of the same issues arise in connection with the data for the developed countries, and there is the additional complication of far greater diversity in the questions asked and in the initial treatment of the data (Economic Commission for Europe, forthcoming). The usual hypothesis relating women's employment to fertility has been that, because of competition for time and personal resources, women who work will have fewer children than those who do not work. Independently of this effect, some types of employment may also result in exposure to innovative ideas and behaviour patterns. As a practical matter, however, it has proved extremely difficult to sort out cause and effect; and, moreover, the possibility of positive as well as negative relationships cannot be ignored. For instance, failure to find hypothesized negative effects of employment on fertility, or weak evidence of such effects, might in some circumstances be due to women going out to work to support their families, a countervailing positive effect of fertility on work.

The results of the multivariate analysis presented in chapter IX indicate that women who have worked in a modern type of occupation since marriage, that is, one typically requiring absence from home and a certain amount of human capital investment, have lower achieved fertility than women who have not been economically active; and this differential increases as the level of socio-economic development of the country rises (chapter IX, figure 72). Work in transitional and mixed occupations also is associated with reduced childbearing once at least an intermediate level of development has been reached. On the other hand, employment in a traditional occupation, which may go on at home and involve few special skills, is not related consistently to fertility at any level of development. The difference in births between women with no recorded work and those who work in modern occupations is also likely to increase as the national level of family planning programme effort rises (chapter IX, figure 74). Although the observations for individual countries vary considerably, it appears that the expected negative association between childbearing and employment since marriage is tied in with change in socio-economic structure and the opening-up to women of occupations in which the obligations, and presumably also the rewards, are significantly greater than in those previously available.

A number of facets of women's employment were examined in the ECE study. Women who were currently employed invariably had fewer children than those who were not working, and almost always women who had never worked had the most children (chapter XIV, table 206).[7] The strength of the current employment relationship overshadowed that of all the other variables included in the multivariate analysis for the developed countries (Economic Commission for Europe, forthcoming, chapter IV). Women who reported themselves as employees had generally had relatively few births, particularly compared with paid family workers. Similarly, the fertility of white-collar workers was usually low and that of women engaged in farm-related activities was usually high. Full-time work was consistently associated with lower childbearing than part-time work, but women who worked away from home had had fewer births than those working at home only in the Northern and Western European countries for which the information was available and not in those in Southern and Eastern Europe. In general, these findings are compatible with the conclusion drawn from the analysis for the developing countries, that reduced fertility is primarily associated with work in the modern sector. On this basis, it seems likely that differentials related to women's employment will be prominent in most parts of the world for some time to come.

Results from the developing countries with respect to the relationship between current contraceptive use and current occupational status confirm concerns posed earlier with respect to the causal chain underlying the observed negative relationship between work in the modern sector and fertility. If work in the modern sector provided an inducement for fertility limitation, a positive relationship between current modern work and current contraceptive use would be expected. While such a positive relationship is observed for most countries even after other socio-economic factors were controlled, it is not usually statistically significant. In addition, the strength and direction of the relationship does not appear to be associated with the level of development, as was the case when fertility differentials were analysed. The inevitable conclusion is that the observed negative relationship between fertility and work in the modern sector may be at least partially explained by the effect of achieved fertility on the likelihood of work. Even in societies with relatively high overall levels of contraceptive use, fertility at the individual level is subject to a significant chance component which can play a role in shaping the type of work experience a woman ultimately develops. Unfortunately, variation in the overall proportions of women currently using a method of contraception according to respondent's employment were not examined in the ECE study. Among contraceptors, however, no consistent pattern was found by wife's work history in the likelihood of using a modern, clinic method (chapter XIV).

D. Conclusion

The preceding comparison of fertility survey data from a sample of developing and developed countries presents a broad picture of concurrent fertility behaviour across the major regions and subregions of the world which is representative of almost the full range of current demographic experience.[8] Although a few of the developing countries included in the sample have contraceptive prevalence that overlaps the range of prevalence observed for the developed countries, the differences between the less and more developed regions of the world in reproductive behaviour remain large in almost all respects, as do important characteristics of the country settings, such as income per capita and educational levels of the population. Change is occurring, however, and this is documented from these samples through the retrospective birth histories as well as through comparisons of the characteristics and behaviour of different birth cohorts within each country. The effects of modernization are clearly reflected in the survey findings. Levels of education are rising, age of marriage is rising and breast-feeding durations are falling. In addition, modern contraceptive methods represent the major means of family planning today in the developing countries, even in the least developed.

The question posed in the introduction of this book related to the relative importance of development, geography and policy in the demographic transition. Although specific causal relationships cannot be identified, given the cross-sectional nature of the data, associations between all three of these macro-level variables and various aspects of reproductive behaviour have been observed for the developing countries, many of which are currently undergoing a demographic transition. The developed countries, which have completed the demographic transition, underwent that process in a northern setting over a long historical period without any deliberate government intervention designed with population policy goals in mind. The absence of government population policy and the unique geographical setting guarantee that the current situation observed among the developed countries cannot be assumed to represent the exact end-point of the process now under way in many of the developing countries observed in this report. While development has been found to be a strong differentiator of reproductive behaviour, many of the findings from the developing countries document the importance of variations in behaviour across countries at similar levels of development. For example, in equally poor countries in Africa and in Asia and Oceania, women expressed very different family size preferences, which are likely to be related to differences between these settings in household organization and institutional arrangements for the rearing of children. The important role of population policy can be seen not only in the role played by modern methods in overall contraceptive practice but in the high levels of contraceptive use achieved in some relatively poor countries with strong family planning programmes.

The importance of development, however, in the transition process cannot be minimized; and throughout the study, this factor, above all others, can be seen to order fertility behaviour across countries in a consistent fashion.

The diffusion of development in the absence of deliberate government intervention is likely to move from those population groups having easy access to the opportunities provided by development to those more removed either because of location, education or skills. Findings in this study provide strong support for the diffusion hypothesis, with fertility differentials by residence and education observed to be small among the least developed and most developed countries and larger for those in the middle. In the process of development, fertility appears to fall first among the more advanced groups but, at a later stage, declines are observed across all groups.

The WFS data also document the important role of family planning programmes in the adoption of modern contraceptives and in the speed of fertility decline. Countries with stronger programmes experienced more rapid fertility decline, higher levels of contraceptive use (in particular, the use of modern methods) and more substantial change among the least advantaged groups. These results suggest that the process of transition has the potential for many variants, possibly even more than those already documented by the WFS data, and that these variants are a collective result of direct government policy as well as of unregulated social, economic and cultural forces.

It is interesting to note, however, that fertility differentials by women's occupation appear to become particularly strong at the highest levels of development, in terms of statistical significance when other socio-economic factors are controlled. While the differential effects of other socio-economic factors on fertility, such as education and residence, can be moderated through modern transport and communications networks as development progresses, women's occupation is indirectly linked to a woman's own personal circumstances and opportunities. The WFS data do not make it possible to sort out the causal paths from which the observed relationship between the type of work women do and fertility derives. It is known, however, that women's participation in the modern sector grows with development. Shifts in the occupational distribution that occur with development require an increasingly complex mix of skills from the labour force in terms of both formal training and job experience. As opportunities grow, so do their implied costs, in terms of both education and work continuity. Thus, a natural consequence of the development process is the growing incompatibility of work with childbearing and child-rearing; the same forces that attract women into the labour market also reduce family size desires. Although the style of development will influence this relationship, it will, none the less, grow stronger as development proceeds.

In the final analysis, the WFS data confirm the inevitability of a demographic transition by documenting common patterns and changes occurring across certain socio-economic groups in a variety of settings. At the same time, these data illustrate the wide range of reproductive behaviour that coexists within any specific phase of development, making a threshold theory of transition questionable. The diversity of policy settings and the adaptability of culture to the modernization process also makes it seem likely that the demographic configuration that will be observed in Africa, Latin America and the Caribbean, and Asia and Oceania will be different from that currently observed in the developed countries when these countries have achieved a similar stage of development. The style of development, the role women play in that process and the cultural setting will be important variables determining the texture of these societies at the point that low fertility is achieved.

Notes

[1] Although China and India, the world's two largest populations, were not covered, smaller countries with cultural and ethnic links to each of them were included.

[2] This is not to say that fertility was decreasing in all the developing countries; the countries where the quality of the WFS data was least satisfactory are also likely to be those where fertility was particularly high and had probably been stable at such levels for some time.

[3] The fact that women aged 45-49 were not included in the samples for the developed countries would tend to reduce exposure and introduce some compensating upward bias into the results for these countries, but this effect should be minimal.

[4] For the developing countries, the excess of actual family size over stated desired family size was used as the measure of unwanted fertility. The number of children desired tends to be usually high in sub-Saharan Africa, and if the sub-Saharan African countries are excluded from the analysis, the relationship between unwanted fertility and level of development or strength of family planning programme effort diminishes markedly. For the developed countries, however, unwanted fertility was measured on the basis of the reported planning status of each birth.

[5] The fact that the tabulations for developed countries were mostly confined to women still in their first marriage, while all currently married women are represented in the tabulations for developing countries, probably does not affect these comparisons appreciably.

[6] The measure of contraceptive use employed excludes contraceptive sterilization.

[7] The combination of a current employment variable with a measure of lifetime fertility adds to the difficulty of disentangling cause and effect.

[8] This refers primarily to the omission of China, which has a unique profile with respect to both recent reproductive behaviour and policy goals.

References

Berent, Jerzy (1982). *Family Planning in Europe and USA in the 1970s*. World Fertility Survey Comparative Studies, No. 20; ECE Analyses of WFS Surveys in Europe and USA. Voorburg, The Netherlands: International Statistical Institute.

_____ (1983). *Family Size Preferences in Europe and USA: Ultimate Expected Number of Children*. World Fertility Survey Comparative Studies, No. 26; ECE Analyses of WFS Surveys in Europe and USA. Voorburg, The Netherlands: International Statistical Institute.

Blake, Judith (1985). The fertility transition: continuity or discontinuity with the past. In *International Population Conference, Florence, 1985*. Liège: International Union for the Scientific Study of Population, vol. 4, 393-405.

Bongaarts, John (1978). A framework for analyzing the proximate determinants of fertility. *Population and Development Review* 4(1):105-132.

_____ (1982). The fertility-inhibiting effects of the intermediate fertility variables. *Studies in Family Planning* 13(6/7):179-189.

Caldwell, John C. (1982). *Theory of Fertility Decline*. London: Academic Press.

Casterline, John B., ed. (1985). *The Collection and Analysis of Community Data*. Voorburg, The Netherlands: International Statistical Institute.

_____ and others (1984). *The Proximate Determinants of Fertility*. World Fertility Survey Comparative Studies, No. 39. Voorburg, The Netherlands: International Statistical Institute.

Cleland, John (1985). Marital fertility decline in developing countries: theories and the evidence. In John Cleland and John Hobcraft, eds., in collaboration with Betzy Dinesen, *Reproductive Change in Developing Countries: Insights from the World Fertility Survey*. Oxford: Oxford University Press, 223-252.

Cochrane, Susan H. (1983). Effects of education and urbanization on fertility. In Rodolfo A. Bulatao and Ronald D. Lee, eds., with Paula D. Hollerbach and John Bongaarts, *Determinants of Fertility in Developing Countries*, vol. 2, *Fertility Regulation and Institutional Influences*. Report of the National Research Council Committee on Population and Demography, Panel on Fertility Determinants. New York: Academic Press, 587-626.

David, Henry P. (1983). Abortion: its prevalence, correlates and costs. In Rodolfo A. Bulatao and Ronald D. Lee, eds., with Paula D. Hollerbach and John Bongaarts, *Determinants of Fertility in Developing Countries*, vol. 2, *Fertility Regulation and Institutional Influences*. Report of the National Research Council Committee on Population and Demography, Panel on Fertility Determinants. New York: Academic Press, 193-244.

Davis, Kingsley and Judith Blake (1956). Social structure and fertility: an analytical framework. *Economic Development and Cultural Change* 4(4): 211-235.

Easterlin, Richard A. (1975). An economic framework for fertility analysis. *Studies in Family Planning* 6(3):54-63.

─────── (1978). The economics and sociology of fertility: a synthesis. In Charles Tilly, ed., *Historical Studies of Changing Fertility*. Princeton, New Jersey: Princeton University Press, 57-133.

Entwisle, Barbara and others (1984). A multilevel model of family planning availability and contraceptive use in rural Thailand. *Demography* 21(4):559-574.

Economic Commission for Europe (forthcoming). *Fertility and Family Planning in the ECE Region: A Comparative Analysis of WFS Surveys*.

Hajnal, John (1965). European marriage patterns in perspective. In D.V. Glass and D.E.C. Eversley, eds., *Population in History: Essays in Historical Demography*. London: Edward Arnold Ltd., 101-143.

Hermalin, Albert I. and William M. Mason (1980). A strategy for the comparative analysis of WFS data, with illustrative examples. In *The United Nations Programme for the Comparative Analysis of World Fertility Survey Data*. New York: United Nations Fund for Population Activities, 90-168.

McCann, Margaret F. and others (1981). *Breast-Feeding, Fertility, and Family Planning*. Population Reports, Series J, No. 24. Baltimore, Maryland: Population Information Program of The Johns Hopkins University.

McNicoll, Geoffrey (1982). Institutional determinants of fertility change. In Charlotte Höhn and Rainer Mackensen, eds., *Determinants of Fertility Trends: Theories Re-Examined*. Proceedings of an International Union for the Scientific Study of Population seminar held at Bad Homburg, Federal Republic of Germany, 14-17 April 1980. Liège: Ordina Editions, 147-168.

Retherford, Robert D. and James A. Palmore (1983). Diffusion processes affecting fertility regulation. In Rodolfo A. Bulatao and Ronald D. Lee, eds., with Paula D. Hollerbach and John Bongaarts, *Determinants of Fertility in Developing Countries*, vol. 2, *Fertility Regulation and Institutional Influences*. Report of the National Research Council Committee on Population and Demography, Panel on Fertility Determinants. New York: Academic Press, 295-338.

Rodríguez, Germán and John Cleland (1981). Socio-economic determinants of marital fertility in twenty countries: a multivariate analysis. In *World Fertility Survey Conference 1980: Record of Proceedings*. London, 7-11 July 1980. Voorburg, The Netherlands: International Statistical Institute, vol. II, 337-414.

Ryder, Norman B. (1983). Fertility and family structure. In *Population Bulletin of the United Nations, No. 15-1983*. New York: United Nations, 15-34.
Sales No. E.83.XIII.4.

Tietze, Christopher (1983). *Induced Abortion: A World Review 1983*. 5th ed. New York: The Population Council.

United Nations (1965). Department of Economic and Social Affairs. Population Division. *Population Bulletin of the United Nations, No. 7-1963, with special reference to conditions and trends of fertility in the world*. New York.
Sales No. E.64.XIII.2.

─────── (1976). *Fertility and Family Planning in Europe around 1970: A Comparative Study of Twelve National Surveys*. Population Studies, No. 58. New York.
Sales No. E.76.XIII.2.

─────── (1983). Department of International Economic and Social Affairs. Population Division. *Relationships between Fertility and Education: A Comparative Analysis of World Fertility Survey Data for Twenty-Two Developing Countries*. Non-sales publication ST/ESA/SER.R/48. New York.

─────── (1984). Department of International Economic and Social Affairs. Statistical Office. *Population and Vital Statistics Report: 1984 Special Supplement*. ST/ESA/STAT/SER.A/149. New York.
Sales No. E/F.84.XIII.2.

─────── (1984a). Population Division. *Recent Levels and Trends of Contraceptive Use as Assessed in 1983*. Population Studies, No. 92. New York.
Sales No. E.84.XIII.5.

─────── (1985). *World Population Trends, Population and Development Interrelations and Policies, 1983 Monitoring Report*, vol. I, *Population Trends*. Population Studies, No. 93. New York.
Sales No. E.84.XIII.10.

─────── (1985a). *World Population Prospects; Estimates and Projections as Assessed in 1982*. Population Studies, No. 86. New York.
Sales No. E.83.XIII.5.

─────── (forthcoming). *Patterns of First Marriage: Concepts and Determinants*. Non-sales publication, series R. New York.

─────── (forthcoming). *Patterns of First Marriage: Levels and Trends*. Non-sales publication, series R. New York.

Vaessen, Martin (1984). *Childlessness and Infecundity*. World Fertility Survey Comparative Studies, No. 31: Cross-National Summaries. Voorburg, The Netherlands: International Statistical Institute.

Westoff, Charles F. (1978). The unmet need for birth control in five Asian countries. *Family Planning Perspectives* 10(3):173-181.

كيفية الحصول على منشورات الأمم المتحدة

يمكن الحصول على منشورات الأمم المتحدة من المكتبات ودور التوزيع في جميع أنحاء العالم . استعلم عنها من المكتبة التي تتعامل معها أو اكتب إلى : الأمم المتحدة ، قسم البيع في نيويورك أو في جنيف .

如何购取联合国出版物

联合国出版物在全世界各地的书店和经售处均有发售。请向书店询问或写信到纽约或日内瓦的联合国销售组。

HOW TO OBTAIN UNITED NATIONS PUBLICATIONS

United Nations publications may be obtained from bookstores and distributors throughout the world. Consult your bookstore or write to: United Nations, Sales Section, New York or Geneva.

COMMENT SE PROCURER LES PUBLICATIONS DES NATIONS UNIES

Les publications des Nations Unies sont en vente dans les librairies et les agences dépositaires du monde entier. Informez-vous auprès de votre libraire ou adressez-vous à : Nations Unies, Section des ventes, New York ou Genève.

КАК ПОЛУЧИТЬ ИЗДАНИЯ ОРГАНИЗАЦИИ ОБЪЕДИНЕННЫХ НАЦИЙ

Издания Организации Объединенных Наций можно купить в книжных магазинах и агентствах во всех районах мира. Наводите справки об изданиях в вашем книжном магазине или пишите по адресу: Организация Объединенных Наций, Секция по продаже изданий, Нью-Йорк или Женева.

COMO CONSEGUIR PUBLICACIONES DE LAS NACIONES UNIDAS

Las publicaciones de las Naciones Unidas están en venta en librerías y casas distribuidoras en todas partes del mundo. Consulte a su librero o diríjase a: Naciones Unidas, Sección de Ventas, Nueva York o Ginebra.

Litho in United Nations, New York   04750   United Nations publication
86-41501—August 1987—5,160   Sales No. E.86.XIII.5
ISBN 92-1-151161-5   ST/ESA/SER.A/100